Contemporary
Endocrinology
Volume 2

Contemporary Endocrinology

(formerly *The Year in Endocrinology*)

A Continuation Order Plan is available for this series. A continuation order will bring delivery of each new volume immediately upon publication. Volumes are billed only upon actual shipment. For further information please contact the publisher.

Contemporary Endocrinology

Volume 2

Edited by

Sidney H. Ingbar, M.D.

William B. Castle Professor of Medicine
Harvard Medical School
Director, Thorndike Laboratory of Harvard Medical School
at the Beth Israel Hospital
Boston, Massachusetts

PLENUM MEDICAL BOOK COMPANY
NEW YORK AND LONDON

The Library of Congress has cataloged this serial title as follows:

Contemporary endocrinology. v. 1-   1979–

New York, Plenum Medical Book Co.

v. ill. 24 cm.

Annual.
Editor: 1979–   S. H. Ingbar.
Supersedes: Year in endocrinology, ISSN 0146-4078.
Key title: Contemporary endocrinology, ISSN 0196-8653.

1. Endocrinology — Periodicals.   I. Ingbar, Sidney H.
[DNLM: W1 CO769MPE]
QP187.A1Y4   612′.4′005
                                                                    80-640369
                                                                    MARC-S

Library of Congress   [8404r84]rev

ISBN-13: 978-1-4684-4819-1   e-ISBN-13: 978-1-4684-4817-7
DOI: 10.1007/978-1-4684-4817-7

© 1985 Plenum Publishing Corporation
Softcover reprint of the hardcover 1st edition 1985

233 Spring Street, New York, N.Y. 10013

Plenum Medical Book Company is an imprint of Plenum Publishing Corporation

Contributors

Edward G. Biglieri, M.D. • Chief, Endocrinology Service of the Medical Services and Director of the Clinical Study Center, San Francisco General Hospital Medical Center; Professor of Medicine, Department of Medicine, University of California School of Medicine, San Francisco, California 94120

Lewis E. Braverman, M.D. • Professor of Medicine; University of Massachusetts Medical School, Worcester, Massachusetts 01605

William H. Daughaday, M.D. • Professor of Medicine; Director, Metabolism Division, Department of Medicine, Washington University School of Medicine, St. Louis, Missouri 63110

Daniel D. Federman, M.D. • Professor of Medicine, Harvard Medical School, Boston, Massachusetts 02115

Charles R. Kleeman, M.D. • Professor of Medicine, Chief Emeritus, Division of Nephrology, Department of Medicine, UCLA Center for the Health Sciences and School of Medicine, Los Angeles, California 90024

Karen E. Kleeman, M.D. • Department of Psychiatry and Biobehavioral Science, UCLA Neuropsychiatric Institute and School of Medicine, Los Angeles, California 90024

Dorothy T. Krieger, M.D. • Professor of Medicine, Director, Division of Endocrinology, Mount Sinai Medical Center, New York, New York 10029

L. Landsberg, M.D. ● Departments of Medicine, Beth Israel Hospital, Charles A. Dana Research Institute, and Thorndike Laboratories, Harvard Medical School, Boston, Massachusetts 02115

Gary R. Robertson, M.D. ● University of Chicago School of Medicine, Chicago, Illinois 60637

Louis M. Sherwood, M.D. ● Baumritter Professor and Chairman, Department of Medicine, Albert Einstein College of Medicine, Bronx, New York 10461

Kenneth A. Woeber, M.D. ● Chief of Medicine, Department of Medicine, Mt. Zion Hospital and Medical Center; Professor of Medicine, University of California School of Medicine, San Francisco, California 94120

J. B. Young, M.D. ● Departments of Medicine, Beth Israel Hospital, Charles A. Dana Research Institute, and Thorndike Laboratories, Harvard Medical School, Boston, Massachusetts 02115

Contents

Chapter 1

Neuroendocrinology

Dorothy T. Krieger

Chapter 2

Prolactin and Growth Hormone in Health and Disease
William H. Daughaday

Chapter 3

The Thyroid

Kenneth A. Woeber and Lewis E. Braverman

Chapter 4

The Testis

Daniel D. Federman

Chapter 5

Aldosterone and Renin

Edward G. Biglieri

Chapter 6

Sympathoadrenal System

L. Landsberg and J. B. Young

Chapter 7

Parathyroid Hormone and Calcitonin

Karen E. Kleeman and Charles R. Kleeman

Chapter 8

Ectopic Hormone Syndromes

Louis M. Sherwood

Chapter 9

Vasopressin

Gary R. Robertson

Neuroendocrinology

Dorothy T. Krieger

1.1. Introduction

Since the last review of this subject, a number of new concepts have emerged in neuroendocrinology. It is increasingly evident that the so-called "hypothalamic releasing factors" have a widespread distribution both within the extrahypothalamic central and peripheral nervous system as well as in nonneural tissues. This is also true for peptides, i.e., vasopressin and oxytocin, previously believed to be exclusively distributed from their site of origin in the magnocellular nuclei to the posterior pituitary. An ever-increasing number of peptides, originally described as originating within the pituitary or the gastrointestinal tract, have now been described within the CNS, with evidence for some that they are synthesized within the CNS as well as in their previously described sites of origin. Questions have arisen concerning the functional significance of these new findings with regard to fundamental physiological processes, and preliminary information suggests multiple interactions between these various peptides as well as with the "classical" CNS neurotransmitters.

From a purely clinical aspect, the increased use of transsphenoidal hypophysectomy for the treatment of functioning pituitary tumors has provided a data base for assessing whether the removal of such tumors can cause complete amelioration of the clinical and pathophysiological

DOROTHY T. KRIEGER • Division of Endocrinology, Mount Sinai Medical Center, New York, New York 10029.

abnormalities present in such patients or whether residual disturbances are present, which would support the suggestion of an extrapituitary etiology of these conditions.

1.2. Biosynthesis of CNS Peptides

Synthesis of secretory proteins is now realized to occur via initial synthesis of precursor forms, which are processed to active peptide fragments by a series of cleavages that take place within specialized subcellular organelles of secretory cells. Recently, this has also been shown to be true for somatostatin, vasopressin, and for brain ACTH, α-MSH, and endorphin.

1.2.1. ACTH and Related Peptides in Brain

Following the report of the presence of ACTH in hypothalamic and extrahypothalamic sites,[1] studies were initiated in an attempt to demonstrate its synthesis in the brain, and to determine, if this proved to occur, whether such synthesis occurred via a precursor molecule as had been demonstrated in the case of pituitary ACTH synthesis.[2,3] Initial studies demonstrated that dispersed cell preparations of hypothalamic tissue rich in arcuate nucleus (the only CNS area in which cell bodies containing ACTH, lipotropin, and α-MSH have been demonstrated) progressively secrete immunoreactive ACTH and β-endorphin-like material in a near-linear fashion without any significant change in their cellular content. Subsequent studies demonstrated the synthesis of ³H-labeled high-molecular-weight material containing both ACTH and β-endorphin antigenic determinants within the same molecule(s) when bovine and rat hypothalamic cells were incubated in the presence of ³H-labeled amino acid.[4–6] Chemical characterization of the brain high-molecular-weight material demonstrated similarity to pituitary-synthesized precursor material, indicating that synthesis of the precursor molecule was similar in both locations. In addition to synthesis of such high-molecular-weight material, products both immunoreactively and physicochemically similar to β-endorphin and α-MSH were also detected, together with lesser amounts of β-lipotropin and ACTH 1–39. This indicates that in the hypothalamus the processing of the precursor molecule more closely resembles that seen in the intermediate lobe rather than that in the anterior lobe (in the anterior pituitary the precursor molecule is processed predominantly to ACTH and β-LPH, whereas in the intermediate lobe ACTH and β-LPH are further processed predominantly to α-MSH and β-endorphin-like material, respectively, so that only small amounts of ACTH and β-LPH are detected in the intermediate lobe).

There are, however, differences in hypothalamic processing from that seen in the intermediate lobe. In the intermediate lobe, immunoreactive β-endorphin-like material is a mixture of several forms (β-endorphin 1–31, β-endorphin 1–27, and their acetylated forms), while in the hypothalamus the major form is authentic β-endorphin 1–31.[7,8] Such differential processing of the precursor molecule provides a fascinating example of a process whereby a single gene product can yield physiologically different molecules depending on the tissue in which the gene is expressed.

1.2.2. Vasopressin, Oxytocin, and Neurophysins

Sachs and Takabatke had suggested in 1964[9] that vasopressin and its accompanying neurophysin were synthesized as part of a large precursor molecule. In 1980, Russell et al.[10] demonstrated the synthesis of two high-molecular-weight proteins ($M_r \sim 20,000$), one of which was apparently associated with vasopressin, the other with oxytocin. In the past year, evidence that this high-molecular-weight protein is a precursor molecule has been presented. Tryptic digestion of these two synthesized high-molecular-weight proteins yields fragments consisting of the neurophysins and vasopressin or oxytocin.[10] Schmale and Richter[11] have demonstrated hypothalamic mRNA-directed synthesis of a polypeptide precursor containing within it the antigenic determinants of neurophysin II and vasopressin. The possibility of a still higher molecular weight form ($M_r \sim 60,000$) has also been suggested,[12] as has the existence of yet a third precursor protein of approximately 20,000 daltons, containing, in addition to a neurophysin-like protein, an uncharacterized neurophysin-binding peptide.[10] By ingenious in vivo labeling experiments, it has been demonstrated that synthesis of the precursor occurs within the cell body, and that processing continues within the secretory granule as it travels along the tuberohypophyseal tract for storage in the posterior pituitary.

1.2.3. Somatostatin

In the past several years, there have been several reports suggesting the presence of high-molecular-weight forms ($M_r \sim 12,500$–$16,000$) of immunoreactive somatostatin in hypothalamic as well as in extrahypothalamic sites (i.e., pancreas, stomach, duodenum, and intestine) of several species.[13–16] Within the past year, there have been major advances in the characterization of this high-molecular-weight protein. Lauber et al.[17] demonstrated the generation of somatostatin-like (M_r 1600) material, as well as forms of intermediate size, from mouse hypothalamic high-molecular-weight immunoreactive somatostatin-like material by proteolytic enzymes that coeluted with the high-molecular-weight form. Such conversion, however, could not be produced by trypsin or trypsin-like proteolytic enzymes. Patzelt et al.[18] demonstrated that similar tryptic fragments could be obtained from prosomatostatin derived either from rat pancreatic islets or from synthetic somatostatin, and also concluded from these studies that the tetradecapeptide somatostatin resides in the C-terminal region of the precursor. Pradayrol et al.[19] and Schally et al.[20] reported the presence of a 28-amino-acid somatostatin consisting of the sequence of the tetradecapeptide with an N-terminal extension of 14 amino acids. The sequence preceding the tetradecapeptide was Arg-Lys, suggesting the possibility of tryptic cleavage at this locus of the 28-amino-acid form to yield the 14-amino-acid form. The 28-amino-acid form has very recently been synthesized[21] and demonstrated to be equipotent with somatostatin on a molar basis in suppressing growth hormone or prolactin release from monolayer cultures of pituitary cells, twice as active on a molar basis in suppressing plasma glucagon concentrations, and ten times as active on a molar basis in suppressing plasma insulin. It has been suggested that the extended form has a longer biological half-life than somatostatin.

The amino acid sequence of the precursor molecule has been deduced from the nucleotide sequence of the cloned angler-fish islet preprosomatostatin. This confirmed the fact that the somatostatin tetradecapeptide is located at the C terminus of a 119-amino-acid precursor ($M_r \sim 12,500$) and also demonstrated identity of the 6 amino acids adjacent to somatostatin in the precursor molecule to those in the 28-amino-acid precursor described above that was isolated from porcine brain and intestine, indicating marked conservation across species.[22] It is felt that the discrepancy in molecular weight calculated for the 119-amino-acid precursor form from the somewhat higher molecular weight (as reported using SDS gel characterization) is secondary to anomalous electrophoretic migration. Two additional pairs of Arg-Arg sequences are present in the precursor molecule, which may represent potential cleavage sites leading to formation of additional, as yet uncharacterized biologically active peptides within this precursor molecule.

1.3. Extrahypothalamic Localization of "Hypothalamic Releasing Factors" and Peptides

1.3.1. ACTH

Previous studies had demonstrated that ACTH,[23–26] β-lipotropin,[27] β-endorphin,[27] and α-MSH[28] are present in human placental extracts. There were also reports of the in vitro biosynthesis of immunoreactive and bioreactive ACTH-like materials by human placental tissue,[23,36] together with the presence of at least one high-molecular-weight immunoreactive ACTH component.[26] Most of these studies were performed prior to the demonstration[2] that ACTH, β-LPH, and β-endorphin are contained within and are posttranslationally derived from a common precursor glycoprotein(s). Recent studies have revealed the presence in placenta of ACTH, LPH, and β-endorphin antigenic determinants in high-molecular-weight material, suggestive of a precursor molecule.[2;9] Furthermore, pulse-labeling of human placental trophoblastic tissue has demonstrated placental synthesis of high-molecular-weight material similar to that found in the human pituitary.[30] It appears, however, that posttranslational processing of this precursor in the placenta differs from that in the anterior pituitary (see Section 1.2.1). The placenta further processes ACTH and β-LPH to α-MSH and β-endorphin, respectively, in a manner qualitatively analogous to processing in the intermediate pituitary lobe.[30] The functional significance of the precursor material and its products in the placenta still remains to be demonstrated.

1.3.2. Vasopressin

Vasopressin-like material not only is present in the paraventricular and supraoptic nuclei and their projections to the median eminence and posterior pituitary, but has also been demonstrated in the suprachiasmatic nucleus,[31] with projections from this latter area to the lateral septum and amygdala.[32] Unlike the magnocellular nuclei and their projections, which also contain oxytocin, only vasopressin is present in the suprachiasmatic nucleus. There are also fiber projections from the paraventricular nucleus to the amygdaloid nuclei; in addition, projections to the spinal cord have also been noted.[33,34] These projections to the limbic system may provide the anatomical basis for the effect of vasopressin on avoidance behavior (since lesions of these limbic system areas block the behavioral effect of vasopressin[35]).

1.3.3. Somatostatin

The extrahypothalamic localization of somatostatin-like immunoreactivity has been demonstrated in axons and nerve cell bodies of primary sensory neurons, sympathetic neurons, intrinsic neurons of the intestine, circumventricular organs, and CNS neurons.[35] Somatostatin-like immunoreactivity has recently been reported in three types of retinal cells in the rat[36] and goldfish[37]; in the latter, uncharacterized high-molecular-weight material was also noted. The relation of such high-molecular-weight material to that described in Section 1.2.3 is unknown. Localization of somatostatin to such cells and their processes in a tissue

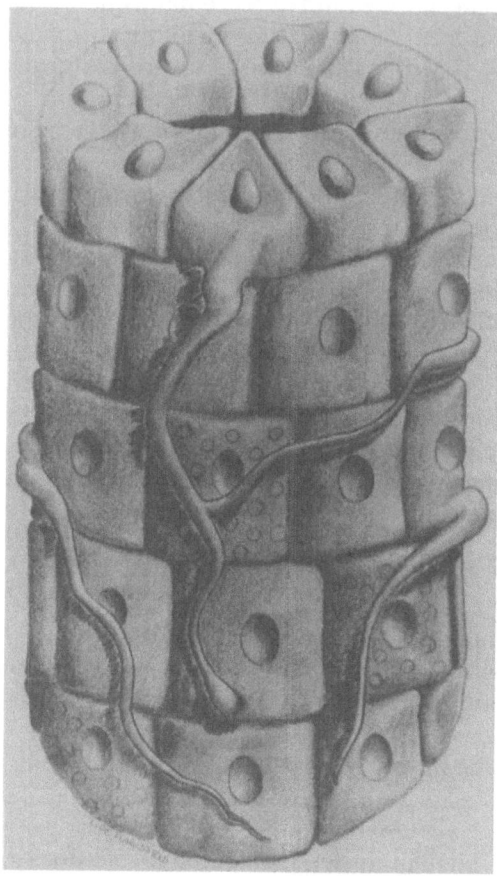

Fig. 1. Schematic drawing showing a three-dimensional arrangement of the somatostatin cells and their processes in an antral gland. Reproduced from Larsson et al.[38] with permission.

in which each of the major cell types has been characterized by intracellular recording, and which is easily isolated and can be maintained in organ culture for prolonged periods, should be of great aid in assessing both its role as a neurotransmitter or neuromodulator and its interaction with other peptides (i.e., TRH, enkephalin, and substance P) that are present in the retina.

Somatostatin is also present in secretory cells of the gastroenteropancreatic system, and it has recently been shown that such cells have long, nonluminal cytoplasmic processes terminating on gastrin-producing and hydrochloric acid-producing cells, suggesting a paracrine function (Fig. 1).[38] Immunoreactive somatostatin is also present in the epithelial and subepithelial layer of the toad urinary bladder and in the renal distal tubules and collecting ducts,[39] areas sensitive to antidiuretic hormone. Somatostatin is reported to inhibit vasopressin-stimulated water flow in the toad urinary bladder.[40]

1.3.4. Gonadotropin-Releasing Hormone (LHRH)

Cytochemical studies have been performed best in the guinea pig brain; these have identified LHRH-containing cell bodies in the medial preoptic area, septum, and olfactory tubercle, in addition to their previously described hypothalamic sites. Projections from these cell bodies have been traced not only to the organum vasculosum of the lamina tuberalis, as previously noted, but also to the limbic system, thalamus, and midbrain.[41] Such projections are not involved in gonadotropin release, and it has been suggested that they may function in the regulation of sexual behavior, since the neurons and terminals are present in areas shown to be involved in lordosis behavior. A number of physiological studies have suggested that there may be species variations in the location of LHRH-containing cell bodies and their function.[42]

Other previous reports had suggested an extra-CNS distribution of LHRH. Such suggestions were based on the observations that LHRH agonists (although in pharmacological amounts) could inhibit gonadal effects of hCG and FSH, decrease the number of testicular LH receptors, and suppress placental hCG and progesterone secretion. Additionally, there have been reports of the presence of specific high-affinity receptors for LHRH in the ovary[43] and testes.[44] In view of the known rapid peripheral degradation of LHRH, these observations suggest the existence of extrahypothalamic sites of LHRH production. This is supported by recent evidence of placental production of LHRH.[45] Ying and Guillemin[46] have demonstrated material in rat ovarian follicular fluid and in the media of cultured rat granulosa cells that is immunologically dissimilar to LHRH but has LHRH-like biological activity, and Sharpe and Fraser[47] have described testicular production of a biologically active LHRH-like factor.

1.3.5. Thyrotropin-Releasing Hormone

In the previous volume (*Contemporary Endocrinology*, Volume 1, p. 10, 1979) there was a citation of a report[48] suggesting that extrahypothalamic immunoreactive TRH differed from synthetic TRH. Two more recent studies, however, have reported identity of extrahypothalamic TRH immunoreactivity to synthetic TRH, as judged by Sephadex gel filtration, thin-layer chromatography, high-pressure liquid chromatography, ion-exchange chromatography, and bioassay.[49,50] In addition to its extrahypothalamic nervous system distribution, TRH, as characterized by these methods, is also present in the pancreas and gastrointestinal tract,[51,52] as well as the placenta.[53] Studies to date suggest a role in gastrointestinal motility and absorption; its role in pancreatic and placental function still remains to be established.

1.4. Possible Functional Homeostatic Significance of Brain Peptides

It is becoming apparent that a number of major homeostatic systems are regulated by a complex interplay of various peptides and neurotransmitters within the CNS. Among these are those concerned with feeding; glucoregulation; pain; temperature; cognitive, emotional, and sexual behaviors; salt and water regulation; blood pressure; and sleep–arousal states. Within the framework of this review, it is not possible to cover all of these areas. The following two examples should give some indication of the nature of progress in this field.

1.4.1. Cognitive Behavior

The behavioral effects of ACTH, α-MSH, and vasopressin were reviewed in *The Year in Endocrinology 1976*. Briefly, the data indicated that these peptides could enhance the rate of acquisition of avoidance behavior (interpreted as memory retention) and inhibit the extinction of such avoidance behavior (interpreted as indicative of persistence of a learned response). ACTH fragments (4–7, 4–10) appear to be involved in short-term memory processes, while vasopressin may be involved in long-term memory. Recent studies have also reported effects of endorphin(s) on avoidance behavior.[54] Both α- and β-endorphin have effects similar to those noted for ACTH, whereas γ-endorphin facilitates extinction. There are a few reports concerning the effect of these peptides on human learning and memory. ACTH 4–10 is reported to improve the attention of mentally retarded subjects,[55] increase visual discrimination in normal men, and augment verbal skills in women.[56] Thus far, however, the number of clinical observations is insufficient to draw any definitive conclusions, and negative findings have also been reported.[57] Vasopressin has been reported to have a beneficial effect in patients suffering from long-term amnesia,[58] in tests of attention and memory in elderly people,[59] and in the ability of children with Lesch–Nyhan syndrome to learn a passive avoidance response.[60] A negative report[61] indicating lack of significant effects in patients with memory defects following severe head trauma may have been the result of inadequate dosage.

1.4.2. Effects on Feeding

A number of peptides reported to be present in the brain have been implicated in the regulation of feeding behavior. In several recent animal studies, cholecystokinin,[62] TRH,[63] and insulin[64] have been reported to decrease food intake. Brain content of CCK is also reported to be low in *ob/ob* mice,[65] and it is suggested that this may be causally related to the hyperphagia present in these animals. Other studies,[66–68] however, have not shown significant alteration in brain CCK concentrations in obese animals. Brain endorphin concentrations are elevated in genetically obese Zucker fatty rats,[69] and concentrations are decreased in starved animals.[70] In view of the serotoninergic, dopaminergic, and adrenergic regulation of feeding that has been reported,[71] and the observations that endorphin administration affects serotonin and dopamine turnover, it is indeed possible that interactions between peptidergic and monoaminergic systems are involved in feeding regulation.

Additional studies implicating neurotensin,[72] bombesin,[73] and CCK[74] in glucoregulation suggest additional influences on feeding behavior. In human subjects, however, physiologically relevant doses of neurotensin (less than those employed in animal studies) have failed to demonstrate a hyperglycemic effect.[75]

1.5. Possible Functions of Opioid-like Peptides

1.5.1. On Prolactin Release

Opiate effects on pituitary hormone secretion are of great interest; the most extensive studies to date have been concerned with prolactin secretion. There is general agreement, based on animal studies, that opiates stimulate prolactin release *in vivo*, and that naloxone administration can depress endogenous prolactin levels (see *Contemporary Endocrinology*, Volume 1, p. 10, 1979). There are contradictory reports as to whether this action occurs at a hypothalamic or a pituitary level. In favor of a pituitary site of origin is the fact that β-endorphin has been reported to be present in high concentrations in pituitary portal blood.[76] Another study[77] has reported high-affinity opiate binding in the posterior and intermediate lobe, and markedly lower receptor density in the anterior pituitary lobe. (It is now realized that at least two types of opiate receptors exist, type I and type II, characterized by their relative affinities for morphine, β-endorphin, and enkephalin, and by whether or not they are antagonized by naloxone. Pituitary receptors have not as yet been so characterized; such characterization would be of aid in defining their natural ligand.)

To date, however, virtually all experiments utilizing pituitary tissue culture[78–81] or administration of endorphin to pituitary stalk-sectioned animals[82] have failed to demonstrate a direct effect of endorphin on pituitary prolactin release. In addition, other studies indicating that endorphin decreases hypothalamic turnover[83,84] and efflux,[85,86] and also affects hypothalamic serotonin concentrations,[87] support a hypothalamic locus of endorphin action. There is one *in vitro* study, however, that found that enkephalin, morphine, and β-endorphin, although not directly affecting pituitary prolactin release, can suppress the inhibitory effect of dopamine on such release in a dose-dependent manner.[81] This reversal of the dopamine effect could be restored by naloxone administration, naloxone alone having no effect on dopamine-induced inhibition. These findings, as well as the lack of observable binding of opiates to dopamine receptors or of dopamine to opiate receptors, would suggest that two independent receptors mediate the action of dopamine and opiates on the pituitary.

Fewer data are available from human studies. Bolus injection of morphine has been reported to elevate plasma prolactin concentrations.[88] The effect of β-endorphin administration has thus far been studied only in two patients with cancer,[89] two uncharacterized psychiatric patients,[90] six depressed psychiatric patients, and four methadone addicts.[91] Mode of administration and dose of β-endorphin differed in these studies, and only the latter study was placebo-controlled double-blind in design. All these studies report an increase in plasma prolactin concentrations following β-endorphin administration. Naloxone, however, is ineffective in suppressing basal prolactin concentrations in normal subjects,[92–94] and also fails to suppress the sleep-associated release of prolactin[95] or its response to insulin-induced hypoglycemia.[92,96,97] Naloxone is also ineffective in suppressing prolactin levels in hyperprolactinemic females.[95,98] In the latter study, however, those patients with low-normal basal LH levels demonstrated a rise in LH levels following naloxone administration, but no effect of naloxone was seen in those hyperprolactinemic patients with significantly depressed basal LH levels. In normal women, naloxone has been reported to increase endogenous LH levels in the late follicular and midluteal phase, but not in the early follicular phase of the menstrual cycle.[99] These findings should be considered in the context of previous reports (*Contemporary Endocrinology*, Volume 1, p. 10, 1979) that in rodents, opioid administration inhibits LH release.

These studies have been cited as examples of the complexity in elucidating the role of opiates in prolactin release; similar considerations apply to reports on the effects of opiates on the release of other pituitary hormones. It is apparent that there are species variations in response, which may be inherent or may reflect differences in doses of agonists and antagonists employed in the various studies. It is also possible that the doses of opiates employed (which have usually been calculated based on their analgesic effect) may not be appropriate for investigation of endocrine responses in which a different type of opiate receptor may possibly be involved. The multifactorial nature of prolactin regulation (neurotransmitter, hormonal) and the effect of endorphin on a number of these factors require more rigorous investigation before the precise relationship of opiates and prolactin can be deciphered.

1.5.2. In Clinical Syndromes

Endorphins have been implicated in addiction, analgesia, seizure disorders, psychiatric disease, learning ability, sexual behavior, and regulation of feeding and temperature. It would be of interest, therefore, to determine β-endorphin concentrations in patients presenting with disorders involving these parameters. However, since β-endorphin is produced both within the pituitary and the CNS, and possibly has different functional roles in these two tissues, the question arises as to which body fluid is best sampled to detect possible abnormalities in endorphin synthesis, secretion, or metabolism. The best evidence to date would imply that CSF endorphin reflects concentrations within the CNS. Concentrations in CSF are greater than those in plasma, and β-endorphin is present in CSF of hypopituitary patients in whom β-endorphin is undetectable in plasma.[100] Reference has already been made to the various forms of endorphins that exist (see Section 1.2.1). Preliminary results[101,102] suggest that in the hypothalamus authentic β-endorphin is the major form present, while other forms may predominate in human plasma. Since different antisera may have different affinities for the various forms of endorphins, this suggests that it may be necessary, when measuring concentrations in plasma, to characterize the various forms present.

With these caveats, it is of interest to assess two clinical reports that have appeared. Dunger et al.[103] described a 13-year-old boy who since age 4½ years developed obesity; abnormal temperature control (with rapid variations in body temperature and periods of profound hypothermia); decreased thirst sensation; reversed circadian pattern of urinary volume excretion; episodes of respiratory depression; decreased pain perception; and alterations in sleep and mood, the latter characterized by episodes of inactivity and euphoria. The predominant endocrine findings were absence of growth hormone responsiveness to insulin-induced hypoglycemia, marked elevation of prolactin concentrations (which normalized spontaneously during the course of the illness), elevated cortisol production rate and absence of cortisol circadian periodicity (again, normalizing during the course of the illness), and decreased thyroxine levels. Neurological examinations, including EEG and tomography, were normal. Met-enkephalin and "immunoreactive" β-endorphin levels in blood and CSF were normal. However, administration of naloxone over an 8-day period was associated with altered pain sensation, restoration of normal circadian variation of urinary volume, and increased basal levels of TSH, FSH, and LH. Basal prolactin levels were not affected, but responsiveness of both prolactin and TSH levels to TRH, which had previously been absent, was restored to normal.

The other case report by Brandt *et al.*[104] was that of a child with "Leigh's syndrome" (subacute necrotizing encephalomyelopathy). Onset was at 8 months of age, with demise at age 23 months. The course was characterized by periods of prolonged apnea, unconsciousness, hypothermia, and restlessness. On four of seven occasions these were reversed by naloxone administration for only a short period of time, with return of symptoms that were unresponsive to further naloxone injection. Serum prolactin was normal in this patient. Neurological examination was also normal, save for abnormal EEGs during and after attacks. CSF was assayed for "endorphin-like" activity, and an increased amount of both fraction I- and fraction II-like activity was reported. (Fraction I has been linked to enkephalin-like activity; fraction II may represent other opiate-like compounds.) Chemical analysis of the brain (autopsy performed 26 hr after death) revealed high levels of Met- and Leu-enkephalin in the cortex, but not in other CNS areas examined. β-Endorphin concentrations were normal.

In both of these studies, the suggestion of alterations in opiate-like activity is inferred from the response to naloxone administration. It should be stressed that this effect may not be specific for opiate-like activity; indeed, in the first case there was no detectable alteration in such activity, and in the second case the long delay between time of death and examination of brain tissue raises questions as to the significance of the results.

1.6. Results of Transsphenoidal Hypophysectomy for Hyperfunctioning Pituitary Adenomas

This subject has been reviewed in the previous two volumes (*The Year in Endocrinology 1977* and *Contemporary Endocrinology*, Volume 1, 1979). As was noted, there is still controversy as to whether acromegaly, hyperprolactinemia, and Cushing's disease represent primary pituitary diseases or are secondary to hyperstimulation of the pituitary by hypothalamic releasing hormones (or to a defect in hypothalamic inhibitory factors). It is also possible that within each classification, subgroups exist in which one or the other etiology might be present. Since this topic was last considered, there have been several series in which large numbers of patients have been studied following transsphenoidal hypophysectomy, with relatively long follow-up periods having elapsed. As will be noted below, however, the findings still have not completely helped to resolve the basic questions asked.

1.6.1. Acromegaly

With continued experience, it has become evident that the criterion of normalization (mean of plasma growth hormone level <5 ng/ml on repeated serial sampling) of basal growth hormone levels may not be adequate to judge the efficacy of surgery, and that such assessment should include dynamic testing of growth hormone responsiveness. A large proportion of patients with acromegaly initially manifest abnormal growth hormone responses to glucose tolerance testing, TRH administration, and circadian release, which should disappear postoperatively if the disease is of pituitary origin. There are two reported series[105,106] in which 8 of 11 and 20 of 28 patients, respectively (72%), for whom prolonged follow-up observation was available, had normal postoperative baseline growth hormone levels according to the above criteria. Five of the eight patients in the first series[105] manifested normal growth hormone responsiveness to glucose administration, TRH, bromocryptine, and normal nocturnal elevation of plasma growth hormone levels in the postoperative period (Figs. 2A–C). In the remaining three patients, follow-up studies of plasma growth hormone levels sampled every 20 min over 24 hr varied from 4.6 to 10.8 ng/ml, in contrast to values of 1.0 to 2.0 ng/ml in the other five patients. These three patients also maintained abnormal responsiveness to all of the tests noted above in the postoperative period, and were subsequently placed on bromocryptine therapy. In the second series,[106] of the 20 patients with normal basal growth hormone levels, seven had abnormal growth hormone responses to at least one of the dynamic tests of growth hormone function; of these, three have subsequently relapsed (the remaining four continue to have abnormal responsiveness over a mean 23-month follow-up) (Fig. 3). It is of interest that six of the seven patients with abnormal dynamics had evidence of extrasellar extension, whereas only one of the 13 with return of normal dynamic growth hormone responsiveness had such evidence. (There appeared to be no correlation between basal growth hormone levels and presence of suprasellar extension.) Therefore, only 62% of patients in this series with normal basal growth hormone levels with adequate follow-up can be said to still be in remission. There are no reports as to efficacy of subsequent surgery in patients who do manifest relapse.

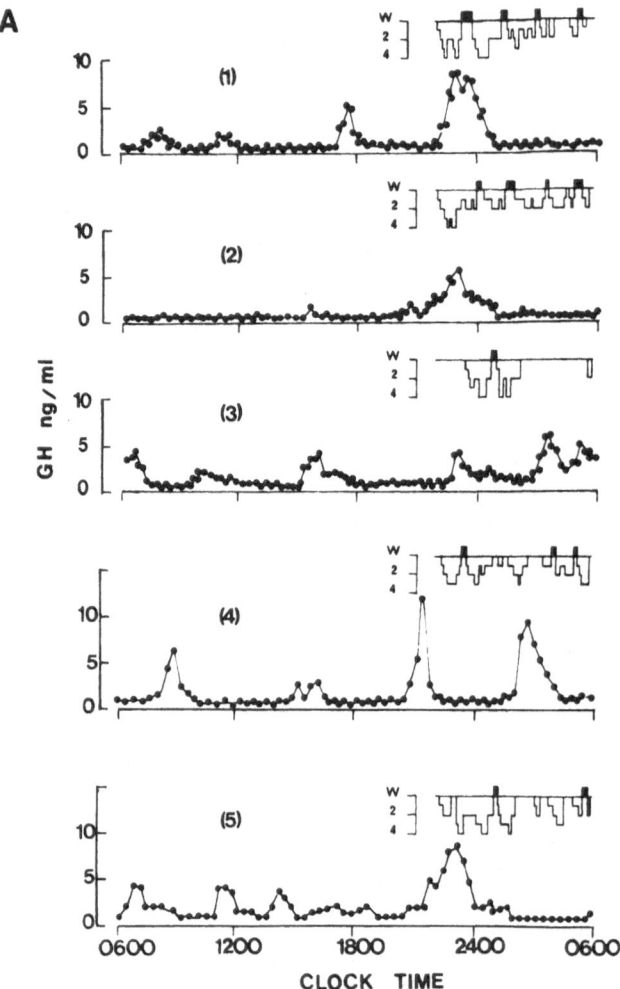

Fig. 2. (A) Twenty-four-hour growth hormone secretory pattern in five postoperative (1–4 years) acromegalic patients with normal growth hormone secretory dynamics. Sleep histograms are shown above each panel. (B) Evolution of the postoperative pattern of growth hormone secretion in patient (5) at intervals following surgery. (C) Abnormal 24-hr secretory patterns of growth hormone secretion in an acromegalic patient who had normal basal growth hormone levels and abnormal responses to dynamic testing 1–4 years after surgery. Reproduced from Jacquet et al.[105] with permission.

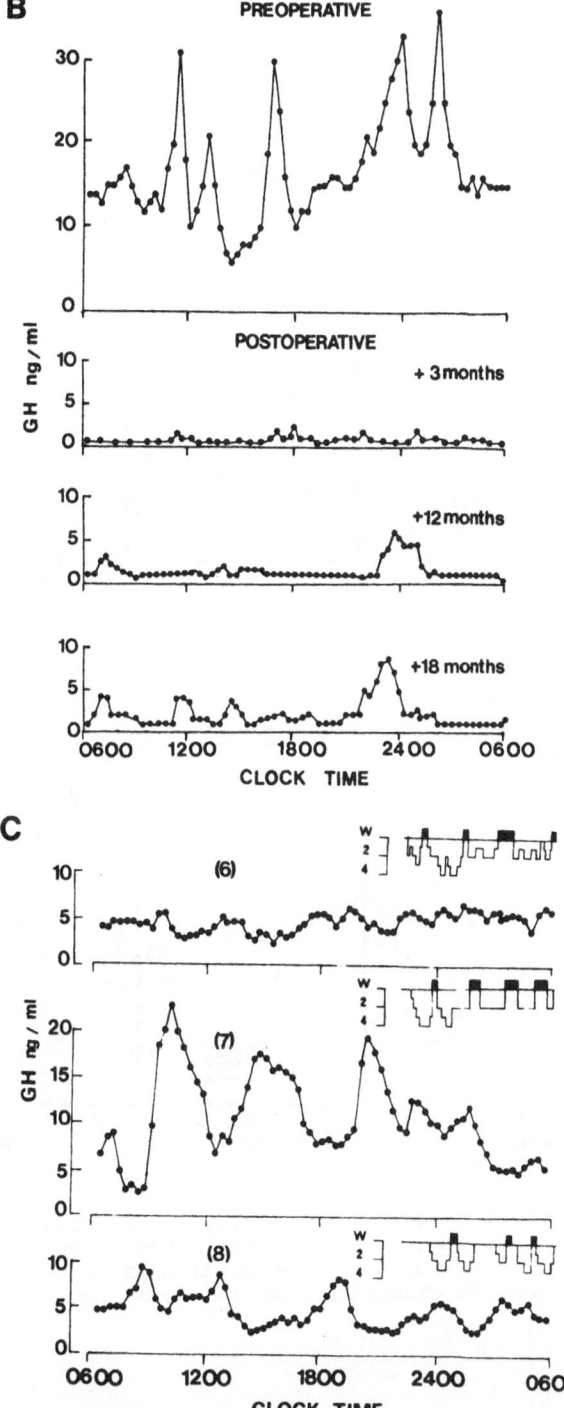

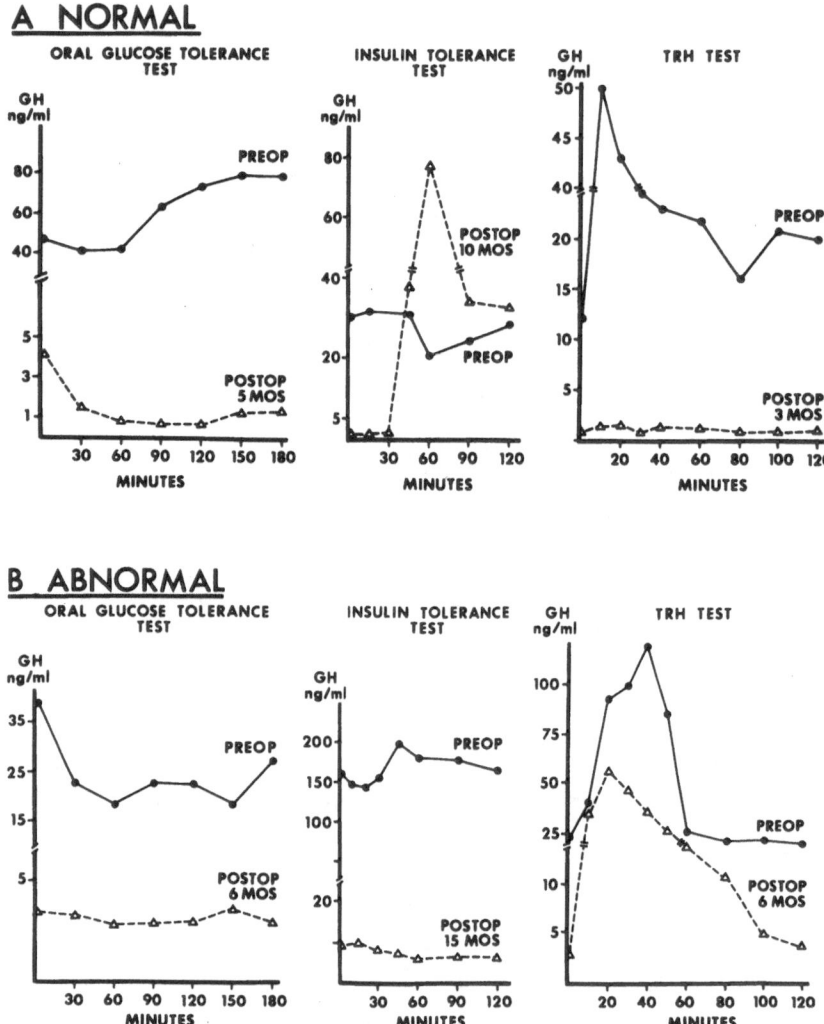

Fig. 3.   Pre- and postoperative growth hormone dynamic studies in five patients.   (A) Restoration of growth hormone dynamics to normal in three patients; (B) persistence of abnormal growth hormone dynamics postoperatively in two patients, despite normal basal growth hormone levels. Reproduced from Arafah et al.[106] with permission.

1.6.2. Prolactinomas

An abnormality in CNS dopaminergic regulation of prolactin secretion has been postulated to be present in patients with prolactin-
secreting pituitary tumors. Fine and Frohman[107] reported that concurrent administration of carbidopa (a peripheral dopa-decarboxylase
inhibitor) and L-dopa does not alter the effect of L-dopa in suppressing prolactin levels in normal subjects. However, in hyperprolactinemic
patients whose prolactin levels were suppressed following L-dopa administration alone, such suppression was not seen with concurrent use
of carbidopa. The authors postulated that such lack of suppression in
hyperprolactinemic patients might be either secondary to a central
impairment in the decarboxylation of dopa to dopamine or to altered
regulation of a prolactin inhibitory factor (if there were one other than
dopamine). Crosignani et al.[108] have demonstrated that nomifensine, a
drug which acts on central dopaminergic receptors, is not effective in
suppressing elevated prolactin levels in hyperprolactinemic patients, although it is effective in normal subjects. Whether these abnormalities in
dopaminergic regulation in patients with hyperprolactinemia represent
a primary abnormality or are secondary to the effects of increased prolactin concentrations on CNS dopamine levels, and, consequently, on
dopamine receptors, still remains to be resolved. (There appears to be
an inverse relationship between dopamine concentrations in hypophyseal portal blood and release of prolactin from the pituitary gland.[109])
If there were a primary abnormality in dopamine receptors, one would
expect similar responses to pre- and postoperative testing. To date, there
are no reports of such repeat testing in patients in whom levels have
normalized following removal of prolactinomas. Possible insights into
mechanisms might also be obtained, however, by comparing the response
of plasma prolactin levels to various stimuli before and after such surgical
removal. In a recent report,[110] TRH, metoclopromide (MCP), chlorpromazine (CPZ), and insulin (ITT) stimulation tests were performed
on 45 such patients (not all tests were performed on all patients) in
whom prolactin concentrations were less than 30 ng/ml following surgery
(mean 11.3 ± 1.4 ng/ml). The patients were studied serially for as long
as 8 years postoperatively. Blunted responses to all of these stimuli were
present at 6 months postoperatively (similar to preoperative testing).
When tested 1 to 8 years postoperatively, a blunted TRH response was
still present in 33% of patients, a blunted CPZ response in 87% of patients, and a blunted response to ITT in 71%. The abnormal responses
to the latter two agents, which act centrally to stimulate prolactin release,
would suggest a persistent hypothalamic deficit in these patients.

It is difficult to give an absolute number for the surgical cure rate
of prolactinomas, since restoration of menses and pregnancy can occur

in patients who have experienced a reduction in serum prolactin levels but in whom normalization of such levels has not occurred. (Indeed, it appears that a similar percentage of postoperative reduction of prolactin levels occurs in all tumors, i.e., to approximately 20% of the initial value.[111])

1.6.3. Cushing's Disease

There are no similar large series of patients with Cushing's disease who have been subjected to dynamic tests of hypothalamic–pituitary–adrenal function following surgery. Four large series, comprising 85 patients in whom microadenectomy was performed, have been reported.[112-115] The reported surgical cure rate varied from 76 to 85% in patients in whom tumors were localized and in whom localized adenectomy was performed. Postoperative adrenocortical insufficiency was reported to occur in most patients in two series,[112,113] but only in a minority of patients in another.[114] The presence of such insufficiency would indicate that at least during the time of observation, there was no evidence of hyperfunction of remaining pituitary tissue. As a result, many patients received prolonged postoperative corticosteroid replacement therapy, making it difficult to assess their subsequent responsiveness to other testing procedures of the hypothalamic–pituitary–adrenal axis. The cortisol response to insulin-induced hypoglycemia remained blunted 12 months postoperatively[116]; circadian periodicity of plasma corticosteroid levels was normal in 14 of 24 postoperative patients.[114,115,117-119] There have been two reports[118,119] of return of normal dexamethasone suppressibility. These reports would suggest that in those instances where normal hypothalamic–pituitary–adrenal function had returned, there was no residual hypothalamic abnormality. There have, however, been reports of recurrences following surgically induced remission. Reports of pathological findings in some operated patients have also indicated the concurrent presence of hyperplasia and adenoma.[120] To date, there have been three reported cases[114,121] of recurrences within 1 to 3 years postoperatively in patients who had exhibited clinical and laboratory evidence of remission, including normal dexamethasone suppressibility and cortisol responsiveness to insulin-induced hypoglycemia.

Submitted January 1981.

References

1. Krieger, D. T., Liotta, A., and Brownstein, M. J., 1977, Presence of adrenocorticotropin in brain of normal and hypophysectomized rats, *Proc. Natl. Acad. Sci. USA* **74:**648–652.

2. Mains, R. E., Eipper, B., and Ling, M., 1977, Common precursor to corticotropins and endorphins, *Proc. Natl. Acad. Sci. USA* **74:**3014–3018.
3. Roberts, J. L., and Herbert, E., 1977, Characterization of a common precursor to corticotropin and β-lipotropin: Identification of β-lipotropin peptides and their arrangement relative to corticotropin in the precursor synthesized in a cell-free system, *Proc. Natl. Acad. Sci. USA* **74:**5300–5304.
4. Liotta, A. S., Gildersleeve, D., Brownstein, M. J., and Krieger, D. T., 1979, Biosynthesis *in vitro* of immunoreactive 31,000-dalton corticotropin/β-endorphin-like material by bovine hypothalamus, *Proc. Natl. Acad. Sci. USA* **76:**1448–1452.
5. Krieger, D. T., Liotta, A. S., Brownstein, M. J., and Zimmerman, E. A., 1980, ACTH, β-lipotropin and related peptides in brain, pituitary, and blood, *Recent Prog. Horm. Res.* **36:**272–344.
6. Liotta, A. S., Loudes, C., McKelvy, J. F., and Krieger, D. T., 1980, Biosynthesis of precursor corticotropin/endorphin, corticotropin, α-melanotropin, β-lipotropin, and β-endorphin like material by cultured neonatal rat hypothalamic neurons, *Proc. Natl. Acad. Sci. USA* **77:**1880–1884.
7. Smyth, D., Massey, D. E., Zakarian, S., and Finnie, M., 1979, Endorphins are stored in biologically active and inactive forms: Isolation of α-N-acetyl peptides, *Nature (London)* **279:**252–254.
8. Liotta, A. S., Yamaguchi, H., and Krieger, D. T., 1981, Biosynthesis and release of β-endorphin, N-acetyl β-endorphin, β-endorphin (1–27), and N-acetyl β-EP (1–27) like peptides by rat pituitary neurointermediate lobe: β-Endorphin is not further processed by anterior lobe, *J. Neurosci.* **1:**585–595.
9. Sachs, H., and Takabatke, Y., 1964, Evidence for a precursor in vasopressin synthesis, *Endocrinology* **75:**943–948.
10. Russell, J. T., Brownstein, M. J., and Gainer, H., 1980, Biosynthesis of vasopressin, oxytocin, and neurophysins: Isolation and characterization of two common precursors (propresophysin and prooxyphysin), *Endocrinology* **107:**1880–1891.
11. Schmale, J., and Richter, D., 1981, Immunological identification of a common precursor to arginine vasopressin and neurophysin II synthesized by *in vitro* translation of bovine hypothalamic mRNA, *Proc. Natl. Acad. Sci. USA* **787:**766–769.
12. Nicholas, P., Camier, M., Lauber, M., Masse, M. O., Mohring, J., and Cohen, P., 1980, Immunological identification of high molecular weight forms common to bovine neurophysin and vasopressin, *Proc. Natl. Acad. Sci. USA* **77:**2587–2591.
13. Arimura, A., Sato, J., Dupont, A., Nishi, N., and Schally, A. V., 1975, Somatostatin: Abundance of immunoreactive hormone in rat stomach and pancreas, *Science* **189:**1007–1009.
14. Noe, B. D., Fletcher, D. J., Bauer, G. E., Weir, G. C., and Patel, Y., 1978, Somatostatin biosynthesis occurs in pancreatic islets, *Endocrinology* **102:**1675–1685.
15. Ensinck, U. W., Laschansky, E. C., Kanter, R. A., Fujimoto, W. Y., Koerker, D. J., and Goodner, C. H., 1978, Somatostatin biosynthesis and release in the hypothalamus and pancreas of the rat, *Metabolism* **27:**1207–1210.
16. Conlon, M. J., Zyznar, E., Vale, W., and Under, R. H., 1978, Multiple

forms of somatostatin-like immunoreactivity in canine pancreas, *FEBS Lett.* **94**:327–330.

17. Lauber, M., Camier, M., and Cohen, P., 1979, Higher molecular weight forms of immunoreactive somatostatin in mouse hypothalamic extracts: Evidence of processing in vitro, *Proc. Natl. Acad. Sci. USA* **76**:6004–6008.

18. Patzelt, C., Tager, H. S., Carroll, R. J., and Steiner, D. F., 1980, Identification of prosomatostatin in pancreatic islets, *Proc. Natl. Acad. Sci. USA* **77**:2410–2414.

19. Pradayrol, L., Jornvall, H., Mutt, V., and Ribert, A., 1980, N-terminally extended somatostatin: The primary structure of somatostatin 28, *FEBS Lett.* **109**:55–58.

20. Schally, A. V., Huang, W.-Y., Chang, R. C. C., Arimura, A., Redding, T., Millar, R. P., Hunkapiller, M. W., and Hood, L. E., 1980, Isolation and structure of pro-somatostatin: A putative somatostatin precursor from pig hypothalamus, *Proc. Natl. Acad. Sci. USA* **77**:4489–4493.

21. Meyers, C. A., Murphy, W. A., Tedding, T. W., Coy, D. H., and Schally, A. V., 1980, Synthesis and biological actions of prosomatostatin, *Proc. Natl. Acad. Sci. USA* **77**:6171–6174.

22. Goodman, R. H., Jacobs, J. W., Chin, W. W., Lund, P. K., Dee, P. C., and Habener, J. F., 1980, Nucleotide sequence of a cloned structural gene coding for a precursor of pancreatic somatostatin, *Proc. Nat. Acad. Sci. USA* **77**:5869–5873.

23. Genazzani, A. R., Hurliman, J., Fioretti, P., and Felber, J. P., 1974, *In vitro* synthesis of an ACTH-like hormone and human chorionic somatomammotrophin by placental and amniotic cells, *Experientia* **30**:430.

24. Genazzani, A. R., Fraioli, F., Hurliman, J., Fioretti, P., and Felber, J. P., 1975, Immunoreactive ACTH and cortisol plasma levels during pregnancy. Detection and partial purification of corticotrophin-like placental hormone: The human chorionic corticotrophin (HCC), *Clin. Endocrinol. (Oxford)* **4**:1–14.

25. Rees, L. H., Burke, C. W., Evans, S. W., and Letchworth, A. T., 1975, Possible placental origin of ACTH in normal human pregnancy, *Nature (London)* **254**:620–622.

26. Liotta, A. S., Osathanondh, R., Ryan, K. J., and Krieger, D. T., 1977, Presence of ACTH in human placenta: Demonstration of *in vitro* synthesis, *Endocrinology* **101**:1552–1558.

27. Nakai, Y., Nakao, K., Oki, S., and Imura, H., 1978, Presence of immunoreactive β-lipotropin and β-endorphin in human placenta, *Life Sci.* **23**:2013–2018.

28. Clark, D., Thody, A. J., Shuster, S., and Bowers, H., 1978, Immunoreactive α-MSH in human plasma in pregnancy, *Nature (London)* **273**:163–164.

29. Odagiri, E., Sherrell, B. J., Mount, C. D., Nicholson, W. E., and Orth, D. N., 1979, Human placental immunoreactive corticotropin, lipotropin, and β-endorphin: Evidence for a common precursor, *Proc. Natl. Acad. Sci. USA* **76**:2027–2031.

30. Liotta, A. S., and Krieger, D. T., 1980, *In vitro* biosynthesis and comparative posttranslational processing of immunoreactive precursor corticotropin/β-

endorphin by human placental and pituitary cells, *Endocrinology* **106:**1504–1511.

31. Vandesande, F., Dierickx, K., and DeMey, J., 1975, Identification of the vasopressin–neurophysin producing neurons of the rat suprachiasmatic nuclei, *Cell Tissue Res.* **156:**377–380.

32. Buijs, R. M., 1980, Immunocytochemical demonstration of vasopressin and oxytocin in the rat brain by light and electron microscopy, *J. Histochem. Cytochem.* **28:**357–360.

33. Ono, T., Nishino, H., Sasaka, K., Muramoto, K., Yano, I., and Simpson, A., 1978, Paraventricular nucleus connections to spinal cord and pituitary, *Neurosci. Lett.* **10:**141–146.

34. Elde, R., and Hökfelt, T., 1978, Distribution of hypothalamic hormones and other peptides in the brain, in: *Frontiers in Neuroendocrinology*, Volume 5 (W. F. Ganong and L. Martini, eds.), pp. 1–34, Raven Press, New York.

35. van Wimersma Greidanus, T. B., Croiset, G., Bakker, E., and Bouman, H., 1979, Amygdaloid lesions block the effect of neuropeptides (vasopressin, ACTH 4–10) on avoidance behavior, *Physiol. Behav.* **22:**291–295.

36. Krisch, B., and Leonhardt, H., 1979, Demonstration of a somatostatin-like activity in retinal cells of the rat, *Cell Tissue Res.* **204:**127–140.

37. Yamada, T., Marshak, D., Basinger, S., Walsh, J., Morley, J., and Stell, W., 1980, Somatostatin-like immunoreactivity in the retina, *Proc. Natl. Acad. Sci. USA* **77:**1691–1695.

38. Larsson, L.-I., Golterman, N., de Magistris, L., Rehfeld, J. F., and Schwartz, T. W., 1979, Somatostatin cell processes as pathways for paracrine secretion, *Science* **205:**1393–1395.

39. Bolaffi, J. L., Reichlin, S., Goodman, D. B. P., and Forrest, J. N., Jr., 1980, Somatostatin: Occurrence in urinary bladder epithelium and renal tubules of the toad, *Bufo marinus, Science* **210:**644–646.

40. Forrest, J. N., Jr., Reichlin, S., and Goodman, D. B. P., 1980, Somatostatin: An endogenous peptide in the toad urinary bladder inhibits vasopressin-stimulated water flow, *Proc. Natl. Acad. Sci. USA* **77:**4984–4987.

41. Silverman, A. J., and Krey, L. C., 1978, The luteinizing hormone-releasing hormone (LH-RH) neuronal networks of the guinea pig brain. 1. Intra- and extra-hypothalamic projections, *Brain Res.* **157:**233–246.

42. Brownstein, M. J., 1980, Distribution of hypothalamic hormones, in: *The Endocrine Functions of the Brain* (M. Motta, ed.), pp. 143–154, Raven Press, New York.

43. Clayton, R. N., Harwood, J. P., and Catt, K. J. 1979, Gonadotropin-releasing hormone analogue binds to luteal cells and inhibits progesterone production, *Nature (London)* **282:**90–92.

44. Clayton, R. N., Katikineni, M., Chan, V., Dufau, M. L., and Catt, K. J., 1980, Direct inhibition of testicular function by gonadotropin-releasing hormone: Mediation by specific gonadotropin-releasing hormone receptors in interstitial cells, *Proc. Natl. Acad. Sci. USA* **77:**4459–4463.

45. Khodr, G. S., and Siler-Khodr, T., 1978, Localization of luteinizing hormone-releasing factor in the human placenta, *Fertil. Steril.* **29:**523–526.

46. Ying. S. Y., and Guillemin, R., 1980, Gonadocrinins: Peptides in ovarian

follicular fluid stimulating the secretion of pituitary gonadotropins, 62nd Annual Meeting of the Endocrine Society, p. 114, Abstract No. 158.

47. Sharpe, R. M., and Fraser, H. M., 1980, HCG stimulation of testicular LHRH-like activity, *Nature (London)* **287**:642–643.

48. Youngblood, W. W., Lipton, M. A., and Kizer, J. S., 1978, TRH-like immunoreactivity in urine, serum, and extrahypothalamic brain: Non-identity with synthetic Pyroglu-His-pro-NH₂ (TRH), *Brain Res.* **151**:99–116.

49. Kreider, M. S., Winokur, A., and Utiger, R. D., 1979, TRH immunoreactivity in rat hypothalamus and brain: Assessment by gel filtration and thin-layer chromatography, *Brain Res.* **171**:161–165.

50. Spindel, E., and Wurtman, R., 1979, Immunoreactive thyrotropin releasing hormone (TRH) outside the hypothalamus really is TRH, *Soc. Neurosci. Abstr.* **5**:539.

51. Morley, J. E., Garvin, T. J., Pekary, A. E., and Hershman, J. M., 1977, Thyrotropin-releasing hormone in the gastrointestinal tract, *Biochem. Biophys. Res. Commun.* **79**:314–318.

52. Leppaluoto, J., Koivulsalo, F., and Kraama, R., 1978, Thyrotropin-releasing factor: Distribution in neural and gastrointestinal tissues, *Acta Physiol. Scand.* **104**:175–179.

53. Gibbons, J. M., Mitnick, M., and Chiefo, V., 1975, In vitro biosynthesis of TSH- and LH-releasing factors by the human placenta, *Am. J. Obstet. Gynecol.* **121**:127–131.

54. de Kloet, R., and de Wied, D., 1980, The brain as target tissue for hormones of pituitary origin: Behavioral and biochemical studies, in: *Frontiers in Neuroendocrinology*, Volume 6 (L. Martini and W. F Ganong, eds.), pp. 157–202, Raven Press, New York.

55. Sandman, C. A., George, J., Walker, B.B., Nolan, J. D., and Kastin, A. J., 1976, Neuropeptide MSH-ACTH 4–10 enhances attention in the mentally retarded, *Pharmacol. Biochem. Behav.* **5**(Suppl. 1):23–28.

56. Sandman, C. A., and Kastin, A. J., 1978, A behavioral strategy for the CNS actions of the neuropeptides, in: *Current Studies of Hypothalamic Function*, Volume 2 (K. Lederis and W. L. Veale, eds.), pp. 163–174, Karger, Basel.

57. Bohus, B., 1979, Effects of ACTH-like neuropeptides on animal behavior and man, *Pharmacology* **18**:113–122.

58. Legros, J. J., Gilot, P., Seron, X., Claessens, J., Adam, A., Moeglen, J. M., Audibert, A., and Berchier, P., 1978, Influence of vasopressin on learning and memory, *Lancet* **1**:41–42.

59. Oliveros, J. C., Jandali, M. K., Timsit-Berthier, M., Remy, R., Benghezal, A., Audibert, A., and Moeglin, J. M., 1978, Vasopressin in amnesia, *Lancet* **1**:42–43.

60. Anderson, L. T., Davis, R., Bonnet, K., and Dancis, J., 1979, Passive avoidance learning in Lesch–Nyhan disease: Effect of 1-desamino-8-arginine vasopressin, *Life Sci.* **24**:905–910.

61. Jenkins, J. S., Mather, H. M., Coughland, A. K., and Jenkins, D. G., 1979, Desmopressin in post-traumatic amnesia, *Lancet* **2**:1245–1246.

62. Gibbs, J., Young, E. C., and Smith, G. P., 1973, Cholecystokinin elicits satiety in rats with open gastric fistulas, *Nature (London)* **245**:323–325.

63. Vijayan, E., and McCann, S. M., 1979, Suppression of feeding and drinking activity in rats following intraventricular injection of thyrotropin releasing hormone (TRH), *Endocrinology* **100:**1727–1730.

64. Woods, S. C., Lotter, E. C., McKay, L. D., and Porte, D., Jr., 1979, Chronic intracerebroventricular infusion of insulin reduces food intake and body weight of baboons, *Nature (London)* **282:**503–505.

65. Straus, E., and Yalow, R. S., 1979, Cholecystokinin in the brains of obese and nonobese mice, *Science* **203:**68–69.

66. Schneider, B. S., Monahan, J. W., and Hirsch, J., 1979, Brain cholecystokinin and nutritional status in rats and mice, *J. Clin. Invest.* **64:**1136–1147.

67. Oku, J., Glick, Z., Shimomura, Y., Inoue, S., Bray, G. A., and Walsh, J., 1980, Cholecystokinin and obesity, *Clin. Res.* **28:**281A.

68. Ho, P., and Hansky, J., 1979, Cholecystokinin (CCK)-like peptide in gut and brain of normal and genetically obese mice, *Gastroenterology* **76:**1155A.

69. Gibson, M. J., and Krieger, D. T., 1980, Altered CNS–pituitary function in Zucker *(fa/fa)* fatty rats: Absent circadian periodicity of activity, feeding, and plasma corticosterone (B) concentrations and elevated brain and pituitary neurointermediate (NI) lobe beta-endorphin (B-EP) concentrations, *Soc. Neurosci. Abstr.* **6:**118.

70. Gambert, S. R., Garthwait, T. L., Pontzer, C. H., and Hagen, T. C., 1980, Fasting associated with decrease in hypothalamic β-endorphin, *Science* **210:**1271–1272.

71. Morley, J. E., 1980, The neuroendocrine control of appetite: The role of the endogenous opiates, cholecystokinin, TRH, gamma-amino-butyric acid and the diazepam receptor, *Life Sci.* **27:**355–368.

72. Carraway, R. E., Demers, L. M., and Leeman, S. E., 1976, Hyperglycemic effect of neurotensin, a hypothalamic peptide, *Endocrinology* **99:**1452–1462.

73. Brown, M., and Vale, W., 1979, Bombesin—A putative mammalian neurogastrointestinal peptide, *Trends Neurosci.* **2:**95–97.

74. Morley, J. E., and Levine, A. S., 1980, Intraventricular cholecystokinin-octapeptide (CCK-8) produces hyperglycemia and hypothermia, *Clin. Res.* **28:**721A.

75. Blackburn, A. M., Fletcher, D. R., Adrian, T. E., and Bloom, S. R., 1980, Neurotensin infusion in man: Pharmacokinetics and effect on gastrointestinal and pituitary hormones, *J. Clin. Endocrinol. Metab.* **51:**1257–1261.

76. Wardlaw, S. L., Wehrenberg, W. B., Ferin, M., Carmel, P. W., and Frantz, A. G., 1980, High levels of β-endorphin in hypophyseal portal blood, *Endocrinology* **106:**1323–1326.

77. Simantov, R., and Snyder, S. H., 1977, Opiate receptor binding in the pituitary gland, *Brain Res.* **124:**178–184.

78. Rivier, C., Vale, W., Ling, N., Brown, M., and Guillemin, R., 1977, Stimulation *in vivo* of the secretion of prolactin and growth hormone by β-endorphin, *Endocrinology* **100:**238–240.

79. Grandison, L., Fratta, W., and Guidotti, A., 1980, Location and characterization of opiate receptors regulating pituitary secretion, *Life Sci.* **26:**1633–1642.

80. Shaar, C. J., Frederickson, R. C. A., Dininger, N. B., and Jackson, L., 1977,

Enkephalin analogues and naloxone modulate the release of growth hormone and prolactin—Evidence for regulation by an endogenous opioid peptide in brain, *Life Sci.* **21**:853–860.

81. Enjalbert, A., Rubert, M., Arancibia, S., Priam, M., and Kordon, C., 1979, Endogenous opiates block dopamine inhibition of prolactin secretion *in vitro*, *Nature (London)* **280**:595–597.

82. Wardlaw, S. L., Wehrenberg, W. B., Ferin, M., and Frantz, A. G., 1980, Failure of β-endorphin to stimulate prolactin release in the pituitary stalk-sectioned monkey, *Endocrinology* **107**:1663–1666.

83. Deyo, S. N., Swift, R. M., and Miller, R. J., 1979, Morphine and endorphins modulate dopamine turnover in rat median eminence, *Proc. Natl. Acad. Sci. USA* **76**:3006–3009.

84. Van Vugt, D. A., Bruni, J. F., Sylvester, P. W., Chen, H. T., Ieiri, T., and Meites, J., 1979, Interaction between opiates and hypothalamic dopamine on prolactin release, *Life Sci.* **24**:2361–2367.

85. Wilkes, M. M., Fulton, S. L., and Yen, S. S. C.,1980, Attenuation by β-endorphin (β-EP) of efflux of dopamine (DA) and its deaminated metabolite from superfused medial basal hypothalamus (MBH) in vitro, 62nd Annual Meeting of the Endocrine Society, p. 152.

86. Gudelsky, G. A., and Porter, J. C., 1978, Morphine- and opioid-induced increase in striatal dopamine turnover, *Life Sci.* **23**:961–970.

87. Spampinato, S., Locatelli, V., Cocchi, D., Vincentini, L., Bajusz, S., Ferri, S., and Muller, E. E., 1979, Involvement of brain serotonin in the prolactin releasing effect of opioid peptides, *Endocrinology* **105**:163–170.

88. Tolis, G., Hickey, J., and Guyda, H., 1975, Effects of morphine on serum growth hormone, cortisol, prolactin and thyroid stimulating hormone in man, *J. Clin. Endocrinol. Metab.* **41**:797–800.

89. Foley, K. M., Inturrisi, C. E., Kourides, I. A., Kaiko, R. F., Posner, J. B., Houde, R. W., and Li, C, H., 1978, Intravenous (iv) and intraventricular (ivt) administration of beta-endorphin (βH-EP) in man: Safety and disposition, in: *Characteristics and Function of Opioids* (J. M. van Ree and L. Terenius, eds.), pp. 421–422, Elsevier/North-Holland, Amsterdam.

90. Lehmann, H., Nair, N. P. V., and Kline, N. S., 1979, β-Endorphin and naloxone in psychiatric patients: Clinical and biological effects, *Am. J. Psychiatry* **136**:762–766.

91. Catlin, D. H., Polane, R. E., Gorelick, D. A., Gerner, R. H., Hui, K. K., Rubin, R. T., and Li, C. H., 1980, Intravenous infusion of β-endorphin increases serum prolactin, but not growth hormone or cortisol, in depressed subjects and withdrawing methadone addicts, *J. Clin. Endocrinol. Metab.* **50**:1021–1025.

92. Wakabayashi, I., Demura, R., Mike, N., Ohmura, E., Miyoshi, H., and Shizume, K., 1980, Failure of naloxone to influence plasma growth hormone, prolactin, and cortisol secretions induced by insulin hypoglycemia, *J. Clin. Endocrinol. Metab.* **50**:597–599.

93. Volavka, J., Bauman, J., Pevnick, J., Reker, D., James, B., and Cho, D., 1980, Short-term hormonal effects of naloxone in man, *Psychoneuroendocrinology* **5**:225–234.

94. Veldhuis, J. D., Worgul, T. J., Monsaert, R., and Hammond, J. M., 1980, A possible role for endogenous opioids in the control of prolactin and luteinizing-hormone secretion in the human, *Clin. Res.* **28:**269A.

95. Martin, J. B., Tolis, G., Woods, I., and Guyda, H., 1979, Failure of naloxone to influence physiological growth hormone and prolactin secretion, *Brain Res.* **168:**210–215.

96. Spiler, I. J., and Molitch, M. E., 1980, Lack of modulation of pituitary hormone stress response by neural pathways involving opiate receptors, *J. Clin. Endocrinol. Metab.* **50:**516–520.

97. Blankstein, J., Reyes, R. I., Winter, J. S. D., and Faiman, C., 1980, Effects of naloxone upon prolactin and cortisol in normal women, *Proc. Soc. Exp. Biol. Med.* **164:**363–372.

98. Quigley, M. E., Sheehan, K. L., Casper, R. F., and Yen, S. S. C., 1980, Evidence for an increased opioid inhibition of luteinizing hormone secretion in hyperprolactinemic patients with pituitary microadenoma, *J. Clin. Endocrinol. Metab.* **50:**427–430.

99. Quigley, M. E., and Yen, S. S. C., 1980, The role of endogenous opiates on LH secretions during the menstrual cycle, *J. Clin. Endocrinol. Metab.* **51:**179–181.

100. Jeffcoate, W. J., Rees, L. H., McLoughlin, L., Ratter, S. J., Hope, J., Lowry, P. J., and Besser, G. M., 1978, β-Endorphin in human cerebrospinal fluid, *Lancet* **2:**119–121.

101. Liotta, A. S., and Krieger, D. T., 1980, Electrophoretic heterogeneity of rat brain and pituitary immunoreactive (immuno) beta-endorphin (EP), 62nd Annual Meeting of the Endocrine Society, p. 221.

102. Liotta, A. S., and Houghten, R., 1980, Charge heterogeneity of human pituitary and plasma immunoreactive (immuno) β-endorphin (β-EP), *Clin. Res.* **28:**480A.

103. Dunger, D. B., Leonard, J. V., Wolff, O. H., and Preece, M. A., 1980, Effect of naloxone in a previously undescribed hypothalamic syndrome, *Lancet* **1:**1277–1281.

104. Brandt, N. J., Terenius, L., Jacobsen, B. B., Klinken, L., Nordius, A., Brandt, S., Blegvad, K., and Yssing, M., 1980, Hyper-endorphin syndrome in a child with necrotizing encephalomyelopathy, *N. Engl. J. Med.* **303:**914–916.

105. Jacquet, P., Guibout, M., Jaquet, C., Grisoli, F., Conte Devolx, B., Dumas, D., and Bert, J., 1980, Circadian regulation of growth hormone secretion after treatment in acromegaly, *J. Clin. Endocrinol. Metab.* **50:**322–328.

106. Arafah, B. M., Brodkey, J. S., Kaufman, B., Velasco, M., Manni, A., and Pearson, O. H., 1980, Transsphenoidal microsurgery in the treatment of acromegaly and gigantism, *J. Clin. Endocrinol. Metab.* **50:**578–585.

107. Fine, S. A., and Frohman, L. A., 1978, Loss of central nervous system component of dopaminergic inhibition of prolactin secretion in patients with prolactin-secreting pituitary tumors, *J. Clin. Invest.* **61:**973–980.

108. Crosignani, P. G., Ferrari, C., Malinverni, A., Barbieri, C., Mattei, A. M., Caldara, R., and Rochetti, M., 1980, Effect of central nervous system dopaminergic activation on prolactin secretion in man: Evidence for a com-

mon central defect in hyperprolactinemia patients with and without radiological signs of pituitary tumors, *J. Clin. Endocrinol. Metab.* **51**:1068–1073.

109. Pilotte, N. S., Gudelsky, G. A., and Porter, J. C., 1976, Relationship of dopamine turnover in the median eminence to dopamine concentration in hypophysial portal plasma and prolactin release, *Soc. Neurosci. Abstr.* **5**:476.

110. St. George Tucker, J., Lankford, H. V., Gardner, D. G., and Blackard, W. G., 1980, Persistent defect in regulation of prolactin secretion after successful pituitary tumor removal in women with the galactorrhea–amenorrhea syndrome, *J. Clin. Endocrinol. Metab.* **51**:968–971.

111. Frantz, A. G., Cogen, P. H., Chang, C. H., and Holub, D. A., 1981, Long-term evaluation of the results of transsphenoidal surgery and radiotherapy in patients with prolactinoma, in: *Endocrinology of Human Infertility: New Aspects* (P. Crosignani and B. L. Rubin, eds.), Grune & Stratton, New York.

112. Tyrrell, J. B., Brooks, R. M., Fitzgerald, P. A., Cofoid, P. B., Forsham, P. H., and Wilson, C. B., 1978, Selective trans-sphenoidal resection of pituitary microadenomas, *N. Engl. J. Med.* **298**:753–758.

113. Salassa, R. M., Laws, E. R., Jr., Carpenter, P. C., and Northcutt, R. C., 1978, Transsphenoidal removal of pituitary microadenoma in Cushing's disease, *Mayo Clin. Proc.* **53**:24–28.

114. Bigos, S. T., Somma, M., Rasio, E., Eastman, R. C., Lanthier, A., Johnston, H. H., and Hardy, J., 1980, Cushing's disease: Management by transsphenoidal pituitary microsurgery, *J. Clin. Endocrinol. Metab.* **50**:348–354.

115. Kuwayama, A., Kageyama, N., Nakane, T., Watanabe, M., and Kanie, N., 1980, Anterior pituitary function after transsphenoidal selective microadenomectomy in Cushing's disease, *Proc. VII Int. Cong. Endocrinol.*, Melbourne, No. 385.

116. Fitzgerald, P. A., Tyrrell, J. B., Brooks, R. M., Forsham, P. H., and Wilson, C. B., 1978, Cushing's disease: Secondary adrenal insufficiency after selective removal of pituitary adenomas, 60th Annual Meeting of the Endocrine Society, p. 250.

117. Boyar, R. M., Witkin, M., Carruth, A., and Ramsey, J., 1979, Circadian cortisol secretory rhythms in Cushing's disease, *J. Clin. Endocrinol. Metab.* **48**:760–765.

118. Lagerquist, L. G., Meikle, A. W., West, D. C., and Tyler, F. H., 1974, Cushing's disease with cure by resection of a pituitary adenoma: Evidence against a primary hypothalamic defect, *Am. J. Med.* **57**:826–830.

119. Schnall, A. M., Brodkey, J. S., Kaufman, B., and Pearson, O. H., 1978, Pituitary function after removal of pituitary microadenomas in Cushing's disease, *J. Clin. Endocrinol. Metab.* **47**:410–417.

120. Carmalt, M. H. B., Dalton, G. A., Fletcher, R. F., and Smith, W. T., 1977, The treatment of Cushing's disease by trans-sphenoidal hypophysectomy, *Q. J. Med.* **46**:119–134.

121. Pont, A., and Gutierrez-Hartman, A., 1979, Cushing's disease: Recurrence after a surgically induced remission, *Arch. Intern. Med.* **139**:938–940.

Prolactin and Growth Hormone in Health and Disease

William H. Daughaday

2.1. Introduction

The pituitary is best considered as five more or less independent endocrine secretory units that happen to be accommodated in the same anatomical location. Because the thyrotropin, corticotropin, and gonadotropin secretory units are more readily considered in relation to their end organ effects, this review focuses on the two secretory units for prolactin and growth hormone (GH) that act without an intermediary endocrine target gland. While prolactin exerts all of its physiologic effects directly, some of the physiologic actions of GH are mediated by the somatomedins (insulin-like growth factors). In this chapter the principal recent contribution to our knowledge of prolactin, GH, and somatomedins as it relates to human physiology and disease will be reviewed. Even with this restricted scope no attempt has been made to include all publications in this area, but those of greatest interest and application will be considered.

WILLIAM H. DAUGHADAY ● Metabolism Division, Department of Medicine, Washington University School of Medicine, St. Louis, Missouri 63110.

2.2. Prolactin

2.2.1. The Prolactin Gene and mRNA

The human prolactin cDNA complementary to the prolactin mRNA has been cloned and its nucleotide sequence established.[1] The prolactin mRNA defined by this sequence codes for a primary translation product of 227 amino acids. This preprolactin contains a signal peptide of 28 amino acids and prolactin itself, which contains 199 amino acids. Knowledge of the mRNA nucleotide sequence allowed recognition of an additional serine in position 28, which was unrecognized in the original peptide sequencing.

The human prolactin gene has been localized to chromosome 6 and is thus separated from the genes and pseudogenes for hGH and somatomammotropin, which are present in linear array on the long arm of chromosome 17.[2] The detailed structure of the human prolactin gene has not yet been established but it is likely that it will have sequences coding for four introns interrupting the five exons of the pre-mRNA.

2.2.2. Prolactin Molecular Heterogeneity

Heterogeneity of circulating peptide hormones is a common phenomenon and it is not unexpected that different molecular forms of prolactin exist in the pituitary and body fluids. Nybert et al.[3] isolated prolactin from frozen human pituitaries using mild chromatographic procedures. The final product was subjected to zonal electrophoresis in 0.17% agarose at alkaline pH. Prolactin immunoreactivity was present in three bands. The most retarded band had a higher relative activity in a radioimmunoassay and a lower prolactin bioactivity in a pigeon crop-sack assay as compared to the initial preparation. The most rapidly moving band had enhanced biologic potency relative to its immunologic reactivity. The intermediate band could be further resolved into two roughly equal components by isoelectric focusing. The difference between these components probably represented a difference in only one net charge.

In addition to this heterogeneity of charge, size heterogeneity of prolactin is known to exist. A "big" prolactin with a molecular weight of about 50,000, about twice that of prolactin monomer, has been demonstrated by gel filtration. This component represents about 9% of serum prolactin immunoactivity. A "big-big" prolactin is also present in the void volume and constitutes about 5% of the total immunoactivity. In patients with prolactinomas, the percentage of "big" prolactin is often increased and in two patients constituted 32 and 40% of the immunoreactivity.[4] In another patient with acromegaly, "big-big" prolactin accounted for 58% of the immunoactivity. In radioreceptor assays, "big" prolactin proved much less active than prolactin monomer. Under certain conditions, "big" prolactin could be converted into "little" prolactin and the suggestion was made that "big" prolactin represents a dimer linked by intermolecular disulfide bonds and is not a true precursor prohormone.

Prolactin is found in spinal fluid in increased amounts in patients with large suprasellar prolactinomas. There is disagreement concerning the size heterogeneity of CSF prolactin. Kiefer and Malarkey[5] reported that there was an increased proportion of "big-big" prolactin, whereas Jordan and Kendall[6] found reduced amounts of this prolactin.

Despite the established size heterogeneity of prolactin, knowledge of the human prolactin mRNA structure rules out a precursor role for "big" and "big-big" prolactin; increased proportions of these larger molecular forms are inconstant findings and not of diagnostic import.

2.2.3. Amniotic Fluid Prolactin

The amniotic fluid contains relatively large amounts of prolactin, particularly in midpregnancy. That the maternal or fetal pituitary is not the source of this prolactin has been shown by bromocriptine administration; this drug, which can suppress maternal and fetal pituitary prolactin secretion, does not lower amniotic fluid prolactin. There is now considerable evidence that this prolactin arises from decidual tissue. Human chorion-decidual tissue contains prolactin mRNA,[7] and several groups showed that fetal membranes with attached decidual tissue released immunoassayable prolactin in vitro. Golander et al.[8] succeeded in completely separating decidual tissue from amniotic or chorionic membranes by using membranes separating dizygotic twins. They obtained chorionic membranes unassociated with decidua from the membranes separating dizygotic twins. These membranes released prolactin only transiently in vitro and did not incorporate labeled amino acids into prolactin. Decidual explants, however, incorporated labeled amino acids into prolactin and had sustained secretion of prolactin in vitro.

Further evidence that decidual tissue can synthesize prolactin has been provided by Maslar and Riddick.[9] In women, decidualization of the uterine endometrium occurs during the second week of the luteal phase of the menstrual cycle. Endometrial biopsy specimens incubated in culture medium released no prolactin in the proliferative or early secretory phases of the menstrual cycle. Small amounts of prolactin were secreted on days 21–24 of the cycle, and much larger amounts of prolactin were released on days 27 and 28. These studies provide further evidence of the decidual source of prolactin, indicating that pregnancy is not a prerequisite for the synthesis of prolactin. The functional significance of decidual prolactin remains to be determined. Maslar and Riddick speculate that decidual prolactin may act at the local tissue level in the uterus or may affect corpus luteal function. Because prolactin has a role in fluid and electrolyte metabolism in fish and some other non-mammalian vertebrates, a possible role in amniotic fluid regulation has been proposed.

Despite the proximity of decidua to the amniotic space, it is not clear how prolactin traverses the fetal membranes to reach very high concentrations in the amniotic fluid. The anatomy suggests that the polarity of secretion would be directed toward the mother and not across the fetal membranes. Fetal membranes with or without attached decidua are unable to transfer significant concentrations of [^{125}I]prolactin in either direction when studied *in vitro* in a two-chamber perfusion apparatus.[10,11] However, prolactin that is formed within attached decidua is transferred freely across the chorionic and amniotic membranes. This transfer could be inhibited by the addition of colchicine, suggesting a role for the microtubular system. Direct cellular contact, perhaps by intercellular bridges, appears to be required.

2.2.4. Pituitary Prolactin Secretion in Pregnancy

In normal human pregnancy, there is a progressive rise in serum prolactin that parallels the increase in serum estrogens. Two studies have addressed the question of whether there is an alteration in prolactin secretory reserve as measured by the response to TRH. In the first study, Ylikorkala et al.[12] found that the thyrotropin and prolactin responses to 200 μg of TRH i.v. were not altered as pregnancy progressed. Kletzky et al.,[13] in a similar study, found an augmentation of the prolactin response during the first trimester and a further rise in the TRH response in the second trimester. No further rise occurred in the third trimester during the period of greatest rise in the basal prolactin levels. Thus, despite the lactotroph hyperplasia that occurs in pregnancy, there is little or no increase in prolactin secretory reserve.

The consequences of excessive lowering of serum prolactin with bromocriptine administration in human pregnancy have been investigated. Ylikorkala et al.[14] gave bromocriptine to 29 women who had requested a "morning-after" contraceptive. Serum prolactin levels were lowered to less than 2 ng/ml. A rise in hCG indicating implantation occurred in five women and legal abortion was performed in three. In two women the putative pregnancy terminated in menstruation. The authors concluded that the abnormally low prolactin levels of these women had not adversely affected implantation and normal early pregnancy.

They did not consider the occurrence of two occult pregnancies excessive.

A possible role for prolactin in controlling the levels of hCG in pregnancy was suggested by Yuen et al.[15] A patient with a prolactinoma was treated with bromocriptine for the first 32 weeks of pregnancy. From day 18 to week 32, the hCG levels in serum were definitely elevated. When bromocriptine was discontinued, prolactin levels rose from 10 to about 70 ng/ml and serum hCG fell to less than half its former level. Subsequent pregnancy and delivery were uneventful. Two other women who received bromocriptine in pregnancy with only slight hypoprolactinemia did not show this hormonal pattern. Although these two studies did not show that bromocriptine adversely affected the course of pregnancy, its safety for mother and infant has not been established. The use of the drug in pregnancy is not authorized by the FDA.

The fetal pituitary, like that of the mother, is exposed to high concentrations of estrogens and responds with an increase in prolactin secretion. Perlman et al.[16] observed that the postnatal fall in serum prolactin was delayed in premature, compared with full-term, newborn infants. However, when comparisons were made according to postmenstrual age, the decline in prolactin levels was similar. The authors suggested that premature infants had not yet established the hypothalamic inhibition of prolactin secretion by prolactin-inhibiting factor (dopamine).

2.2.5. Physiologic Secretion of Prolactin and Functional Abnormalities

Normally there is a circadian rhythm of prolactin secretion, a significant rise in serum levels occurring in the later hours of sleep. Polleri et al.[17] have shown that the normal adult pattern is established in children at 3 to 6 years of age. In boys with gynecomastia, both daytime and nighttime secretion of prolactin are modestly increased.[18] This increase correlated with the estrogen–androgen imbalance that exists in gynecomastia. The elevation of prolactin appeared to account for the one case of transient galactorrhea associated with gynecomastia in this series.

Conflicting reports have appeared concerning the secretion of prolactin in primary and secondary hypogonadism. Spitz et al.[19] studied pituitary function following the administration of TRH and LRH in six patients with isolated gonadotropin deficiency and six patients with primary testicular failure. These latter patients had elevated gonadotropins but relatively normal estrogen and testosterone levels. Although baseline prolactin levels were not different between the groups, the prolactin response to TRH was greatly impaired in the patients with hypogonadotropic hypogonadism. A greater than normal prolactin response was observed in patients with primary testicular failure, perhaps because of disturbed estrogen–androgen balance. Treatment of patients with go-nadotropin deficiency with hCG restored the prolactin response to TRH.

In contrast to the above report, Turksoy[20] described a case of Kall-mann's syndrome in a young woman whose prolactin response to TRH was normal but whose response to chlorpromazine administration was absent.

The secretion of prolactin in hypothyroidism has been studied in the past. In general, some but not all investigators found basal levels of prolactin to be elevated in individual patients and the response to TRH exaggerated. An occasional hypothyroid patient will have galactorrhea. Two recent studies extend information on this subject. Suter et al.[21] measured basal and TRH-stimulated serum prolactin in 43 normal chil-dren, 41 children with primary hypothyroidism, and 28 children with idiopathic thyrotropin deficiency. Sixty-eight percent of the children with primary hypothyroidism had elevated serum prolactin levels (i.e., >15 ng/ml). The serum prolactin in children with hypothalamic thy-rotropin deficiency was lower than in children with primary hypothy-roidism. In confirmation of earlier findings, the response to TRH was exaggerated. The authors conclude that in primary hypothyroidism, both increased endogenous TRH secretion and increased lactotroph sensitivity to TRH are present. In children with hypothalamic hypothy-roidism, decreased secretion of dopamine might be involved.

Honbo et al.[22] conducted a similar study of hypothyroidism in adults. Basal prolactin levels were elevated in 39% of patients and this elevation was more common in women. In fact, the mean serum prolactin level in hypothyroid men was not higher than that in the euthyroid control group. A significant correlation between the log of serum prolactin and the log of serum TSH was evident. Galactorrhea was not present in any of the 39 hypothyroid women. In another study of 50 hypothyroid women, Contreras et al.[23] found a linear correlation between the serum prolactin and the duration of hypothyroidism and a logarithmic correlation be-tween serum prolactin and TSH levels. The 7 patients with spontaneous hypothyroidism and galactorrhea were younger and had higher serum prolactin levels than in 20 hypothyroid patients without galactorrhea (69 ± 8.9 ng/ml vs. 42.9 ± 2.2 ng/ml).

In a provocative article, Ben-David and Schenker[24] proposed that transient hyperprolactinemia can affect fertility in women with normal menstrual cycles. In a group of 48 women with long-standing idiopathic infertility and normal menses, 45 were found to have transitory rises of serum prolactin to 27–70 ng/ml associated with the preovulatory rise in estradiol. When bromocriptine was given in doses sufficient to suppress this transitory hyperprolactinemia, pregnancy occurred in 18 women within 3 months. The authors suggest that transient hyperprolactinemia might impair fertilization or implantation. It is possible that bromocriptine might have affected fertility by a mechanism independent of prolactin suppression.

2.2.6. Hyperprolactinemia in Uremia

A number of alterations of pituitary function occur in chronic renal failure (see review by Tolis et al.[25]). Prolactin secretion has been carefully investigated because of the frequent occurrence of decreased gonadal function and galactorrhea. About 60% of men and 90% of women with chronic renal failure have elevated serum prolactin concentrations. Hemodialysis is not effective in lowering serum prolactin, but successful renal transplantation will restore normal prolactin concentrations. In uremia the rise in serum prolactin following TRH administration is markedly decreased. The elevation of prolactin in uremia has commonly been attributed to decreased renal clearance of prolactin, although the net contribution of the kidneys to total prolactin clearance is unresolved. In a study by Lim et al.,[26] oral administration of 0.5 g of L-dopa did not significantly lower prolactin levels. This failure could not be attributed to impaired decarboxylation of L-dopa because dopamine infusions were equally ineffective in acutely lowering serum prolactin levels. The authors concluded that the chronic hyperprolactinemia in this condition was the result of a hypothalamic defect. In addition, the impaired responses to TRH and dopamine suggested that the lactotroph response to regulatory substances was abnormal. This abnormality could exist at the receptor or postreceptor level.

In another study of patients with renal insufficiency, Gomez et al.[27] confirmed the impaired prolactin response to TRH and the impaired acute inhibitory response to the dopaminergic agent, bromocriptine. However, with more prolonged bromocriptine administration in a daily dose of 3.75–5.0 mg/day, they did succeed in lowering serum prolactin levels by 60% in patients undergoing hemodialysis. The effect was observed at 10 days and was sustained for the 30 days of the study. Surprisingly, the four women with galactorrhea continued to have galactorrhea despite a 90% reduction of serum prolactin. Three of the ten women had resumption of menstruation during bromocriptine treatment. No improvement in potency was observed in five men.

2.2.7. Prolactin Effects on Androgens

There are conflicting reports concerning the concentration of dehydroepiandrosterone sulfate (DHA-S) and 17-ketosteroids in women with hyperprolactinemia. A number of recent contributions to this field have appeared. Vermeulen and Ando[28] found that DHA and DHA-S were elevated in young women with prolactinomas. In three postmenopausal women with prolactinomas, DHA was elevated in each and DHA-S was elevated in two. In men with prolactinomas, DHA-S but not DHA was elevated. Bromocriptine therapy lowered serum levels of prolactin, DHA, and DHA-S. The metabolic clearance rate of DHA-S was found to be normal in patients with prolactinomas. The elevations in DHA-S thus could not be attributed to reduced metabolism of the steroid.

In contrast to these findings, Parker et al.[29] found no difference in serum cortisol, DHA, Δ^4 androstenedione, and DHA-S in five men and eight women with prolactinomas. The two studies differ in the severity of the hyperprolactinemia, which averaged 198.8 ng/ml in the patients studied by Parker et al. but was in excess of 900 ng/ml in the patients studied by Vermeulen and Ando. In addition, Parker et al. did not separately analyze their results by age and sex.

In a reexamination of this question, Lobo et al.[30] studied 21 women with the hyperprolactinemia (mean 257 ng/ml), amenorrhea, galactorrhea syndrome. The mean plasma DHA-S was 2.54 ± 0.2 μg/ml, compared with 1.78 ± 0.1 μg/ml in 41 normal control women. While the results in the hyperprolactinemic women closely resembled those obtained by Parker et al., the control results that Lobo et al. obtained in women were considerably lower than found by Parker et al. in men and women.

From these various studies, one can conclude that with proper matching of control groups it is possible to observe an increase in DHA and DHA-S in severely hyperprolactinemic women.

An acute effect of hyperprolactinemia on plasma testosterone has been studied by Rubin and collaborators in a series of publications. They reported that hyperprolactinemia induced by a single dose of the dopamine-blocking agent, haloperidol, produced a relative increase in serum testosterone.[31] This increase was unassociated with changes in serum LH. In a second study, they found no synergistic effect of hLH administration and haloperidol-induced hyperprolactinemia in elevating plasma testosterone.[32] To rule out the possibility that haloperidol might be affecting plasma testosterone by mechanisms other than by elevating serum prolactin, they increased prolactin levels by the administration of a long-acting TRH analog, N^{31m}-methylthyrotropin releasing hormone. The serum testosterone level of young men receiving methyltestosterone was increased; however, it is likely that more prolonged administration of methyl-TRH might lead to decreased testosterone by prolactin suppression of gonadotropin secretion.

2.2.8. Effects of Pharmacologic Agents on Prolactin Secretion

The number of agents that can affect prolactin secretion is very large, indicative of the multiple CNS mediators that control its secretion. While the role of hypothalamic and pituitary dopaminergic agents has been extensively studied, agents that modify other mediators have not been extensively studied. Pontiroli and Pozza[33] reported that histamine infusions stimulated prolactin secretion in normal male volunteers, though histidine was ineffective. This effect of histamine is not mediated by H_2 receptors because cimetidine is known to elicit prolactin secretion. Diphenhydramine, an H_1 blocker, has no effect on prolactin secretion,[34] but it is not known whether it can block the stimulatory effect of histamine secretion. Pontiroli et al.[35] found that cimetidine did not modify the effect of L-dopa in suppressing prolactin secretion, suggesting that an antidopaminergic mechanism was not involved. We must conclude at this time that the mechanism of action of histamine on prolactin secretion has not been resolved. Perhaps the stimulatory response to histamine represents a nonspecific stress response.

The role of serotonin in the regulation of prolactin secretion has attracted continued investigation. Earlier work in humans established that administration of serotonin precursors, such as 1-tryptophan or 5-hydroxytryptophan, stimulated prolactin secretion, and administration of methysergide is known to suppress nocturnal prolactin secretion. In a more recent study, Golstein, et al.[36] administered 4 mg of cyproheptadine every 6 hr for 3 days to four young men. This treatment suppressed nocturnal prolactin secretion but was without effect on TSH secretion. Cyproheptadine did not decrease the prolactin response to TRH. Masala et al.[37] observed that the drug fluoxetine, which blocks serotonin reuptake in the CNS, did not affect basal prolactin serum levels or the response to hypoglycemia. The effects of the drug on nocturnal prolactin secretion were not examined.

Morphine administration leads to increased prolactin secretion in man. The administration of the natural opioid compound β-endorphin either i.v. or intraventricularly resulted in prolactin secretion in patients with cancer.[38] These studies have been extended by Schulz et al.,[39] who administered 10, 14, and 15 mg of β-endorphin to drug-free schizophrenic patients under controlled conditions. Prolactin secretion was stimulated at all doses. No effect on GH secretion was observed.

The possibility that γ-aminobutyric acid (GABA) helps to regulate prolactin secretion was investigated by Tamminga et al.[40] Because GABA does not cross the blood–brain barrier, muscimol, a GABA agonist, was administered to patients with Huntington's disease or schizophrenia.

Serum prolactin and GH were elevated, but TSH and cortisol remained unchanged. The authors considered direct effects of muscimol on the pituitary unlikely from experiments on isolated rat pituitaries. An action on the hypothalamus was postulated.

An unexpected effect of parathyroid hormone on prolactin secretion was reported by Isaac et al.[41] These workers administered parathyroid extract and synthetic 1–34 bovine PTH to normal volunteers. A two- to sixfold acute rise in serum prolactin was observed. The authors speculated that prolactin might mediate the effect of PTH in stimulating 1,25-dihydroxycholecalciferol formation by the kidney. This suggestion seems a bit fanciful because there is no evidence that changes of PTH within the physiologic range do in fact alter serum prolactin levels or that modest alterations of prolactin are in fact the determinant of 1-hydroxylation of 25-hydroxycholecalciferol.

2.2.9. Provocative Tests of Prolactin Secretion

Pontiroli et al.[42] have examined the reproducibility of the prolactin response to a number of provocative stimuli repeated after 3–6 days. The response to arginine infusion and benzerazide (an inhibitor of extracerebral dopa-decarboxylase) was identical when repeated. The prolactin response to a second insulin-induced hypoglycemia was reduced whereas the response to a second sulpiride dose was increased. These observations should make investigators cautious in planning or interpreting the results of repetitive application of the same prolactin-stimulating agent.

Two dopamine antagonists related to procainamide, metoclopramide and sulpiride, have been used to study the physiologic effects of hyperprolactinemia. The acute effects of a single injection of sulpiride have been studied by L'Hermite et al.[43] A four- to fivefold rapid rise in serum prolactin occurred and was maintained for 7 hr of study. Despite the rise in serum prolactin, there were no significant changes in the serum concentrations of LH and FSH. Sulpiride pretreatment greatly suppressed the prolactin-inhibiting action of L-dopa.

In a more extended study, Healy and Burger[44] administered metoclopramide, 10 mg tid, for a week. A sustained hyperprolactinemia was achieved, with higher levels in women (42 ± 6.5 ng/ml) than in men (24.3 ± 5.2 ng/ml). When these patients were challenged with a single dose of 10 mg of metoclopramide, there was little additional rise in serum prolactin. The prolactin response to TRH was decreased in women but not in men. The pattern of response in men also differed in that it was sustained during 120 min of study. The authors concluded that in drug-induced hyperprolactinemia the responses to TRH and additional metoclopramide challenge were similar to those that are observed in patients with hyperprolactinemia.

2.2.10. Etiology of Prolactinomas

The wide application of prolactin radioimmunoassays has led to increased recognition of pituitary tumors in women, but not in men. In Olmsted County, Minnesota, Annegers et al.[45] reported that in women aged 15 through 44 the annual incidence of pituitary tumors, which was 0.7/100,000 for the years 1935 through 1969, rose to 7.1/100,000 for 1970–1977. This rise was largely the result of the increased number of patients with microprolactinomas. There was no evidence of a comparable rise in macroprolactinomas, which suggests that microadenomas do not often progress to macroadenomas. The authors were unable to find a relationship between the development of pituitary tumors and the use of contraceptive steroids.

Sherman et al.[46] arrived at a different conclusion. In their series of 42 women with prolactinomas, 74% developed amenorrhea and/or galactorrhea associated either with contraceptive steroid use or with pregnancy. They suggested that estrogens could be responsible for activating previously silent microadenomas, which may be present in as many as 19% of the population.

Shy et al.[47] have provided a possible explanation why some have found an association between oral contraceptive use and the development of prolactinomas. They made a comprehensive study of the oral contraceptive use of all patients with diagnosed prolactinomas in a three-county area of Washington over a 5-year period. Seventy-two patients were identified and compared with 303 appropriately selected control women. For the entire population, the relative risk of developing a prolactinoma for women taking the pill was 2.0, but for those women who started oral contraceptive pills because of menstrual disorders, the risk was 7.7; for women who used the pills for contraceptive purposes only, the relative risk was only 1.3. In view of the chronicity and insidious onset of symptoms of prolactinomas, it is possible that the menstrual disturbances for which the pill was taken could have been an early manifestation of a microadenoma. Estrogens might also act to stimulate the growth and secretory activity of a preexisting subclinical prolactinoma. Some observers report that microscopic prolactinomas may be present in as many as 10% of the population.

It is now recognized that prolactinomas are a frequent feature of the multiple endocrine adenomatosis, Type 1, syndrome. Carlson et al.[48]

described three men with this association. Prosser et al.[49] surveyed three unrelated families with the MEA 1 syndrome and found four patients with hyperprolactinemia and probable prolactinoma.

2.2.11. Hypothalamic Function Associated with Prolactinoma

If dopamine is the physiologic prolactin-inhibiting factor, one might anticipate that dopamine secretion should be stimulated by autonomous prolactin hypersecretion. Continued secretion and growth of a prolactinoma would suggest, therefore, that a tumor was partially or totally resistant to dopamine. Prolactin-secreting tumors in rats do seem to be resistant to dopamine; but there is conflicting evidence for human prolactinomas. Reschini et al.[50] compared the responses to dopamine infusions (5 μg/kg per min) in 271 patients with prolactinomas and 21 control subjects. No significant difference was observed in the suppression of prolactin achieved in each group.

Evidence of relative dopamine resistance has been obtained, however, when graded doses were given to hyperprolactinemic subjects. In the study of Bansal et al.,[51] dopamine was given at rates of 1, 2, 4, and 8 μg/kg per min to hyperprolactinemic patients and control subjects. In the hyperprolactinemic subjects, the regression line of serum prolactin versus dopamine required to cause a 50% decrease in prolactin was higher than in control subjects.

In a further study by Serri et al.,[52] dopamine was administered at a rate of 20 ng/kg per min for 180 min to 10 normal subjects, 13 patients with microprolactinomas, 8 patients with macroprolactinomas, and 4 nonsecretory macroadenomas. The percentage fall of serum prolactin was lowest with the microprolactinomas, intermediate with the two varieties of macroadenoma, and highest with the control subjects.

Webb et al.[53] have restudied this question by administering successive infusions of dopamine at rates of 4, 40, and 400 ng/kg per min to 17 women with hyperprolactinemia and to 19 control women. At the lowest rates of infusion, the fractional suppression of prolactin secretion in the control women was substantially greater than in the hyperprolactinemic women. The latter were also less responsive to domperidone (2 mg i.v.) and bromocriptine (2.5 mg p.o.).

All three studies with dopamine infusions provide some evidence that resistance to the agent exists in most patients with hyperprolactinemia. As most of the patients studied probably had prolactinomas, resistance to portal vein dopamine might account for the sustained hypersecretion. What is missing in this argument is knowledge of human pituitary blood dopamine concentration and how this corresponds to the levels attained by i.v. infusion.

After successful removal of a prolactin-secreting microadenoma, some but not all measures of normal prolactin regulation return. Tucker *et al.*[54] observed that 2–6 months after adenomectomy, the increases in prolactin response to TRH and metoclopramide were usually normal, but the responses to chlorpromazine- and insulin-induced hypoglycemia had rarely returned. Even 1–8 years after surgery, responses to chlorpromazine and insulin were blunted. The stimuli that were ineffective in stimulating prolactin secretion required hypothalamic participation, but the exact mechanism of the hypothalamic dysfunction was not determined. Other measures of pituitary function were not abnormal.

2.2.12. Clinical Manifestations of Prolactinomas

Altered gonadal function is the most common endocrine manifestation of prolactinomas.[55] Between 11 and 23% of women with secondary amenorrhea for more than 6 months have hyperprolactinemia. Not so well recognized is anovulatory oligomenorrhea, which is also associated with hyperprolactinemia. In the series of Wolf *et al.*,[56] this occurred in 26 of 138 cases. In the same study, primary amenorrhea occurred in only 2 of 60 cases. Galactorrhea is an inconstant manifestation of hyperprolactinemia, only occurring in about one-quarter of the cases. At the present time, parasellar manifestations of prolactinoma growth are infrequent in women but a relatively common presenting manifestation in men, reflecting the much higher percentage of macroadenomas in men. Loss of libido and potency are common in men with prolactinomas.

The major abnormality responsible for decreased gonadal function in patients with microprolactinomas is a decreased secretion of gonadotropin-releasing hormone (LRH). In women the response of serum LH and FSH to administered LRH is usually normal or increased. In men with macroprolactinomas and compression of normal pituitary tissue, the response of LH and FSH after LRH administration is often subnormal.

A possible role of endogenous opioids in inhibiting GnRH secretion in patients with hyperprolactinemia has been suggested by Quigley *et al.*[57] They administered naloxone, a competitive inhibitor of opioid binding, to ten hyperprolactinemic women with microprolactinomas and five normal women in the follicular phase of the menstrual cycle. In the normal individuals, no change in LH occurred in a 4-hr period, but there was a definite rise in LH in six of the ten patients with prolactinomas. In these patients, the characteristic pulsatile pattern of LH secretion returned. Four patients did not respond to naloxone. These patients differed in having a lower initial LH level. No changes in serum FSH or prolactin in either the normal or the hyperprolactinemic patients occurred after naloxone. The authors suggest that hyperprolactinemia increases hypothalamic endogenous opioids which in turn inhibit GnRH secretion. The failure of four patients to respond to naloxone could not be attributed to impaired pituitary responsiveness because the patients responded to GnRH with a normal rise in serum LH. It would appear that in these patients, opioid-induced hypothalamic changes were more severe and less promptly reversed.

The possibility that hyperprolactinemic patients might be subject to accelerated osteoporosis is suggested by a clinical study by Klibanski *et al.*[58] of 14 women between the ages of 20 and 40 years who had suffered from sustained hyperprolactinemia, bone density, measured by photon absorptiometry, was significantly reduced compared with that in a control group of 16 premenopausal women. The lowest bone densities were found in patients with the lowest serum estradiol levels. In this series, the hyperprolactinemic patients resembled the postmenopausal control group. Levels of calcium, phosphorus, alkaline phosphatase, PTH, and 25-OH-vitamin D were normal in the hyperprolactinemic women. The authors suggest that hyperprolactinemia leads to hypoestrogenemia, which in turn permits accelerated osteoporosis. In view of the high person-to-person variation in bone densitometry readings and the fact that the study groups were small, confirmation in a larger series is needed. It is also notable that half of the patients had had amenorrhea for 2 years or less. This period of hypoestrogenemia would seem too brief to produce easily measured osteopenia.

The effect of hyperprolactinemia on glucose tolerance and insulin secretion has been studied. Landgraf *et al.*[59] found that patients with prolactin-secreting adenomas had decreased glucose tolerance and increased insulin response. These changes were reversed by effective bromocriptine treatment.

Johnston *et al.*[60] have extended these studies. Glucose, insulin, lactate, pyruvate, alanine, 3β-hydroxybutyrate, and glycerol were carefully monitored during a 12-hr period with normal meal ingestion in 9 hyperprolactinemic subjects and 14 control patients. Fasting and postprandial glucose levels were unchanged in the hyperprolactinemic subjects, but the insulin response to meals was exaggerated. Lactate, pyruvate, and alanine responses to meals were increased, a change that was attributed to the hyperinsulinism. Glycerol and 3β-hydroxybutyrate levels were reduced. The results are consistent with a mild diabetogenic effect of prolactin.

2.2.13. Diagnosis of Prolactinomas

The diagnostic challenge facing the clinician is to distinguish patients with functional hyperprolactinemia from those with microprolactinomas. In those patients with serum prolactin concentrations greater than

200 ng/ml and radiologic abnormalities of the sella, little problem exists. In the remaining cases, clinicians have employed stimulatory tests with centrally acting dopaminergic blocking agents, such as chlorpromazine or TRH. The response of hyperprolactinemic patients with radiologic evidence of prolactinoma to these stimuli has almost invariably been blunted, but so has been the response of patients without evidence of prolactinomas by X-ray tomography. This has led to conflicting conclusions, some authors concluding that these tests are useful and others reaching the opposite conclusion.

Fine and Frohman[61] observed that in normal and puerperal individuals, L-dopa inhibition of prolactin secretion could not be inhibited by carbidopa, a drug that inhibits conversion of L-dopa to dopamine in the pituitary but not within the hypothalamus above the median eminence. The persistence of the L-dopa effect in the presence of carbidopa is therefore indicative of L-dopa activation of central dopaminergic pathways, presumably, in the hypothalamus. They found that patients with prolactinomas had a marked reduction of central dopaminergic inhibition of prolactin secretion while retaining pituitary responsiveness to dopamine derived from L-dopa.

Still another pharmacologic approach to the problem of the diagnosis of prolactinomas was proposed by Müller et al.[62] They employed nomifensine, a drug that appears to act by increasing hypothalamic dopamine release by blocking its reuptake in secretory vesicles. When nomifensine was given to normal or puerperal women, a fall in serum prolactin occurred over a 5-hr period. When the drug was administered to 47 patients with hyperprolactinemia, only 11 patients had a fall in serum prolactin. Ten of these had radiologically normal sellas and serum prolactin levels less than 50 ng/ml. Of the 36 nonresponders to nomifensine, all but five had sellar abnormalities. All 22 patients who underwent surgery had prolactinomas.

Despite the elegant rationale for these two procedures, subsequent investigation has shown that they are not reliable discriminators between functional and neoplastic hyperprolactinemia. Ferrari et al.[63] found that the nomifensine test was plagued with many false-positive and false-negative responses. Four patients with obvious tumors responded to the drug. Moriondo et al.[64] conducted a more extensive comparison of the nomifensine and L-dopa–carbidopa tests. They found significant inhibition of prolactin levels in 20% of patients with proven prolactinomas given nomifensine and in 25% given L-dopa and carbidopa. Of interest is the fact that the same patients tended to respond to both tests, suggesting that these tumors were subject to endogenous dopaminergic control. When tested, many of these patients also responded to TRH. In the patients without radiologic evidence of pituitary tumor, only 15%

responded to nomifensine and 40% responded to L-dopa–carbidopa. One patient with hyperprolactinemia with hypothyroidism failed to respond to either test until her hypothyroidism was corrected by treatment.

What is the clinician to conclude concerning the usefulness of these tests in establishing the presence or absence of a prolactinoma? Of undoubted value is the level of baseline prolactin measured on multiple occasions by a reliable laboratory. If the hyperprolactinemia is in excess of 100 ng/ml, a prolactinoma is usually present, unless the patient is receiving antidopaminergic drugs or has overt hypothalamic pathology. With values of less than 100 ng/ml, possible pregnancy, hypothyroidism, medications, and hypothalamic disease should be thoroughly considered. Radiologic techniques have greatly improved in recent years. Conventional radiographs of the sella do not provide adequate screening for pituitary tumors. Hypocycloidal tomography greatly improves recognition of localized changes in the sellar floor, but reveals little parenchymal detail. CT scanning, particularly with the new high-resolution equipment, has provided the most information about pituitary parenchyma, and small adenomas are frequently seen on contrast scans. With current CT techniques, air or metrizamide contrast studies are rarely required to establish the extent of suprasellar extension. Despite these advances, the diagnosis of microadenoma is primarily an endocrine diagnosis and the radiologic examination serves to confirm the diagnosis and guide the neurosurgeon. It should not be overlooked that microadenomas can exist in the presence of an otherwise "empty sella."

2.2.14. Pituitary Function in Patients with Prolactinoma

In addition to establishing the presence of hyperprolactinemia, the clinician wishes to know the extent to which other pituitary functions might be impaired. Two recent studies have addressed this question. Hagen et al.[65] studied 42 patients with pituitary tumors unassociated with acromegaly or Cushing's disease. Sixty-nine percent of these patients had hyperprolactinemia. GH deficiency was present in 78%, and gonadal insufficiency occurred in 77%. Laboratory evidence of adrenal insufficiency was less common (31%), and thyroid deficiency was still less common (21%). In a second study restricted to patients with hyperprolactinemia, Klijn et al.[66] found that tumors with a lateral area in excess of 3 cm^2 were most likely to have deficiencies of other pituitary hormones.

2.2.15. Treatment with Dopaminergic Agents

From the work of many authors, it is established that dopaminergic drugs will lower serum prolactin levels to normal in most patients with prolactinomas. Except in women with the very largest pituitary tumors, bromocriptine has usually led to the prompt resumption of menses and the restoration of fertility. Most men respond with a rise in serum testosterone, correction of impotence, and improvement in libido. While these short-term responses are impressive, the role of bromocriptine in the long-term treatment of this condition remains in contention. Many, including nearly all neurosurgeons, prefer removal of neoplastic tissue by the safe transsphenoidal route. Others prefer to use dopaminergic agents on a chronic basis. Unfortunately, no controlled study directly comparing drug therapy with surgical treatment has been conducted.

A prospective study of bromocriptine treatment of 18 patients with prolactinoma and 1 patient with a nonsecretory adenoma for 3 to 22 months led to objective reduction in tumor size as evaluated by contrast CT studies in 12 patients (63%).[67] Seven of nine patients with initial visual field defects had improvement and secretory defects in other pituitary hormones improved in nine and became normal in three. While most patients sustain reduction in tumor size and suppression of prolactin secretion, exceptions have been reported. In a patient reported by Breidahl et al.,[68] there was evidence of tumor regrowth by CT and a rising serum prolactin despite increased dosage after a period of tumor regression and partial correction of hyperprolactinemia. In another patient reported by Dallabonzana et al.,[69] sudden increase in tumor size in a patient who had had an initial good response to bromocriptine was attributable to a pituitary hemorrhage. In a second patient, hormonal escape and slight increase in tumor size by CT may have been due to treatment of an intercurrent infection with spiramycin. A drug interaction, perhaps on absorption of bromocriptine, may have occurred.

Tumor shrinkage with bromocriptine can occur with remarkable rapidity, often over days to a few weeks but the tumor can reexpand equally rapidly after the discontinuance of bromocriptine.[70] Tindall et al.[71] conducted an important morphologic study of the effects of bromocriptine. Six patients with macroprolactinomas were studied prior to surgery. Two were untreated; two received 7.5 mg of bromocriptine per day for 4–6 weeks; and two patients received bromocriptine for 4 weeks and discontinued medication for 1 and 2 weeks. All patients were subjected to transsphenoidal adenomectomy. The reduction in tumor size that occurred in the bromocriptine-treated patients could not be attributed to cells necrosis, infarction, or vascular injury. There was a significant reduction of both the cryptoplasmic, nuclear, and nucleolar areas of the tumor cells treated with bromocriptine. The percentage volumes of the rough endoplasmic reticulum and Golgi were reduced. In contrast, the percentage area occupied by secretory granules was increased. In the prolactinomas where bromocriptine therapy had been discontinued,

the changes were intermediate between the untreated and the uninter-
rupted treatment cases. There was depletion of prolactin immunostain-
ing of these two tumors, suggesting secretory depletion of these prolactinoma cells. There was also a two- to fourfold increase in relative nucleolar
area, which might reflect a great acceleration of RNA synthesis. These
observations lead to the conclusion that bromocriptine-induced reduction in prolactinoma size is not the result of a cytolytic action of bromocriptine but due to a profound loss in cell volume. Likewise, the rapid
regrowth of some tumors after stopping bromocriptine is not due to cell
proliferation but the restoration of original cell volume.

One measure of the long-term effects of bromocriptine is the course
of serum prolactin after treatment with the drug is stopped. Eversmann
et al.[72] reported on 37 patients treated for periods between 2 and 30
months. In 8 patients with microprolactinomas, the serum prolactin rose
to within 62% of the initial level after treatment was discontinued. In
women with macroadenomas, the serum prolactin rose to 52% of the
initial value, and in male patients rose to 43% of the initial value. On
the basis of this very limited evidence the authors concluded that the
antiproliferative action of bromocriptine "seems to be specific for the
prolactin secreting cells in macroprolactinomas with high proliferation
rate and high prolactin turnover." They suggested that macroprolactinomas might be treated with bromocriptine preoperatively to transform
an invasive tumor into a surgically resectable tumor.

This study by Eversmann et al. addressed an important question.
Unfortunately, it is flawed by its retrospective nature and the lack of
uniform treatment and posttreatment observation periods. The statistical analysis does not clearly establish the lack of regression of microprolactinomas after bromocriptine treatment. Clearly, a prospective controlled study is needed to answer the important clinical questions that
have been raised.

While bromocriptine therapy has repeatedly been found to improve
visual field defects and reduce suprasellar extension, a rare patient may
develop complications from acelerated tumor regression. In a patient
observed by Aronoff et al.,[73] bromocriptine therapy led to normalization
of serum prolactin and the appearance of rhinorrhea on two occasions
in a woman with an invasive macroadenoma. They interpreted this development as indicating leak of CSF around the regressing tumor. Two
similar patients have been described by Wilson et al.[74]

The long-term results of dopaminergic therapy are still not completely defined. Zarate et al.[75] have reported their experience with 16
women with prolactinomas who were treated for at least 2 years and
followed for an additional 2 years after discontinuation of bromocriptine.
Serum prolactin levels were maintained with normal limits in 14 of the

women during treatment and remained normal in 6 of these women after stopping treatment. The remaining 10 patients had a return of amenorrhea and galactorrhea within 3 months of stopping treatment. In this series, no significant expansion of tumor size was observed after stopping the drug. It should be noted that others have not noted as frequent apparent cures or the absence of tumor reexpansion.

Treatment of most young women with amenorrhea and hyperprolactinemia with bromocriptine will restore ovulation and fertility. If pregnancy ensues, most authorities recommend that bromocriptine be discontinued as soon as pregnancy is confirmed. The subsequent course of pregnancy and delivery is generally uneventful and there is no convincing evidence that bromocriptine is teratogenic. Enlargement of a prolactinoma during pregnancy with development of parasellar signs of visual field impairment or hemorrhagic infarction is rare. In the series of Thorner et al.[76] including 92 pregnancies in 76 hyperprolactinemic patients, this occurred in only 2 patients both of whom had macroprolactinomas. Sixteen other patients with macroprolactinomas had no difficulty although 14 of these had received radiation therapy before pregnancy. In a study from Sweden of 28 patients during 31 pregnancies, no serious complications were observed without radiation treatment.[77] Radiologically demonstrable enlargement of the pituitary occurred during pregnancy in 4 cases but regressed in all after delivery.

While not generally recommended, Konopka et al.[78] continued bromocriptine treatment throughout pregnancy in nine cases with grade II and III sellar enlargement. In two additional cases, bromocriptine treatment was instituted during the 5th and 7th months because of bitemporal hemianopia and resulted in prompt normalization. In all cases the course of pregnancy and delivery was normal. The infants were normal at birth and physical and mental development were normal when observed up to 6 years. This study would suggest that continuous bromocriptine therapy during pregnancy is a possible approach to women with macroprolactinomas.

Most authors have reported on the effects of bromocriptine in the treatment of prolactinomas; however, it is clear that other dopaminergic drugs such as lisuride or pergolide are effective. Franks et al.[79] reported their experience with pergolide in 25 patients with hyperprolactinemia treated for 6–20 months. Most patients received 50–150 μg daily in a single dose but larger doses were administered to some patients with macroprolactinomas. The side effects of pergolide were similar to those of bromocriptine and included occasional nausea, vomiting, and hypotension. The advantage of the drug would appear to be the convenience of once-a-day treatment.

2.2.16. Neurosurgical Treatment

The reports of surgical treatment of prolactinomas in the larger clinics have shown similar short-term results.[80,81] If the patient has a microprolactinoma and the serum prolactin is less than 100 ng/ml, normal serum prolactin levels will be achieved in 80–90% of cases. The results are less favorable with higher initial serum prolactin levels or with macroprolactinomas. Few patients with invasive prolactinomas have had endocrine cure after transsphenoidal adenomectomy.

Unfortunately, there have been few long-term follow-up reports of patients treated by transsphenoidal adenomectomy. Particularly disturbing has been the experience of an excellent neurosurgical clinic with 44 surgically treated patients who were followed for 5 to 10 years after operation.[82] Twenty-four of twenty-eight patients with microprolactinomas had an immediate return to normal serum prolactin levels but in the follow-up period hyperprolactinemia recurred in 12 of these patients. The results with macroprolactinomas were even less favorable. Only 5 of 16 patients had immediate return to normal serum prolactin levels and in 4 of the 5 cases hyperprolactinemia returned during the follow-up period. Radiographic evidence of tumor recurrence was not recognized in any case, although the high-resolution CT techniques were probably not employed. If similar disappointing long-term results appear from other clinics, it will force a reconsideration of the ultimate role of neurosurgical treatment in this disease.

2.3. GH

2.3.1. GH Genes and mRNA

We now have detailed information about the GH gene and mRNA.[83] Initially, mRNA from a human pituitary tumor was extracted and the appropriate size mRNAs were used to synthesize cDNA, which was subsequently introduced into plasmids by recombinant methods.[84] The plasmids were introduced into *E. coli* and cloned. The GH cDNA was recognized and its structure determined. This allowed the structure of the GH mRNA to be deduced. GH mRNA codes for a pre-GH, which contains a 29-amino-acid signal peptide and the 191 amino acids of GH itself. The signal peptide is cleaved as the peptide enters the vesicular space of the rough endoplasmic reticulum. Cloning of the GH cDNA has made possible the bacterial synthesis of a GH with a structure identical to native GH except for an additional methionine at the N-terminus of the molecule.[85] The bacterially synthesized GH appears to have the same receptor and biologic properties of the native hormone.[86] Although the methionine group is believed to be buried within the molecule, a question remains whether or not methionyl-GH is more antigenic in man than the native hormone.

The availability of a labeled hGH cDNA probe has made possible the recognition of the GH gene in a human gene library. The gene has been cloned and its structure established. It, as well as other members of the GH family, has its five coding regions interrupted by four introns.[83] It is now likely that a 20K variant of GH lacking amino acids 32–46, found in human pituitaries to the extent of about 10%, arises by aberrant splicing of the β intron.[87]

The human GH gene has been localized to the long arm of chromosome 17 where it is associated with at least four other related genes or pseudogenes.[2,88] After the GH gene on chromosome 17, there is a choriosomatomammotropin (hCS) pseudogene; the hCS A gene, which is expressed; an hGH variant pseudogene; and an hCS β gene, which is normally expressed. The two hCS genes differ only in their noncoding regions and are structurally extremely similar to the hGH gene. It is likely the hCS arose by genic exchange from the hGH gene in relatively recent evolutionary time.[89]

2.3.2. GH Heterogeneity

In addition to the 20K variant, other variants of hGH have been recognized. Of potential significance are forms of GH that have been enzymatically cleaved at various positions between residues 134 and 150 of the large loop of the molecule. The two peptide chains of hGH so generated are still held together by a disulfide bond. The GH potency of this modified molecule is actually increased in certain experimental systems. While this variant of GH is not found in GH isolated from pituitaries soon after death, it may be formed after secretion because immunologic evidence of its existence in plasma has been obtained. Lewis *et al.*[90] speculated that the uncleaved GH might represent a prohormone that requires enzymatic cleavage to a two-chain hormone for full activity. This hypothesis would make GH activation analogous to the conversion of proinsulin to insulin. Thus far, demonstration that this putative enzymatic cleavage is important *in vivo* is lacking.

Lewis *et al.*[90] have also recognized other GH variants in hGH preparations. A form with a blocked N-terminal sequence, a form with an interchain disulfide dimer, and various slow-migrating forms have all been found. The biologic significance of all of these molecular forms of hGH is unknown.

2.3.3. Homologous Radioreceptor Assays for hGH

Progress has been made in the development of practical radiore-ceptor assays (RRAs) for hGH that employ human receptors. Prior RRAs had utilized receptors obtained from pregnant rabbit or rat liver mem-branes. While these membranes possessed high concentrations of sites that bound [^{125}I]hGH, there is concern that some of the binding occurred on prolactin- rather than on GH-preferring sites. More importantly, it is known that primates respond only to primate GH, whereas the rat and rabbit liver membranes bind primate and nonprimate GHs. Three groups have now reported RRAs utilizing hGH-binding sites on IM-9 lymphocytes, a cell line previously proven to be richly endowed with hGH-binding sites. Eastman et al.[91] found that when IM-9 cells were incubated with varying concentrations of unlabeled hGH for 4½ hr at 30°C before the addition of [^{125}I]hGH, the sensitivity of the RRA could be increased sevenfold compared with that of a simple competitive assay conducted for 1½ hr. The increased sensitivity results from the decreased number of binding sites, which is the result of the preliminary 4½ hr incubation (down-regulation) and is not simply a phenomenon of oc-cupancy. The observed potency of different GH and placental lactogen preparations in the receptor modulation assay correlated well with the known biologic potencies of the peptides.

Rosenfeld and Hintz[92] applied the principle of receptor modulation to the RRA of GH in human serum. In their method, IM-9 lymphocytes were preincubated with GH standards or aliquots of human serum for 4 hr at 37°C. At the end of this period the cells were sedimented and resuspended in fresh buffer containing [^{125}I]hGH. In this way they avoided some of the nonspecific serum effects that often plague RRAs. When they compared the results obtained with the hGH, IM-9 lymphocyte RRA and the RIA in serum from patients with acromegaly, and from newborns and older children after provocative stimulation of GH se-cretion, they found almost identical results with each assay.

Gavin et al.[93] have applied a similar IM-9 RRA to sera from short children with normal GH secretion but low somatomedin levels. In four of five cases the RRA appeared to give inappropriately low results. This finding supports the hypothesis that defective circulating GH may be responsible for certain cases of growth failure.

2.3.4. GH Regulation by Somatostatin

Studies in rats have provided new evidence concerning the regu-lation of GH secretion. In this animal, GH is secreted in major secretory bursts occurring every 4 hr, with intervening periods of minimal secre-tion. Many types of stress, which in humans act to stimulate GH secretion, suppress GH secretion in the rat. Because of this response to stress, it is important to study GH secretion in unanesthetized, unrestrained rats with chronic inlying catheters for use in administering test substances and withdrawing blood. Using such methods, Tannenbaum et al.[94] found that starvation markedly inhibited GH secretion, but that the administration of somatostatin antisera restored GH secretion in starved rats. These and other experiments clearly establish a role for somatostatin in the regulation of GH secretion in the rat.

A number of studies suggest that circulating GH may regulate its own secretion by increasing somatostatin secretion. Patel[95] found that the somatostatin concentration in the rat hypothalamus was increased by GH administration. In hypophysectomized rats, the hypothalamic somatostatin was decreased. Tannenbaum[96] has provided direct evidence that feedback inhibition occurs in vivo: the normal pulsatile pattern of GH secretion was suppressed by injection of 15 µg of GH into the cerebral ventricles. The inhibition of secretion persisted during the subsequent 3 hr of study.

There is accumulating evidence that GH inhibits its own secretion by increasing hypothalamic somatostatin secretion. Sheppard et al.[97] measured the release of somatostatin by hypothalamic explants in vitro and showed that the secretion was increased by the presence in the medium of rGH in concentrations as low as 50 ng/ml. TSH did not affect somatostatin secretion. These findings have been confirmed by Berelowitz et al.[98]

An additional pathway of feedback inhibition of GH secretion appears to exist. There is considerable evidence that GH exerts its effects on skeletal cartilage and perhaps on some other tissues by stimulating the hepatic release of somatomedin. Sheppard et al.[99] found that a partially purified preparation of somatomedin A stimulated the release of somatostatin by isolated rat hypothalamic explants in a dose-related fashion. A significant stimulation was observed with as little as 0.1 U/ml (the amount of somatomedin in 0.1 ml of serum). Berelowitz et al.[100] have confirmed these observations by showing that a highly purified preparation of somatomedin C stimulated somatostatin release from rat hypothalamic explants. In addition, they found that preincubation of primary rat pituitary cell cultures with somatomedin C for 24 hr markedly decreased subsequent GH response to a GH-releasing peptide. This would suggest an additional site of feedback control of GH secretion.

2.3.5. GH Regulation by Somatocrinin (GHRH)

There has been rapid progress in our understanding of the regulation of GH secretion. Two groups succeeded in establishing almost simultaneously the structure of the elusive GH-releasing hormone (somatocrinin, GHRF) from pancreatic islet tumors in clinically acromegalic patients.[101,102] Both isolated GHRHs are simple single-chain peptides of 41 and 44 residues of similar amino acid sequence except that one peptide had three additional C-terminal amino acids.

The cDNA derived from GHRF mRNA has been cloned and its nucleic acid sequence determined.[103] The primary translation product of the GHRF mRNA includes a signal peptide whose structure is still incompletely known divided by an Arg–Arg cleavage site from the 44 amino acids of GHRF and a terminal peptide of 31 amino acids, which is cleaved in the formation of the final hormone.

GRF has been identified in the hypothalamus by immunohisto-chemical techniques.[104] The arcuate nucleus in monkeys and humans contains cell bodies that react intensely against anti-hp GRF serum. Fibers were seen projecting to the median eminence and ending in contact with portal vessels.

GRF regulates the release of GH from the pituitaries of experimental animals both *in vitro* and *in vivo*. Its potency in man has been established.[105,106] A single i.v. injection of as little as 0.5 μg/kg results in a near-maximal response. The response is rapid with significant increases of serum GH within 5 min. Maximal responses occurred between 30 and 60 min and persisted for 120–180 min.

Administration of GRF was associated with facial flushing and a feeling of warmth, and a slight rise in blood pressure has been observed with larger doses.

2.3.6. GH Regulation in Men

It is known from earlier work that there is a considerable increase in GH secretion at the time of puberty in both boys and girls. Pieters *et al.*[107] found that glucose administration at this age failed to suppress GH secretion in 66% of the adolescents tested and in many cases led to a paradoxical rise of GH secretion at 30 min. This pattern has previously been reported only in pathologic states, including acromegaly, anorexia nervosa, and chronic renal failure. The neuroendocrine significance of the paradoxical response to glucose remains unknown, but the phenomenon should not be overlooked if glucose supression tests are used in adolescent patients suspected of hypersomatotropism.

It is widely appreciated that the GH response of obese subjects to provocative stimuli is frequently impaired. Surprisingly, Copinschi *et al.*[108] found the hourly integrated level of serum GH was not significantly lower in awake obese subjects, but that the sleep-related portion of GH secretion was decreased, though it was restored by prolonged wakefulness. In contrast, the sleep-related secretion of prolactin was retained in obese subjects, but occurred at an earlier hour. The pattern of cortisol secretion in obesity was normal. The failure of obese subjects to respond to acute provocative stimuli, such as L-dopa, may reflect increased adrenergic tone in the hypothalamus. Pretreatment of obese subjects with 40 mg of propranolol p.o. 2 hr before L-dopa ingestion resulted in normal GH secretion.

The integrated concentration of GH was also measured in young insulin-dependent diabetics by the continuous blood withdrawal method.[108a] Samples collected over 30-min periods were pooled. When compared to suitable nondiabetic control subjects, both male and female, diabetics had integrated GH secretion more than twice normal. No comparable increase in integrated GH secretion was noted in 43 nonketotic newly diagnosed insulin-dependent diabetics. No correlation was observed between GH secretion and the absolute blood sugar, but variability of blood sugar was positively correlated with GH secretion. This carefully performed study appears to resolve conflicting results obtained in earlier, less well-controlled studies.

A major secretory peak of GH occurs 60–90 min after the onset of stage 3 and 4 sleep in normal individuals. Clark et al.[109] investigated the extent to which this normal pattern is disturbed in patients with sleep disorders. Patients with excessive drowsiness and narcolepsy, without other neurologic diseases, frequently did not exhibit sleep-related GH peaks. The nocturnal pattern of prolactin secretion was retained but reduced. Subnormal GH responses to L-dopa and arginine were also common in these patients. The authors attributed these disorders of GH and prolactin secretion to possible abnormalities of hypothalamic catecholamines.

2.3.7. GH Effects on Calcium and Phosphorus Metabolism

Golde et al.[110] had previously reported that hGH can stimulate normal erythropoiesis in vitro. They have now found that hGH in doses as small as 0.1 ng/ml can stimulate increased cloning of murine erythroleukemic cells. In this subsequent study, they found that hGH, but not bovine GH, stimulated a cell line of human erythroleukemic cells.[111] Both cell lines also responded to insulin.

The lack of effect of GH on isolated cartilage of many species and the ability of somatomedins to stimulate cartilage matrix synthesis and mitosis have led to the general view that GH actions are mediated by somatomedins. This view has been challenged by Isaksson and his colleagues. In one study, they injected 10 μg of hGH directly into the proximal tibial growth plate on three occasions.[112] Two weeks after the first hGH injection, the animals were killed and bone growth was determined by a tetracycline labeling technique. An increase in bone growth was observed in the injected tibia but not in the other tibia.

In a subsequent study, it was shown that ear chondrocytes of rabbits bound [^{125}I]hGH specifically but costal cartilage of young rabbits bound no [^{125}I]hGH specifically and epiphyseal cartilage bound [^{125}I]hGH minimally.[113] These observations suggest that cartilage is not totally insensitive to GH but do not establish the significance of direct actions of GH on cartilage tissue. They also do not rule out the possibility that GH may be acting by stimulating local production of somatomedins.

It is well known that the administration of GH to hypopituitary subjects will produce a transient hypercalciuria, an increase in the intestinal absorption of calcium, an increase in renal tubular reabsorption of phosphorus, and an increase in the rate of bone formation.

Several studies have focused on the effects of GH on vitamin D metabolism and parathyroid function. Hypophysectomized rats have a considerable decrease in plasma $1\alpha,25(OH)_2D_3$ that can be partially restored by GH treatment.[114] This occurs without significant change in PTH levels. Ovine prolactin has no significant effect on $1\alpha,25(OH)_2D_3$. In a similar study, Yeh and Aloia[115] fed intact and hypophysectomized rats a D-deficient diet for 14 days. Subsequently the rats were treated with GH for 12 days. During the last 6 days of GH treatment, [^{3}H]-25-OH-D_3 was injected. At the completion of the experiment the distribution of D metabolites was determined. In the hypophysectomized animals [^{3}H]-1,25(OH)$_2$D$_3$ was decreased and [^{3}H]-24,25(OH)$_2$D$_3$ was increased in plasma and kidney. The concentration of unmetabolized [^{3}H]-25-OH-D_3 was increased. These abnormalities were largely corrected by GH treatment. Probably as a consequence of the increase in $1,25(OH)_2D_3$ levels, treatment also increases the concentration of calcium-binding protein in the intestinal mucosa of hypophysectomized rats.[116]

In humans the effects of GH on vitamin D metabolism are less clear. Gertner et al.[117] studied nine children with hypopituitarism before and after 3 months of GH administration. The expected increases in growth rate, renal tubular reabsorption of phosphate, and intestinal calcium absorption were observed. These changes were unassociated, however, with any changes in 25-OH-D_3, 24,25(OH)$_2$D$_3$, or 1,25(OH)$_2$D$_3$. Similar results were obtained by Chipman et al.[118] in a study of seven hypopituitary children treated for 5–14 months. In these patients, 1,25(OH)$_2$D$_3$ actually decreased under GH treatment.

It has been long known that serum phosphorus is elevated in acromegaly and that GH administration increases the renal reabsorption of phosphorus in dogs. Direct evidence has now been presented by Hammerman et al.[119] that GH acts on the brush border of the renal proximal tubule to stimulate phosphate transport. In their experiments, brush border vesicles from GH-treated dogs exhibited a rate of Na^+-dependent phosphate transport that was 34% greater than that of vesicles prepared from kidneys of control dogs. PTH decreased phosphate transport in both control and GH-treated dogs.

2.3.8. Pituitary Pathology in Acromegaly

Melmed et al.[120] have reviewed the anatomic findings in acromegalic patients and have provided a useful classification of causes of hypersomatotropism. A simplified version of this classification is provided in Table 1. Most cases of acromegaly and gigantism are associated with somatotroph cells producing only GH; these cells may be either sparsely or densely granulated. Less frequently, the adenoma contains both separate GH-containing cells and prolactin-containing cells identifiable by immunohistochemical methods. Less frequently, an adenoma contains, in addition to somatotroph cells, cells of the basophilic stem cell line associated with ACTH, TSH, LH, and FSH in various combinations. Some adenomas contain both GH and prolactin within the same cells. If the cells appear immature and are rapidly growing, the authors refer to this adenoma as a stem cell adenoma. If the adenoma contains more mature and slowly growing cells, it is referred to as a mammosomatotroph cell adenoma. True somatotroph cell carcinomas are extremely rare. This diagnosis cannot be made on the basis of morphology and local invasiveness alone but requires the existence of distant metastases.

Extrasellar causes of GH excess are rare but of great interest. Adenomas have been reported to have arisen in ectopic pituitary tissue in

Table 1. The Etiology of Hypersomatotropism[a]

Pituitary
   GH cell adenoma
   Mixed GH and prolactin cell adenoma
   Plurihormonal adenoma
   Mammosomatotroph stem cell adenoma
   Mammosomatotroph cell adenoma
   GH cell carcinoma
   GH cell hyperplasia
Extrapituitary
   Eutopic GH cell adenoma (sphenoid sinus, parapharyngeal)
   Extopic GH-producing tumor (lung, ovary, breast, carcinoid)
      Eutopic (hypothalamic hamartoma, choristoma)
      Ectopic (islet and carcinoid tumors)

[a] Modified from Melmed et al.[120]

the sphenoid sinus or parapharyngeal tissue. Ectopic production of GH by nonpituitary tumors has been described in breast, ovarian, and bronchial cancers. In general, GH has been demonstrated in the tumor by RIA and immunohistochemistry. Elevations of serum GH have usually been very modest and clinical manifestations of acromegaly absent.

The newest development has been the recognition of cases of GH excess as the result of oversecretion of GHRF. In the cases associated with carcinoid or islet cell tumors, this is referred to as ectopic GHRF secretion. In a well-studied case of Thorner et al.,[121] a 21-year-old girl with Turner's syndrome and acromegaly was found at transsphenoidal operation to have no pituitary adenoma but hyperplasia of densely granulated somatotroph cells. The operation failed to correct the elevated serum GH levels. Because of the pituitary findings, an ectopic source of GHRF was suspected, an extensive search was made, and eventually a pancreatic islet cell tumor was found and removed. The islet cell tumor contained GH-releasing activity when tested on rat pituitaries in vitro. Subsequently, GHRF 1–40 was isolated from the tumor and its amino acid sequence determined.

Leveston et al.[122] described a somewhat similar case of GH excess. Their patient, a young black male with gigantism, was eventually shown to have a metastatic duodenal carcinoid. His course was complicated by the sudden onset of severe hyperadrenal corticism and he eventually died of myocardiopathy. At autopsy the pituitary was greatly enlarged, weighing 10 g. Histologically, the pituitary had some features of nodular hyperplasia and some of adenoma. The somatotroph cells were well differentiated and densely granulated. The metastatic carcinoid tumor in the liver was shown to contain both GHRF and somatostatin. In addition, immunohistologic studies established the presence of scattered cells densely staining for GH and ACTH. This tumor, therefore, had the unusual ability to make and store both GHRF and GH.

A number of cases of acromegaly have been associated with hypothalamic hamartoma or choristoma.[123] The suspicion that these tumors arose from neuroendocrine cells has been supported by finding immunoreactive GHRF. Because this peptide is not foreign to these cells, Melmed et al.[120] refer to "eutopic" GHRF secretion.

2.3.9. Control of GH Secretion in Acromegaly

It is well recognized that GH secretion in many patients with acromegaly is not fixed, but can be modified by adrenergic agents, dopaminergic agents, and hypophysiotropic hormones. Hanew et al.[124] conducted a systematic study of 15 patients whose GH responses to TRH, LRH, and arginine infusion were measured. Ten of these patients (group

I) responded to one or more of these stimuli. A GH response to TRH was most commonly present. Group I patients responded to somatostatin infusion with a greater fall in GH than nonresponders (group II). Four of five patients in group I responded to bromocriptine with a fall in serum GH, whereas none of the patients of group II responded. The authors attributed the difference between responders and nonresponders with respect to these test procedures to differences in tumor receptors. They suggested that the response to TRH, LRH, or arginine might be helpful in selecting patients for bromocriptine therapy.

There is considerable evidence that dopamine acts directly at the pituitary level. Camanni et al.[125] found that L-dopa administration to eight acromegalic patients lowered GH and prolactin levels. When carbidopa was given, blocking the pituitary decarboxylation of L-dopa to dopamine, the inhibition of GH and prolactin levels was markedly decreased. It should be recalled that carbidopa cannot cross the blood–brain barrier and so does not block dopamine formation in much of the hypothalamus.

2.3.10. Disturbed Organ Physiology in Acromegaly

It has been known from earlier reports that acromegaly is associated with increased lung volumes. Perhaps this is a direct effect on growth of the lung parenchyma, but it also may result from increased chest volume resulting from continued costal chondral growth. Harrison et al.[126] conducted a careful study of lung function in a series of 30 acromegalic patients. They confirmed the frequent presence of increased lung volumes. In addition, they found extrathoracic airway narrowing at the level of the glottis in five men. Fourteen patients showed evidence of small airway narrowing. In eight cases this may have been the result of pulmonary venous hypertension and/or kyphosis. The small airway obstruction in the remaining six patients appeared to correlate with disease of more than 9 years' duration.

In a less extensive study, Luboshitzky and Barzilai[127] reported that 8 of 11 acromegalic patients had hypoxemia, with partial pressures of O_2 of 58 to 90 mm Hg. This appeared to be related to ventilation–perfusion defects in 4 of the 5 patients studied. Hypoxemia was positively associated with duration of acromegaly.

Daytime somnolence or excessive snoring are common in acromegaly, being present in 5 of the 11 patients studied by Perks et al.[128] Affected patients had more severe GH hypersecretion. Sleep apnea in these patients is frequent and may be central, obstructive, or mixed. Cadieux et al.[129] endoscoped 2 acromegalic patients with severe sleep apnea and observed that the soft tissue of the posterior and lateral hypopharynx invaginated into the laryngeal vestibule on inspiration before any posterior movement of the tongue. Both patients were relieved by trachectomy.

The heart is affected in acromegaly, leading to increased mortality from cardiovascular diseases. Because of the rarity of acromegaly, there has not been general agreement concerning the pathologic anatomy of the heart present in this disease. For this reason, a recent study by Lie and Grossman[130] of 27 autopsied cases from the Mayo Clinic is valuable. Cardiomegaly was common (22 of 27 cases) and was not dependent on the presence of hypertension. Cardiomegaly appeared to progress with increasing duration of acromegaly. In patients who died within 10 years of onset of clinical symptoms, the mean cardiac weight was 348 g, whereas the cardiac weight of patients who lived more than 10 years after onset of clinical symptoms was 618 g. Cardiomegaly could not be attributed to diabetes, accelerated atherosclerosis, or valvular disease. Histologic evidence of myocardial fiber hypertrophy and interstitial fibrosis was common. Mononuclear cell infiltration, and other evidence of myocarditis, was found in 59% of the cases. Although these findings are impressive, the authors did not commit themselves as to whether their pathologic evidence constituted a specific acromegalic cardiomyopathy.

Additional information about the heart in acromegaly has come from two conflicting echocardiographic studies. Smallridge et al.[131] studied 27 acromegalic patients and found that 6 had evidence of asymmetric septal hypertrophy and 8 had concentric left ventricular hypertrophy. GH levels were higher in patients with left ventricular hypertrophy.

However, among the 25 acromegalic patients studied by Savage et al.,[132] only 1 was considered to have asymmetric septal hypertrophy although septal thickening was present in 16 other patients but was not considered asymmmetric and was associated with concentric left ventricular wall thickening. In this series, no correlation between the degree of serum GH elevation and cardiac hypertrophy was found.

While valvular lesions are uncommon in acromegaly, myxomatous involvement of the mitral and aortic valve can lead to click-murmur syndrome and aortic valvular insufficiency. A case reported by Ondreyco et al.[133] is of interest because the patient had myxomatous degeneration of all four cardiac valves and cystic medial necrosis of the aorta and pulmonary artery.

The pathogenesis of hypertension in acromegaly has been under scrutiny. Mantero et al.[134] compared seven hypertensive patients with nine normotensive acromegalic patients. Plasma renin activity (PRA) was lower in the hypertensive acromegalic subjects under baseline conditions, after fludrocortisone administration, and after furosamide diuresis. Urinary aldosterone was in the high-normal range and failed to suppress by more than 50% with fludrocortisone administration. Subsequent exploration of two patients established a diagnosis of aldosteronoma in one case and macronodular hyperplasia in the other case.

Ogihara et al.[135] infused saralasin, an inhibitor of angiotensin-converting enzyme, into five hypertensive and three normotensive acromegalic patients. All patients had a significant pressor response. Baseline PRA and plasma aldosterone levels were lower than in normal controls. The authors attributed the pressor response to saralasin to prior suppression of the renin–angiotensin–aldosterone system, which allowed the weak agonist action of saralasin to be evident.

A more extensive investigation of hypertension in acromegaly was conducted by Moore et al.[136] They compared the response to sodium restriction in 10 hypertensive and 4 normotensive acromegalics to that in 26 normal subjects. In an upright posture, plasma aldosterone rose less in acromegalic subjects than it did in the normal controls. When angiotensin II was infused, the increment of plasma aldosterone was also lower in the acromegalic patients than in the controls, but the rise in blood pressure was greater. When saralasin was given, both blood pressure and plasma aldosterone rose in the acromegalic subjects, but fell in the normal subjects. When the two groups of subjects were compared on a 200 mEq sodium diet, the responses to angiotensin II and saralasin were similar. The authors suggest that acromegalic patients remain volume-expanded even in the face of sodium restriction. The studies of Ogihara et al.[135] and Moore et al.[136] suggest that this volume expansion is not caused by increase in the PRA–angiotensin II–aldosterone system, but the study of Mantero et al.[134] suggests some increase in aldosterone excretion.

The long-term complications of untreated gigantism became evident in a follow-up of all the patients seen in Manchester, England.[137] Of the 10 patients so diagnosed, 9 were still living. Four of these patients had developed severe kyphosis and the others had frequent disabling complaints. The development of severe peripheral neuropathy has been noted by other authors.[138]

2.3.11. Diabetes and Acromegaly

A number of studies provide new insights into the disorders of carbohydrate metabolism in acromegaly. Wass et al.[139] found that 13 of 69 acromegalic patients had symptomatic diabetes, and an additional 26 had asymptomatic diabetes. It was remarkable that a family history of diabetes was no more common in the acromegalic patients who had diabetes than those who did not. In addition, there were no significant disturbances in the frequency of HLA types and no patient had serum antibodies reactive with islet cells.

Maneschi et al.,[140] in a kinetic study of insulin distribution and clearance after injection of [^{125}I]insulin and glucose-induced endogenous insulin secretion, concluded that all acromegalic patients have an increased initial distribution volume for insulin, an increased rate of metabolic clearance, and increased basal and glucose-stimulated posthepatic insulin secretion. The acromegalic patients with diabetes have an increase in the total distribution volume, perhaps reflecting increased vascular permeability to insulin. They also have a marked decrease of the early phase of insulin secretion and an additional factor of insulin resistance.

A study by Muggeo et al.[141] on the binding of [^{125}I]insulin by circulating monocytes in acromegaly provides more information about the insulin resistance seen in this disease. They selected 11 patients with normal or only slightly impaired carbohydrate tolerance. Compared with monocytes from 22 normal control patients, the monocytes from acromegalic patients had a decrease in the total number of insulin-binding sites in proportion to the chronic hyperinsulinemia. There was, however, an increase in affinity of the empty receptors (limiting high-affinity state) but no change in affinity of the filled receptors (limiting low-affinity state). All these changes correlated well with the degree of insulin resistance and the magnitude of the GH elevation.

2.3.12. Treatment of Acromegaly

Several reports of the results of transsphenoidal hypophysectomy allow generalization of the strengths and limitations of this form of therapy. Hardy and Somma[142] have described their experience with 160 patients. Nearly all cases with noninvasive adenomas had GH levels lowered to less than 5 ng/ml, the authors' criterion of cure. Only in instances of invasive adenomas (grade III and IV of Hardy's classification) were there significant numbers of operative failures. In general, the height of the preoperative serum GH concentration correlated with the size and extent of the tumor. The only death occurred as a result of carotid vasospasm in a patient with an invasive tumor. The overall hormonal cure (serum GH <5 ng/ml) in this series was 79% in previously untreated cases. In 76% of the patients, postoperative pituitary function was unimpaired.

Laws et al.[143] and Tucker et al.[144] have also reported the results of transsphenoidal hypophysectomy in an additional 82 and 32 patients with acromegaly, respectively. In these series, there were no deaths. Endocrine cure as defined by basal GH levels less than 10 or 5 ng/ml was achieved in about the same frequency as in the series of Hardy and Somma.

Despite the fact that most neurosurgeons have been satisfied that basal GH levels less than 5 or 10 ng/ml in the postoperative state are indicative of endocrine cure, there is evidence that this may not always be the case. Clemmons *et al.*[145] have shown that in some of these patients, evidence of active disease may persist and elevations of serum somatomedin C may be present. It was proposed that somatomedin C measurements provide a more sensitive index of excess GH secretion than serum GH measurements.

As noted, acromegalic patients may respond preoperatively to glucose, L-dopa, TRH, and LRH in an aberrant manner. The persistence of these responses in the postoperative period despite "normal" basal GH secretion may be indicative of eventual relapse. Faglia *et al.*[146] reported the relapse of one patient with persistent response to TRH 10 months after surgery.

The efficacy of bromocriptine in the treatment of acromegaly remains controversial. This form of therapy has found little favor in the USA, but has been used extensively abroad. Wass *et al.*[147] treated 73 acromegalic patients for 3 to 25 months. The usual dose was 20 mg/day, but doses as high as 60 mg/day were sometimes employed. Clinical improvement was reported in 71 patients, and GH was lowered significantly in 79%, but in only 20% were the levels of GH lowered to less than 5 ng/ml. Shalet *et al.*[148] have evaluated the response to bromocriptine with somatomedin measurements as well as GH measurements. In only 2 of 6 patients was there an excellent response by these parameters. A third patient was improved, but 3 patients were unresponsive. Unfortunately, the somatomedin measurements in this study were performed by the porcine cartilage disk bioassay and were not clearly abnormal before treatment.

Not all authors have found bromocriptine an effective agent in acromegaly. Lindholm *et al.*[149] conducted a controlled study of 18 acromegalic patients who were given bromocriptine or placebo alternately for 3 months. The dose of bromocriptine was increased progressively to 20 mg/day. No significant change in serum GH levels was observed during bromocriptine treatment. Only one mild case appeared to respond. Moreover, no improvement in symptoms or glucose tolerance was observed. The failure of this group of patients to respond to bromocriptine is difficult to explain. Initial serum GH levels were higher than in other series, 11 of 18 being greater than 50 ng/ml. In addition, the maximum dose of bromocriptine was lower than that employed by the British groups.

The excellent results of transsphenoidal hypophysectomy in the treatment of most patients with acromegaly make it unlikely that bromocriptine will ever find extensive use in the primary treatment of this condition. There are however, patients who are not cured by surgery, with or without radiation. Pelkonen *et al.*[150] selected 11 such patients for bromocriptine treatment. In 7 patients whose baseline GH values were less than 30 ng/ml, 6 responded with a lowering of serum GH to values less than 10 ng. The 3 patients whose serum GH was in excess of 50 ng/ml did not respond satisfactorily to bromocriptine. In this study, as in others, the clinical symptoms of many patients improved despite absence of objective hormone improvement. The response in these patients may represent a placebo effect.

Despite the success of transsphenoidal adenomectomy in most patients with acromegaly, there appears to be a place for radiation treatment. The favorable response to proton beam therapy has been well documented and the response to conventional supravoltage (4000–5000 rads) is often satisfactory. This form of treatment has been preferred by the group at the NIH. In a recent follow-up report on the treatment of 47 patients, 73% had serum GH levels below 10 ng/ml after 5 years, and 81% were less than 10 ng/ml after 10 years.[151] In no case was extrasellar extension of the tumor documented after irradiation. The disadvantages of this form of treatment are: (1) the relatively slow development of maximal hormonal improvement, which may take years; (2) the high incidence of hypopituitarism, which exceeds 50% after 10 years; and (3) the occasional patient who has progressive visual loss due to optic nerve radiation damage. Radiation damage to other cranial nerves, and even to the frontal lobe, may occur.[152]

2.4. Hypopituitarism

2.4.1. Etiology

While the pathologic processes that cause hypopituitarism are well recognized, recent studies have emphasized that the distinction between hypopituitarism resulting from destruction of the pituitary (primary) and hypopituitarism resulting from impaired neuroendocrine control (secondary) is often blurred and that both may exist together. Evidence for this has been the increased secretion of TSH after TRH administration and of gonadotropins after GnRH administration. In the patients with pituitary infarction and apoplexy reviewed by Veldhuis and Hammond,[153] little evidence of hypothalamic pathology was found. They suggested that hypothalamic dysfunction was due to impaired neurohypophyseal vasculature with inadequate delivery of releasing factors to the adenohypophysis. Such appeared to be the case in a patient with Sheehan's syndrome reported by Jordan et al.[154] This patient had clinical evidence of adrenal insufficiency and absent ACTH response to hypoglycemia. When vasopressin was administered, however, there was a marked ACTH response. At postmortem, the hypothalamus displayed only mild gliosis. The pituitary was greatly reduced in size with small islands of tissue in dense fibrous scar. In Hand–Schiller–Christian disease (histiocytosis), the major defect may be hypothalamic. Rothman et al.[155] described a case in which GnRH infusions given for 4 hr daily for a week restored the normal LH response to GnRH. Hypothalamic deficiency is probably the major cause of panhypopituitarism after head trauma.[156]

In sarcoidosis, in contrast, hypopituitarism is often the result of pituitary damage. None of ten patients studied by Stuart et al.[157] responded to TRH and GnRH with an increase in serum TSH and LH.

In some cases of hypopituitarism it is possible to demonstrate hypothalamic atrophy of unknown etiology. The case described by Hendricks et al.[158] responded briskly to releasing factor administration with a rise of serum TSH and gonadotropins. Pneumoencephalography demonstrated downward bulging of the third ventricle and enlargement of the infundibular recess. One cause of hypothalamic injury may be viral meningoencephalitis. Kupari et al.[159] described three cases of partial hypopituitarism that followed meningoencephalitis. There was serologic evidence of infection with influenza A in two cases and with herpes simplex in the third case.

It is well known that a number of midline developmental defects can lead to hypopituitarism. The syndrome of optic nerve hypoplasia with absent septum pellucidum in association with hypopituitarism is now well known. The defect in the septum pellucidum can be established by CT scanning.[160] Even such a common condition as cleft lip or palate is associated with an increased incidence of GH deficiency. Of 200 such children examined by Rudman et al.,[161] 24 were below the third percentile in height. Of these short children, 4 were judged to have total GH deficiency and 4 had partial GH deficiency (peak value of GH after provocative testing between 2 and 7 ng/ml).

An unusual form of familial hypopituitarism with enlarged sella turcica, in the absence of radiologic evidence of pituitary tumor or empty sella, was described by Parks et al.[162] Two sisters and a brother were affected. The parents were unrelated and had normal sellar volume. Rapid growth followed treatment with thyroxine and GH. The pituitary pathology was not established.

A survey of the possible etiologic factors in idiopathic GH deficiency, conducted by Rona and Tanner[163] in England and Wales, indicated a high frequency of breech and difficult deliveries. These basic associations have been confirmed and extended by studies of 151 cases in the Netherlands by Steendijk[164] and of 93 cases in France by Calzada et al.[165] In the Dutch study, breech delivery occurred in 37.1%, as compared to only 2.8% in the general population. As in other series, boys were affected more often than girls. Unlike the British study, idiopathic GH deficiency was not more common in firstborn children. Four families with multiple cases were encountered. The prevalence of GH deficiency in children between the ages of 4 and 19 years was estimated to be 1 : 19,000 (1 : 14,000 in boys and 1 : 32,000 in girls). The French experience was similar, with 38% breech deliveries. They did observe that boys and girls were equally affected by isolated GH deficiencies. This suggested that genetic factors might have been important in these cases.

2.4.2. Familial Isolated GH Deficiency

Two types of familial isolated GH deficiency have been described, transmitted as a Mendelian recessive trait. Affected individuals exhibit the manifestations of severe GH deficiency but differ in their response to GH treatment. In one type, originally recognized in Switzerland, the initial response to GH treatment is excellent but refractoriness to GH develops over a period of several months associated with the development of high titers of neutralizing antibodies in the serum. This led Illig[166] to postulate that these patients were completely devoid of endogenous GH and that the administered GH was treated by the immune system as a foreign protein. This hypothesis has been confirmed by Phillips et al.[167] They used a specific [^{32}P]hGH cDNA probe to study the GH genes in these patients and found that there was a 7.5-kb deletion, which included the entire GH gene but did not include the GH variant pseudogene. This observation provides direct evidence that this GH variant gene cannot substitute for the normal gene. Studies in three families established transmission as a recessive trait.

The more common type of familial isolated GH deficiency responds normally to exogenous GH suggesting reduced but not absent GH secretion, and limited pathologic studies suggest the presence of GH in the pituitaries of affected individuals. Studies of the GH genes of affected families with this type of dwarfism were conducted by Phillips et al.[168] Polymorphism of the GH gene after specific endonuclease digestion was recognized with the [^{32}P]hGH cDNA probe. This allowed determination by deduction of the individual chromosome 17 carrying the GH gene which was transmitted from parent to offspring. No correlation could be established between the specific parental chromosomes inherited by affected and unaffected siblings and the development of GH deficiency. The defect in this type of dwarfism may reside in the synthesis and/or secretion of GHRF.

2.4.3. Hormonal Studies in Hypopituitary Children

The diagnosis of GH deficiency is most often made after one or more provocative stimuli fail to cause a rise in serum GH to above some arbitrary level, variously considered to be between 5 and 10 ng/ml. Plotnick et al.[169] have examined how well the response to standard stimulation tests correlates with the integrated serum concentration of GH (ICGH) in 30 short children. The stimulation tests employed were the sequential arginine–insulin tolerance test in 28 cases and consecutive L-dopa and insulin hypoglycemia tests in 2. In general, the ICGH correlated with the results of the two stimulation tests. However, 5 patients who had low responses to provocative tests had normal ICGH values. Also, 3 patients wih borderline GH stimulation responses (10–12 ng/ml) had normal ICGH values. These results indicate that the stimulation tests do not reflect spontaneous GH secretion in an important minority of cases.

The most appropriate way to stimulate GH secretion remains in contention. Fass et al.[170] measured serum GH 60–90 min after sleep onset, after the administration of L-dopa, and after L-dopa with propranolol in a large number of short children. In all three procedures, a positive response was considered to be a rise of serum GH to greater than 7 ng/ml. Patients who failed these tests were primed for 3 days with diethylstilbestrol and challenged with sequential insulin hypoglycemia and arginine infusion. Lack of response to this rigorous test was considered diagnostic of pituitary dwarfism. It was found that sleep GH measurements had a 31% false-positive rate, L-dopa alone had a 20% false-positive rate, and L-dopa–propranolol had a false-positive rate of 5.2%.

In view of the shortcomings of GH provocation tests, additional agents continue to be proposed. Gil-Ad et al.[171] gave a single oral dose of 0.15 mg/m^2 of clonidine, a central α-adrenergic agonist, to 18 healthy, short children and 7 patients with hypopituitarism diagnosed by other provocative tests. The serum GH rose between 60 and 120 min to 34.3 ± 4.5 ng/ml in the normal individuals. In the hypopituitary subjects, no significant change of serum GH occurred. Despite a fall of 20–25 mm of systolic blood pressure, the authors reported that the procedure was well tolerated and a useful test. Clonidine may not be a consistent stimulus for GH secretion in adults.[172]

There is reason to believe that the provocative tests that are generally used to diagnose GH deficiency may exclude individuals who have partial GH deficiency and might benefit from GH treatment. Spiliotis et al.[173] have selected a group of very short children with retarded bone age and with somatomedin levels that were low for their age but who responded normally to GH provocative tests. They evaluated the physiologic secretion of GH by measurement every 20 min for a 24-hr period. The integrated GH concentration of these children was 2.1 ng/ml as compared to 5.5 ng/ml in a control group and 1.6 ng/ml in patients fulfilling the usual requirements for a diagnosis of pituitary dwarfism. A deficiency of physiologic GH secretion but with normal responses to provocative tests was termed "neurosecretory dysfunction." The authors went on to show that these patients responded to GH treatment with a doubling of growth velocity over the first year.

Some patients with thyroid hormone levels that are initially normal may become hypothyroid during GH treatment. In a study by Demura et al.,[174] this occurred in 10 of 26 patients. In an additional 8 patients who were hypothyroid before treatment, T_4 decreased further. Initially, these patients exhibited a delayed TSH response to TRH; after hGH treatment, the pattern was exaggerated. It was suggested that GH increases T_4 metabolism and brings out or exacerbates TRH deficiency. Unfortunately, this study did not separate patients with IGHD from those with MPHD. While it has been generally accepted that the response of the serum prolactin and TSH to TRH is indicative of hypothalamic damage, the pathologic evidence for this is skimpy at best. There is a realization that response to TRH and GnRH can occur in some patients with Sheehan's syndrome and other primary disorders of the pituitary. The usual explanation is that residual pituitary tissue may be sequestered in scar tissue and inaccessible to hypophysiotropic hormones transmitted by the portal vessels.

2.4.4. GH Treatment

The general effectiveness of hGH in the treatment of pituitary dwarfism is well established. The experience in the treatment of 642 patients in Great Britain over 18 years is summarized by Milner et al.[175] They estimate that pituitary dwarfism is present in about 1 in 10,000 children. Despite a well-organized hGH treatment program in a socialized medical system, the mean chronological age at the start of treatment of IGHD was 8.1 ± 0.6 years. Earlier recognition and treatment would improve growth responses. The British have had adequate supplies of hGH and have found that superior growth was obtained with doses of 5 IU three times weekly. This is a larger dose than that usually employed in the U.S. With hGH prepared by the Wilhelmi method, antibody formation inhibited growth response in 2–3% of the children. The authors argued that this constituted a reason for not attempting hGH treatment in children who are not GH deficient.

In the U.S., where GH supplies have been limited, studies have been conducted to define therapeutic regimens requiring less GH. In one study by Kirkland and Clayton,[176] hGH was given at 1 IU/day for 12–36 days four times yearly. Simultaneously, the children received 1–2 mg of fluoxmesterone daily. On this regimen, the mean growth velocity was 6.4 cm/year without evidence of accelerated bone maturation. Rosenbloom et al.[177] studied the response of 29 hypopituitary patients to a single weekly dose of hGH of 2.5 IU. The growth velocity during treatment was 7.2 ± 0.5 cm/year, which compared favorably to the studies of Kirkland and Clayton and to the more conventional dose of 2 U three times weekly. These two studies suggest that significant growth stimulation can be achieved with small doses of hGH with and without androgen supplementation. No claim is made that these low-dose regimens are superior.

2.4.4.1. GH Refractoriness

Laron dwarfism is characterized by short stature and other features suggesting GH deficiency. Nevertheless, in this disorder, serum GH levels are high and no abnormalities of immunologic or receptor binding properties of the serum GH have been observed. Resistance to endogenous GH is suggested by the invariably low serum somatomedin concentration, which remains low despite the administration of exogenous GH. Other metabolic actions of GH are either blunted or absent. Significant stimulation of skeletal height does not follow GH treatment. Golde et al.[178] have provided in vitro evidence of GH resistance. Stimulation of peripheral blood erythrogenic stem cells from two patients with this condition by physiologic concentrations of GH in vitro was impaired, whereas cells from normal individuals and normal hypopituitary dwarfs had an increase in erythrogenic burst-forming units. However, these results would have been more conclusive if the presence of Laron dwarfism had been better documented. The first patient did not exhibit increased GH levels and somatomedin levels were not reported. The second patient was observed to have a somatomedin concentration of 0.7 U/ml, which makes the diagnosis of Laron dwarfism doubtful.

Eshet et al.[179] have now provided convincing evidence of a defect in the GH receptor in Laron-type dwarfism. The binding of [^{125}I]hGH to liver membranes was measured in two patients with Laron-type dwarfism obtained at open biopsy and in six kidney transplant donors. In the normal individuals, specific binding of [^{125}I]hGH varied from 7.3 to 24.1% while the specific binding in the membranes from the Laron-type dwarfs was 0.1 and 0.5%.

2.5. Somatomedins

2.5.1. Structure

The nature of the circulating somatomedins has been greatly clarified by the isolation and structural characterization of the two principal somatomedins, insulin-like growth factor I (IGH-I) and insulin-like growth factor II (IGF-II) by Rinderknecht and Humbel.[180,181] According to Klapper et al.,[182] the amino acid sequence of somatomedin C (Sm C) is identical to IGF-I. It is now generally believed that SmA is not a separate peptide but a mixture of peptides derived from IGF-I and IGF-II. Another peptide fraction derived from serum that has mitogenic activity in human glial cells was called somatomedin B. This name is now known to be inappropriate because the mitogenic activity of SmB preparations is attributable to its epidermal growth factor content.[183]

2.5.2. Measurement of Somatomedins

There is disagreement whether or not serum binding proteins interfere with direct RIAs of SmC/IGF-I. Furlanetto et al.[184] attempted to avoid interference by prolonged incubation of the antibody with serum before adding tracer [^{125}I]-IGF-I/SmC. Bala and Bhaumick[185] found that brief acidification of serum increased the measured somatomedin level and improved parallelism of serum dilutions and standards. Clemmons et al.[186] found that addition of heparin further increased the SmC detectable in acidified serum. They presented evidence that heparin inhibited the binding of SmC by serum binding protein. Zapf et al.[187] have avoided any interference with binding protein by acid gel filtration of serum, which separates free IGFs from the binding protein. Because this gel filtration is laborious, Daughaday et al.[188] have developed a simple method of acid–ethanol extraction that extracts SmC/IGF-I and IGF-II nearly quantitatively and precipitates most of the binding protein. After centrifugation, the supernatant is merely neutralized and is then added directly to RIAs or RRAs. The values obtained with radioligand assays with such sera are nearly three times those obtained with assays on unextracted sera. While the direct assays have correlated well with the GH status of most patients, there is much certainty concerning what is actually being measured. Serious discrepancies result if direct assays are applied to rat serum or to human serum with altered somatomedin-binding protein.

Specific assays have now been developed for IGF-II. Daughaday et al.[189] found that rat placentas are rich in receptors for IGF-II and deficient in receptors for IGF-I. They have described an RRA utilizing rat placental membranes and [^{125}I]-IGF-II.[190] Cross-reaction with IGF-I is less than 1%. IGF-II can easily be detected in acid–ethanol extracts of human serum. Hintz and Liu[191] have developed an antibody against the portion of the IGF-II molecule analogous to the connecting peptide of proinsulin. The RIA with this antiserum also cross-reacts negligibly with IGF-I. Zapf et al.[187] have raised an antibody against IGF-II, and utilized this antibody in an RIA. In their assay, IGF-I has about 10% of the immunologic potency of IGF-II.

Clinical studies with these assays have established that the GH dependence of IGF-II is less than that of IGF-I. In hypopituitarism, the levels of IGF-II are not as low as those of IGF-I. In acromegaly, no elevation of IGF-II occurs, whereas there is marked elevation of IGF-I.

2.5.3. Somatomedin-Binding Proteins of Serum

Progress has been made in the unraveling of the complex nature of the transport of somatomedin peptides in serum. Furlanetto[192] confirmed the findings of earlier workers that nearly all the SmC of human serum is carried in a protein complex that by neutral gel filtration had an apparent molecular size equivalent to that of IgG (Stokes radius 43 Å). After ammonium sulfate precipitation and DEAE-Sephadex chromatography, most of the endogenous somatomedin appeared in the second of three protein peaks. The SmC in this peak was associated with smaller complexes with Stokes radii of 36 and 14 Å. The third peak of the DEAE fractionation lacked SmC, but when recombined with the second peak reconstituted a complex similar in size to that present in native serum. Exposure of serum to acid conditions irreversibly converts the large somatomedin complex into the small-molecular-size complex (Stokes radius 36 Å). Addition of the third peak to this acid-treated serum fraction also regenerated the large native somatomedin–protein complex. These observations have given rise to the formulation that somatomedin in serum is bound to a specific binding protein that is acid-stable. The complex includes a third acid-labile component present in the third fraction of the DEAE separation. This binding component was retained in Con A-Sepharose columns, which suggests that it is a glycoprotein.

In hypopituitarism, there is little somatomedin present as the large molecular complexes, but after GH treatment this complex reappears.[193] Both acid-stable and acid-labile components of the IgG-sized somatomedin-binding complex are decreased in hypopituitarism.[192]

When labeled somatomedin is added to native serum, it does not equilibrate with endogenous somatomedins, but a fraction is bound as a protein complex smaller than albumin. Furlanetto[192] found that this complex, unlike the acid-stable binding protein, did not increase in size after the addition of DEAE fraction 3. This suggests that this native somatomedin-binding protein is not identical to the acid-stable somatomedin-binding protein. Hintz et al.[194] have studied the binding protein of serum accessible to exogenous [^{125}I]-SmC; they call this unsaturated somatomedin-binding protein (SmBP). They found that plasma SmBP of hypopituitary patients actually bound more [^{125}I]-SmC/IGF-I than it did in normal plasma. Scatchard analysis suggested that the difference was due to an increased affinity rather than a change in receptor number. This difference disappeared after GH treatment of the hypopituitary children.

2.5.4. Variation in Normal Serum Somatomedin Levels

There is a rise in IGF-I/SmC levels during pregnancy. Furlanetto et al.[195] found the levels to be increased 60% between the weeks 31 and 42 of pregnancy when measured by RIA. Using a similar RIA, Bala et al.[196] found an 80% rise in somatomedin concentration in late pregnancy as compared to normal nonpregnant individuals. Wilson et al.[197] reported that the elevated IGF-I levels of late pregnancy fell abruptly after delivery. They also observed that there was a modest rise in IGF-II levels during pregnancy with a fall after delivery. Most observers have found that IGF-I/SmC and IGF-II levels in cord serum as measured by RIA are substantially lower than maternal levels.

In the newborn infant, IGF-I levels in serum fall rapidly to very low concentrations on day 1–3 of life.[196] During infancy, SmC/IGF-I levels remain low, which has been variously interpreted as meaning that the rapid growth at this age is unrelated to somatomedins or alternatively that the tissue sensitivity to somatomedins is so great that low concentrations suffice. After infancy, there is a progressive rise in SmC/IGF-I levels until adult levels are reached just before puberty. A marked rise in IGF-I/SmC levels occurs at puberty and persists for 3–4 years.[196,198] Thereafter, levels fall to the normal adult level.

SmC/IGF-I levels gradually fall in the elderly. In a study by Rudman et al.,[199] the mean SmC level of 10 normal individuals between 20 and 29 years of age was 1.43 U/ml with 95% confidence limits of 0.64–2.22. In contrast, 6 of 12 individuals between 60 and 79 years of age had SmC levels that were below normal limits for the third decade. The lower SmC levels were attributed to decreased GH secretion in the elderly.

Familiarity with the changes in SmC/IGF-I serum concentrations at various ages is important for clinicians using these assays. Before the age of 4 years, the difference between normal and hypopituitary dwarfs with respect to serum SmC/IGF-I is small and the test has little diagnostic value. Similarly, it is difficult to distinguish the physiologically elevated serum SmC/IGF-I puberty from that due to excess GH secretion.

Most workers have found somatomedin levels relatively uniform throughout the day. A thorough study of SmC levels by RIA was reported by Minuto et al.[200] These workers found little change in SmC levels during waking hours, but a mean drop of 24% occurred after the onset of sleep. This period is associated, of course, with a peak of GH secretion. The relationship between these SmC and GH changes remains conjectural.

2.5.5. Somatomedin Levels in Malnutrition and Uncontrolled Diabetes Mellitus

Malnutrition, especially protein calorie malnutrition, has been found to be associated with low levels of somatomedin bioactivity despite normal or elevated serum GH levels. In a study by Hintz et al.[201] of 27 young children with protein calorie malnutrition in Thailand, serum GH was inversely related to somatomedin bioactivity. Following refeeding, normal GH and somatomedin levels were attained by day 29.

The effects of fasting on serum SmC/IGF-I concentrations have studied under controlled conditions by Clemmons et al.[202] The serum SmC/IGF-I of obese male volunteers before fasting averaged 0.83 U/ml and fell to 0.21 U/ml after 10 days of fasting. Refeeding restored the serum SmC/IGF-I rapidly. In a subsequent study from the same laboratory, individuals of normal weight were fasted for 5 days with a fall in SmC/IGF-I levels from 1.85 ± 0.39 U/ml to 0.67 ± 0.16 U/ml.[203] Full dietary restoration led to a rapid recovery of SmC/IGF-I, but recovery was delayed when an isocaloric diet was restricted to 0.43 g protein/kg per day. When the low-protein diet was combined with caloric restriction to 552–799 calories/day, there was a continued fall in serum SmC/IGF-I. These studies emphasize the great importance of normal nutrition in maintaining somatomedin levels. This becomes of importance in the interpretation of results obtained in clinical applications of somatomedin measurements.

Anorexia nervosa is an unusual condition in childhood. Rappaport et al.[204] found that the somatomedin bioactivity was reduced in 8 of 12 patients despite elevated GH levels. Six children who responded to dietary treatment had a rise in somatomedin bioactivity. One anorexia nervosa patient treated with GH failed to respond.

Growth failure may occur in uncontrolled diabetes. The role of somatomedin deficiency in this condition is controversial. Winter et al.[205] reported low somatomedin bioactivity in a case of poorly controlled diabetes mellitus, growth failure, and hepatomegaly—the Mauriac syndrome. Levels rose with improved diabetic control. Nash[206] could not confirm this finding in 4 diabetic children with growth failure. In a larger study of 40 diabetic children, Winter et al.[207] found an inverse relationship between somatomedin bioactivity and hemoglobin A_{1c}. The correlation, although significant, was relatively poor.

Tamborlane et al.[208] investigated the effect of intensive treatment of eight poorly controlled insulin-dependent diabetics for 16 weeks with the insulin pump. Before treatment, basal and exercise-provoked serum GH levels were increased. Serum SmC by RRA and RIA was within the normal limits. It could be argued that normal somatomedins could only be maintained in these subjects by increased GH levels. Following normalization of blood sugar by the insulin pump, serum GH levels fell and somatomedin levels rose. In two adolescents, growth velocity doubled during 13 and 15 months of pump therapy.

Neonatal diabetes mellitus is a transient condition associated with hyperglycemia, glycosuria, and impaired growth. In studies of a patient with this disorder, Blethen et al.[209] found low SmC/IGF-I levels by RIA before insulin therapy. After insulin was instituted, weight increased promptly, but SmC/IGF-I levels rose more slowly. With spontaneous acquisition of normal endogenous insulin secretion, SmC/IGF-I RIA levels were normal for her age. Throughout this child's course, IGF-II by RRA was normal.

2.5.6. Somatomedins in Chronic Renal Failure

Chronic renal failure impairs growth in children by mechanisms as yet uncertain. In the past, a number of investigators have reported that somatomedin bioactivity is reduced in this condition. Phillips et al.[210] have indicated that some of the apparent low results reported could have been due to the elevated sulfate present in uremic serum. This sulfate would dilute the $^{35}SO_4$ in the bioassay procedures. They found corrected mean results before hemodialysis to be slightly lower than normal, with a rise after hemodialysis. Removal of an inhibitor by hemodialysis was suggested.

Takano et al.[211] measured SmA by RIA and RRA of unextracted serum in 57 adult patients with chronic renal failure. Levels were elevated to about 2.5 times normal with both analytic techniques. When Goldberg et al.,[212] using acid–ethanol extracts, measured SmC/IGF-I by RIA in uremic sera, the levels were reduced. They postulated that abnormalities existed in protein binding in uremia that artifactually elevated results with unextracted serum.

Schiffrin et al.[213] did extract uremic serum prior to assay with an RRA using placental membranes and an ^{125}I-labeled acidic somatomedin preparation. They found a mean elevation of 70% in apparent somatomedin in nine uremic children. This assay, however, probably detects both IGF-I and IGF-II. When Goldberg, et al.[212] measured IGF-II in acid–ethanol extracts by a specific IGF-II RRA, this peptide was found to be elevated to about 3 times normal. In conclusion, it appeared to these authors that the actual level of IGF-I is reduced in uremia and that the level of IGF-II is increased. Abnormalities of serum binding are also present.

2.5.7. Somatomedin Levels in Hypopituitarism

Copeland et al.[214] measured by RIA the effect of GH on SmC levels in serum. They confirmed earlier bioassay data that a rise in serum somatomedin was delayed 6–8 hr after GH treatment. The authors interpreted this to mean that there was no store of previously synthesized somatomedin to be rapidly released by GH. Twenty-eight hypopituitary patients were started on GH treatment; for 8 of these patients, treatment was restarted after a long interval. Thirty-six paired serum samples were obtained before and at least 4 months after hGH treatment had been started. In 28 studies, a rise of SmC to normal adult levels or more was noted. Six other studies showed a subnormal rise to adult levels, but no attempt was made to compare results with those in age-appropriate controls. In 2 studies, no significant rise in SmC was found. The authors were surprised that, despite the subnormal SmC levels, all patients were growing normally. The authors noted that these children tended to be underweight and had poor appetites. Two children who had gained 4–5 pounds before retesting had a normal somatomedin response. The authors speculated that impaired nutrition might have resulted in a selective failure to manufacture binding protein. In such a case, the serum levels would not accurately reflect tissue delivery of somatomedin.

Low serum somatomedin is characteristic of children with GH deficiency, yet low somatomedin occurs in other conditions, such as nutritional failure and Laron-type GH resistance. Kowarski et al.[215] described 2 patients with growth failure and low serum somatomedin bioactivity whose GH secretion to provocative testing was entirely normal. Unlike patients with Laron-type dwarfism, there was a prompt rise in serum somatomedin bioactivity in response to GH treatment and continued GH treatment stimulated accelerated skeletal growth. Preliminary evidence of an abnormal circulating GH was obtained by comparison of radioreceptor assayable GH with the results obtained by RIA. Apparently, the 2 patients had circulating GH with impaired radioreceptor activity detected by the pregnant rabbit liver membrane GH receptor. Similar patients were identified by Rudman et al.[216] in a study of 21 children exhibiting normal variant short stature. All children had birth weights greater than 2.5 kg and were below the third percentile in height. No organic or emotional cause for growth retardation existed. Pituitary dwarfism was excluded by serum GH levels more than 12 ng/ml after provocative testing. All children were challenged with two 10-day courses of hGH. Nitrogen retention and linear growth were measured. Three of the children were hyperresponsive to both the anabolic and growth-promoting actions of GH, and 2 of the children were partially responsive. These children had low levels of serum SmC by RIA and normal noctural GH secretion. The ratio of GH by RRA to GH by RIA was 0.22 and 0.38 in the two GH-responsive groups. An abnormality in circulating GH was postulated in these patients. The defect appears to be identical to that previously reported by Kowarski et al.,[215] cited above. The GH gene in such patients is under current investigation.

In a subsequent paper, Rudman et al.[217] treated 20 children of normal variant short stature for 6 months with 0.08 U hGH/kg body wt daily for 6 months. In the 11 children who originally were resistant or refractory to the anabolic effects of GH (authors' subgroups 1 and 2) and had normal mean somatomedin levels, little or no long-term stimulation of growth occurred. In the subjects who exhibited an anabolic response to GH and had low somatomedin levels (subgroups 3 and 4), prolonged GH treatment restored normal somatomedin levels, and growth velocity was accelerated fivefold. On the basis of these studies, the authors concluded that the best predictor of subsequent increased growth velocity during GH treatment is a low initial somatomedin level and a rise in somatomedin (>0.5 U/ml) after short-term GH administration.

References

1. Cooke, N. E., Coit, D., Shine, J., Baxter, J. D., and Martial, J. A., 1981, Human prolactin: cDNA structural analysis and evolutionary comparisons, *J. Biol. Chem.* **256:**4007–4016.
2. Barsh, G. S., Seeburg, P. H., and Gelinas, R. E., 1983, The human growth hormone gene family: Structure and evolution of the chromosomal locus, *Nucleic Acid Res.* **11:**3939–3958.
3. Nybert, F., Roos, P., and Wide, L., 1980, Human pituitary prolactin: Isolation and characterization of three isohormones with different bioassay and radioimmunoassay activities, *Biochim. Biophys. Acta* **625:**255–265.
4. Garnier, P. E., Aubert, M. L., Kaplan, S. L., and Grumbach, M. M., 1978, Heterogeneity of pituitary and plasma prolactin in man: Decreased affinity of "big" prolactin in a radioreceptor assay and evidence for its secretion, *J. Clin. Edocrinol. Metab.* **47:**1273–1281.
5. Kiefer, K. A., and Malarkey, W. B., 1978, Size heterogeneity of human prolactin in CSF and serum: Experimental conditions that alter gel filtration patterns, *J. Clin. Endocrinol. Metab.* **46:**119–124.
6. Jordan, R. M., and Kendall, J. W., 1978, Dissociation of plasma and CSF prolactin heterogeneity, *Acta Endocrinol. (Copenhagen)* **89:**38–47.
7. Pochet, R., Martial, J., and Pasteels, J. L., 1982, Detection and characterization of human prolactin messenger RNA in chorion-decidua, *DNA* **1:**193.
8. Golander, A., Hurley, T., Barrett, J., Hizi, A., and Handwerger, S., 1978, Prolactin synthesis by human chorion-decidual tissue: A possible source of prolactin in the amniotic fluid, *Science* **202:**311–313.
9. Maslar, I. A., and Riddick, D. H., 1979, Prolactin production by human

endometrium during the normal menstrual cycle, *Am. J. Obstet. Gynecol.*
135:751–754.

10. Riddick, D. H., and Maslar, I. A., 1981, The transport of prolactin by human fetal membranes, *J. Clin. Endocrinol. Metab.* **52:**220–224.

11. McCoshen, J. A., Tagger, O. Y., Wodzicki, A., and Tyson, J. E., 1982, Choriodecidual adhesion promotes decidual prolactin transport by human fetal membrane, *Am. J. Physiol.* **243:**R552–557.

12. Ylikorkala, O., Kivinen, S., and Reinila, M., 1979, Serial prolactin and thyrotropin responses to thyrotropin-releasing hormone throughout normal human pregnancy, *J. Clin. Endocrinol. Metab.* **48:**288–292.

13. Kletzky, O. A., Marrs, R. P., Howard, W. F., McCormick, W., and Mishell, D. R., Jr., 1980, Prolactin synthesis and release during pregnancy and puerperium, *Am. J. Obstet. Gynecol.* **136:**545–550.

14. Ylikorkala, O., Huhtaniemi, I., Tuimala, R., and Seppala, M., 1979, Subnormal postconceptional levels of prolactin do not interfere with the early events of human pregnancy, *Fertil. Steril.* **32:**286–288.

15. Yuen, B. H., Cannon, W., Lewis, J., Sy, L., and Woolley, S., 1980, Possible role for prolactin in the control of human chorionic gonadotropin and estrogen secretion by the fetoplacental unit, *Am. J. Obstet. Gynecol.* **136:**286–291.

16. Perlman, M., Schenker, J., Glassman, M., and Ben-David, M., 1978, Prolonged hyperprolactinemia in preterm infants, *J. Clin. Endocrinol. Metab.* **47:**894–897.

17. Polleri, A., Masturzo, P., Vignola, G., Barreca, T., and Gallamini, A., 1978, Sleep–wake differences in serum prolactin levels in children, *J. Endocrinol. Invest.* **1:**347–350.

18. Large, D. M., Anderson, D. C., and Laing, I., 1980, Twenty-four hour profiles of serum prolactin during male puberty with and without gynaecomastia, *Clin. Endocrinol.* **12:**293–302.

19. Spitz, I. M., Zylber, E., Cohen, H., Almaliach, U., and Leroith, D., 1979, Impaired prolactin response to thyrotropin-releasing hormone in isolated gonadotropin deficiency and exaggerated response in primary testicular failure, *J. Clin. Endocrinol. Metab.* **48:**941–945.

20. Turksoy, R. N., 1979, Dissociation of prolactin responsiveness to thyrotropin-releasing hormone and chlorpromazine in a female with Kallmann's syndrome, *Fertil Steril.* **32:**228–229.

21. Suter, S. N., Kaplan, S. L., Aubert, M. L., and Grumbach, M. M., 1978, Plasma prolactin and thyrotropin and response to thyrotropin-releasing factor in children with primary and hypothalamic hypothyroidism, *J. Clin. Endocrinol. Metab.* **47:**1015–1020.

22. Honbo, K. S., van Herle, J. J., and Kellett, K. A., 1978, Serum prolactin levels in untreated primary hypothyroidism, *Am. J. Med.* **64:**782–787.

23. Contreras, P., Generini, G., Michelsen, H., Pumarino, H., and Campino, C., 1981, Hyperprolactinemia and galactorrhea—Spontaneous versus iatrogenic hypothyroidism, *J. Clin. Endocrinol. Metab.* **53:**1036–1039.

24. Ben-David, M., and Schenker, J. G., 1983, Transient hyperprolactinemia: A correctable cause of idiopathic female infertility, *J. Clin. Endocrinol. Metab.* **57:**442–444.

25. Tolis, G., Goltzman, D., Guyda, H., and Mountokalakis, T., 1980, Hormonal derangements in uremia, *J. Endocrinol. Invest.* **3:**83–97.
26. Lim, V. S., Lim, S. C., Kathpalia, S. C., and Frohman, L. A., 1979, Hyperprolactinemia and impaired pituitary response to suppression and stimulation in chronic renal failure: Reversal after transplantation, *J. Clin. Endocrinol. Metab.* **48:**101–107.
27. Gomez, F., Delacueva, R., Wauters, J. P., and Lemarchandberaud, T., 1980, Endocrine abnormalities in patients undergoing long-term hemodialysis— The role of prolactin, *Am. J. Med.* **68:**522–530.
28. Vermeulen, A., and Ando, S., 1978, Prolactin and adrenal androgen secretion, *Clin. Endocrinol.* **8:**295–304.
29. Parker, L. N., Chang, S., and Odell, W. D., 1978, Adrenal androgens in patients with chronic marked elevation of prolactin, *Clin. Endocrinol.* **8:**1–6.
30. Lobo, R. A., Kletzky, O. A., Kaptein, E. M., and Goebelsmann, U., 1980, Prolactin modulation of dehydroepiandrosterone sulfate secretion, *Am. J. Obstet. Gynecol.* **138:**632–636.
31. Rubin, R. T., Poland, R. E., Sobel, I., Tower, B. B., and Odell, W. D., 1978, Effects of prolactin and prolactin plus luteinizing hormone on plasma testosterone levels in normal adult men, *J. Clin. Endocrinol. Metab.* **47:**447–456.
32. Rubin, R. T., Poland, R. E., Sowers, J. R., and Hershman, J. M., 1978, Influence of methyl-TRH-induced prolactin increase on serum testosterone levels in normal adult men, *J. Clin. Endocrinol. Metab.* **46:**830–833.
33. Pontiroli, A. E., and Pozza, G., 1978, Histamine stimulates prolactin release in normal men, *Acta Endocrinol. (Copenhagen)* **88:**23–28.
34. Carlson, H. E., and Ippoliti, A. F., 1977, Cimetidine, an H_2-antihistamine, stimulates prolactin secretion in man, *J. Clin. Endocrinol. Metab.* **45:**367–370.
35. Pontiroli, A. E., Pellicciotta, G., Alberetto, M., DePasqua, A., Girardi, A. M., and Pozza, G., 1979, Cimetidine and L-dopa in the control of prolactin secretion in man, *Horm. Metab. Res.* **11:**257–258.
36. Golstein, J., Vanhaelst, L., Bruno, O. D., and L'Hermite, M., 1979, Effect of cyproheptadine on thyrotrophin and prolactin secretion in normal man, *Acta Endocrinol. (Copenhagen)* **92:**205–213.
37. Masala, A., Delitala, G., Devilla, L., Alagna, S., and Rovasio, P. P., 1979, Enhancement of insulin-induced prolactin secretion by fluoxetine in man, *J. Clin. Endocrinol. Metab.* **49:**350–352.
38. Foley, K. M., Kourides, I. A., Inturrisi, C. E., Kalko, R. F., Zaroulis, C. G., Posner, J. B., Houde, R. W., and Li, C. H., 1979, Beta endorphin analgesic and hormonal effects in humans, *Proc. Natl. Acad. Sci. USA* **76:**5377–5381.
39. Schulz, S. C., Wagner, R., Van Kammen, D. P., Rogol, A. D., Davies, G. C., Wyatt, R. J., Pickar, D., Bunney, W. E., Jr., and Li, C. H., 1980, Prolactin response in beta-endorphin in man, *Life Sci.* **27:**1735–1742.
40. Tamminga, C. A., Neophytides, A., Chase, T. N., and Frohman, L. A., 1978, Stimulation of prolactin and growth hormone secretion by muscimol, a γ-aminobutyric acid agonist, *J. Clin. Endocrinol. Metab.* **47:**1349–1351.
41. Isaac, R., Merceron, R. E., Caillens, G., Raymond, J-P., and Ardaillou, R., 1978, Effect of parathyroid hormone on plasma prolactin in man, *J. Clin. Endocrinol. Metab.* **47:**18–23.
42. Pontiroli, A. E., Gala, R. R., Pellicciotta, G., DePasqua, A., Girardi, A. M.,

and Pozza, G., 1979, Study on the reproducibility of human prolactin response to sulpiride, benserazide, insulin hypoglycaemia and arginine infusion *Acta Endocrinol (Copenhagen)* **91:**410–420.

43. L'Hermite, M., Denayer, P., Golstein, J., Virasoro, E., Vanhaelst, L., Copinschi, G., and Robyn, C., 1978, Acute endocrine profile of sulpiride in the human, *Clin. Endocrinol.* **9:**195–204.

44. Healy, D. L., and Burger, H. G., 1978, Sustained elevation of serum prolactin by metoclopramide: A clinical model of idiopathic hyperprolactinemia, *J. Clin. Endocrinol. Metab.* **46:**709–714.

45. Annegers, J. F., Coulam, C. B., Abboud, C. F., Laws, E. R., Jr., and Kurland, L. T., 1978, Pituitary adenoma in Olmsted County, Minnesota, 1935–1977: A report of increasing incidence of diagnosis in women of childbearing age, *Mayo Clin. Proc.* **53:**641–643.

46. Sherman, B. M., Harris, C. E., Schlechte, J., Duello, T. M., Halmi, N. S., Van Gilder, J., Chappler, F. K., and Granner, D. K., 1978, Pathogenesis of prolactin-secreting pituitary adenomas, *Lancet* **2:**1019–1021.

47. Shy, K. K., McTiernan, A. M., Daling, J. R., and Weiss, N. S., 1983, Oral contraceptive use and the occurrence of pituitary prolactinoma, *J. Am. Med. Assoc.* **249:**2204–2207.

48. Carlson, H. E., Levine, G. A., Goldberg, N. J., and Hershman, J. M., 1978, Hyperprolactinemia in multiple endocrine adenomatosis, type I, *Arch. Intern. Med.* **138:**1807–1808.

49. Prosser, P. R., Karam, J. H., Townsend, J. J., and Forsham, P. H., 1979, Prolactin-secreting pituitary adenomas in multiple endocrine adenomatosis, type-1, *Ann. Intern. Med.* **91:**41–43.

50. Reschini, E., Ferrari, C., Peracchi, M., Fadini, R., Meschia, M., and Crosignani, P., 1980, Effect of dopamine infusion on serum prolactin concentration in normal and hyperprolactinaemic subjects, *Clin. Endocrinol.* **13:**519–524.

51. Bansal, S., Lee, L. A., and Woolf, P. D., 1981, Abnormal prolactin responsivity to dopaminergic suppression in hyperprolactinemic patients, *Am. J. Med.* **71:**961–966.

52. Serri, O., Kuchel, O., Bun, N. T., and Somma, N., 1983, Differential effects of a low dose dopamine infusion on prolactin secretion in normal and hyperprolactinemic subjects, *J. Clin. Endocrinol. Metab.* **56:**255–259.

53. Webb, C. B., Thominet, J. L., Barowsky, H., Berelowitz, M., and Frohman, L. A., 1983, Evidence for lactotroph dopamine resistance in idiopathic hyperprolactinemia, *J. Clin. Endocrinol. Metab.* **56:**1089–1093.

54. Tucker, H. S. G., Lankford, H. V., Gardner, D. F., and Blackard, W. G., 1980, Persistent defect in regulation of prolactin secretion after successful pituitary tumor removal in women with the galactorrhea–amenorrhea syndrome, *J. Clin. Endocrinol. Metab.* **51:**968–971.

55. Nabarro, J. D. N., 1982, Pituitary prolactinomas, *Clin. Endocrinol.* **17:**129–156.

56. Wolf, A. S., Musch, K., and Lauritzen, C., 1979, Hyperprolactinemia in anovulatory women: Incidence and endocrine features, *J. Endocrinol. Invest.* **2:**5–11.

57. Quigley, M. E., Sheehan, K. L., Casper, R. F., and Yen, S. S. C., 1980, Evidence for an increased opioid inhibition of luteinizing hormone secre-

tion in hyperprolactinemic patients with pituitary microadenoma, *J. Clin. Endocrinol. Metab.* **50:**427–430.

58. Klibanski, A., Neer, R. M., Beitins, I. Z., Ridgway, E. C., Zervas, N. T., and McArthur, J. W., 1980, Decreased bone density in hyperprolactinemic women, *N. Engl. J. Med.* **303:**1511–1514.

59. Landgraf, R., Landgraf-Leurs, M. M. C., Weismann, A., Horl, R., Von Warder, K., and Scriba, P. C., 1977, Prolactin: A diabetogenic hormone, *Diabetologia* **13:**99–104.

60. Johnston, D. G., Alberti, K. G. M. M., Nattrass, M., Burrin, J. M., Blesa-malpica, G., Hall, K., and Hall, R., 1980, Hyperinsulinaemia in hyperpro-lactinamic women, *Clin. Endocrinol.* **13:**361–368.

61. Fine, S. A., and Frohman, L. A., 1978, Loss of central nervous system component of dopaminergic inhibition of prolactin secretion in patients with prolactin-secreting tumors, *J. Clin. Invest.* **61:**973–980.

62. Müller, E. E., Genazzani, A. R., and Murru, S., 1978, Nomifensine: Di-agnostic test in hyperprolactinemic states, *J. Clin. Endocrinol. Metab.* **47:**1352–1357.

63. Ferrari, C., Crosignani, P. G., Caldara, R., Picciotti, M. C., Malinverni, A., Barattini, B., Rampini, P., and Telloli, P., 1980, Failure of nomifensine administration to discriminate between tumorous and nontumorous hy-perprolactinemia, *J. Clin. Endocrinol. Metab.* **50:**23–26.

64. Moriondo, P., Travaglini, P., Nissim, M., and Faglia, G., 1980, Evaluation of two inhibitory tets (nomifensine and L-dopa carbidopa) for the diagnosis of hyperprolactinaemic states, *Clin. Endocrinol.* **13:**525–534.

65. Hagen, C., Lindholm, J., Suenson, E., Riishede, J., Hummer, L., and Ja-cobsen, H-H., 1979, Relationship between plasma prolactin concentration and pituitary function in patients with a pituitary adenoma, *Clin. Endocrinol.* **11:**671–679.

66. Klijn, J. G. M., Lamberts, W. J., De Jong, F. H., Docter, R., Van Dongen, K. J., and Birkenhager, J. C., 1980, The importance of pituitary tumour size in patients with hyperprolactinaemia in relation to hormonal variables and extrasellar extension of tumour, *Clin. Endocrinol.* **12:**341–355.

67. Wass, J. A. H., Williams, J., Charlesworth, M., Kingsley, D. P. E., Halliday, A. M., Doniach, I., Rees, L. H., McDonald, W. I., and Besser, G. M., 1982, Bromocriptine in management of large pituitary tumours, *Br. Med. J.* **284:**1908–1911.

68. Breidahl, H. D., Topliss, D. J., and Pike, J. W., 1983, Failure of bromo-criptine to maintain reduction in size of a macroprolactinoma, *Br. Med. J.* **287:**451–452.

69. Dallabonzana, D., Spelta, B., Oppizzi, G., Tonon, C., Luccarelli, G., Chiod-ini, P. G., and Liuzzi, A., 1983, Reenlargement of macroprolactinomas during bromocriptine treatment report of two cases, *J. Endocrinol. Invest.* **6:**47–50.

70. Thorner, M. O., Perryman, R. L., Rogol, A. D., Conway, B. P., MacLeod, R. M., Login, I. S., and Morris, J. L., 1981, Rapid changes of prolactinoma volume after withdrawal and reinstitution of bromocriptine, *J. Clin. En-docrinol. Metab.* **53:**480–483.

71. Tindall, G. T., Kovacs, K., Horvath, E., and Thorner, M. O., 1982, Human prolactin-producing adenomas and bromocriptine: A histological immunocytochemical, ultrastructural and morphometric study, *J. Clin. Endocrinol. Metab.* **55:**1178–1183.

72. Eversmann, T., Fahlbusch, R., Rjosk, H. K., and Von Werder, K., 1979, Persisting suppression of prolactin secretion after long-term treatment with bromocriptine in patients with prolactinomas, *Acta Endocrinol. (Copenhagen)* **92:**413–427.

73. Aronoff, S. L., Daughaday, W. H., and Laws, E. R., Jr., 1979, Bromocriptine treatment of prolactinomas, *N. Engl. J. Med.* **300:**1391–1392.

74. Wilson, J. D., Newcombe, R. L. G., and Long, F. L., 1983, Cerebrospinal fluid rhinorrhoea during treatment of pituitary tumours with bromocriptine, *Acta Endocrinol. (Copenhagen)* **103:**457–460.

75. Zarate, A., Canales, E. S., Cano, C., and Pilonieta, C. J., 1983, Follow-up of patients with prolactinomas after discontinuation of long-term therapy with bromocriptine, *Acta Endocrinol. (Copenhagen)* **104:**139–142.

76. Thorner, M. O., Edwards, C. R. W., Charlesworth, M., Dacie, J. E., Moult, P. J. A., Rees, L. H., Jones, A. E., and Besser, G. M., 1979, Pregnancy in patients presenting with hyperprolactinaemia, *Br. Med. J.* **2:**1771–1774.

77. Bergh, T., Nillius, S. J., Larsson, S.-G., and Wide, L., 1981, Effects of bromocriptine-induced pregnancy on prolactin-secreting pituitary tumours, *Acta Endocrinol. (Copenhagen)* **98:**333–338.

78. Konopka, P., Raymond, J. P., Merceron, R. E., and Seneze, J., 1983, Continuous administration of bromocriptine in the prevention of neurological complications in pregnant women with prolactinomas, *Am. J. Obstet. Gynecol.* **146:**935–937.

79. Franks, S., Horrocks, P. M., Lynch, S. S., Butt, W. R., and London, D. R., 1983, Effectiveness of pergolide mesylate in long term treatment of hyperprolactinaemia, *Br. Med. J.* **286:**1177–1178.

80. Landolt, A. M., 1981, Surgical treatment of pituitary prolactinomas: Postoperative prolactin and fertility in seventy patients, *Fertil. Steril.* **35:**620–625.

81. Randall, R. V., Laws, E. R., Jr., Abboud, C. F., Ebersold, M. J., Kao, P. C., and Scheithauer, B. W., 1983, Transsphenoidal microsurgical treatment of prolactin-producing pituitary adenomas: Results in 100 patients, *Mayo Clin. Proc.* **58:**108–121.

82. Serri, O., Rasio, E., Beauregard, H., Hardy, J., and Somma, M., 1983, Recurrence of hyperprolactinemia after selective transsphenoidal adenomectomy in women with prolactinoma, *N. Engl. J. Med.* **309:**280–283.

83. Miller, W. L., and Eberhardt, N. L., 1983, Structure and evolution of the growth hormone gene family, *Endocrine Rev.* **4:**97–130.

84. Martial, J. A., Hallewell, R. A., Baxter, J. D., and Goodman, H. M., 1979, Human growth hormone: Complementary DNA cloning and expression in bacteria, *Science* **205:**602–606.

85. Miozzari, G. F., 1981, Strategies for obtaining expression of peptide hormones in E. coli, in: *Insulins, Growth Hormone and Recombinant DNA Technology* (J. L. Gueriguian, ed.), pp. 13–31, Raven Press, New York.

86. Rosenfeld, R. G., Wilson, D. M., and Hintz, R. L., 1982, Biological activity

of recombinant DNA-derived human growth hormone in humans: In vitro and in vivo studies, in: Hormone Drugs, Proceedings of the FDA-USP Workshop on Drug and Reference Standards for Insulins, Somatotropins and Thyroid-axis hormones, United States Pharmacopeial Convention, Inc., Rockville, Md., pp. 352–362.

87. Wallis, M., 1980, Growth hormone: Deletions in the protein and introns in the gene, *Nature (London)* **284:**512.

88. Owerbach, D., Rutter, W. J., Martial, J. A., Baxter, J. D., and Shows, T. B., 1980, Genes for growth hormone, chorionic somatomammotropin, and growth hormone-like gene on chromosome 17 in humans, *Science* **209:**289–292.

89. Wallis, M., 1981, The molecular evolution of pituitary growth hormone, prolactin and placental lactogen: A protein family showing variable rates of evolution, *J. Mol. Evol.* **17:**10–18.

90. Lewis, U. J., Singh, R. N. P., Tutwiler, G. F., Sigel, M. B., Vanderlaan, E. F., and Vanderlaan, W. P., 1980, Human growth hormone—A complex of proteins, *Recent Prog. Horm. Res.* **36:**477–508.

91. Eastman, R. C., Lesniak, M. A., Roth, J., Demeyts, P., and Gorden, P., 1979, Regulation of receptor by homologous hormone enhances sensitivity and broadens scope of radioreceptor assay for human growth hormone, *J. Clin. Endocrinol. Metab.* **49:**262–268.

92. Rosenfeld, R. G., and Hintz, R. L., 1980, Modulation of homologous receptor concentrations—Sensitive radioassay for human growth hormone in acromegalic, newborn, and stimulated plasma, *J. Clin. Endocrinol. Metab.* **50:**62–69.

93. Gavin, J. R., Trivedi, B., and Daughaday, W. H., 1979, Homologous radioreceptor and receptor modulation assays for human serum growth hormone: A screening method for growth hormone in serum, *Clin. Res.* **27:**655A.

94. Tannenbaum, G. S., Epelbaum, J., Colle, E., Brazeau, P., and Martin, J. B., 1978, Antiserum to somatostatin reverses starvation-induced inhibition of growth hormone but not insulin secretion, *Endocrinology* **102:**1909–1914.

95. Patel, Y. C., 1979, Growth hormone stimulates hypothalamic somatostatin, *Life Sci.* **24:**1589–1594.

96. Tannenbaum, G. S., 1980, Evidence for autoregulation of growth hormone secretion via the central nervous system, *Endocrinology* **107:**2117–2120.

97. Sheppard, M. C., Kronheim, S., and Pimstone, B. L., 1978, Stimulation by growth hormone of somatostatin release from the rat hypothalamus *in vitro*, *Clin. Endocrinol.* **9:**583–586.

98. Berelowitz, M., Firestone, S. L., and Frohman, L. A., 1981, Effects of growth hormone excess and deficiency on hypothalamic somatostatin content and release and on tissue somatostatin distribution, *Endocrinology* **109:**714–719.

99. Sheppard, M., Pimstone, B., Hendricks, S., Kronheim, S., and Shapiro, B., 1979, Somatomedin A effect on somatostatin release from rat hypothalamus and growth hormone release from perifused pituitary, in: *Molecular Endocrinology* (I. MacIntyre and M. Szelke, eds.), pp. 141–144, Elsevier/North-Holland, Amsterdam.

100. Berelowitz, M., Szabo, M., Frohman, L. A., Firestone, S., and Chu, L.,

1981, Somatomedin-C mediates growth hormone negative feedback by effects on both the hypothalamus and the pituitary, *Science* **212**:1279–1281.

101. Guillemin, R., Brazeau, P., Bohlen, P., Esch, F., Ling, N., and Wehrenberg, W. B., 1982, Growth hormone-releasing factor from a human pancreatic tumor that caused acromegaly, *Science* **218**:585–587.

102. Spiess, J., Rivier, J., Thorner, M., and Vale, W., 1982, Sequence analysis of a growth hormone releasing factor from a human pancreatic islet tumor, *Biochemistry* **21**:6037–6040.

103. Mayo, K. E., Vale, W., Rivier, J., Rosenfeld, M. G., and Evans, R. M., 1983, Expression-cloning and sequence of a cDNA encoding human growth hormone-releasing factor, *Nature (London)* **306**:86–88.

104. Bloch, B., Brazeau, P., Ling, N., Bohlen, P., Esch, F., Wehrenberg, W. B., Benoit, R., Bloom, F., and Guillemin, R., 1983, Immunohistochemical detection of growth hormone-releasing factor in brain, *Nature (London)* **301**:607.

105. Gelato, M. C., Pescovitz, O., Cassorla, F., Loriaux, D. L., and Merriam, G. R., 1983, Effects of a growth hormone releasing factor in man, *J. Clin. Endocrinol. Metab.* **57**:674–676.

106. Rosenthal, S. M., Schriock, E. A., Kaplan, S. L., Guillemin, R., and Grumbach, M. M., Synthetic human pancreas growth hormone-releasing factor (hpGRF)$_{1–44}$-NH$_2$) stimulates growth hormone secretion in normal men, *J. Clin. Endocrinol. Metab.* **57**:677–679.

107. Pieters, G. F. F. M., Smals, A. G. H., and Kloppenborg, P. W. C., 1980, Defective suppression of growth hormone after oral glucose loading in adolescence, *J. Clin. Endocrinol. Metab.* **51**:265–270.

108. Copinschi, G., DeLaet, M.-H., Brion, J. P., Leclercq, R., L'Hermite, M., Robyn, C., Virasoro, E., and Van Cauter, E., 1978, Simultaneous study of cortisol, growth hormone and prolactin nyctohemeral variations in normal and obese subjects: Influence of prolonged fasting in obesity, *Clin. Endocrinol.* **9**:15–26.

108a. Hayford, J. T., Danney, M. M., Hendrix, J. A., and Thompson, R. G., 1979, Integrated concentration of growth hormone in juvenile-onset diabetes, *Diabetes* **29**:391–398.

109. Clark, R. W., Schmidt, H. S., and Malarkey, W. B., 1979, Disordered growth hormone and prolactin secretion in primary disorders of sleep, *Neurology* **29**:855–861.

110. Golde, D. W., Bersch, N., and Li, C. H., 1978, Growth hormone modulation of murine erythroleukemia cell growth *in vitro*, *Proc. Natl. Acad. Sci. USA* **75**:3437–3439.

111. Gauwerky, C., Golde, D. W., and Li, C. H., 1980, Growth hormone polypeptides stimulate proliferation of K562 human erythroleukemia cells, *J. Clin. Endocrinol. Metab.* **51**:1208–1210.

112. Isaksson, O. G. P., Jansson, J.-O., and Gause, I. A. M., 1982, Growth hormone stimulates longitudinal bone growth directly, *Science* **216**:1237–1238.

113. Eden, S., Isaksson, O. G. P., Madsen, K., and Friberg, U., 1983, Specific binding of growth hormone to isolated chondrocytes from rabbit ear and epiphyseal plate, *Endocrinology* **112**:1127–1129.

114. Spanos, E., Barrett, D., MacIntyre, I., Pike, J. W., Safilian, E. F., and Haussler, M. R., 1978, Effect of growth hormone on vitamin D metabolism, *Nature (London)* **273:**246–247.

115. Yeh, J. K., and Aloia, J. F., 1979, The influence of growth hormone on vitamin D metabolism, *Biochem. Med.* **21:**311–322.

116. Bruns, M. E. H., Vollmer, S. S., Bruns, D. E., and Overpeck, J. G., 1983, Human growth hormone increases intestinal vitamin D-dependent calcium-binding protein in hypophysectomized rats, *Endocrinology* **113:**1387–1392.

117. Gertner, J. M., Horst, R. L., Broadus, A. E., Rasmussen, H., and Genel, M., 1979, Parathyroid function and vitamin-D metabolism during human growth hormone replacement, *J. Clin. Endocrinol. Metab.* **49:**185–188.

118. Chipman, J. J., Zerwekh, J., Nicar, M., and Marks, J., 1980, Effect of growth hormone administration—Reciprocal changes in serum 1-alpha, 25-dihydroxyvitamin D and intestinal calcium absorption, *J. Clin. Endocrinol. Metab.* **51:**321–324.

119. Hammerman, M. R., Karl, I. E., and Hruska, K. A., 1980, Regulation of canine renal vesicle P_i transport by growth hormone and parathyroid hormone, *Biochim. Biophys. Acta* **603:**322–335.

120. Melmed, S., Braunstein, G. D., Horvath, E., Ezrin, C., and Kovacs, K., 1983, Pathophysiology of acromegaly, *Endocrine Rev.* **4:**271–290.

121. Thorner, M. O., Perryman, R. L., Cronin, M. J., Rogol, A. D., Draznin, M., Johanson, A., Vale, W., Horvath, E., and Kovacs, K., 1982, Somatotroph hyperplasia: Successful treatment of acromegaly by removal of a pancreatic islet tumor secreting a growth hormone-releasing factor, *J. Clin. Invest.* **70:**965–977.

122. Leveston, S. A., McKeel, D. W., Jr., Buckley, P. J., Deschryver, K., Greider, M. H., Jaffe, B. M., and Daughaday, W. H., 1981, Acromegaly and Cushing's syndrome associated with a foregut carcinoid tumor, *J. Clin. Endocrinol. Metab.* **53:**682–689.

123. Asa, S. L., Bilbao, J. M., Kovacs, K., and Linfoot, J. A., 1980, Hypothalamic neuronal hamartoma associated with pituitary growth hormone cell adenoma and acromegaly, *Acta Neuropathol.* **52:**231–234.

124. Hanew, K., Kokubun, M., Sasaki, A., Mouri, T., and Yoshinaga, K., 1980, The spectrum of pituitary growth hormone responses to pharmacological stimuli in acromegaly, *J. Clin. Endocrinol. Metab.* **51:**292–297.

125. Camanni, F., Picotti, G. B., Massara, F., Molinatti, G. M., Mantegazza, P., and Muller, E. E., 1978, Carbidopa inhibits the growth hormone- and prolactin-suppresive effect of L-dopa in acromegalic patients, *J. Clin. Endocrinol. Metab.* **47:**647–652.

126. Harrison, B. D. W., Millhouse, K. A., Harrington, M., and Nabarro, J. D. N., 1978, Lung function in acromegaly, *Q. J. Med.* **47:**517–532.

127. Luboshitzky, R., and Barzilai, D., 1980, Hypoxemia and pulmonary function in acromegaly, *Am. Rev. Respir. Dis.* **121:**471–476.

128. Perks, W. H., Horrocks, P. M., Cooper, R. A., Bradbury, S., Allen, A., Baldock, N., Prowse, K., and Van't Hoff, W., 1980, Sleep apnoea in acromegaly, *Br. Med. J.* **280:**894–896.

129. Cadieux, R. J., Kales, A., Santen, R. J., Bixler, E. O., and Gordon, R.,

1982, Endoscopic findings in sleep apnea associated with acromegaly, *J. Clin. Endocrinol. Metab.* **55:**18–22.

130. Lie, J. T., and Grossman, S. J., 1980, Pathology of the heart in acromegaly—Anatomic findings in 27 autopsied patients, *Am. Heart J.* **100:**41–52.

131. Smallridge, R. C., Rajfer, S., Davia, J., and Schaaf, M., 1979, Acromegaly and the heart: An echocardiographic study, *Am. J. Med.* **66:**22–27.

132. Savage, D. D., Henry, W. L., Eastman, R. C., Borer, J. S., and Gorden, P., 1979, Echocardiographic assessment of cardiac anatomy and function in acromegalic patients, *Am. J. Med.* **67:**823–829.

133. Ondreyco, S. M., Lewis, H. D., and Hartman, C. R., 1980, Myxomatous degeneration and cystic medial necrosis associated with acromegaly, *Arch. Intern. Med.* **140:** 547–549.

134. Mantero, F., Opocher, G., Armanini, D., Paviotti, G., Boscaro, M., and Muggeo, M., 1979, Plasma renin activity and urinary aldosterone in acromegaly, *J. Endocrinol. Invest.* **2:**13–18.

135. Ogihara, T., Hata, T., Maruyama, A., Mikami, H., Nakamaru, M., Okada, Y., and Kumahara, Y., 1979, Blood pressure response to an angiotensin II antagonist in patients with acromegaly, *J. Clin. Endocrinol. Metab.* **48:**159–162.

136. Moore, T. J., Theinwai, W., Dluhy, R. G., Dawson-Hughes, B. F., Hollenberg, N. K., and Williams, G. H., 1980, Abnormal adrenal and vascular response to angiotensin-II and an angiotensin antagonist in acromegaly, *J. Clin. Endocrinol. Metab.* **51:**215–222.

137. Whitehead, E. M., Shalet, S. M., Davies, D., Enoch, B. A., Price, D. A., and Beardwell, C. G., 1982, Pituitary gigantism: A disabling condition, *Clin. Endocrinol.* **17:**271–278.

138. Daughaday, W. H., 1977, Extreme gigantism, *N. Engl. J. Med.* **297:** 1267–1269.

139. Wass, J. A. H., Cudworth, A. G., Bottazzo, G. F., Woodrow, J. C., and Besser, G. M., 1980, An assessment of glucose intolerance in acromegaly and its response to medical treatment, *Clin. Endocrinol.* **12:**53–60.

140. Maneschi, F., Navalesi, R., Pilo, A., and Paci, A., 1978, [^{125}I] hGH metabolism in acromegaly: Effects of chronic treatment with 2-Br-α-ergocryptine, *J. Clin. Endocriol. Metab.* **47:**110–118.

141. Muggeo, M., Bar, R. S., Roth, J., Kahn, C. R., and Gorden, P., 1979, The insulin resistance of acromegaly: Evidence for two alterations in the insulin receptor on circulating monocytes, *J. Clin. Endocrinol. Metab.* **48:**17–25.

142. Hardy, J., and Somma, M., 1979, Acromegaly: Surgical treatment by transsphenoidal microsurgical removal of the pituitary adenoma, in: *Clinical Management of Pituitary Tumors* (G. T. Tindall and W. F. Collins, eds.), pp. 209–217, Raven Press, New York.

143. Laws, E. R., Jr., Piepgras, D. G., Randall, R. V., and Abboud, C. F., 1979, Neurosurgical management of acromegaly: Results in 82 patients treated betwen 1972 and 1977, *J. Neurosurg.* **50:**454–461.

144. Tucker, H. S. G., Grubb, S. R. Wigand, J. P., Watlington, C. O., Blackard, W. G., and Becker, D. P., 1980, The treatment of acromegaly by transsphenoidal surgery, *Arch. Intern. Med.* **140:**795–803.

145. Clemmons, D. R., Van Wyk, J. J., Ridgway, E. C., Kliman, B., Kjellberg,

R. N., and Underwood, L. E., 1979, Evaluation of acromegaly by radioimmunoassay of somatomedin-C, *N. Engl. J. Med.* **301:**1138–1142.

146 Faglia, G., Paracchi, A., Ferrari, C., and Beck-Peccoz, P., 1978, Evaluation of the results of trans-sphenoidal surgery in acromegaly by assessment of the growth hormone response to thyrotrophin-releasing hormone, *Clin. Endocrinol.* **8:**373–380.

147. Wass, J. A. H., Thorner, M. O., Morris, D. V., Rees, L. H., Mason, A. S., Jones, A. E., and Besser, G. M., 1977, Long-term treatment of acromegaly with bromocriptine, *Br. Med. J.* **2:**875–878.

148. Shalet, S. M., Price, D. A., Beardwell, C. G., Mindel, A., and MacFarlane, I. A., 1980, Growth hormone and somatomedin levels in acromegalics treated with bromocriptine, *Horm. Res.* **12:**121–129.

149. Lindholm, J., Rushede, J., Vestergaard, S., Hummer, L., Faber, O., and Hagen, C., 1981, No effect of bromocriptine in acromegaly, *N. Engl. J. Med.* **304:**1450–1454.

150. Pelkonen, R., Ylikahri, R., and Karonen, S-L., 1980, Bromocriptine treatment of patients with acromegaly resistant to conventional therapy, *Clin. Endocrinol.* **12:**219–224.

151. Eastman, R. C., Gorden, P., and Roth, J., 1979, Conventional supervoltage irradiation is an effective treatment for acromegaly, *J. Clin. Endocrinol. Metab.* **48:**931–940.

152. Atkinson, A. B., Allen, I. V., Gordon, D. S., Hadden, D. R., Maguire, C. J. F., Trimble, E. R., and Lyons, A. R., 1979, Progressive visual failure in acromegaly following external pituitary irradiation, *Clin. Endocrinol.* **10:**469–480.

153. Veldhuis, J. D., and Hammond, J. M., 1980, Endocrine function after spontaneous infarction of the human pituitary: Report, review, and reappraisal, *Endocr Rev.* **1:**100–107.

154. Jordon, R. M., Cook, D. M. McDonald, W. J. Houghton, D. C., and Kendall, J. W., 1980, Corticotrophin, growth hormone and prolactin deficiencies with hypoaldosterone and corticosteroid-reversible hypothyroidism in Sheehan's syndrome—Clinical and anatomical correlations, *Acta Endocrinol. (Copenhagen)* **95:**12–22.

155. Rothman, J. G., Snyder, P. J., and Utiger, R. D., 1978, Hypothalamic endocrinopathy in Hand-Schuller-Christian disease, *Ann. Intern. Med.* **88:**512–513.

156. Jambart, S., Turpin, G., and de Gennes, J. L., 1980, Panhypopituitarism secondary to head trauma: Evidence for a hypothalamic origin of the deficit, *Acta Endocrinol. (Copenhagen)* **93:**264–270.

157. Stuart, C. A., Neelon, F. A., and Lebovitz, H. E., 1978, Hypothalamic insufficiency the cause of hypopituitarism in sarcoidosis, *Ann. Intern. Med.* **88:**589–594.

158. Hendricks, S. A., Lippe, B. M., Kaplan, S. A., and Bentson, J. R., 1981, Hypothalamic atrophy with progressive hypopituitarism in an adolescent girl, *J. Clin. Endocrinol. Metab.* **52:**563–564.

159. Kupari, M., Pelkonen, R., and Valtonen, V., 1980, Post-encephalitic hypothalamic–pituitary insufficiency, *Acta Endocrinol. (Copenhagen)* **94:**433–438.

160. Krause-Brucker, W., and Gardner, D. W., 1980, Optic nerve hypoplasia associated with absent septum pellucidum and hypopituitarism, *Am. J. Ophthalmol.* **89:**113–120.

161. Rudman, D., Davis, G. T., Priest, J. H., Patterson, J. H., Kutner, M. H., Heymsfield, S. B., and Bethel, R. A., 1978, Prevalence of growth hormone deficiency in children with cleft lip or palate, *J. Pediatr.* **93:**378–382.

162. Parks, J. S., Tenore, A., Bongiovanni, A. M., and Kirkland, R. T., 1978, Familial hypopituitarism with large sella turcica, *N. Engl. J. Med.* **298:**698–702.

163. Rona, R. J., and Tanner, J. M., 1977, Aetiology of idiopathic growth hormone deficiency in England and Wales, *Arch. Dis. Child.* **52:**1197–1208.

164. Steendijk, R., 1980, Diagnostic and aetiologic features of idiopathic and symptomatic growth hormone deficiency in the Netherlands—A survey of 176 children, *Helv. Paediatr. Acta* **35:**129–139.

165. Calzada, L.-D., Chaussain, J.-L., and Job, J.-C., 1978, Etiologie et associations du nanisme hypophysaire, *Arch. Fr. Pediatr.* **35:**144–150.

166. Illig, R., 1970, Growth hormone antibodies in patients treated with different preparations of human growth hormone (HGH), *J. Clin. Endocrinol. Metab.* **31:**679–692.

167. Phillips, J. A., Hjelle, B. L., Seeburg, P. H., and Zachmann, M., 1981, Molecular basis for familial isolated growth hormone deficiency, *Proc. Natl. Acad. Sci. USA* **78:**6372–6375.

168. Phillips, J. A., III, Parks, J. S., Hjelle, B. L., Herd, J. E., Plotnick, L. P., Migeon, C. J., and Seeburg, P. H., 1982, Genetic analysis of familial isolated growth hormone deficiency type I, *J. Clin. Invest.* **70:**489–495.

169. Plotnick, L. P., Lee, P. A., Migeon, C. J., and Kowarski, A. A., 1979, Comparison of physiological and pharmacological tests of growth hormone function in children with short stature, *J. Clin. Endocrinol. Metab.* **48:**811–815.

170. Fass, B., Lippe, B. M., and Kaplan, S. A., 1979, Relative usefulness of 3 growth hormone stimulation screening tests, *Am. J. Dis. Child.* **133:**931–933.

171. Gil-Ad, I., Topper, E., and Laron, Z., 1979, Oral clonidine as a growth hormone stimulation test, *Lancet* **2:**278–279.

172. Ferrari, C., Caldara, R., Testori, G. P., Crossignani, R., and Barbieri, C., 1979, Clonidine and growth-hormone secretion, *Lancet* **2:**796.

173. Spiliotis, B. E., August, G. P., Hung, W., Sonis, W., Meldelson, W., and Bercu, B. B., 1984, Growth hormone neurosecretory dysfunction, *J. Am. Med. Assoc.* **251:**2223–2230.

174. Demura, R., Yamaguchi, H., Wakabayashi, I., Demura, H., and Shizume, K., 1980, The effect of hGH on hypothalamic–pituitary–thyroid function in patients with pituitary dwarfism, *Acta Endocrinol (Copenhagen)* **93:**13–19.

175. Milner, R. D. G., Fraser, T. R., Brook, C. G. D., Cotes, P. M., Farquhar, J. W., Parkin, J. M., Preece, M. A., Snodgrass, G. J. A. I., Mason, A. S., Tanner, J. M., and Vince, F. P., 1979, Experience with human growth hormone in Great Britain: The report of the MRC working party, *Clin. Endocrinol.* **11:**15–38.

176. Kirkland, R. T., and Clayton, G. W., 1979, Growth increments with low dose intermittent growth hormone and fluoxymesterone in 1st year of therapy in hypopituitarism, *Pediatrics* **63:**386–388.

177. Rosenbloom, A. L., Riley, W. J., Silverstein, J. H., Garnica, A. D., Netzloff, M. L., and Weber, F. T., 1980, Low dose single weekly injections of growth hormone—Response during 1st year of therapy of hypopituitarism, *Pediatrics* **66:**272–276.

178. Golde, D. W., Bersch, N., Kaplan, S. A., Rimoin, D. L., and Li, C. H., 1980, Peripheral unresponsiveness to human growth hormone in Laron dwarfism, *N. Engl. J. Med.* **303:**1156–1159.

179. Eshet, R., Laron, Z., Pertzelan, A., Arnon, R., and Dintzman, M., 1984, Defect of human growth hormone receptors in the liver of two patients with Laron-type dwarfism, *Isr. J. Med. Sci.* **20:**8–11.

180. Rinderknecht, E., and Humbel, R. E., 1978, The amino acid sequence of human insulin-like growth factor I and its structural homology with proinsulin, *J. Biol. Chem.* **253:**2769–2776.

181. Rinderknecht, E., and Humbel, R. E., 1978, Primary structure of human insulin-like growth factor II, *FEBS Lett.* **89:**283–286.

182. Klapper, D. G., Svoboda, M. E., and Van Wyk, J. J., 1983, Sequence analysis of somatomedin-C: Confirmation of identity with insulin-like growth factor I, *Endocrinology* **112:**2215–2217.

183. Heldin, C.-H., Wasteson, A., Fryklund, L., and Westermark, B., 1981, Somatomedin B: Mitogenic activity derived from contaminant epidermal growth factor, *Science* **213:**1122–1123.

184. Furlanetto, R. W., Underwood, L., Van Wyk, J. J., and D'Ercole, A. J., 1977, Estimation of somatomedin-C levels in normals and patients with pituitary disease by radioimmunoassay, *J. Clin. Invest.* **60:**648–657.

185. Bala, R. M., and Bhaumick, B., 1979, Radioimmunoassay of a basic somatomedin: Comparison of various assay techniques and somatomedin levels in various sera, *J. Clin. Endocrinol. Metab.* **49:**770–779.

186. Clemmons, D. R., Underwood, L. E., Chatelain, P. G., and Van Wyk, J. J., 1983, Liberation of immunoreactive somatomedin-C from its binding proteins by proteolytic enzymes and heparin, *J. Clin. Endocrinol. Metab.* **56:**384–389.

187. Zapf, J., Walter, H., and Froesch, E. R., 1981, Radioimunological determination of insulin-like growth factors I and II in normal subjects and in patients with growth disorders and extrapancreatic tumor hypoglycemia, *J. Clin. Invest.* **68:**1321–1330.

188. Daughaday, W. H., Mariz, I. K., and Blethen, S. L., 1980, Inhibition of access of bound somatomedin to membrane receptor and immunobinding sites: A comparison of radioreceptor and radioimmunoassay of somatomedin in native and acid-ethanol-extracted serum, *J. Clin. Endocrinol. Metab.* **51:**781–788.

189. Daughaday, W. H., Mariz, I. K., and Trivedi, B., 1981, A preferential binding site for insulin-like growth factor II in human and rat placental membranes, *J. Clin. Endocrinol. Metab.* **53:**282–288.

190. Daughaday, W. H., Trivedi, B., and Kapadia, M., 1981, Measurement of insulin-like growth factor II by a specific radioreceptor assay in serum of normal individuals, patients with abnormal growth hormone secretion, and patients with tumor-associated hypoglycemia, *J. Clin. Endocrinol. Metab.* **53:**289–294.

191. Hintz, R. L., and Liu, R., 1981, Insulin-like growth factor-II radioimmunoassay based on an antiserum against the synthetic C-peptide segment, *Clin. Res.* **29**:408A.

192. Furlanetto, R. W., 1980, The somatomedin-C binding protein: Evidence for a heterologous subunit structure, *J. Clin. Endocrinol. Metab.* **51**: 12–19.

193. White, R. M., Nissley, S. P., Moses, A. C., Rechler, M. M., and Johnsonbaugh, R. E., 1981, The growth hormone dependence of a somatomedin-binding protein in human serum, *J. Clin. Endocrinol.* **53**:49–57.

194. Hintz, R. L., Liu, F., Rosenfeld, R. G., and Kemp, S. F., 1981, Plasma somatomedin-binding proteins in hypopituitarism: Changes during growth hormone therapy, *J. Clin. Endocrinol. Metab.* **53**:100–104.

195. Furlanetto, R. W., Underwood, L. E., Van Wyk, J. J., and Handwerger, S., 1978, Serum immunoreactive somatomedin-C is elevated late in pregnancy, *J. Clin. Endocrinol. Metab.* **47**:695–698.

196. Bala, R. M., Lopatka, J., Leung, A., McCoy, E., and McArthur, E., 1981, Serum immunoreactive somatomedin levels in normal adults, pregnant women at term, children at various ages, and children with constitutionally delayed growth, *J. Clin. Endocrinol. Metab.* **52**:508–512.

197. Wilson, D. M., Bennett, A., Adamson, G. D., Nagashima, R. J., Liu, F., DeNatale, M. L., Hintz, R. L., and Rosenfeld, R. G., 1982, Somatomedins in pregnancy: A cross-sectional study of insulin-like growth factors I and II and somatomedin peptide content in normal human pregnancies, *J. Clin. Endocrinol. Metab.* **55**:858–861.

198. Hall, K., Enberg, G., Ritzen, M., Svan, H., Fryklund, L., and Takano, K., 1980, Somatomedin-A levels in serum from healthy children and from children with growth hormone deficiency or delayed puberty, *Acta Endocrinol. (Copenhagen)* **94**:155–165.

199. Rudman, D., Kutner, M. H., Rogers, C. M., Lubin, M. F., Fleming, G. A., and Bain, R. P., 1981, Impaired growth hormone secretion, *J. Clin. Invest.* **67**:1361–1369.

200. Minuto, F., Underwood, L. E., Grimaldi, P., Furlanetto, R. W., Van Wyk, J. J., and Giordano, G., 1981, Decreased serum somatomedin-C concentrations during sleep: Temporal relationship to the nocturnal surges of growth hormone and prolactin, *J. Clin. Endocrinol. Metab.* **52**:399–403.

201. Hintz, R. L., Suskind, R., Amatayakul, K., Leitzmann, C., and Olson, R. E., 1978, Somatomedin and growth hormone in children with protein calorie malnutrition, *J. Pediatr.* **92**:153–156.

202. Clemmons, D. R., Klibanski, A., Underwood, L. E., McArthur, J. W., Ridgway, E. C., Beitins, I. Z., and Van Wyk, J. J., 1981, Reduction of plasma immunoreactive somatomedin C during fasting in humans, *J. Clin. Endocrinol. Metab.* **53**:1247–1250.

203. Isley, W. L., Underwood, L. E., and Clemmons, D. R., 1983, Dietary components that regulate serum somatomedin-C concentrations in humans, *J. Clin. Invest.* **71**:175–182.

204. Rappaport, R., Prevot, C., and Czernichow, P., 1980, Somatomedin activity and growth hormone secretion. I. Changes related to body weight in anorexia nervosa, *Acta Paediatr. Scand.* **69**:37–42.

205. Winter, R. J., Phillips, L. S., Green, O. C., and Traisman, H. S., 1980, Somatomedin activity in the Mauriac syndrome, *J. Pediatr.* **97:**598–600.

206. Nash, H., 1979, Growth failure, somatomedin and growth hormone levels in juvenile diabetes mellitus: A pilot study, *Aust. N.Z. J. Med.* **9:**245–249.

207. Winter, R. J., Phillips, L. S., Klein, M. N., Traisman, H. S., and Green, O. C., 1979, Somatomedin activity and diabetic control in children with insulin-dependent diabetes, *Diabetes* **28:**952–954.

208. Tamborlane, W. V., Hintz, R. L., Bergman, M., Genel, M., Felig, P., and Sherwin, R. S., 1981, Insulin-infusion-pump treatment of diabetes, influence of improved metabolic control on plasma somatomedin levels, *N. Engl. J. Med.* **305:**303–307.

209. Blethen, S. L., White, N. H., Santiago, J. V., and Daughaday, W. H., 1981, Plasma somatomedins, endogenous insulin secretion and growth in transient neonatal diabetes mellitus, *J. Clin. Endocrinol. Metab.* **52:**144–147.

210. Phillips, L. S., Pennisi, A. J., Belosky, D. C., Uittenbogaart, C., Ettenger, R. B., Malekzaden, M. H., and Fine, R. N., 1978, Somatomedin activity and inorganic sulfate in children undergoing hemodialysis, *J. Clin. Endocrinol. Metab.* **46:**165–168.

211. Takano, K., Hall, K., Kastrup, K. W., Hizuka, N., Shizume, K., Kawai, K., Akimoto, M., Takuma, T., and Sugino, N., 1979, Serum somatomedin-A in chronic renal failure, *J. Clin. Endocrinol. Metab.* **48:**371–376.

212. Goldberg, A. C., Trivedi, B., Delmez, J. A., Harter, H. R., and Daughaday, W. H., 1981, Uremia reduces serum insulin-like growth factor-I concentration but markedly increases serum insulin-like growth factor-II concentration, *Clin. Res.* **29:**770A.

213. Schiffrin, A., Guyda, H., Robitaille, P., and Posner, B., 1978, Increased plasma somatomedin reactivity in chronic renal failure as determined by acid gel filtration and radioreceptor assay, *J. Clin. Endocrinol. Metab.* **46:**511–514.

214. Copeland, K. C., Underwood, L. E., and Van Wyk, J. J., 1980, Induction of immunoreactive somatomedin-C in human serum by growth hormone: Dose–response relationships and effect on chromatographic profiles, *J. Clin. Endocrinol. Metab.* **50:**690–697.

215. Kowarski, A. A., Schneider, J., Ben-Galim, E., Weldon, V. V., and Daughaday, W. H., 1978, Growth failure with normal serum RIA-GH and low somatomedin activity: Somatomedin restoration and growth acceleration after exogenous GH, *J. Clin. Endocrinol. Metab.* **47:**461–464.

216. Rudman, D., Kutner, M. H., Goldsmith, M. A., Kenny, J., Jennings, H., and Bain, R. P., 1980, Further observations on four subgroups of normal variant short stature, *J. Clin. Endocrinol. Metab.* **51:**1378–1384.

217. Rudman, D., Kutner, M. H., Blackson, R. D., Cushman, R. A., Bain, R. P., and Patterson, J. H., 1981, Children with normal-variant short stature: Treatment with human growth hormone for six months, *N. Engl. J. Med.* **305:**123–131.

The Thyroid

Kenneth A. Woeber and Lewis E. Braverman

3.1. Hypothalamic–Pituitary–Thyroid Interrelationships

In the years that have elapsed since the publication of the first volume, some strides have been made in defining certain aspects of the localization, metabolic clearance, and disposition of thyrotropin-releasing hormone (TRH). This is due in large part to the increasing availability of improved methods for the radioimmunoassay (RIA) of TRH. A detailed review on all aspects of TRH physiology has recently been published.[1]

Previous work has indicated that TRH is distributed widely throughout the CNS, as well as in extraneural sites such as the placenta, gastrointestinal tract, and pancreas. A recent study has now provided a more precise localization of TRH in the human hypothalamus.[2] The hypothalamus and upper pituitary stalk obtained from victims of sudden death were serially biopsied by a micropunch technique, and TRH was sought in the tissue extracts by RIA. The median eminence and arcuate nucleus yielded the highest concentrations of TRH, suggesting that these areas in man, as in the laboratory animal, are those principally concerned with TSH regulation. Smaller concentrations were found in other hypothalamic nuclei, suggesting that TRH may fulfill functions in addition to the regulation of TSH secretion. Discrete hypothalamic lesions in the

KENNETH A. WOEBER • Department of Medicine, Mt. Zion Hospital and Medical Center and the University of California School of Medicine, San Francisco, California 94120. LEWIS E. BRAVERMAN • Department of Medicine, University of Massachusetts Medical School, Worcester, Massachusetts 01605.

rat indicate, however, that only the immediate area of the paraventricular nucleus is important for TSH secretion.[3] Studies in the neonatal rat suggest that TRH immunoreactivity in the plasma, pancreas, and gastrointestinal tract is indistinguishable from that of synthetic TRH, and that pancreatic secretion is the major source of circulating TRH in the neonate.[4]

A material (or materials) with TSH-releasing activity has been extracted from human placenta, though its nature is uncertain. While the initial study reporting the presence of this material suggested that it was TRH, based on its immunologic and chromatographic behavior,[5] more recent work suggests that the biologic and immunologic activities are distinct from TRH and from one another.[6] Further work is needed to elucidate the nature of this placental activity. Whether it could subserve a regulatory function in the fetus with respect to the developing pituitary–thyroid axis is in doubt, however, since evidence noted elsewhere suggests that TRH is not important in the development of the axis in the fetus.

Similar uncertainty prevails concerning the nature of the material extracted from human urine with anti-TRH antiserum. This material is reactive in the TRH RIA, but differs from TRH in its chromatographic behavior. It does not react in the RIA for deamidated TRH.[7] On the other hand, unextracted human urine does contain another material that reacts in the RIA for deamidated TRH and that coelutes with deamidated TRH on gel filtration chromatography.[7] Since some tissues, such as brain, pituitary, and liver, possess TRH-deamidase activity, deamidated TRH in urine may be the product of the metabolism of TRH. However, the percentage of TRH produced in the brain that undergoes deamidation there *in vivo* is small.[8] Another product of TRH metabolism in brain is histidyl-proline diketopiperazine (HPD), which can be detected by a specific RIA.[9] Although earlier reports had suggested that this metabolite might inhibit prolactin release, more recent data do not support the concept that HPD is a physiological prolactin-inhibitory factor.[10]

TRH is rapidly cleared from plasma. In man, the constant infusion technique has revealed a plasma half-disappearance time of approximately 6 min and a plasma clearance rate of 1.5 liters/min.[11] The more potent analog methyl-TRH is cleared more slowly, with a plasma half-disappearance time of 11.5 min and a clearance rate of 0.78 liter/min. This may contribute to its greater biologic potency relative to TRH.[11] The rapid clearance of TRH is due at least in part to its degradation in plasma. A recent study has examined the degradation of TRH and deamidated TRH by human plasma using specific RIAs for quantification.[12] The degradation of TRH was found to greatly exceed that of deamidated TRH, and the latter was not generated in plasma as a product of TRH degradation. Moreover, the degradative activity of plasma from thyrotoxic patients was found to be no greater than that of normal plasma. The latter observation is noteworthy in view of the several studies with rat plasma,[13] as well as a previous study with human plasma, that seemed to show a direct relationship between thyroid functional state and the TRH-degradative activity of plasma.

cAMP has been invoked as the factor responsible for mediating the action of TRH on TSH release. Previous work with hemipituitaries and pituitary tumor cell lines has provided evidence both for and against this suggestion. A recent study has reexamined this question by measuring the cAMP, cGMP, TSH, and prolactin responses to TRH in short-term cultures of normal rat pituitary cells.[14] TRH induced the release of both TSH and prolactin. In the presence of a phosphodiesterase inhibitor, the TRH-induced release of both hormones was augmented, and the intracellular content of both cAMP and cGMP increased. Dibutyryl-cAMP, but not dibutyryl-cGMP, increased prolactin release, whereas both cyclic nucleotides were found to increase TSH release. These observations support the view, therefore, that both cAMP and cGMP are involved in mediating the stimulatory effect of TRH on TSH release. However, the same authors have more recently reported that when anterior pituitary cells from 15-day-old female rats are separated into mammotrophs and thyrotrophs, cAMP is involved in TRH-induced release of prolactin whereas cGMP is involved in TRH-induced release of TSH.[15]

In certain clinical situations, such as acromegaly, hypothyroidism, diabetes mellitus, depression, anorexia nervosa, and chronic renal and liver diseases, TRH administration evokes a nonspecific release of GH. TRH has now been demonstrated to stimulate the secretion of GH in the term fetus following its administration to the mother.[16] TRH also provokes abnormal FSH and LH responses in men who have pituitary adenomas and FSH hypersecretion.[17] Two intriguing reports have suggested that TRH may have therapeutic value in improving neurologic recovery after spinal trauma in cats[18] and cardiovascular function in experimental endotoxic and hemorrhagic shock in rats.[19]

It is now well established that TSH secretion is subject to both brief episodic and circadian variations. The latter variation is characterized by a nocturnal surge that antecedes the onset of sleep[20] and appears not to be determined by the circadian rhythm of cortisol secretion or by fluctuations in T_4 or T_3 concentrations. In pubertal boys, the nyctohemeral maximum TSH secretion occurred after sleep.[21] It has been proposed that this nocturnal surge in TSH secretion is due to fluctuations in endogenous TRH. A recent study does not support this view, however.[22] In this study, normal subjects were given a continuous infusion of a low dose of TRH over 48 hr. while 4-hr measurements of serum TSH and prolactin concentrations were made. The nocturnal increases of both TSH and prolactin persisted during the period of the infusion. Had the nocturnal surge of TSH been due to fluctuations in endogenous TRH, the continuous infusion of exogenous TRH should have damped or abolished it. The observations suggest, therefore, that some other factor, whether it be variations in the intrinsic sensitivity of the pituitary to TRH or inverse fluctuations in a release-inhibiting factor, is responsible for the nocturnal surge of TSH.

It has been proposed that T_3 rather than T_4 is the principal arbiter of the negative feedback regulation of pituitary TSH secretion, and that this regulatory action requires the nuclear binding of T_3. Studies in pituitary tumor cells demonstrate that the thyroid hormones also regulate pituitary TRH receptors, and that this may play a role in modifying the pituitary responsiveness to TRH.[23] The nuclear binding view is based on the observation of a close correlation between the extent of inhibition of TSH release and the nuclear T_3 content within the pituitary following administration of either T_3 or T_4.[24] Since the bulk of nuclear T_3 is generated within the pituitary through in situ 5'-deiodination of T_4, it has further been proposed that intrapituitary conversion of T_4 to T_3 is the mechanism principally responsible for the acute inhibition of TSH release that T_4 induces.[24] Support for the latter is now provided by a recent study in which the effect of iopanoic acid, a radiographic contrast agent that inhibits the 5'-deiodination of T_4, was examined in the hypothyroid rat.[25] Administration of this agent was shown both to decrease qreatly the pituitary nuclear T_3 generated in situ from T_4 and to prevent the acute decrease in TSH secretion that follows an injection of T_4. Over the longer term, of course, T_3 generated peripherally from T_4 and reaching the pituitary in the perfusing blood also contributes to the regulation of TSH secretion. This is evident in a recent study involving euthyroid human subjects.[26] Administration of iopanoic acid led to an increase in the TSH response to TRH, but this increase could be prevented if the decline in serum T_3 concentration that iopanoic acid induced was offset by the administration of exogenous T_3. (The feedback regulation of TSH secretion by thyroid hormones has been extensively reviewed this year.[27])

It is now well recognized that TSH secretion is also under dopaminergic control since dopamine administration decreases TSH release and the administration of dopamine receptor-blocking drugs, such as metoclopramide, is followed by the acute release of TSH. The increase in TSH release induced by metoclopramide declines in magnitude with increasingly severe hypothyroidism, suggesting that endogenous dopamine inhibition of TSH release also declines.[28] It has been proposed that thyroid hormones may affect the regulation of TSH secretion by increasing hypothalamic dopaminergic inhibition of TSH release.[29] Corticosteroids also decrease TSH secretion. Recent findings in the rat under stress-free conditions confirm the fact that physiological concentrations of corticosterone decrease the TSH response to TRH.[30] It has also been observed that GH is a determinant in regulating the TSH response to TRH in patients with hypothalamic–pituitary disease.[31] The presence of endogenous GH in these patients is associated with a depressed TSH response, possibly through the mediation of somatostatin.

The effect of the nonhalogenated analog 3,5-dimethyl-3'-isopropyl-L-thyronine (DIMIT) on the regulation of TSH secretion has now been examined in man.[32] DIMIT was found to decrease basal serum TSH and the TSH response to TRH in euthyroid subjects, as well as in a patient with diminished thyroid reserve. The effect of DIMIT was relatively prolonged since it could still be demonstrated several days after a single oral dose. This demonstration that DIMIT has thyroid hormone-like activity in man is important. Since DIMIT has been shown to cross the placenta much more readily than T_3 or T_4, it may eventually have clinical utility in treating hypothyroidism in the human fetus.

3.2. Thyroid Hormone and Thyroglobulin Synthesis and Release

Thyroglobulin is present in the serum of all normal subjects and its concentration is almost always increased in patients with toxic, nontoxic, and endemic iodine deficiency goiter due to excess release of thyroglobulin from the gland. Studies of the interaction of thyroglobulin, TSI, and TSH on human thyroid plasma membranes *in vitro* using an adenylate cyclase assay system have revealed that thyroglobulin inhibits basal and TSI- or TSH-stimulated adenylate cyclase activity. Thus, thyroglobulin might regulate thyroid adenylate cyclase sensitivity *in vivo* by a short-loop counter-regulation system.[33] In contrast to thyroglobulin, cholera toxin activates thyroid adenylate cyclase and stimulates cAMP generation even in thyroid tissue that is resistant to TSH-stimulated cAMP formation because of prior *in vivo* or *in vitro* exposure to excess TSH.[34,35] Cholera toxin also was shown to potentiate the action of TSI and TSH on cAMP generation.[36]

Ericson and colleagues have continued their studies on the stimulatory effects of TSH on thyroid function as viewed by anatomical changes. Their previous studies had demonstrated that TSH affected a transfer of membrane from exocytotic vesicles to the apical plasma membrane and then to endocytotic structures. More recent findings indicate that exocytosis represents the first step in the redistribution of membranes in the apical part of the follicle cell in response to TSH and that membranes of the exocytotic vesicles serve as the membrane reserve to produce endocytotic structures.[37] An increase in rough endoplasmic reticulum of the endothelium of capillaries and pericytes occurs in the TSH-stimulated hyperplastic rat thyroid, suggesting that these structures have protein synthetic and secretory functions of an unknown nature.[38] In a series of elegant studies, Laurberg has employed an *in situ* perfused canine thyroid model to study iodothyronine release before, during, and after TSH stimulation.[39–41] T_4, T_3 rT_3, and $3,3'-T_2$ were readily identified in the effluent, and a considerable portion of the T_3, rT_3, and $3,3'-T_2$ originates from T_4, T_3, and rT_3 deiodination, respectively, during secretion. There was no evidence, however, of any modification of intrathyroidal iodothyronine deiodination during prolonged TSH stimulation.

The effects of iodide on various aspects of thyroid hormone synthesis and secretion continue to be of interest to many investigators. It is paradoxical that iodide is essential for the synthesis of the iodothyronines yet may transiently inhibit iodothyronine synthesis and release. The iodination of thyroglobulin occurs in the follicular lumen, probably at the apical surface of the follicular cells, in both normal and hyperplastic rat thyroids.[42] The peroxidase required for this iodination resides in the apical plasma membrane. It has been reemphasized that two iodide pools exist in the thyroid, one resulting from the active transport of iodide from blood (external pool) and the other from the deiodination of the iodinated tyrosines within the thyroid (internal pool). This iodotyrosine deiodinase appears to be a flavoprotein, which has now been partially purified and characterized.[43] The internal iodide pool apparently passes through a stage in which it is not available for organic-binding before it mixes with the external pool, which is the source of active iodine.[44] The internal iodide pool is generated in the follicular cell and transported to the site of organic-binding, the follicular lumen, by a perchlorate-sensitive system.[45] Transient inhibition of the organic binding of iodide in the thyroid with a subsequent decrease in the synthesis of the thyroid hormones following a large iodide load has been recognized since the 1940s (acute Wolff–Chaikoff effect). Many explanations have been offered for this phenomenon. Most recently, this inhibition of organic-binding of iodine has been ascribed to a diminished generation or a decreased availability of hydrogen peroxide.[46] Finally, the effect of iodide enrichment on the adenylate cyclase–cAMP system of slices of normal and Graves' thyroid glands has been studied.[47] The increase in cAMP responsiveness of TSH was not affected by excess iodide in normal thyroid tissue, but was inhibited in tissue from patients with Graves' disease. This effect was not due to the higher iodine uptake in Graves' glands.

The sympathetic nervous system exerts some control of thyroid function by way of adrenergic innervation of the thyroid follicle cells. Exogenously administered catecholamines have been reported to inhibit, to stimulate, or not to affect thyroid function, depending on the animal species employed. *In vitro* studies using cat thyroid have demonstrated that epinephrine and norepinephrine (NE) reduce TSH-stimulated cAMP generation, suggesting an inhibitory role of the catecholamines on TSH-mediated thyroid function.[48] *In vivo* studies have revealed similar findings. MMI-induced goiters are significantly larger in superior cervical ganglionectomized than in sham-operated rats, indicating that the cervical sympathetics exert a negative effect on thyroid function.[49] Maayan *et al.* have carried out an extensive study of the effects of NE and TSH on various aspects of the function of the mouse thyroid *in vitro* and have reached the following conclusions. TSH stimulation of iodide organification, hormone release, and cAMP formation is not exerted through adrenergic receptors; NE stimulates organification and inhibits TSH-stimulated thyroid hormone release through α-adrenergic receptors but stimulates cAMP generation through β-receptors; cAMP may not be the mediator of all TSH actions on the thyroid.[50] Cholinergic nerve fibers also reach follicle cells in the normal human thyroid, and cholinergic agents enhance cGMP accumulation in the thyroid, supporting a role of the parasympathetic nervous system in the regulation of thyroid function in man.[51] A fascinating study by Ahren and co-workers has demonstrated that the thyroid of several species is supplied with VIP-containing nerve fibers and that mouse neuronal VIP may regulate thyroid secretion via cAMP.[52]

The control of thyroglobulin synthesis and secretion has been thoroughly reviewed by Van Herle *et al.*[53] This area of thyroid research has been of great interest, but continues to be extremely complex. Thyroglobulin mRNA is not selectively increased relative to the other thyroid RNAs in response to chronic endogenous TSH stimulation suggesting the possibility of a preexisting maximum concentration of thyroglobulin mRNA in response to physiological levels of TSH.[54] In this regard, TSH deficiency is associated with a decrease in thyroglobulin mRNA greater than that for other thyroid mRNAs and TSH administration to these rats stimulates the reaccumulation of thyroglobulin mRNA.[54] The substructure of thyroglobulin is highly dependent on the degree of TSH stimulation and this appears to be a more important determinant of thyroglobulin substructure than the degree of iodination of the protein.[55] It has been suggested that poorly iodinated thyroglobulin is more susceptible to dissociation and hydrolysis. Schneider and his colleagues and others have postulated two mechanisms for the release of thyroglobulin from the thyroid into the circulation. One is that thyroglobulin already in the colloid is released and the other is that a portion of newly synthesized, poorly iodinated thyroglobulin is secreted directly into the circulation before it enters the colloid. Data supporting the latter possibility have now been reported. Thyroglobulin in the circulation appears to arise from the direct release of poorly iodinated, newly synthesized thyroglobulin.[56] Release of thyroglobulin from the human thyroid into the circulation can be stimulated by the administration of bTSH, and the half-life of this released thyroglobulin has been estimated to be approximately 4 days.[57] As noted below in Section 3.8 on thyroid cancer, an elevated serum thyroglobulin is a useful marker for residual thyroid tissue or recurrent thyroid carcinoma following surgery and ablative ^{131}I therapy. However, a major problem in the measurement of serum thyroglobulin by RIA is the presence of antithyroglobulin antibodies in approximately 20% of these patients. These antibodies interfere with the RIA, producing falsely high or falsely low values. An immunoradiometric assay for serum thyroglobulin permits a semiquantitative measurement of serum thyroglobulin in antithyroglobulin-positive sera.[58] It is most important that a thyroglobulin assay be developed that eliminates this problem. Serum thyroglobulin is almost always elevated in patients with hyperthyroidism. A failure to detect thyroglobulin in the serum of patients with thyrotoxicosis is a useful diagnostic test in the detection of thyrotoxicosis facticia, since the synthesis and release of thyroglobulin would be suppressed in these patients.[59] Finally, a gastric peroxidase has been isolated from the fundic region of the mouse stomach that catalyzes the formation of mono- and diiodotyrosine and is capable of synthesizing T_4 and T_3 in proteins such as thyroglobulin or albumin.[60]

3.3. Peripheral Metabolism, Action, and Serum Protein Binding of the Thyroid Hormones

Since the first demonstration in 1970 that the major source of the circulating T_3 in man is the outer ring monodeiodination of T_4 in peripheral tissues,[61] a major area of basic and clinical research has been concerned with various aspects of the peripheral metabolism of the thyroid hormones. Over the past 8 years, RIAs for rT_3, and three T_2s, $3'-T_1$,[62] the acetic acid derivatives of T_4 and T_3, tetrac and triac, respectively, and the proprionic acid derivative of T_3 (triprop) have been described, and thyronine has been quantified in the urine by gas chromatography.[63] As reported earlier for rT_3, almost all the circulating T_2s and $3'-T_1$ are generated by sequential deiodination of their precursor iodothyronines. The urinary excretion of free and the glucuronide and sulfate conjugates of T_4, T_3, rT_3, $3',5'-T_2$, and $3,3'-T_2$ has been assessed in euthyroid subjects and patients with hypo- and hyperthyroidism.[64] Significant amounts of the T_4 and T_3 sulfate conjugates could not be demonstrated in any of the groups, and the excretion of free and conjugated iodothyronines was increased in hyperthyroidism and decreased in hypothyroidism. The amounts of free iodothyronines excreted in the urine varied considerably, suggesting active renal handling; this was partially confirmed by Faber *et al.* who observed that the renal production of $3,3'-T_2$ and $3',5'-T_2$ in man exceeds the degradation and urinary excretion. A model of the distribution kinetics and metabolism of T_4 and T_3 in man employing thin-layer chromatography of serum samples after the pulse injection of both $[^{131}I]-T_4$ and $[^{125}I]-T_3$ eliminates some of the problems inherent in other methods.[66] The conversion ratio of T_4 to T_3 in euthyroid man can more accurately be assessed by sampling urine rather than plasma following the administration of $[^{125}I]-T_4$ and $[^{131}I]-T_3$.[67] This method offers a significant technical improvement in the extremely difficult task of determining T_4 conversion to T_3 *in vivo*.

It has generally been accepted that the free or unbound thyroid hormones in plasma are available to the cell for metabolic action as well as further metabolism, and that the protein-bound hormone does not readily enter the cell. Recently, Pardridge has suggested that, as with albumin-bound steroids, albumin-bound T_4 and T_3 do enter the cell.[68] *In vivo* studies of the influx of thyroid hormones into rat liver during a single initial pass have suggested that T_4 and T_3 traverse the liver cell membrane by free diffusion and that albumin-bound T_4 and T_3, as well as approximately 50% of TBG-bound T_3 but not TBG-bound and TBPA-bound T_4), are cleared by liver cells.[69] The albumin-bound fraction of T_4 far exceeds the dialyzable fraction measured *in vitro* and both fractions vary inversely with the concentration of TBG and TBPA. Thus, the *in vitro* measurement of free T_4 would accurately reflect in a qualitative way the quantity of T_4 available for transport *in vivo*. However, since TBG-bound T_3 does enter the liver *in vivo* and the dialyzable fraction of T_3 measured *in vitro* is affected by TBG, measurements of free T_3 *in vitro* would not accurately predict the fraction of T_3 available for transport into the liver *in vivo*. These, however, are single-pass studies with isotopic hormones, and do not reflect net fluxes. It should be pointed out, in addition, that the capillary wall–liver cell interface is unique, and this model may not be applicable to other organs. In this regard, an increase in the plasma free T_3 concentration measured by equilibrium dialysis is accompanied by an elevation of intracellular (human erythrocyte) free hormone, suggesting that the free T_3 concentration in the red cell does reflect plasma free T_3 concentration.[70] Studies of red cell free T_3 in the presence of alterations in plasma TBG would be of interest.

A wide variety of drugs have been demonstrated to inhibit both inner and outer ring deiodination of the iodothyronines. Most studies have been primarily concerned with the effects of these drugs on the serum concentrations of T_3 and rT_3. Following the administration of such drugs as the X-ray contrast dyes (Telepaque® and Oragrafin®), corticosteroids, propranolol, propylthiouracil, and amiadarone, serum T_3 concentration is decreased and rT_3 concentration increased. It is generally believed that these findings result from decreased outer ring deiodinase activity, producing a decrease in T_3 generation from T_4 and a decrease in rT_3 deiodination to yield $3,3'-T_2$. The cholecystographic agents also impair the hepatic binding of T_4, which could further explain the decrease in T_3 generation from T_4.[71] Iopanoic acid (Telepaque®) inhibits outer ring deiodination of T_4 in all tissues studied, including the pituitary, resulting in a marked decrease in T_3 generation. The low serum T_3 that occurs during Telepaque® administration does not reduce the basal metabolic rate nor does the dye affect the metabolic rate in T_3-treated subjects.[72] Amiadarone is a potent antiarrhythmic drug containing 37.2% iodine by weight. It is used extensively in Europe for the treatment of cardiac arrhythmias and angina and, like other iodine containing medications, has been reported to induce Jod–Basedow's syndrome (iodine-induced thyrotoxicosis) in European countries where daily iodine intake is often marginally low.[73] Amiadarone also inhibits outer ring deiodination of the iodothyronines and a recent prospective study in the United States has revealed that it produces the following abnormalities in thyroid function tests: increases in T_4, free T_4, and rT_3, a decrease in T_3, and an increase in basal and TRH-stimulated TSH secretion.[74] After amiadarone was discontinued, return to baseline values was prolonged. Although no patients in this series developed thyrotoxicosis, it appears likely that this might occur if more patients are treated. Sodium salicylate can now be added to the growing list of drugs that inhibit outer ring monodeiodination of T_4 and rT_3 in the liver.[75] Chronic and acute administration of ritalin to developing rats reduces serum concentrations of T_4 and T_3 by accelerating their clearance from the blood, and the maturational rise in basal serum TSH is permanently depressed after ritalin treatment has been withdrawn.[76] These findings may have relevance in man, since ritalin is used as a psychotropic stimulant in the management of hyperkinesis in elementary school children. A thorough review of the effects of drugs on the distribution and metabolism of the thyroid hormones has recently been published.[77]

Earlier studies demonstrated that serum T_3 is decreased and rT_3 increased in many patients with nonthyroidal illness (NTI), changes believed to be due to impaired outer ring deiodination of T_4 to T_3 and of rT_3 to $3,3'-T_2$. The serum T_4 concentration may also be low in critically ill patients, who are most often being treated in intensive care units. The free thyroxine index (FTI) is also decreased in these severely ill patients, whereas the percent free T_4 measured by equilibrium dialysis is often elevated, frequently resulting in a normal free T_4 concentration (% free $T_4 \times$ total T_4). It has been suggested that a nondialyzable inhibitor of T_4 binding, less effective against the binding of T_3, is present in the sera and extrathyroidal tissues of these ill patients. Thus, the decreased hormone binding is not as readily detected by the resin T_3 uptake as it is by equilibrium dialysis of T_4.[78] Since dopamine administration decreases basal and TRH-stimulated TSH concentrations in normal subjects, its frequent use in the treatment of severely ill patients in shock would further contribute to the low serum T_4 by decreasing TSH secretion and the subsequent release of T_4 from the thyroid.[79] An extremely low serum T_4 concentration is associated with a high mortality rate.[80] Studies of thyroxine metabolism in these ill patients with a low serum T_4 concentration have revealed a two- to threefold increase in both the free fraction in serum and the metabolic clearance rate of T_4. This resulted in T_4 disposal rates that were within the normal 95% confidence limits, although the mean was significantly below normal.[81] A normal early T_4 distribution phase, despite defective serum T_4 binding, suggested an additional abnormality of deficient extravascular T_4 bindings, perhaps due to the tissue inhibitor noted above. In contrast, other observations of the bioavailability of T_4 (and T_3) in ill patients with a low serum T_4 (and T_3) concentration, using the effects of normal and sick sera on the first-pass extraction of labeled T_4 and T_3 by rat liver, have suggested that the amount of T_4 or T_3 that is available for transport into the liver is markedly reduced in NTI and is proportional to the decrease in total plasma hormone concentrations.[82] rT_3 kinetics in NTI have also been evaluated and, as observed earlier in starvation, outer ring deiodination of rT_3 is reduced and inner ring deiodination is normal.[83]

The availability of at least four new commercial kits to measure serum free T_4 by RIA has led to a series of papers evaluating the efficacy of these kits in measuring free T_4 concentration in patients with thyroid disease, abnormalities in TBG, and NTI. All of the commercial methods gave consistent and accurate values for FT_4 (RIA), as compared to FT_4 measured by equilibrium dialysis in patients with hypo- and hyperthyroidism and in those with abnormalities in TBG,[84–88] except for one method that resulted in a low FT_4 (RIA) in many euthyroid patients during the third trimester of pregnancy.[89] In contrast to the reliable results in such patients, FT_4 (RIA) values were frequently low in patients with a low serum T_4 concentration secondary to NTI when measured by three of the four methods.[85,87,88] On the other hand, this method failed to detect true hypothyroidism in two ill patients whose FT_4 (RIA) values were normal.[90] It is evident, therefore, that FT_4 measured by RIA in patients with severe NTI must be interpreted with some caution. This problem is most evident when FT_4 is measured by equilibrium dialysis and by some of the RIA kits in sick patients with a normal or, far less common, an elevated serum T_4 concentration. In these patients, the serum FT_4, even by dialysis, is often elevated,[85,86,91] raising the possibility of concurrent hyperthyroidism. This latter diagnosis could be excluded by a normal TRH test or, as recently suggested, by the finding of a normal or low FT_3I.[92] An absent TSH response to TRH and an elevated serum FT_3I would be consistent with true hyperthyroidism in a sick patient. Patients with acute psychiatric illness may also present with an elevation of the serum T_4 and FT_4I, which returns to normal within a few weeks of hospitalization.[93,94] The serum T_3 is normal in these patients, although the initial TSH response to TRH may be blunted.[95] These findings in acutely psychotic patients resemble the recently described abnormality in the pituitary–adrenal axis, evident in an abnormal overnight dexamethasone suppression test in depressed patients, and suggest that acute mental illness may be associated with a wide variety of neuroendocrine abnormalities.

Abnormalities in thyroid function tests in hepatic and renal diseases, and in diabetes mellitus, continue to be evaluated. Serum T_4 and TBG concentrations are elevated, resulting in a normal FTI; serum T_3 is decreased; and serum TSH is normal during the acute phase of hepatitis B virus infection.[96] The rise in serum TBG correlated with the rise in serum aspartate aminotransferase, suggesting a nonspecific release of both proteins from the injured hepatocytes. All tests returned to normal after recovery from the hepatitis. Kinetic studies of T_4, T_3, rT_3, $3',5'$-T_2, $3,3'$-T_2, and $3'$-T_1 metabolism have been carried out in patients with liver cirrhosis.[97] A general inhibition of outer ring deiodinations and no alteration in inner ring deiodination occurred, suggesting the existence of a common outer ring deiodinase and a common inner ring deiodinase for the sequential deiodination of the iodothyroinines. Further data have been reported concerning thyroid function in patients with the nephrotic syndrome[98] and in patients with chronic renal disease treated by hemodialysis.[99] In nephrotic patients, most values were in the normal range, although the serum T_3 and TBG concentrations were significantly decreased. Urinary excretion of T_4 and T_3, and urinary protein and TBG were markedly increased, but the only correlation seen was between daily urinary protein excretion and urinary T_4. Serum T_4, FT_4I, T_3, and FT_3I concentrations are frequently low in patients treated by hemodialysis and, as in most patients with NTI, the serum TSH concentration is usually normal. These abnormalities in the circulating thyroid hormones do not explain the abnormal lipids and premature atherosclerosis that frequently occur in patients on chronic maintenance dialysis. A uremic rat model has been employed to determine whether tissue hypothyroidism occurs in uremia. A reduced liver T_3 content and a decrease in α-glycerophosphate dehydrogenase (GPD) and malic dehydrogenase (MDH) activity in uremic rats, with restoration of enzyme activities toward normal levels after T_3 administration, strongly suggest the presence of hypothyroidism at the tissue level.[100] A decrease in hepatic nuclear T_3 receptors in the uremic rat has also been observed,[101] which certainly correlates well with the reduced liver T_3 content and enzyme activity noted above. This reduction in hepatic nuclear T_3 receptors is similar to that observed in starvation and after partial hepatectomy. As in other systemic illnesses, serum T_3 is decreased and rT_3 increased in diabetic patients who are not well controlled, suggesting the possibility that the reduction in T_3 production may be an adaptation to limit catabolism in these patients.[102] Serum T_3 and rT_3 values return to normal several days after good diabetic control has been achieved. Thus, a normal T_3/rT_3 ratio may be a reliable indicator of good diabetic control. The marked decrease in the peripheral conversion of T_4 to T_3 will result in normal serum T_3 concentrations in patients who have both diabetic ketoacidosis and severe thyrotoxicosis, including thyroid storm.[103,104] Studies in the streptozotocin-induced diabetic rat and mouse have revealed abnormalities in the hypothalamic–pituitary–thyroid axis manifested by a decreased plasma and pituitary TSH and hypothalamic TRH content, a diminished TSH response to thyroidectomy,[105] and a decreased thyroid response to TSH beyond the generation of cAMP.[106] Conflicting data on the effect of streptozotocin-induced diabetes on hepatic nuclear T_3 receptor content have been reported. In accord with reduced hepatic T_3 receptors observed in starvation and the state of intracellular starvation present in untreated diabetes, hepatic T_3 receptor content was reduced in the diabetic rat in one study.[107] In contrast, no change was observed in another.[108] It is evident that further studies are necessary to resolve these conflicting findings. Reduced nuclear T_3-binding capacity in rat lung occurs in diabetes and might be related to the depressed level of pulmonary lipogenic enzyme activities that is also present in these diabetic rats.[109]

In patients with NTI and low serum T_4 and T_3 concentrations, the serum TSH concentration is almost always normal. It has been suggested that a normal serum TSH may not always be a reliable index of the euthyroid state in these sick patients. Thus, decreases in serum T_4 and T_3 concentrations induced by iodide administration to sick patients resulted in an enhanced TSH response to TRH in only half of the patients.

This is in contrast to a consistent increase in the TSH response in healthy subjects given iodides.[110] The TSH response to TRH may be blunted in a small proportion of patients with NTI and a low serum T_4 concentration, suggesting an abnormal pituitary feedback set point in some of these patients.[111] To further study the regulation of TSH secretion in NTI, a tumor-bearing rat model has been employed.[112] The findings of decreased serum T_4 and T_3 concentrations and normal basal and stimulated TSH values resemble the findings most often observed in critically ill patients. The pituitary production of T_3 from T_4 was increased two-fold in the tumor-bearing rats, but this was not sufficient to restore pituitary T_3 content to normal. The fact that TSH regulation appears relatively normal in the face of decreased pituitary nuclear T_3 suggests a shift in the normal feedback regulation of TSH secretion so that a relatively normal biological TSH response occurs in the presence of decreased pituitary T_3 content.

The localization and properties of the outer and inner ring deiodinases in rat liver have been extensively studied by many workers. There is general agreement that the 5'-deiodinase that converts T_4 to T_3 and that converts rT_3 to $3,3'$-T_2 is probably one enzyme,[113–115] except perhaps in the pituitary and cerebral cortex.[116,117] There is, however, some disagreement as to the subcellular localization of the two enzymes in liver fractions. The microsomal fraction contains both inner and outer ring deiodinases,[118] although an earlier report suggested that 5-deiodinase activity resided in the soluble cytosol fraction.[119] Both enzymes appear to be associated with the endoplasmic reticulum, and not with the plasma membranes,[120] though these were reported by others to be rich in enzyme activity.[121] Solubilization and partial characterization of the hepatic deiodinases have now been achieved,[122,123] and Leonard and Rosenberg have found similar enzyme specificity, localization, and sulfhydryl requirements for the rat kidney 5'-deiodinase for rT_3.[124] The pituitary is a rich source of 5'-deiodinase activity.[125] In contrast to the findings in liver and kidney homogenates, DTT is required to demonstrate conversion of T_4 to T_3 in pituitary homogenates and activity is decreased in hyperthyroidism and increased in hypothyroidism. The anatomical distribution and kinetics of brain inner and outer ring deiodinase activity have also been described and, as in the anterior pituitary, hypothyroidism increases 5'-deiodination of T_4 to T_3 and DTT is required.[126–128] This increase is 5'-deiodinase induced by hypothyroidism is rapidly abolished (within 4 hr) by a single intravenous injection of T_3.[129] Human spinal fluid rT_3 is probably produced from brain T_4 and a transport mechanism may regulate free rT_3 in the spinal fluid.[130] The production of GH in cultured nonthyrotropic rat pituitary cells is enhanced by T_4 and this T_4 effect is at least in part related to the GSH-dependent intracellular 5'-monodeiodination of T_4 to T_3.[131] The placenta is an active site for DTT-dependent inner ring deiodination and may, at least in part, be responsible for the placental barrier for the passage of T_4 and T_3 from mother to fetus in both man and rat.[132,133] Unlike the case in other tissues, rT_3 is not further deiodinated, suggesting the possibility that the placenta and the fetal membranes may be a major source of amniotic fluid rT_3,[134] since the rT_3 content in amniotic fluid is more dependent on maternal than fetal thyroid function.[135] Inner and outer ring iodothyronine deiodinase activity has been demonstrated in rat thyroid tissue,[136] and enhanced conversion of T_4 to T_3 occurs in Graves' thyroids as compared with normal thyroid tissue.[137] An immunosequestration technique has been described that should make possible more valid studies of the generation of iodothyronine metabolites that are themselves rapidly degraded; specific antibodies are employed to sequester these metabolites as they are formed, thereby blocking their further degradation.[138]

Many studies have been carried out to determine the effect of starvation on the peripheral metabolism of the thyroid hormones; the mechanism(s) responsible for the reduced outer ring deiodinase activity consistently observed in starved man and rat; and the effect of starvation on the responsiveness of the pituitary to T_3. Nonetheless, there continue to be gaps in our understanding of the complex events that occur during starvation and that might influence various aspects of the control of hypothalamic–pituitary–thyroid function. Starvation does induce a marked decrease in the production of T_3 from T_4 (impaired outer ring deiodination of T_4), resulting in a decrease in the serum T_3 concentration. The increase in serum rT_3 concentration is primarily due to a decrease in the clearance of rT_3 (impaired outer ring deiodination of rT_3), although a small increase in rT_3 and tetrac production has also been found.[139] Most of the confusion concerning the role of reduced thiols in the impaired outer ring deiodinase activity induced by starvation can be attributed to variations among different studies as to the length of time of starvation, whether the rats were supplemented with T_4, and finally of greatest importance, whether the effects of starvation were compared to glucose or Purina Chow (protein-rich diet) feeding. Earlier reports[140,141] challenging the important role of a decrease in reduced thiols[142–145] in the impaired outer ring deiodinase activity observed in starved as compared to Purina-fed rats have been questioned.[146] Gavin and co-workers have now confirmed the earlier observations that enrichment of liver homogenates from T_4-treated starved rats with thiol-reducing agents reverses the decrease in T_3 generation from T_4, that hepatic nonprotein sulfhydryls and reduced glutathione are decreased in starvation, and that hepatic T_4 inner ring deiodinase activity is neither impaired or enhanced.[146] Their earlier observations that glucose feeding increases the hepatic content of active enzyme and that reduced thiols do not play a role in this increased 5'-deiodinase activity were again noted, emphasizing the importance of dietary constituents in the regulation of iodothyronine deiodination. Confirmatory and conflicting results have also been obtained in cultured rat hepatocytes, which contain both inner and outer ring deiodinases, as well as in cultured monkey hepatocarcinoma cells, which contain only inner ring deiodinase. In the rat hepatocytes, glucose did not alter deiodinase activity, insulin stimulated activity, and glucagon blocked this insulin action but had no effect in the absence of insulin.[147] In contrast, the constant infusion of glucagon in the rat does not affect thyroid hormone metabolism.[148] Hepatocarcinoma cells incubated in the absence of glucose (starvation) generated increased quantities of rT_3 from T_4,[149] suggesting that the increase in serum rT_3 observed in starvation might be secondary to enhanced production of rT_3 rather than decreased rT_3 clearance. This *in vitro* observation was in contrast to the findings that glucose feeding enhanced both inner and outer ring deiodinase activity. From data obtained in both cultured liver cell systems, it has been suggested that reduced glutathione (GSH) is so abundant that hepatocytes can tolerate a greater than 90% reduction in GSH without any impairment of inner or outer ring deiodinase activity.[150] The decrease in outer ring deiodinase activity during prolonged starvation in the rat also appears to be due to a decrease in the enzyme itself secondary to hypothyroidism, since T_4 treatment of starved animals partly reverses the decreased deiodinase activity.[144,145,151] It is probable that both cofactors and enzyme are altered during starvation and that both play a role in the multiple changes in the peripheral metabolism of the thyroid hormones that have been reported to occur in man and rat.[152]

Conflicting reports have also appeared concerning the effectiveness of T_3 in suppressing the TSH response to TRH during starvation in man. Burger *et al.* reported a diminished effectiveness of T_3 in inhibiting TSH secretion during starvation, consistent with the hypothesis of a generalized resistance of target organs to T_3 during starvation.[153] In contrast, Gardner *et al.* observed that administered T_3 was more effective in suppressing the TSH response to TRH during starvation, and concluded that fasting is accompanied by a lower set point of TSH secretion, which could explain the failure of serum TSH to increase despite the low serum T_3 that occurs during fasting.[154]

In a series of related studies on the interaction of starvation, carbohydrate administration, and T_3 on the synthesis of labile protein and hepatic lipogenic enzymes, Oppenheimer and his colleagues have made the following observations[155–159]: T_3 is essential for the generation of the labile protein pool serving as the immediate source of amino acids for gluconeogenesis and protein synthesis during acute starvation; the acute lowering of T_3 does not result in a protein-sparing effect in the rat; α-GPD, but not malic enzyme (ME), is preserved during the first 3 days of starvation; T_3 and carbohydrate induce ME within 2 hr, making it unlikely that either stimulus is secondary to the other; thyroid hormone interacts with a product or an intermediate of carbohydrate metabolism in stimulating ME; and in cultured rat hepatocytes, an increased concentration of glucose per se can induce ME.

It is generally agreed that the thyroid hormones exert many of their metabolic effects through nuclear events initiated by specific binding to nuclear chromatin. It is beyond the scope of this review to discuss the multiple effects of the thyroid hormones in stimulating the synthesis and activity of a wide variety of enzymes and hormones mediated by the production of nuclear RNA. However, a few specific observations will be noted. Both T_4 and GH are involved in maintaining normal hepatic RNA content, but do not restore the RNA to normal levels in hypophysectomized rats, suggesting the possibility that unidentified pituitary factors may be required.[160] T_4 stimulates both submaxillary gland nerve growth factor (NGF) and epidermal growth factor (EGF) in adult female mice, but only NGF in adult males. These preferential effects are not dependent on testosterone or corticosterone, suggesting separate regulatory mechanisms for T_4, testosterone, and corticosterone on these two growth factors.[161] A decline in renal cortical Na^+—K^+ ATPase has been noted with age in the rat and it has been shown that this decline is thyroid hormone dependent and that age decreases the enzyme response to thyroid hormone.[162] The thyroid hormones exert effects on behavior and on the activity of the autonomic nervous system. Support for these thyroid hormone actions on nervous tissue has been further enhanced by the demonstration that nerve cells and neuropil from adult rat brain concentrate and retain intravenously administered $[^{125}I]$-T_3.[163]

Some questions have recently been raised concerning the early *in vivo* binding of labeled T_3 to the nucleus. Goldfine and associates were unable to detect significant nuclear localization of $[^{125}I]$-T_3 in cultured GH_1 cells as determined by quantitative EM autoradiographs.[164] The $[^{125}I]$-T_3 initially bound to the plasma membrane, was rapidly internalized, and subsequently interacted with mitochondria, outer nuclear structures, and the nucleolus. A large pool of data suggest that the thyroid hormones exert their effects at sites other than the nucleus, specifically the mitochondrion[165] and plasma membrane.[166] T_3 promptly stimulates the accumulation of certain amino acids and the inward transport of glucose analogs in the isolated rat thymocyte *in vivo,* responses independent of new protein synthesis and, therefore, negating a role for nuclear events in this plasma membrane-mediated process.[166] Further support for the importance of the plasma membrane as a possible site of thyroid hormone action is the recent confirmation of earlier data identifying specific binding of T_3 to a plasma membrane protein receptor on the cell surface of cultured mouse fibroblasts.[167]

A thyronine-binding protein that migrates in the TBG zone appears in the serum of young rats fed a low-protein diet,[168] explaining the unique observation that in these protein-deficient rats, serum T_3 is increased, the percent free T_3 assessed by equilibrium dialysis is decreased, and the FT_3 concentration is unchanged.[168,169] Since TBPA is a potent binder of T_4, but not of T_3, and TBG is not present in rats fed a normal diet, the presence of TBG will affect T_3 binding much more than T_4 binding. Thus, serum T_4 and free T_4 concentrations are normal in these rats. Although serum thyronine binding studies have not been carried out in rats fed the nutritionally deficient Remington diet, it is unlikely that similar binding changes occur since the increase in serum T_3 in these rats is associated with an increase in serum FT_3 measured by equilibrium dialysis.[170] Hepatic cellular uptake is decreased in the Remington diet-fed rats, which could explain the fact that no change in oxygen consumption was observed in spite of the increase in free T_3 concentration.[171]

A series of papers has described a new hereditary autosomal dominant syndrome characterized by serum T_4 and FT_4I elevations due to an abnormal serum albumin. This protein binds T_4 with a much greater affinity for T_4, relative to its affinity for T_3, than does TBG.[172–175] Patients with this syndrome are clinically euthyroid, as indicated by normal TRH and thyroid suppression tests, normal free T_4 measured by equilibrium dialysis, and a normal or only slightly elevated serum T_3 concentration.[175] This syndrome has been termed familial dysalbuminemic hyperthyroxinemia (FDH). FDH may be more common than originally suspected. Since both serum T_4 and FT_4I are increased, this syndrome may be mistaken for hyperthyroidism. Familial euthyroid hyperthyroxinemia due to increased T_4 binding by TBPA has been reported in one family.[176] Heavy amphetamine use may also increase the serum T_4 and FT_4I, with a normal serum T_3, and the proposed mechanism is an enhanced TSH secretion.[177] Antibodies to T_4 or T_3 will result in abnormal concentrations of these iodothyronines, depending on the RIA method employed: low values when nonspecific separation methods, such as use of polyethylene glycol or charcoal, are used, and elevated values with double-antibody or solid-phase RIA methods.[178,179]

It has been proposed that microheterogeneity of TBG is caused by differences in N-acetylneuraminic acid content and that variations in TBG patterns in native sera may reflect altered TBG synthesis or degradation.[180] A genetically related microheterogeneity of TBG could not be demonstrated. A low serum TBG concentration occurs secondary to L-asparaginase therapy in patients with acute lymphocytic leukemia.[181] Eleven patients with Graves' disease and an increase in serum TBG concentration (often familial) have been described, suggesting that this combination is not rare.[182] It is important to recognize such patients in the early thyrotoxic state to avoid overtreatment of the Graves' disease with antithyroid drugs. Another study reveals that serum free T_4 concentration assessed by equilibrium dialysis tends to be in the low-normal range or slightly low in patients with familial TBG deficiency. The serum TSH is normal in these euthyroid patients. New data suggest that euthyroidism and a normal serum TSH is maintained by a subtle equilibrium between low FT_4 and high FT_3 concentrations.[183]

3.4. Fetal and Neonatal Thyroid Function

A superb, thorough, and detailed review of thyroid development and disorders of thyroid function in the newborn has appeared.[184] In view of the high incidence of neonatal hypothyroidism detected by screening programs, studies related to fetal and neonatal thyroid function assume great importance. Over the past few years, a large number of reports concerned with the function of the hypothalamic–pituitary–thyroid axis in the fetus and newborn have appeared. Severe hypothyroidism in the pregnant rat results in some alterations in pituitary–thyroid function in their progeny during development: a decrease in serum T_4 and T_3 within the first 30 days, and a decrease and then increase in serum TSH that persists into adult life.[185] The high TSH values in the adult progeny were not seen when hypothyroid dams were treated with GH during pregnancy. GH content in rat pituitaries progressively increases from birth to 60 days of age and is unaffected by T_3 administration, suggesting that the rate of formation of GH is already maximal during early life or that the pituitary T_3 receptors are saturated during development.[186] As in the adult, hypothyroidism in the neonate is associated with a marked reduction in pituitary GH content that is rapidly restored by T_3 administration. In a careful study of cultured bovine fetal thyroids, Avivi *et al.* reported that the thyroids of fetuses that have reached a crown–rump length of 3 cm produce both T_4 and T_3, and that T_4 is the dominant hormone.[187] The administration of TRH antiserum to neonatal rats from birth to 5 days did not decrease serum TSH as it does in rats 10 days and older,[188] confirming earlier observations by Theodoropoulos[189] and Greer[190] and their co-workers that fetal and neonatal pituitary function in the rat is not physiologically dependent on TRH secretion. This axis reaches complete maturity by 5 to 7 weeks after birth, when the hypothalamic–pituitary–thyroid response to acute cold exposure attains an adult pattern.[191] The TSH response to exogenous TRH is greater in the young neonatal rat than in the more mature rat[192] and, as in the fetal lamb,[193] the effect of exogenous T_3 on the TSH response to TRH is markedly reduced, suggesting immaturity of the negative feedback system for the control of TSH release. A recent study in man also demonstrates that the fetal TSH response to TRH administered to the mother is greater than that induced in the adult.[194] Serum thyroglobulin concentrations are higher in cord blood than in maternal serum, increase during the first few days of life, and gradually fall to adult levels by 1 year of age.[195,196] A fascinating observation that suckling rat pups, but not weaned rats, respond to perorally administered bTSH with increases in serum T_3 and T_4 concentrations suggests that the characteristics of the gastric secretion and intestinal epithelium in the adult prevent absorption of the polypeptide hormone.[197]

During the transition from fetal to adult life, changes in iodothyronine metabolism also occur. During fetal life, the hepatic outer ring deiodinase activity that results in the conversion of T_4 to T_3 is relatively reduced, and inner ring deiodination of T_4 to the inactive iodothyronine rT_3 is relatively enhanced. These observations, as well as those noted earlier that the placenta is a rich source of inner ring deiodinase activity, suggest that the fetus is protected from the possible adverse effects of the active thyroid hormones on fetal development. Similar findings have now been described in the chick embryo, in which maturation of iodothyronine metabolism occurs during the last 2 days *in ovo*.[198] The availability of T_3 at this time may be important for the final stages of development from embryo to newborn chick. In like manner, the conversion of T_4 to T_3 is always evident in tadpoles either undergoing or having just completed metamorphic climax.[199] The outer ring 5′-deiodinase system can be induced in premetamorphic tadpoles by injecting them with either T_4 or T_3, indicating that this enzyme is under the control of the thyroid hormones. In further studies in the tadpole, Galton has described T_3 receptors in hepatic nuclei that appear to be near saturation in late premetamorphosis and during climax at a time when the serum thyroid hormones increase.[200] Unlike the situation in mammals, T_4 can exert a physiological effect (increase hepatic carbamyl phosphate synthetase activity) in premetamorphic tadpoles without being converted to T_3.[201]

The development of the human and rat lung and the synthesis of surfactant may be influenced by the thyroid hormones. High-affinity T_3 nuclear receptors are present in human lung as early as the second trimester.[202] In the rat, T_3 is preferentially taken up by the perinatal rat lung and there is a burst of T_3-concentrating capacity in the early post-natal period, suggesting a role for T_3 in surfactant regulation during the perinatal period.[203] As noted in Section 3.1, DIMIT has thyromimetic activity, readily crosses the placenta, and has been recommended as a possible therapeutic agent in the treatment of fetal hypothyroidism. DIMIT administration to pregnant rabbits accelerates maturation of the surfac-tant system in fetal lung, a finding that further supports the role of thyroactive hormones in surfactant synthesis.[204]

It is well known that immunoglobulins readily traverse the placenta from mother to fetus. The transplacental passage of thyroid-stimulating IgG induces neonatal Graves' disease. Transient neonatal hypothyroid-ism due to maternal TSH-binding inhibitor immunoglobulins has now been reported.[205] Falsely elevated serum TSH concentrations in new-born infants may occur secondary to the presence of heterophilic anti-bodies that interfere with the TSH RIA in the plasma of the infants and their mothers.[206] This problem is especially important when the serum TSH is used as the primary screening test for neonatal hypothyroid-ism.[207]

3.5. Hyperthyroidism

Methods to detect the thyroid-stimulating antibodies or immuno-globulins (stimulation of cAMP, TSAb) and the thyrotropin-binding in-hibitory immunoglobulins (TBII) in the sera of patients with Graves' disease have continued to be of great interest to many investigators. Multiple terms for these immunoglobulins (IgGs) have been used and it is now essential that consistent abbreviations be employed—TSAb or TSI for the stimulatory IgGs and TBII for the TSH-binding inhibitory IgGs. Unfortunately, there is little correlation of values for TSAb and TBII in the sera of patients with untreated Graves' disease,[208,209] al-though the majority of patients with this disorder have both TSAb and TBII in their serum; this frequent discrepancy between TSAb and TBII may be due to the methods employed. A receptor-purification method to purify Graves' IgG has recently been described in which guinea pig fat cell membranes absorb Graves' IgG and this is followed by elution with acid–glycine.[210] By this technique, as much as 150-fold enrichment of biological activity has been achieved. Further purification may result in the development of an RRA for Graves'-specific IgG. Guinea pig fat cells have also been used as a source of TSH receptors for TBII assays.[211] Similarly, porcine thyroid may be substituted for human tissue in the TBII assay.[212] Newer methods to detect TSAb include a cytochemical bioassay based on the quantification of staining after the exposure of guinea pig[213] or human[214] thyroid tissue preparations to a chromogenic substrate, leucine-2-naphthylamide, for the lysosomal enzyme leucine-2-naphthylamidase; the stimulation of cAMP in cultured human thyroid cells[215,216] or its release into the incubation medium from human thyroid slices[217]; and the measurement of the thyroid hormone concentration in the dialysis fluid following incubation of thyroid slices with serum in a two-compartment dialysis pot.[218] Sera from many patients with untreated Graves' disease were assayed for TBII, LATS, and LATS-protector and only the latter assay was positive in all sera.[219] Evidence of *in vivo* stimulation of the thyroid by circulating TSAb has been documented by the finding of increased cAMP concentration in surgical specimens of Graves' thyroid tissue as compared to normal thyroid tissue.[220,221] Doniach and co-workers have described thyroid growth-stimulating IgGs in some goitrous diseases; these are distinct from TSAb and TBII and it is proposed that these IgGs may be responsible for euthyroid, colloid goiters.[222]

Although assays for TSAb and TBII are not as yet available in clinical laboratories, they do appear to be clinically helpful in predicting remission and recurrence of Graves' disease in patients receiving antithyroid drug therapy. Over the past few years, many studies have been reported[223–228] that strongly suggest that the disappearance of the abnormal Graves' IgGs during thionamide drug therapy is associated with prolonged remission, and persistence of TSAb or TBII predicts recurrence of thyrotoxicosis after drug withdrawal. However, recurrence of thyrotoxicosis almost always occurs in patients with the histocompatibility antigen HLA-DRw3, irrespective of the persistence or disappearance of TBII.[229] The thionamide drugs apparently have a direct inhibitory effect on lymphocyte production of IgG, since both serum TBII and antimicrosomal antibodies may decrease shortly after their administration to patients with Graves' disease.[230,231] A direct immunosuppressive effect of the thionamides has also been demonstrated in cultured lymphocytes from euthyroid subjects and from patients with Graves' disease or Hashimoto's thyroiditis.[232,233]

The role of circulating thyroglobulin–antithyroglobulin immune complexes (CIC) in autoimmune thyroid disease has received considerable attention recently. Such immune complex deposits have been detected along the follicular basement membrane in Graves' disease thyroids.[234] A highly sensitive solid-phase enzyme-linked immunoassay has been developed to detect CIC, and a greater frequency, with higher concentrations, was observed in patients with Graves' disease as compared to those with Hashimoto's thyroiditis.[235] A fascinating study has appeared suggesting that CIC are significantly more common in Graves' disease patients with a negative TBII, that the frequent development of CIC during drug treatment is associated with the disappearance of TBII, and that later in the course of the disease, when CIC can no longer be detected, TBII do not reappear.[236] Thus, the development of CIC could be viewed as the reestablishment of a natural tolerance to TSH receptors in patients with Graves' disease. Finally, the occasional association of glomerulonephritis and Graves' disease or Hashimoto's thyroiditis has now been attributed to the deposition of CIC in the glomeruli.[237,238]

Cell-mediated immunity (CMI), as assessed by production of migration-inhibition factor, by peripheral T lymphocytes (MIF) in Graves' disease and Hashimoto's thyroiditis has been further demonstrated in a series of papers by Volpé and colleagues.[239–242] However, the postulate of a generalized defect of suppressor cell function in these disorders proposed by these workers has recently been challenged.[243] Further work related to the role of CMI in these autoimmune disorders is needed to resolve this problem.

It is well recognized that Graves' disease is a hereditary disorder, raising the possibility that relatives of patients with this disorder might have an increased incidence of thyroid abnormalities. In this regard, studies of siblings and first-degree and other relatives of patients with Graves' disease have been reported. Serum antithyroid antibodies and the thyroid glands of siblings of patients and those of patients without a family history of Graves' disease were evaluated. An increased incidence of serum antithyroglobulin but not anti-M antibodies and increased lymphocytic infiltration in the thyroids, were detected in the siblings. These findings further suggest the close relationship between Hashimoto's thyroiditis and Graves' disease.[244] In two large studies, TSAb, TBII, LATS, and CIC were not detected in any euthyroid relatives of patients with Graves' disease,[245] and only a small increase in the incidence of laboratory or physical exam abnormalities was present in the euthyroid children of Graves' disease patients.[246] In contrast to these studies, which really did not present convincing evidence for a "pre-Graves' disease state" or frequent abnormalities in relatives, a long-term follow-up study of changes in thyroid function in 69 euthyroid subjects with a family history of Graves' disease revealed that many abnormalities in TRH and T_3 suppression tests developed in these patients, including nonsuppressibility of thyroid function and both hyper- and hypo-TSH responses to TRH.[247] The increased frequency of HLA-B8 and HLA-Dw3 in patients with Graves' disease is well recognized. A reduced frequency of HLA-B12 has now been reported, and the increased incidence of HLA-B8 is apparently due to haplotype 1-8.[248]

Ophthalmopathy continues to be a major problem in Graves' disease. Inflammatory disease (primarily Graves' disease) was the etiology of unilateral exophthalmos in 50% of 342 consecutive patients evaluated by ultrasonography, computerized tomography, and radiography, and the combination of ultrasound and CT scan resulted in a 98% correct diagnosis of all types of orbital disease.[249] The etiology of Graves' ophthalmopathy remains an enigma. Employing a vesicle containing eye muscle membrane protein, Kriss and Mehdi have demonstrated that lymphocytes from patients with Graves' disease cause cell-mediated vesicle lysis.[250] A depression of the percentages and absolute numbers of thymus-derived active (A-RFC) and total (T-RFC) rosette-forming cells occurs in some patients with severe Graves' ophthalmopathy, and prednisone therapy was frequently associated with both clinical improvement and a significant increase to normal in the T-cell concentrations.[251] In contrast, patients who were therapeutically resistant to prednisone therapy presented with elevated A-RFC and normal T-RFC. These observations suggest a potential method to determine which patients will respond to steroid therapy and to monitor their response immunologically. The initial enthusiasm for the use of supervoltage orbital irradiation for severe Graves' ophthalmopathy has been somewhat damped by recent results reported by Teng et al. that only 35% of their patients showed some response, that improvement was primarily in soft tissue swelling, that proptosis decreased in only 4 of 20 patients and ophthalmoplegia in one, and that the benefit with treatment was, therefore, not impressive.[252] Although immunosuppressive agents such as cyclophosphamide have been used with some success in the treatment of severe Graves' eye disease,[253,254] the recognized side effects of such drugs preclude their use except under the most critical circumstances, such as severe, progressive loss of vision resistant to steroids and/or radiation therapy. The frequency of exophthalmos in Graves' disease has been carefully evaluated in 61 patients with thyrotoxic Graves' disease and the findings suggest that almost all patients have exophthalmos, although frequently it is mild.[255] The syndrome of nontumor-related exophthalmos in euthyroid patients without other recognized causes of the eye disease has been termed euthyroid Graves' disease. Many of these patients have one or more of the following abnormalities: positive antithyroglobulin and/or anti-M antibodies and TSAb and/or TBII in their serum, as well as abnormal T_3 suppression and/or TRH tests.[256] In 27 patients followed for 3 years, nine became thyrotoxic and two hypothyroid. Five of six patients who had Hashimoto's thyroiditis and exophthalmos were T_3 and TRH nonresponsive.

Antithyroid drug therapy has traditionally been the treatment of choice of Graves' disease in children and adolescents, but surgery and ^{131}I have been used with increasing frequency over the past few years. Although the reported results of treatment with propylthiouracil or methimazole are variable, with relapse occurring in 30 to 70% of patients, Buckingham *et al.* recently reported far more dismal results in 107 children treated with antithyroid drugs.[257] Serious drug complications occurred in 36%, and the sustained remission rate in children treated with drugs as sole therapy for an average of 3 years was only 30%. In the patients with smaller goiters and a considerable reduction in goiter size during drug therapy, a far more successful outcome was achieved. Surgery was eventually carried out in 78 of the 107 children. Minor complications occurred in 9%, but this was markedly reduced when an experienced thyroid surgeon operated. A large proportion (62%) became hypothyroid and only 9% recurred, since only small thyroid remnants were left. [131]I therapy was used in another series of 51 children with Graves' disease and 92% became hypothyroid over a mean follow-up period of 15 years.[258] Cancer, nodules, and recurrent goiter did not occur in these patients, most likely owing to the fact that large cumulative doses of ^{131}I were used (mean 14.1 mCi). Thus, although antithyroid drug therapy continues to be the primary mode of therapy of children and adolescents with Graves' disease, it is evident that many children will require ablative therapy with surgery or [131]I. We would favor surgery in children in whom drug therapy has failed for one reason or another because of the extremely high rate of hypothyroidism which the patient will have for a lifetime and the uneasiness (not based on fact as yet) that many of us feel about administering ^{131}I to children.

Propranolol has continued to be recommended as sole preoperative preparation of patients with thyrotoxicosis, but it should be recognized that the surgeons in those centers reporting favorable results have had vast experience in thyroid surgery.[259] There is considerable variation in plasma levels of propranolol and the degree of β blockade achieved after standard doses, especially in thyrotoxic patients, in whom systemic clearance is enhanced.[260,261] Adequate β blockade preoperatively can be achieved by inducing a greater than 25% reduction in the exercise heart rate.[262] In severely thyrotoxic patients, divided doses of greater than 160 mg propranolol daily, with an average daily dose of 330 mg, are frequently required. These larger doses of propranolol have been associated with small but significant decreases in serum calcium concentrations.[257] The administrations of iodides for 10 to 14 days prior to surgery in patients receiving propranolol has been recommended, since serum T_4 and T_3 concentrations decreased into the normal range at the time of surgery.[263] The efficacy of this combination of propranolol and iodides suggests the possibility of synergism of the two drugs on impairing thyroid hormone synthesis and release, since iodide administration alone for 2 weeks frequently does not restore thyroid function to normal.[264] Further studies of this therapeutic regimen should be carried out. One disturbing finding associated with the use of large doses of propranolol preoperatively is the decreased endocrine response to surgical stress: lowered plasma concentrations of glucose, ACTH, and cortisol.[265] Similar clinical improvement can be obtained with the selective β_1 blocker metoprolol, suggesting that the effects of propranolol are due to β_1 block.[266] In contrast to the response to propranolol, no inhibition of outer ring deiodination of T_4 to T_3 is observed with metoprolol. The propranolol withdrawal syndrome comprises an increased adrenergic activity and a rebound rise in the serum T_3 concentration to peak levels 60 hr after abrupt withdrawal of propranolol treatment in thyrotoxic, but not euthyroid, subjects. The rise in serum T_3 may contribute to the rebound increase in adrenergic activity after propranolol withdrawal in thyrotoxic patients.[267]

A great deal of controversy exists concerning the safety of propranolol therapy in thyrotoxic pregnant women, since this drug readily crosses the placenta and has been associated with both delayed cervical effacement and adverse effects of β blockade in the newborn. In a comprehensive review on the use of β blockers in pregnancy, no increase in fetal anomalies or morbidity was observed in newborns whose mothers received β blockers for hypertension, as compared with the offspring of hypertensive mothers who did not.[268] However, both groups of mothers were hypertensive and therefore these very favorable results cannot necessarily be extrapolated to those that would result from the use of propranolol in eutensive pregnant women with hyperthyroidism.

Thyroid surgery is still recommended for many young adults with Graves' disease whose disease has recurred after antithyroid drug withdrawal, who developed drug toxicity, whose goiter is very large, or who prefer surgery to [131]I. In contrast to the high incidence of hypothyroidism after near-total thyroidectomy in children noted above, 94% of adult patients were euthyroid for up to 4 years after subtotal thyroidectomy when approximately 10 g of tissue was preserved and the inferior thyroid arteries were not ligated.[269] Transient hypocalcemia frequently occurs in patients following subtotal thyroidectomy; this may be related to a transient increase in serum thyrocalcitonin,[270] although transiently impaired parathyroid function seems a more likely cause. Temporary hypothyroidism is not infrequent for 6 months following surgery. It has been recommended, therefore, that liothyronine (T_3) be given for 12 months after subtotal thyroidectomy to avoid the symptoms of transient hypothyroidism.[271] An increased incidence of permanent hypothyroidism was not seen in those patients treated with liothyronine.

For adult patients with thyrotoxicosis ^{131}I therapy remains the treatment of choice in most clinics. The major complication is the high incidence of hypothyroidism. Hypothyroidism within the first 4 months after ^{131}I treatment of Graves' disease may also be transient, and treatment should be withheld during this period unless the patients are very symptomatic.[272] TRH tests and T_3 suppression tests were carried out every 6 months for 2 years after ^{131}I therapy of Graves' disease, and the frequency of normal tests increased, reaching 50% by 2 years.[273] The tests at 6 months were not prognostic, since latent hypothyroidism occurred within 2 years in patients with normal serum T_4 and T_3 concentrations, and failure to suppress or respond to TRH did not indicate the need for further ^{131}I therapy.

Many aspects of antithyroid drug therapy for Graves' disease have been considered over the past few years. Although skin rashes are relatively common during thionamide drug therapy, cutaneous vasculitis does occur[274] and might be overlooked in patients presenting with a skin rash. PTU-induced hepatic dysfunction has been well documented in two patients,[275] and it is likely that mild drug-induced abnormalities in hepatic function tests are more common than has been suspected. The initial report by Greer et al.[276] that the thionamide-induced remission rate in Graves' disease after a 4- to 6-month course of drug therapy was similar to that observed after 1 to 2 years of therapy has not been confirmed by Tamai and Hoffenberg and their associates, who reported a much higher incidence of relapse in patients with Graves' disease treated with the thionamides for 4 to 6 months compared to 1 to 2 years.[277,278] Long-term thionamide drug therapy (mean 4.4 years) was associated with an extremely high remission rate of 76% over a mean follow-up period of 7.6 years, suggesting that drug therapy for many years is a reasonable alternative to ablative therapy with ^{131}I or surgery.[279] It would be most interesting to continue the long-term evaluation of these patients in order to determine whether the incidence of progressive thyroid failure would be even greater than the 25% incidence reported by Wood and Ingbar when patients were reevaluated 20 to 27 years after a single course of propylthiouracil of indeterminant length.[280] The latter findings certainly indicate that hypothyroidism is not infrequently the end result of Graves' disease, and that ablative therapy merely shortens the natural history of the progressively developing hypothyroidism. As noted above, disappearance of TSAb or TBII from the serum during drug treatment of Graves' disease almost always indicates remission of the disease. However, since these tests are not as yet readily available, the T_3 suppression test remains the most practical method to predict remission or persistence of Graves' disease. The T_3 suppression test employing the 20-min ^{123}I uptake has again been evaluated in two large series of patients with Graves' disease receiving thionamide drug therapy. Remission was present if the ^{123}I uptake was less than 10% on one occasion or 10 to 15% on two occasions 6 months apart,[281] or if the ^{123}I uptake was suppressed by more than 50% at 5 months and remained suppressed.[282] Almost all patients in the latter study relapsed if the thyroid ^{123}I uptake was not suppressed during the first 5 months of thionamide treatment. A long-term follow-up study of the natural history of Graves' disease following drug withdrawal indicates that serum thyroglobulin and TBII were poor predictors of recurrent thyrotoxicosis and that thyrotoxicosis was commonly seen when both T_3 suppression and TRH tests became or remained abnormal.[283]

The development of an RIA for PTU has permitted a more accurate assessment of its absorption and metabolism. PTU appears in the plasma 5 min after ingestion, has a shorter half-life in thyrotoxic patients than in euthyroid subjects (75 vs. 90 min), and peak plasma levels are similar in both groups.[284] No age-dependent changes in PTU kinetics were observed, but in studies in which PTU in plasma was measured spectrophotometrically, the absorption rate constant was 3 times higher in younger subjects.[285] When plasma methimazole (MMI) is measured by HPLC after ingestion of MMI or carbimazole (converted to MMI) by thyrotoxic patients, there are large individual variations in the plasma MMI levels achieved especially after carbimazole ingestion, probably due to incomplete and variable absorption of the drug.[286] In another study, the serum MMI concentration after a fixed dose of carbimazole also differed a great deal among individuals, and the response to the antithyroid drug was primarily dependent on the severity of the Graves' disease as reflected in the serum T_3 concentration.[287]

The results of therapy of Graves' disease with carbimazole, surgery, and ^{131}I in 837 patients from the "Land of Graves," Dublin, Ireland, and with thionamides and ^{131}I in 187 patients from Lexington, Kentucky, are summarized in two comprehensive reports.[288,289] In both studies, the relapse rate after thionamide therapy was very high, 91 and 84%, respectively, unless therapy was continued for more than 2 years, when the relapse rate was somewhat reduced to 62%. In both studies, the relapse rate following ^{131}I was low, and the occurrence of hypothyroidism high, especially in the American study. As reported previously, patients who were pretreated with thionamide drugs required a higher total dose of ^{131}I to achieve a cure, but the incidence of hypothyroidism was lower in these patients (54 vs. 73%). The relapse rate after surgery was small and the cumulative incidence of hypothyroidism at 10 years was 18%. Unfortunately, nine patients (3.4%) had permanent vocal cord paralysis and five (1.9%) permanent hypocalcemia.

The etiology of the hyperthyroidism caused by trophoblastic tumors has continued to be pursued and it is now generally believed that human chorionic gonadotropin (hCG) is probably the thyroid stimulator in this disorder. However, the demonstration that crude preparations of hCG have greater activity than purified hCG is displacing ^{125}I-labeled bovine TSH from receptor in human and bovine thyroid membranes, that desialylation of hCG greatly enhances the affinity of hCG for binding to sites in human thyroid receptors suggesting that the greater potency of crude hCG may be due to the presence of partially or fully desialylated hCG molecules,[290] and that partial digestion of the hCG molecule with carboxypeptidase markedly enhances human thyroid adenylate cyclase-stimulating activity[291] raise the possibility that pure hCG itself may not be responsible for the hyperthyroidism of trophoblastic disease. On the other hand, similar effects of crude and pure hCG in inhibiting [^{125}I]-TSH binding by human thyroid membranes have been reported,[292,293] and pure hCG stimulated human thyroid adenylate cyclase activity though only very slightly.[294]

The term "silent thyroiditis" has been used to define a constellation of findings consisting of the signs and symptoms, elevated serum T_4 and T_3 levels, a nontender diffuse goiter or no goiter, a low thyroid radioiodine uptake, lymphocytic thyroiditis on needle biopsy, and spontaneous remission after 2 to 5 months, often followed by transient hypothyroidism. Most investigators agree that this disease is different from painful, subacute thyroiditis; in the latter disorder, the patient frequently is systemically ill and has fever, the thyroid biopsy reveals giant cells, granulomatous changes, and far fewer lymphocytes, and the sedimentation rate is always elevated. Furthermore, in a long-term follow-up study of patients with these two disorders, the painful variety rarely led to permanent thyroid disease while painless thyroiditis was associated with a 50% incidence of goiter and/or hypothyroidism.[295] The histological abnormalities of extensive lymphocytic infiltration and degeneration of follicular cells are reversible and follow the clinical course of the disorder.[296] A very similar, if not identical, syndrome has been described in postpartum women.[297] Approximately 5.5% of postpartum women in Japan have been reported to develop transient hyper- and/or hypothyroidism 3 to 8 months after delivery. Many of these patients had positive serum thyroid antibodies and a surprising finding was the far higher frequency in women who delivered females (4 : 1). It has also been observed that this syndrome may recur following each delivery. Since the hyperthyroidism of silent thyroiditis is due to destruction of the thyroid follicles rather than enhanced secretion from hyperplastic follicles as seen in Graves' disease, the T_4/T_3 ratio has been used to differentiate silent thyroiditis from Graves' disease. In the former, the serum T_4/T_3 ratio is above 20, in contrast to values below 20 seen in patients with Graves' disease unless associated complications such as concurrent illness are present.[298] The other causes of destruction-induced hyperthyroidism (painful subacute thyroiditis and postpartum transient thyroid dysfunction) are also associated with a high T_4/T_3 ratio. The incidence of silent thyroiditis as a cause of hyperthyroidism is variable, probably reflecting the enthusiasm of the physician in searching carefully for this diagnosis. It is, however, extremely important to differentiate silent thyroiditis from Graves' disease, since the former is a self-limited disorder requiring only treatment with β blockers to relieve the symptoms of hyperthyroidism.

Although the syndrome is rare, hyperthyroidism can be caused by increased secretion of TSH. The etiology of the enhanced pituitary secretion of TSH remains unknown in a few patients but is due to selective pituitary resistance to T_4 and T_3 in some patients and a TSH-secreting pituitary tumor in others.[299] TBII were not present in the serum of 13 patients with TSH-mediated hyperthyroidism,[300] although Graves' disease has developed in two such patients.

A series of 349 patients with a solitary autonomously functioning thyroid nodule ("hot nodule") has been reviewed.[301] Sixty-two patients were hyperthyroid: 46% of these were T_3-toxic, the nodule was greater than 3 cm in diameter in almost all, and most patients were elderly. In contrast to findings in earlier studies, hyperthyroidism did develop within 1 to 6 years in approximately 8% of euthyroid patients, especially those with nodules greater than 3 cm in diameter. Hemiaplasia of the thyroid with thyrotoxicosis may be confused with hyperthyroidism secondary to an autonomous nodule.[302] A TSH stimulation test is essential to make this differentiation, although the presence of TBII or TSAb would also be helpful in distinguishing a toxic adenoma from Graves' disease with hemiaplasia. A subtle difference on thyroid scan is also helpful, since uptake would be seen in both the single lobe and isthmus (hockey stick sign) in patients with hemiaplasia, but only in the nodule in patients with a hot nodule.[303]

The mortality rate from thyroid storm has decreased markedly in recent years, owing to prompt treatment with iodides, the thionamide antithyroid drugs, β blockers, corticosteroids, and, more recently, the iodine-containing X-ray contrast dyes, Oragrafin® and Telepaque®.[304] Corticosteroids and the X-ray dyes are potent inhibitors of the peripheral conversion of T_4 to T_3 which explains their efficacy in the treatment of thyroid storm. The contrast dyes also have the added advantage of containing iodine, and the iodide released from these agents will result in a decrease in thyroid hormone release from the thyroid. Sudden death has been described in three patients following the ingestion of large quantities of L-thyroxine.[305] Ventricular fibrillation occurred and focal myocarditis was observed at autopsy examination. Accidental ingestion of various thyroid preparations is not uncommon, since so many patients are now being treated with thyroid hormone, especially L-thyroxine.

There is often a marked discrepancy between the striking elevation of the serum thyroid hormone concentrations and the mild clinical manifestation of thyrotoxicosis in patients who ingest large doses of thyroxine.[306]

It is well known that hyperthyroidism results in abnormalities in other organ systems. Over the years, many studies of the effects of hyperthyroidism on the endocrine pancreas, on the heart and catecholamines, and on calcium metabolism have been carried out, but with controversial results. Kabadi and Perez and their co-workers have recently reported a series of studies on various aspects of glucose metabolism in hyperthyroid patients.[307–309] Previous data had demonstrated increased, normal, or decreased insulin responses to an oral glucose load. In the more recent studies, oral glucose tolerance tests were carried out, and the hyperthyroid patients demonstrated an elevated 30-min plasma glucose with a delayed return, an increased plasma fasting insulin with an exaggerated insulin response, a decreased insulinogenic index and insulin–glucose coefficient, and a less pronounced drop in plasma glucagon after the glucose load. Thus, both decreased glucagon suppression and insulin resistance could be responsible for the abnormal glucose tolerance seen in hyperthyroidism. A protein meal stimulates both α and β cells of the pancreas. In thyrotoxic patients, a protein meal results in an elevation rather than a decrease in plasma glucose, a blunted glucagon response, and an enhanced insulin response, strongly suggesting a decreased sensitivity of the α cells and a hypersensitivity of the β cells. The glucoregulatory responses to physiological infusions of epinephrine or glucagon were also studied in hyperthyroid and normal subjects. Hyperthyroid patients had a reduced glycemic response to epinephrine and glucagon, a sustained response of glucose production to epinephrine and glucagon, and a lack of epinephrine-induced suppression of glucose clearance, most likely due to an exaggerated response of insulin secretion to epinephrine.

As in the case of glucose metabolism, the reported effects of hyperthyroidism on catecholamines and the heart have been extremely variable. There is no evidence that enhanced catecholamine production or release occurs in hyperthyroidism, and this is further indicated by the fact that insulin-induced hypoglycemia evokes a similar rise in plasma catecholamines in euthyroid and hyperthyroid subjects.[310] In studies in rat[311] and man,[312] conclusive evidence has recently been presented that hyperthyroidism induces an increase in cardiac and mononuclear leukocyte β receptors, respectively, providing a plausible mechanism for the enhanced responsiveness of the cardiovascular system to endogenous catecholamines in patients with hyperthyroidism. Mitral valve prolapse is now frequently diagnosed in the general population. It occurs even more frequently in patients with the autoimmune thyroid diseases, Graves' disease[313] and Hashimoto's thyroiditis,[314] and is unrelated to the level of thyroid function.

Hyperthyroidism results in a variety of changes in bone and mineral metabolism. These include decreased bone mineral content and muscle mass, as determined by neutron activation analysis of calcium and measurement of natural ^{40}K by whole body counting, respectively;[315] decreased plasma parathyroid hormone and 1,25-dihydroxyvitamin D, with normal plasma 25-hydroxyvitamin D, concentrations;[316] decreased absorption of ^{47}Ca at 24 hr;[317] and elevated plasma alkaline phosphatase concentration (bone and liver), with a further marked increase in the fraction derived from bone when the hyperthyroidism is treated, most likely due to bone repair and increased osteoblastic activity.[318] All of these effects appear to be mediated by excess thyroid hormone and not by abnormalities in parathyroid gland function.

Hypergastrinemia in patients with hyperthyroidism has been reported from Holland[319] and Japan,[320] and is not fully explained by decreased gastric acid output, but may be due to a hypersensitivity of the catecholamine β-adrenergic stimulus for gastrin release. In contrast, serum gastrin concentration was not elevated in hyperthyroid patients studied in the United States.[321]

A comprehensive review of the neurological manifestations of hyper- and hypothyroidism is now available.[322] Approximately 16% of thyrotoxic patients with myopathy have abnormal neuromuscular transmission similar to that observed in myasthenia gravis.[323] This observation is of great interest in view of the increased concurrence of these two disorders in an individual patient. The relationship between hyperthyroidism and emotional disturbances has been reexamined to determine whether patients who develop thyrotoxic Graves' disease have any underlying psychiatric abnormalities. Certain neurotic emotional disturbances and abnormal social interactions were present as assessed by psychological testing while these patients were hyperthyroid, but these abnormalities disappeared when the patients were euthyroid. The findings strongly suggest that the emotional problems were not indicative or underlying personality traits.[324] The prompt treatment of neonatal hypothyroidism almost always results in normal mental development. This does not appear to be the case with neonatal thyrotoxicosis, since craniosynostosis with impaired mental development is often seen in spite of therapy (5 of 7 patients),[325] a frequency of impaired mental development that is far greater than that reported in an earlier study.[326]

A thorough study of the hypothalamic–pituitary–testicular axis in adult males with thyrotoxicosis revealed a constellation of findings that indicate partial Leydig cell failure: normal serum free testosterone; increased serum LH and an enhanced LH response to LHRH; an increased serum estradiol (E_2) concentration; and a diminished sperm count that varied inversely with serum E_2.[327]

3.6. Hypothyroidism

Decreased thyroid reserve and frank primary hypothyroidism are frequently associated with immunologic and sometimes clinical features of other diseases, such as pernicious anemia and idiopathic adrenal atrophy (Schmidt's syndrome), in which autoimmunity plays a role. Type I diabetes mellitus is that variety in which autoimmune features, such as the presence of islet cell antibodies and a particular HLA association (Dw3), are likely to be found. Patients with Type I diabetes are much more likely than normal to harbor antithyroid-microsomal antibodies. In a recent study of several hundred patients with Type I or insulin-dependent diabetes mellitus, the prevalence of diminished thyroid reserve, as judged by an increase in serum TSH concentration, was found to be 12%.[328] This figure is about twice that reported for the general population and for patients with Type II diabetes mellitus. The prevalence in women alone was even greater (17%) and increased further with increasing age of onset of the diabetes.

A similar overlap exists with primary biliary cirrhosis. In a recent study of 95 patients with this disease,[329] 25 were found to have circulating antithyroid antibodies. Of these, approximately one-half displayed evidence of diminished thyroid reserve or frank hypothyroidism. Interestingly, the presence of antithyroid antibodies in this group of patients correlated in a highly significant fashion with coexisting lacrimal gland dysfunction. Thyroid gland fibrosis and hypothyroidism, possibly on an autoimmune basis, are also frequent and often unsuspected findings in patients with progressive systemic sclerosis.[330]

The association between Down's syndrome and thyroid autoimmunity is well established. In a recent survey,[331] 30 to 101 patients with Down's syndrome were found to have circulating antithyroid antibodies, and 16, of whom most were antibody-positive, displayed evidence of diminished thyroid reserve or frank hypothyroidism. Recognition of this association is important because the clinical features of hypothyroidism may be difficult to discern in a patient with Down's syndrome, and thyroid hormone replacement will result in a significant improvement in the quality of life.

Attention has recently been drawn to the association between hypothyroidism and occupational exposure to brominated hydrocarbons.[332] These agents, which are used as fire retardants, may interfere with the oxidation and organic-binding of intrathyroid iodide. It is note-worthy that those workers who displayed evidence of hypothyroidism were also found to have high titers of circulating antithyroid-microsomal antibodies, suggesting that preexisting thyroid autoimmunity may render the gland more susceptible to the antithyroid effect of the brominated hydrocarbons. Scattered reports in the past have called attention to the induction of hypothyroidism following mantle irradiation therapy for lymphoma or head and neck carcinoma. Two recent comprehensive studies have emphasized the high incidence of hypothyroidism (more than two-thirds) occurring within 5 years of X-ray treatment.[333,334]

The role of maternal antithyroid antibodies in the pathogenesis of congenital hypothyroidism in the child has been uncertain. A recent study undertaken by the Quebec Provincial Network for Genetic Medicine has helped to resolve this uncertainty.[335] Antimicrosomal antibodies were measured in paired maternal and cord blood samples and in blood samples that had been collected as part of the screening program for congenital hypothyroidism. The results were correlated with values for T_4 and TSH concentrations. Although there was an excellent correlation between maternal and neonatal antibody titers in the paired samples, there was no difference in antibody prevalence in the normal or low T_4 neonatal groups or in the neonatal group with frank hypothyroidism. These findings confirm that antimicrosomal antibodies cross the placenta, but strongly suggest that such antibodies are not implicated in the pathogenesis of congenital hypothyroidism. Although there is some question whether severe untreated maternal hypothyroidism will result in fetal abnormalities or impaired somatic and mental development, a recent study by Mestman and co-workers did not reveal any abnormalities in the fetus or in subsequent development that could be attributed to the presence of the maternal hypothyroidism.[336]

A significant proportion of patients with antithyroid antibodies, but without clinical evidence of thyroid dysfunction, display increased serum TSH concentrations, reflecting the presence of diminished thyroid reserve. A recent study involving 60 such asymptomatic patients with antithyroid antibodies provides evidence for a graded diminution of thyroid reserve.[337] Of these 60 patients, 10 were found to have increased basal serum TSH concentrations, 29 had a normal basal serum TSH concentration but displayed enhanced TSH responsiveness to TRH, and the remainder had entirely normal TSH-secretory dynamics. Although all values for serum T_4 concentration were within the normal range, the values were lowest in the group with increased basal serum TSH, intermediate in the group with normal basal TSH but enhanced responsiveness to TRH, and highest in the group with entirely normal TSH dynamics. The overall prevalence of diminished thyroid reserve in the 60 patients in this study was 65%.

Programs for screening neonates for congenital hypothyroidism have been established in various regions of the United States and Canada over the last several years. An ad hoc committee on newborn screening established by the American Thyroid Association has recently presented the results of screening of more than 1 million neonates.[338] The overall prevalence of congenital hypothyroidism was found to be 1 in 3684 live births and, in almost 90% of instances, was determined to be primary in nature. Of utmost importance was the finding that only in very rare instances had the hypothyroidism been suspected clinically before the results of the screening became available. In view of the fact that early treatment prevents mental retardation, the cost of screening approximately 4000 neonates (about $6000) to detect one infant with congenital hypothyroidism is extremely favorable.

Measurement of the concentration of rT_3 in amniotic fluid has been suggested as a means of evaluating thyroid function in the fetus. This is predicated on the evidence that the rT_3 in amniotic fluid is of fetal origin. A recent report suggests, however, that amniotic fluid rT_3 concentrations may not be a reliable indicator of fetal hypothyroidism.[339] Two women who had previously given birth to infants with congenital hypothyroidism underwent amniocentesis during the second trimester. In the one case in which amniotic fluid rT_3 concentrations were low, a normal infant was delivered. In the other case, amniotic fluid rT_3 concentrations were quite normal for the stage of pregnancy, but a hypothyroid infant was subsequently delivered.

A cardiomyopathy is not an uncommon accompaniment of severe myxedema. Nonetheless, there was until recently little, if any, published data concerning its echocardiographic characteristics. This deficiency is beginning to be corrected. In a recent study, echocardiographic evaluation was undertaken in 19 consecutive patients with hypothyroidism.[340] Surprisingly, 17 of the 19 displayed evidence of asymmetric septal hypertrophy and some, in addition, displayed evidence of left ventricular outflow tract obstruction, features reminiscent of idiopathic hypertrophic subaortic stenosis (IHSS). These abnormalities disappeared after a euthyroid state had been restored by treatment. The hemodynamic impact of such a cardiomyopathy is uncertain, however. Systolic time intervals in patients with hypothyroidism are the converse of those found in patients with IHSS, i.e., the preejection period is prolonged and the left ventricular ejection time shortened.[341] In view of this apparent discordance, as well as the potential clinical implications of an obstructive cardiomyopathy, additional studies are needed in which both hemodynamic and echocardiographic characteristics are evaluated.

A relatively high frequency of subclinical hypothyroidism (approximately 20%) was detected in healthy persons over age 60,[342] and an association between borderline low thyroid function, thyroid autoimmunity, and coronary heart disease unrelated to serum cholesterol has been observed.[343] Since the frequency of hypothyroidism in elderly patients is quite high, it is inevitable that some patients requiring coronary bypass surgery will also be overtly hypothyroid. Surprisingly, these patients do not require replacement therapy prior to or shortly after surgery to ensure good surgical results.[344] It is suggested, therefore, that doses of L-thyroxine that restore the serum TSH to normal are not required in these patients preoperatively.

The rate of bone resorption is decreased in hypothyroidism, but the serum calcium concentration usually remains within the range of normal. The maintenance of a normal serum calcium concentration has been ascribed to a compensatory increase in parathyroid hormone secretion with resulting increased 1,25-dihydroxyvitamin D_3 generation. This indeed appears to be the case; recent work has demonstrated that the serum concentration of 1,25-dihydroxyvitamin D_3, as well as that of parathyroid hormone, is increased in hypothyroid patients.[316]

The mechanisms of edema formation in myxedema have finally been carefully studied. The extravascular accumulation of albumin and probably other plasma proteins is important in the generalized edema, and inadequate lymphatic drainage also explains the formation of exudates in the serous cavities frequently present in myxedema.[345] Severe hypothyroidism is also associated with obstructive sleep apnea,[346] muscle stiffness and pseudohypertrophy (Hoffman's syndrome),[347] and multiple cutaneous focal mucinoses.[348] Elevated serum CEA concentrations are present in myxedema, probably due to decreased degradation of the tumor marker;[349] thus, an elevation in CEA in patients with hypothyroidism does not necessarily indicate malignancy.

An increase in serum cholesterol concentration is the most commonly recognized abnormality of lipid metabolism in primary hypothyroidism and has been shown to be comprised of an increase in low-density lipoprotein (LDL) cholesterol. A recent report corroborates the increase in LDL cholesterol and, in addition, demonstrates that high-density lipoprotein (HDL) cholesterol is reduced in patients with hypothyroidism.[350] Interestingly, HDL cholesterol was also found to be reduced to an even greater extent in patients with hyperthyroidism. In both states, the values for HDL cholesterol returned toward normal with treatment. D-Thyroxine has been used in the management of hyperlipidemia. This was predicated on an alleged dissociation between cholesterol-lowering and metabolism-stimulating activities. A recent study does not support such a dissociation of activities, at least in patients with hypothyroidism.[351] In this study, the effects of L- and D-thyroxine were compared with respect to reduction in serum cholesterol concentration, suppression of serum TSH concentration, and stimulation of the BMR.

The dosage of D-thyroxine that produced a decrease in serum cholesterol concentration comparable to that produced by L-thyroxine also resulted in a comparable decrease in serum TSH concentration and a comparable increase in BMR. The approximate dosage equivalence was 4 mg of D-thyroxine to 0.15 mg of L-thyroxine. This study provides further support for the view that D-thyroxine has little use in the management of hypercholesterolemia in euthyroid individuals.

Some interesting observations have been made over the past few years concerning L-thyroxine therapy of hypothyroidism. In contrast to earlier studies, replacement doses of L-thyroxine sufficient to suppress the serum TSH are often associated with serum T_4 values above the normal range.[352] Patients such as these are clinically euthyroid, probably owing to the fact that the serum T_3 concentrations are normal. L-Thyroxine replacement doses for treating hypothyroidism decrease with age from a mean of 158 μg T_4/day in younger patients to 118 μg/day in elderly patients.[353] These findings do offer some help in the therapy of hypothyroidism and suggest that the serum T_4 concentration may be misleading in the management of primary hypothyroid patients. The serum TSH and, perhaps, the serum T_3 concentration appear to be of greater value.

Finally, in the past few years two excellent reviews dealing with certain aspects of hypothyroidism have appeared. One is a useful review of hypothyroidism in childhood[354] and the other is a comprehensive discussion of thyroid ontogeny and thyroid dysfunction in the neonate.[184]

3.7. Nontoxic Goiter

A comprehensive review of simple goiter and its variants has recently been published by Studer and Ramelli[355] and the diagnostic approach to the solitary thyroid thoroughly discussed in a recent UCLA Conference.[356] TSAb do not appear to be etiologic factors in the development of nonautonomous, autonomous, or toxic nodular goiter.[357] The important role of TSH in the genesis of nontoxic goiter has been reemphasized in a study of the pituitary–thyroid axis after hemithyroidectomy for a solitary cold nodule in euthyroid subjects. In these patients, the serum TSH concentration rose significantly (but still within the normal range) by the 30th postoperative day and remained elevated for 90 days.[358] Three years later, all parameters of thyroid function were similar to preoperative values. Although Blichert-Toft and colleagues observed similar rises in serum TSH after surgery for uninodular or multinodular goiter, they did not recommend thyroid suppression therapy after surgery and did not observe recurrent goiter, but the time of observation was only 1 year.[359] We do not agree with this recommendation, since recurrent goiter can be seen years after surgery for nontoxic goiter, and we recommend that these patients receive suppressive doses of L-thyroxine indefinitely. However, thyroid suppression therapy is not effective in preventing the recurrence of benign thyroid cysts after initial aspiration.[360]

Topographical studies of the cAMP, iodine, and DNA contents, as well as the heterogeneity of thyroglobulin, from different regions of 12 surgically removed multinodular goiters have strongly suggested that the pathogenesis of nodular goiters involves a metabolic disorder at the level of the follicular cells, with a wide variation among different follicles.[361] cAMP phosphodiesterase activity and the regulation of cAMP and prostaglandin formation have been evaluated in normal thyroid glands and in various thyroid disorders.[362,363] Goiters due to inborn errors of thyroid hormone synthesis continue to be described: the iodide trapping defect in one patient appeared to be due to an impairment in the specific iodide carrier system,[364] and poorly iodinated thyroglobulin from a goitrous cretin with no detectable peroxidase activity was similar to normal thyroglobulin in its secondary, tertiary, and quaternary structures.[365] A kindred with nodular goiter due to a leak of nonhormonal iodide has been reported, and two of these patients developed metastatic follicular carcinoma years after subtotal thyroidectomy.[365] These two subjects had not received suppressive therapy with thyroid hormone after surgery.

Bacterial contamination of drinking water has been implicated as a causal factor in endemic deficiency goiter in some areas. In western Columbia, sedimentary rocks rich in organic matter may be the source of water borne goitrogens. Gaitan *et al.* also evaluated the role of bacterial contamination of water in goiter formation in this area.[367] Overall concentration of bacteria in the feeder pipeline was marginally related to goiter prevalence, whereas the presence of *K. pneumoniae* in the water was associated with a lower prevalence of goiter. It was suggested that the lower goiter incidence associated with *K. pneumoniae* contamination may be due to biodegradation of the organic contaminants derived from the sedimentary rocks. An association between autoimmune thyroid disease and an inordinate frequency of humoral and cell-mediated immunity against *Yersinia enterocolitica* was reported a few years ago. Very recently, Ingbar and colleagues have described TSH receptors in the plasma membranes of *Yersinia* and *E. coli*, suggesting a possible link between these organisms and the pathogenesis of these thyroid disorders.[368]

3.8. Thyroid Carcinoma

The fine-needle aspiration technique for the cytologic evaluation of the thyroid nodule is being used with increasing frequency in selecting patients for thyroid surgery. Recent reports further corroborate the reliability of this procedure. In a study of 300 patients with thyroid nodules, aspiration cytology correctly predicted the presence of thyroid carcinoma in 19 of the 23 patients so afflicted.[369] A false-positive result was obtained in only 4 of the 277 cases of benign disease. As part of another study, the results obtained with fine-needle aspiration cytology were compared with those obtained by coarse-needle biopsy in relation to the findings at surgery.[370] Although the frequency of a false-positive result was greater with the former technique and somewhat higher than that reported in other series, the frequency of false-negative results was very low and, most importantly, the same with both techniques (~4%). A more recent report by the same workers confirms the efficacy of fine-needle aspiration biopsy in the diagnosis of papillary thyroid cancer.[371] In view of its simplicity and virtual lack of complications, the fine-needle aspiration technique is to be preferred, in the author's view. Cytologic interpretation by an experienced cytologist is, of course, of paramount importance, and accordingly, this procedure should not be undertaken as a *diagnostic* maneuver in a setting where such expertise is not available.

The clinical usefulness of serum calcitonin measurement as a tumor marker in medullary thyroid carcinoma is well established. A retrospective, longitudinal analysis of serum calcitonin concentrations, both basal and stimulated, has recently been undertaken in 32 patients with medullary thyroid carcinoma who had such measurements made before and after various forms of therapy.[372] Several interesting findings emerged. Delay in implementing therapy was accompanied by a gradual increase in the serum calcitonin concentration. Following total thyroidectomy, the serum calcitonin concentration fell in the immediate postoperative period, but took from 1 month to as long as 6 years to reach its nadir. (The mechanism underlying this delay in further decline is unclear.) Thereafter, the serum calcitonin concentration began to increase, even though clinical or radiologic evidence of disease was absent. This increase may have reflected the presence of occult metastases. With clinically overt recurrence of metastases, the serum calcitonin concentration was usually increased distinctly and to a greater extent than in the group with clinically silent disease, although overlap did occur. Noteworthy is the observation that total thyroidectomy was uniformly followed by a decline in the serum calcitonin concentration, whereas this was not the case with radiotherapy or chemotherapy, indicating that surgical removal is the most effective form of treatment. The clinical characteristics seen in a large series of patients with familial, as compared with sporadic medullary carcinomas, revealed that the familial variety was often bilateral, had C-cell hyperplasia in thyroid tissue distant from the primary cancer, and was associated with other endocrine tumors and nonendocrine malignancies.[373] An unusual familial syndrome of medullary and papillary thyroid carcinoma in the same gland, together with one sibling who had papillary cancer and another sibling who had medullary cancer, has been described.[374] Medullary thyroid carcinomas elaborate a variety of biologically active materials, some of which produce distinctive clinical syndromes. In a recent study, an immunohistologic technique was exploited to examine tumor content of β-endorphin, ACTH, and somatostatin, in addition to that of calcitonin.[375] Among the 19 human medullary thyroid carcinomas and 2 C-cell hyperplastic lesions studied, all contained calcitonin. Fifteen of sixteen studied were found to be positive for β-endorphin, 7 of 9 for ACTH, and 3 of 6 for somatostatin. These findings suggest that a close association exists among these peptides in C-cell lesions.

Although there is a clear association between low-dose radiation and the later development of thyroid carcinoma (which may continue to appear for up to 60 months in patients with negative scans when initially observed[376]), high-dose radiation, i.e., radiation in excess of 2000 rads, does not appear to be associated with thyroid carcinoma. This has been ascribed to impairment by high-dose radiation of the replicative potential of thyroid cells. A recent report suggests, however, that patients who have received high-dose radiation may indeed be at increased risk for the development of thyroid carcinoma, though much less so than following low-dose radiation.[377] Of 544 patients with Hodgkin's lymphoma who underwent mantle radiation over a 10-year period, 3 developed differentiated thyroid carcinoma, a figure that is far in excess of the incidence rate of thyroid carcinoma in the nonirradiated population. Since high-dose external radiation induces diminished thyroid reserve in a significant proportion of patients, it was suggested that prolonged hyperstimulation by TSH of cells that still possess replicative potential may be a factor in the development of carcinoma.

Primary lymphoma of the thyroid is rare and may resemble small cell carcinoma histologically. A recent study describes the clinical and histopathologic features of primary lymphoma of the thyroid.[378] The patients were usually elderly women who presented with a rapidly enlarging thyroid and symptoms due to compression of adjacent structures. Features that portended a favorable prognosis included confinement of the disease to the thyroid and a plasmacytoid cell type. Noteworthy was the finding that in most instances the thyroid was the seat of lymphocytic thyroiditis, suggesting that the lymphoma may have had its origins in a preexisting autoimmune disorder of the thyroid.

Some uncertainty has existed concerning the characteristics of TSH-binding and adenylate cyclase stimulation in thyroid carcinoma. Accordingly, a recent study examined TSH-binding and TSH stimulation of cAMP production in crude membrane fractions prepared from a large number of diverse thyroid carcinomas.[379] In general, it was found that well-differentiated follicular carcinoma resembled normal tissue with respect to TSH-binding and stimulatory characteristics. Moderately differentiated follicular and papillary carcinomas differed significantly from normal tissue in displaying a decreased number of TSH-binding sites and a decreased cAMP response to TSH. Undifferentiated carcinoma and medullary thyroid carcinoma were characterized by absence of TSH-binding and response to TSH stimulation. Thus, in general, a correlation was shown to exist between the degree of dedifferentiation of thyroid carcinoma and the extent to which TSH-binding and stimulatory characteristics were altered.

Evaluation for the presence of residual or metastatic differentiated thyroid cancer should include measurements of serum thyroglobulin, since many studies now suggest that serum thyroglobulin may be elevated even in the presence of negative thyroid and total body ^{131}I scans.[380–383] There is no question that thyroid cancer remains if the serum thyroglobulin is elevated while the patient is receiving L-thyroxine after thyroidectomy and ablative ^{131}I therapy. If the serum thyroglobulin is undetectable while the patient is receiving L-thyroxine therapy, liothyronine should be substituted for L-thyroxine for approximately 1 month and then discontinued. Approximately 2 to 4 weeks later, serum thyroglobulin is measured, and an ^{131}I total body scan is obtained. Occasionally, the scan will be negative and the serum thyroglobulin readily detectable. In this situation, it is very likely that thyroid cancer is present, but treatment with ^{131}I is probably not justified since no ^{131}I uptake is detected. These patients should be observed more frequently, however.

The recurrence of papillary and follicular thyroid cancer is less frequent in patients treated with a combination of total thyroidectomy, postoperative ^{131}I, and thyroid hormone, except in those patients with small papillary cancers (<1.5 cm) in whom less than total thyroidectomy and postoperative therapy with thyroid hormone alone gives results similar to those following more aggressive therapy.[384 385] The dose of ^{131}I that should be used in the treatment of thyroid cancer is now open to some debate. Many patients can be adequately treated with 30 mCi ^{131}I, which can be administered on an outpatient basis, decreases the total body radiation dose, and eliminates the expense of hospitalization.[386] External beam irradiation can be effective therapy for recurrent thyroid cancer and metastatic lesions that do not concentrate ^{131}I.[387]

3.9. Miscellaneous

The previously reported association of thyroid hormone adminis-tration and breast cancer has been thoroughly refuted by two recent studies that found absolutely no relationship between the incidence of breast cancer and the use of thyroid supplements.[388,389] Although thy-roid hormone receptors have been detected in human breast cancer tissue, the T_3 receptor concentration was not correlated with age or endocrine status of the patient or with extension or histologic grading of the tumor.[390] The presence of an increased-molecular-weight TSH with impaired biologic activity has been described in a euthyroid sub-ject.[391] This abnormal TSH was immunoreactive, resulting in an elevated serum TSH by RIA, and bound normally to the TSH receptor, but showed decreased stimulation of adenylate cyclase in human thyroid membranes.

A series of studies in various animal and fish models has called attention to some unusual aspects of thyroid physiology. A new auto-somal recessive mutation causing hypothyroidism has been identified in mice.[392] The thyroids are hypoplastic and unresponsive to TSH. The nude mouse has proven to be a possible model for the transplantation of human thyroid tissue. This transplanted tissue continues to maintain its structural and functional properties.[393] The hereditary insulin-de-pendent diabetic BB/W rat not only has lymphocytic infiltration with subsequent destruction of the islet β cells but also associated lymphocytic thyroiditis.[394] This rat model is similar, therefore, to man, in whom there is an association of diabetes mellitus and autoimmune thyroid disease.

ACKNOWLEDGMENT

Supported in part by Grant AM-18919 from the NIAMDD.

References

1. Jackson, I. M. D., 1982, Thyrotropin-releasing hormone, *N. Engl. J. Med.* **306**:145–155.

2. Kubek, M., Wilber, J. F., and George, J. M., 1979, The distribution and concentration of thyrotropin-releasing hormone in discrete human hypothalamic nuclei, Endocrinology **105**:537–540.

3. Aizawa, T., and Greer, M. A., 1981, Delineation of the hypothalamic area controlling thyrotropin secretion in the rat, *Endocrinology* **109**:1731–1738.

4. Engler, D., Scanlon, M. F., and Jackson, I. M. D., 1981, Thyrotropin-releasing hormone in the systemic circulation of the neonatal rat is derived from the pancreas and other extraneural tissues, *J. Clin. Invest.* **67**:800–808.

5. Shambaugh, G., III, Kubek, M., and Wilber, J. F., 1979, Thyrotropin-releasing hormone activity in the human placenta, *J. Clin. Endocrinol. Metab.* **48**:483–486.

6. Youngblood, W. W., Humm, J., Lipton, M. A., and Kizer, J. S., 1980, Thyrotropin-releasing hormone-like bioactivity in placenta: Evidence for the existence of substances other than Pyroglu-His-Pro-NH$_2$ (TRH) capable of stimulating pituitary thyrotropin release, *Endocrinology* **106**:541–546.

7. Bhandaru, L., and Emerson, C. H., 1980, Evidence for the presence of the putative TRH metabolite, deamido-TRH, in human urine, *J. Clin. Endocrinol. Metab.* **51**:410–412.

8. Emerson, C. H., Vogel, W., Currie, B. L., and Okal, T., 1980, Concentrations of thyrotropin-releasing hormone (TRH) and deamido-TRH, and TRH deamidase activity in brain, *Endocrinology* **107**:443–449.

9. Yanagisawa, T., Prasad, C., and Peterkofsky, A., 1980, The subcellular and organ distribution and natural form of histidyl-proline diketopiperazine in rat brain determined by a specific radioimmunoassay, *J. Biol. Chem.* **255**:10290–10298.

10. Emerson, C. H., Alex, S., Braverman, L. E., and Safran, M. S., 1981, A study of the effect of the thyrotropin-releasing hormone metabolite, histidyl proline diketopiperazine, on prolactin in vivo, *Endocrinology* **109**:1375–1379.

11. Morley, J. E., Garvin, T. J., Pekary, A. E., Utiger, R. D., Nair, M. G., Baugh, C. M., and Hershman, J. M., 1979, Plasma clearance and plasma half-disappearance time of exogenous thyrotropin-releasing hormone and pyroglutamyl-N^{3im}-methyl-histidyl prolineamide, *J. Clin. Endocrinol. Metab.* **48**:377–380.

12. Emerson, C. H., Mishal, A., Mahabeer, H. L., and Currie, B. L., 1979, Lack of evidence for thyrotropin-releasing hormone deamidation in normal and hyperthyroid human sera, *J. Clin. Endocrinol. Metab.* **49**:138–140.

13. Jackson, I. M. D., Papapetrou, P. D., and Reichlin, S., 1979, Metabolic clearance of thyrotropin-releasing hormone in the rat in hypothyroid and hyperthyroid states: Comparison with serum degradation in vitro, *Endocrinology* **104**:1292–1298.

14. Naor, Z., Snyder, G., Fawcett, C. P., and McCann, S. M., 1980, Pituitary cyclic nucleotides and thyrotropin-releasing hormone action: The relationship of adenosine 3′,5′-monophosphate and guanosine 3′,5′-monophosphate to the release of thyrotropin and prolactin, *Endocrinology* **106**:1304–1310.

15. Snyder, G., Naor, Z., Fawcett, C. P., and McCann, S. M., 1981, Action of thyrotropin-releasing hormone on mammotrophs and thyrotrophs, *Am. J. Physiol.* **241**:E298–E304.
16. Roti, E., Gnudi, A., Robuschi, G., Emanuele, R., Benassi, L., and Braverman, L. E., 1982, Response of growth hormone (GH) to thyrotropin-releasing hormone (TRH) during fetal life, *J. Clin. Endocrinol. Metab.* **54**:1255–1257.
17. Snyder, P. J., Muzyka, R., Johnson, J., and Utiger, R. D., 1980, Thyrotropin-releasing hormone provokes abnormal follicle-stimulating hormone (FSH) and luteinizing hormone responses in men who have pituitary adenomas and FSH hypersecretion, *J. Clin. Endocrinol. Metab.* **51**:744–748.
18. Faden, A. I., Jacobs, T. P., and Holaday, J. W., 1981, Thyrotropin-releasing hormone improves neurologic recovery after spinal trauma in cats, *N. Engl. J. Med.* **305**:1063–1067.
19. Holaday, J. W., D'Amato, R. J., and Faden, A. I., 1981, Thyrotropin-releasing hormone improves cardiovascular function in experimental endotoxic and hemorrhagic shock, *Science* **213**:216–218.
20. Parker, D. C., Pekary, A. E., and Hershman, J. M., 1976, Effect of normal and reversed sleep–wake cycles upon nyctohemeral rhythmicity of plasma thyrotropin: Evidence suggestive of an inhibitory influence in sleep, *J. Clin. Endocrinol. Metab.* **43**:318–329.
21. Minuto, F., Bagnasco, M., Giusti, M., Grimaldi, G., Biassoni, P., Ferrini, O., and Giordano, G., 1981, Twenty-four hour profile of integrated TSH concentration in puberty, *J. Endocrinol. Invest.* **4**:7–10.
22. Spencer, C. A., Greenstadt, M. A., Wheeler, W. S., Kletzky, O. A., and Nicoloff, J. T., 1980, The influence of long-term low dose thyrotropin-releasing hormone infusions on serum thyrotropin and prolactin concentrations in man, *J. Clin. Endocrinol. Metab.* **51**:771–775.
23. Hinkle, P. M., Perrone, M. H., and Schonbrunn, A., 1981, Mechanism of thyroid hormone inhibition of thyrotropin-releasing hormone action, *Endocrinology* **108**:199–205.
24. Silva, J. E., and Larsen, P. R., 1978, Contributions of plasma triiodothyronine and local thyroxine monodeiodination to triiodothyronine to nuclear triiodothyronine receptor saturation in pituitary, liver, and kidney of hypothyroid rats, *J. Clin. Invest.* **61**:1247–1259.
25. Larsen, P. R., Dick, T. E., Markovitz, B. P., Kaplan, M. M., and Gard, T. G., 1979, Inhibition of intrapituitary thyroxine to 3,5,3′-triiodothyronine conversion prevents the acute suppression of thyrotropin release by thyroxine in hypothyroid rats, *J. Clin. Invest.* **64**:117–128.
26. Kleinmann, R. E., Vagenakis, A. G., and Braverman, L. E., 1980, The effect of iopanoic acid on the regulation of thyrotropin secretion in euthyroid subjects, *J. Clin. Endocrinol. Metab.* **51**:399–403.
27. Larsen, P. R., 1982, Feedback regulation of thyrotropin secretion by thyroid hormones, *N. Engl. J. Med.* **306**:23–32.
28. Scanlon, F., Chan, V., Heath, M., Pourmand, M., Rodriguez-Arnao, M. D., Weightman, R., Lewis, M., and Hall, R., 1981, Dopaminergic control of thyrotropin α-subunit, thyrotropin β-subunit, and prolactin in euthy-

roidism and hypothyroidism: Dissociated responses to dopamine receptor blockade with metoclopramide in hypothyroid subjects, *J. Clin. Endocrinol. Metab.* **53:**360–365.

29. Feek, C. M., Sawers, J. S. A., Brown, N. S., Seth, J., Irvine, W. J., and Toft, A. D., 1980, Influence of thyroid status on dopaminergic inhibition of thyrotropin and prolactin secretion: Evidence for an additional feedback mechanism in the control of thyroid hormone secretion, *J. Clin. Endocrinol. Metab.* **51:**585–589.

30. Pamenter, R. W., and Hedge, G. A., 1980, Inhibition of thyrotropin secretion by physiological levels of corticosterone, *Endocrinology* **106:**162–166.

31. Cobb, W. E., Reichlin, S., and Jackson, I. M. D., 1981, Growth hormone secretory status is a determinant of the thyrotropin response to thyrotropin-releasing hormone in euthyroid patients with hypothalamic–pituitary disease, *J. Clin. Endocrinol. Metab.* **52:**324–329.

32. Tamagna, E. I., Hershman, J. M., and Jorgensen, E. C., 1979, Thyrotropin suppression by 3,5-dimethyl-3'-isopropyl-L-thyroxine in man, *J. Clin. Endocrinol. Metab.* **48:**196–200.

33. Bech, K., Feldt-Rasmussen, U., and Madsen, S. N., 1981, Influence of thyroglobulin on basal and stimulated human thyroid adenylate cyclase activity, *J. Clin. Endocrinol. Metab.* **53:**264–269.

34. Zakarija, M., Witte, A., and McKenzie, J. M., 1980, Influence of cholera toxin on in vitro refractoriness to thyrotropin of thyroids from rats fed propylthiouracil, *Endocrinology* **107:**2045–2050.

35. Holmes, S. D., Titus, G., Chou, M., and Field, J. B., 1980, Effects of thyrotropin and cholera toxin on the thyroidal adenylate cyclase–adenosine 3',5'-monophosphate system, *Endocrinology* **107:**2076–2081.

36. Zakarija, M., and McKenzie, J. M., 1980, Influences of cholera toxin on thyroid stimulation by thyrotropin and thyroid-stimulating antibody, *Endocrinology* **107:**2051–2054.

37. Engström, G., and Ericson, L. E., 1981, Effect of graded doses of thyrotropin on exocytosis and early phase of endocytosis in the rat thyroid, *Endocrinology* **108:**399–405.

38. Ericson, L. E., and Wollman, S. H., 1980, Increase in the rough endoplasmic reticulum in capillary endothelial cells and pericytes in hyperplastic rat thyroid glands, *Endocrinology* **107:**732–737.

39. Laurberg, P., 1981, Iodothyronine secretion from perfused dog thyroid lobes after prolonged thyrotropin treatment in vivo, *Endocrinology* **109:**1560–1565.

40. Laurberg, P., 1980, Iodothyronine release from the perfused canine thyroid following cessation of stimulation, *J. Clin. Invest.* **65:**488–495.

41. Laurberg, P., 1980, Secretion of 3,3'-diiodothyronine by the perfused canine thyroid isolated in situ, *Endocrinology* **107:**989–993.

42. Wollman, S. H., and Ekholm, R., 1981, Site of iodination in hyperplastic thyroid glands deduced from autoradiographs, *Endocrinology* **108:**2082–2085.

43. Rosenberg, I. N., and Goswami, A., 1979, Purification and characterization of a flavoprotein from bovine thyroid with iodotyrosine deiodinase activity, *J. Biol. Chem.* **254:**12318–12325.

44. Hildebrandt, J. D., and Halmi, N. S., 1980, Intrathyroidally generated iodide: The role of propylthiouracil-sensitive processes in its production, *Endocrinology* **107**:830–838.

45. Hildebrandt, J. D., and Halmi, N. S., 1981, Intrathyroidally generated iodide: The role of transport in its utilization, *Endocrinology* **108**:842–849.

46. Chiraseveenuprapund, P., and Rosenberg, I. N., 1981, Effects of hydrogen peroxide-generating systems on the Wolff–Chaikoff effect, *Endocrinology* **109**:2095–2101.

47. Uchimura, H., Chiu, S. C., Kuzaya, N., Ikeda, H., Ito, K., and Nagataki, S., 1980, Effect of iodine enrichment in vitro on the adenylate cyclase–adenosine 3′,5′-monophosphate system in thyroid glands from normal subjects and patients with Graves' disease, *J. Clin. Endocrinol. Metab.* **50**:1066–1070.

48. Sherwin, J. R., and Mills, I., 1980, Epinephrine inhibits thyrotropin-stimulated adenosine 3′,5′-monophosphate accumulation in cat thyroid tissue, *Endocrinology* **106**:28–34.

49. Pisarev, M. A., Cardinali, D. P., Juvenal, G. J., Vacas, M. I., Barontini, M., and Boado, R. J., 1981, Role of the sympathetic nervous system in the control of the goitrogenic response in the rat, *Endocrinology* **109**:2202–2207.

50. Maayan, M. L., Volpert, E. M., and From, A., 1981, Norepinephrine and thyrotropin effects on the thyroid in vitro: Simultaneous stimulation of iodide organification and antagonism of thyroxine release, *Endocrinology* **109**:930–934.

51. Van Sande, J., Dumont, J. E., Melander, A., and Sundler, F., 1980, Presence and influence of cholinergic nerves in the human thyroid, *J. Clin. Endocrinol. Metab.* **51**:500–502.

52. Ahren, B., Alumets, J., Ericsson, M., Fahrenkrug, J., Fahrenkrug, L., Håkanson, R., Hedner, P., Loren, I., Melander, A., Rerup, C., and Sundler, F., 1980, VIP occurs in intrathyroidal nerves and stimulates thyroid hormone secretion, *Nature (London)* **287**: 343–345.

53. Van Herle, A. J., Vassart, G., and Dumont, J. E., 1979, Control of thyroglobulin synthesis and secretion, *N. Engl. J. Med.* **301**:307–314.

54. Scherberg, N. H., Vassart, G., Lecocq, R., Dumont, J. E., and Refetoff, S., 1981, Modulation of thyroglobulin messenger RNA accumulation in the rat thyroid, *Endocrinology* **109**:1650–1656.

55. Haeberli, A., Kneubuehl, F., and Studer, H., 1981, Changes in the polypeptide assembly of guinea pig thyroglobulin induced by thyrotropin-regulated thyroid activity, *Endocrinology* **109**:523–529.

56. Ikekubo, K., Kishihara, M., Sanders, J., Sutton, J., and Schneider, A. B., 1981, Differences between circulating and tissue thyroglobulin in rats, *Endocrinology* **109**:427–432.

57. Unger, J., Van Heuverswyn, B., Decoster, C., Cantraine, F., Mockel, J., and Van Herle, A., 1980, Thyroglobulin and thyroid hormone release after intravenous administration of bovine thyrotropin in man, *J. Clin. Endocrinol. Metab.* **51**:590–594.

58. Bayer, M. F., and Kriss, J. P., 1979, Immunoradiometric assay for serum thyroglobulin: Semiquantitative measurement of thyroglobulin in antithyroglobulin-positive sera, *J. Clin. Endocrinol. Metab.* **49**:557–564.

59. Mariotti, S., Martino, E., Cupini, C., Lari, R., Giani, C., Baschieri, L., and Pinchera, A., 1982, Low serum thyroglobulin as a clue to the diagnosis of thyrotoxicosis factitia, *N. Engl. J. Med.* **307**:410–412.

60. Banerjee, R. K., and Datta, A. G., 1981, Gastric peroxidase—Localization, catalytic properties and possible role in extrathyroidal thyroid hormone formation, *Acta Endocrinol. (Copenhagen)* **96**:208–214.

61. Braverman, L. E., Ingbar, S. H., and Sterling, K., 1970, Conversion of thyroxine (T_4) to triiodothyronine (T_3) in athyreotic human subjects, *J. Clin. Invest.* **49**:855–864.

62. Chopra, I. J., 1980, A radioimmunoassay for measurement of 3'-monoiodothyronine, *J. Clin. Endocrinol. Metab.* **51**:117–123.

63. Willets, P., Crossley, D. N., Ramsden, D. B., and Hoffenberg, R., 1979, The role of thyronine in thyroid hormone metabolism, *J. Clin. Endocrinol. Metab.* **49**:658–660.

64. Faber, J., Busch-Sørensen, M., Rogowski, P., Kirkegaard, C., Siersbaek-Nielsen, K., and Friss, T., 1981, Urinary excretion of free and conjugated 3',5'-diiodothyronine and 3,3'-diiodothyronine, *J. Clin. Endocrinol. Metab.* **53**:587–593.

65. Faber, J., Faber, O. K., Lund, B., Kirkegaard, C., and Wahren, J., 1980, Hepatic extraction and renal production of 3,3'-diiodothyronine and 3',5'-diiodothyronine in man, *J. Clin. Invest.* **66**:941–945.

66. McGuire, R. A., and Hays, M. T., 1981, A kinetic model of human thyroid hormones and their conversion products, *J. Clin. Endocrinol. Metab.* **53**:852–862.

67. Warren, D. W., LoPresti, J. S., and Nicoloff, J. T., 1981, A new method for measurement of the conversion ration of thyroxine to triiodothyronine in euthyroid man, *J. Clin. Endocrinol. Metab.* **53**:1218–1222.

68. Pardridge, W. M., 1981, Transport of protein-bound hormones into tissues in vivo, *Endocr. Rev.* **2**:103–123.

69. Pardridge, W. M., and Mietus, L. J., 1980, Influx of thyroid hormones into rat liver in vivo—differential availability of thyroxine and triiodothyronine bound by plasma proteins, *J. Clin. Invest.* **66**:367–374.

70. Yoshida, K., and Davis, P. J., 1980, Estimation of intracellular free triiodothyronine in man, *J. Clin. Endocrinol. Metab.* **50**:667–669.

71. Felicetta, J. V., Green, W. L., and Nelp, W. B., 1980, Inhibition of hepatic binding of thyroxine by cholecystographic agents, *J. Clin. Invest.* **65**:1032–1040.

72. Acheson, K. J., and Burger, A. G., 1980, A study of the relationship between thermogenesis and thyroid hormones, *J. Clin. Endocrinol. Metab.* **51**:84–89.

73. Emrich, D., and Weinheimer, B. (eds.), 1980, *Thyroid 1979*, *J. Mol. Med.* **4**:3–258, 1980.

74. Melmed, S., Nademanee, K., Reed, A. W., Hendrickson, J. A., Singh, B. N., and Hershman, J. M., 1981, Hyperthyroxinemia with bradycardia and normal thyrotropin secretion after chronic amiodarone administration, *J. Clin. Endocrinol. Metab.* **53**:997–1001.

75. Chopra, I. J., Solomon, D. H., Teco, G. N. C., and Nguyen, A. H., 1980, Inhibition of hepatic outer ring monodeiodination of thyroxine and 3,3',5'-triiodothyronine by sodium salicylate, *Endocrinology* **106**:1728–1734.

76. Greeley, G. H., Jr., Jahnke, G., Nicholson, G. F., and Kizer, J. S., 1980, Decreased serum 3,5,3'-triiodothyronine and thyroxine levels accompanying acute and chronic ritalin treatment of developing rats, *Endocrinology* **106:**898–904.

77. Cavalieri, R. R., and Pitt-Rivers, R., 1981, The effects of drugs on the distribution and metabolism of thyroid hormones, *Pharm. Rev.* **33:**55–80.

78. Chopra, I. J., Solomon, D. H., Teco, G. N. C., and Eisenberg, J. B., 1982, An inhibitor of the binding of thyroid hormones to serum proteins is present in extrathyroidal tissues, *Science* **215:**407–409.

79. Kaptein, E. M., Spencer, C. A., Kamiel, M. B., and Nicoloff, J. T., 1980, Prolonged dopamine administration and thyroid hormone economy in normal and critically ill subjects, *J. Clin. Endocrinol. Metab.* **51:**387–393.

80. Slag, M. F., Morley, J. E., Elson, M. K., Crowson, T. W., Nuttall, F. Q., and Shafer, R. B., 1981, Hypothyroxinemia in critically ill patients as a predictor of high mortality, *J. Am. Med. Assoc.* **245:**43–45.

81. Kaptein, E. M., Grieb, D. A., Spencer, C. A., Wheeler, W. S., and Nicoloff, J. T., 1981, Thyroxine metabolism in the low thyroxine state of critical nonthyroidal illnesses, *J. Clin. Endocrinol. Metab.* **53:**764–771.

82. Pardridge, W. M., Slag, M. F., Morley, J. E., Elson, M. K., Shafer, R. B., and Mietus, L. J., 1981, Hepatic bioavailability of serum thyroid hormones in nonthyroidal illness, *J. Clin. Endocrinol. Metab.* **53:**913–916.

83. Geola, F. L., Chopra, I. J., and Geffner, D. L., 1980, Patterns of 3,3',5'-triiodothyronine monodeiodination in hypothyroidism and nonthyroid illnesses, *J. Clin. Endocrinol. Metab.* **50:**336–340.

84. Braverman, L. E., Abreau, C. M., Brock, P., Kleinmann, R., Fournier, L., Odstrchel, G., and Schoemaker, H. J. P., 1980, Measurement of serum free thyroxine by RIA in various clinical states, *J. Nucl. Med.* **21:**233–239.

85. Chopra, I. J., Van Herle, A. J., Teco, G. N. C., and Nguyen, A. H., 1980, Serum free thyroxine in thyroidal and nonthyroidal illnesses: A comparison of measurements by radioimmunoassay, equilibrium dialysis, and free thyroxine index, *J. Clin. Endocrinol. Metab.* **51:**135–143.

86. Bayer, M. F., and McDougall, I. R., 1980, Radioimmunoassay of free thyroxine in serum: Comparison with clinical findings and results of conventional thyroid-function tests, *Clin. Chem.* **26:**1186–1192.

87. Kaptein, E. M., MacIntyre, S. S., Weiner, J. M., Spencer, C. A., and Nicoloff, J. T., 1981, Free thyroxine estimates in nonthyroidal illness: Comparison of eight methods, *J. Clin. Endocrinol. Metab.* **52:**1073–1077.

88. Melmed, S., Geola, F. L., Reed, A. W., Pekary, A. E., Park, J., and Hershman, J. M., 1982, A comparison of methods for assessing thyroid function in nonthyroidal illness, *J. Clin. Endocrinol. Metab.* **54:**300–306.

89. Boss, A. M. B., and Kingstone, D., 1981, Further observations on serum free thyroxine concentrations during pregnancy, *Br. Med. J.* **283:**584.

90. Slag, M. F., Morley, J. E., Elson, M. K., Labrosse, K. R., Crowson, T. W., Nuttall, F. Q., and Shafer, R. B., 1981, Free thyroxine levels in critically ill patients—A comparison of currently available assays, *J. Am. Med. Assoc.* **246:**2702–2706.

91. Kaplan, M. M., Larsen, P. R., Crantz, F. R., Dzau, V. J., Rossing, T. H.,

and Haddow, J. E., 1982, Prevalence of abnormal thyroid function test results in patients with acute medical illnesses, *Am. J. Med.* **72:**9–16.

92. Gavin, L. A., Rosenthal, M., and Cavalieri, R. R., 1979, The diagnostic dilemma of isolated hyperthyroxinemia in acute illness, *J. Am. Med. Assoc.* **242:**251–253.

93. Cohen, K. L., and Swigar, M. E., 1979, Thyroid function screening in psychiatric patients, *J. Am. Med. Assoc.* **242:**254–257.

94. Levy, R. P., Jensen, J. B., Laus, V. G., Agle, D. P., and Engel, I. M., 1981, Serum thyroid hormone abnormalities in psychiatric disease, *Metabolism* **30:**1060–1064.

95. Pont, A., Spratt, D. I., McDougall, I. R., Miller, M. B., McLaughlin, W. T., and Bayer, M. F., 1981, Hyperthyroxinemia in acute psychiatric patients, Program of the American Thyroid Association, 57th Annual Meeting, p. T-4.

96. Gardner, D. F., Carithers, R. L., Jr., and Utiger, R. D., 1982, Thyroid function tests in patients with acute and resolved hepatitis B virus infection, *Ann. Intern. Med.* **96:**450–452.

97. Faber, J., Thomsen, H. F., Lumholtz, I. B., Kirkegaard, C., Siersbaek-Nielsen, K., and Friss, T., 1981, Kinetic studies of thyroxine, 3,5,3'-triiodothyronine, 3,3',5'-triiodothyronine, 3',5'-diiodothyronine, 3,3'-diiodothyronine, and 3'-monoiodothyronine in patients with liver cirrhosis, *J. Clin. Endocrinol. Metab.* **53:**978–984.

98. Afrasiabi, M. A., Vaziri, N. D., Gwinup, G., Mays, D. M., Barton, C. H., Ness, R. L., and Valenta, L. J., 1979, Thyroid function studies in the nephrotic syndrome, *Ann. Intern. Med.* **90:**335–338.

99. Felicetta, J. V., Green, W. L., Haas, L. B., Kenny, M. A., Sherrard, D. J., and Brunzell, J. D., 1979, Thyroid function and lipids in patients with chronic renal disease treated by hemodialysis: With comments on the "free thyroxine index," *Metabolism* **28:**756–763.

100. Lim, V. S., Henriquez, C., Seo, H., Refetoff, S., and Martino, E., 1980, Thyroid function in a uremic rat model—Evidence suggesting tissue hypothyroidism, *J. Clin. Invest.* **66:**946–954.

101. Thompson, P., Jr., Burman, K. D., Lukes, Y. G., McNeil, J. S., Jackson, B. D., Latham, K. R., and Wartofsky, L., 1980, Uremia decreases nuclear 3,5,3'-triiodothyronine receptors in rats, *Endocrinology* **107:**1081–1084.

102. Fujii, S., Akai, T., Tanaka, S., Nakatani, K., Kinoshita, M., Seki, J., and Wada, M., 1981, Thyroid hormone abnormalities in patients with diabetes mellitus, *J. Endocrinol. Invest.* **4:**71–74.

103. Mayfield, R. K., Sagel, J., and Colwell, J. A., 1980, Thyrotoxicosis without elevated serum triiodothyronine levels during diabetic ketoacidosis, *Arch. Intern. Med.* **140:**408–410.

104. Ahmad, N., and Cohen, M. P., 1981, Thyroid storm with normal serum triiodothyronine level during diabetic ketoacidosis, *J. Am. Med. Assoc.* **245:**2516–2517.

105. Gonzalez, C., Montoya, E., Jolin, T., and Gonzalez, M., 1980, Effect of streptozotocin diabetes on the hypothalamic–pituitary–thyroid axis in the rat, *Endocrinology* **107:**2099–2103.

106. Bagchi, N., Brown, T. R., Shivers, B., Lucas, S., and Mack, R. E., 1981, Decreased thyroidal response to thyrotropin in diabetic mice, *Endocrinology* **109:**1428–1432.

107. Wiersinga, W. M., Frank, H. J. L., Chopra, I. J., and Solomon, D. H., 1982, Alterations in hepatic nuclear binding of triiodothyronine in experimental diabetes mellitus in rats, *Acta Endocrinol. (Copenhagen)* **99:**79–85.

108. Las, M. S., and Surks, M. L., 1981, Dissociation of serum triiodothyronine concentration and hepatic nuclear triiodothyronine-binding capacity in streptozotocin-induced diabetic rats, *Endocrinology* **109:**1259–1263.

109. Das, D. K., and Ganguly, M., 1981, Diabetes, hypophysectomy, or thyroidectomy reduces nuclear L-triiodothyronine-binding capacity of rat lung, *Endocrinology* **109:**296–300.

110. Maturlo, S. J., Rosenbaum, R. L., Pan, C., and Surks, M. I., 1980, Variable thyrotropin response to thyrotropin-releasing hormone after small decreases in plasma free thyroid hormone concentrations in patients with nonthyroidal diseases, *J. Clin. Invest.* **66:**451–456.

111. Wood, D. G., and Samols, E., 1982, Impaired thyroid stimulating hormone secretion with decreased free T_4 in nonthyroidal illness, *Clin. Res.* **30:**494A.

112. Kumara-Siri, M. H., Lee, K., and Surks, M. I., 1981, Regulation of thyrotropin secretion in rats bearing the Walker 256 carcinoma, *Endocrinology* **109:**1760–1768.

113. Eisenstein, Z., Balsom, A., Garber, J. R., and Ingbar, S. H., 1980, A study of the properties of the enzyme in rat liver that deiodinates 3,3′,5′-triiodothyronine to 3,3′-diiodothyronine, *Endocrinology* **107:**530–537.

114. Heinen, E., Basler, M., Herrmann, J., Hafner, D., and Krüskemper, H. L., 1980, Enzyme kinetic and substrate-binding studies of the thyroxine to 3,5,3′-triiodothyronine converting enzyme in the rat liver microsomal fraction, *Endocrinology* **107:**1198–1204.

115. Chopra, I. J., 1981, Characteristics of outer ring (5′- or 3′-) monodeiodination of 3′,5′- and 3,3′-diiodothyronine: Evidence suggesting one outer ring monodeiodinase for various iodothyronines, *Endocrinology* **108:**464–471.

116. Visser, T. J., Leonard, J. L., Kaplan, M. M., and Larsen, P. R., 1982, Molecular mechanisms of thyroid hormone 5′-deiodination in rat brain and pituitary, 64th Annual Meeting of the Endocrine Society, p. 132.

117. Maeda, M., and Ingbar, S. H., 1982, Evidence that the 5′-monodeiodinases for thyroxine (T_4) and for 3,3′,5′-triiodothyronine (reverse T_3, rT_3) are separate enzymes, 64th Annual Meeting of the Endocrine Society, p. 133.

118. dem Brinke, D. A., Köhrle, J., Ködding, R., and Hesch, R.-D., 1980, Subcellular localization of thyroxine-5-deiodinase in rat liver, *J. Endocrinol. Invest.* **3:**73–76.

119. Cavalieri, R. R., Gavin, L. A., and Bui, F., 1977, Conversion of thyroxine to 3,3′,5′-triiodothyronine (reverse-T_3) by a soluble enzyme system of rat liver, *Biochem. Biophys. Res. Commun.* **79:**897–902.

120. Fekkes, D., Overmeeren-Kaptein, E. V., Docter, R., Hennemann, G., and Visser, T. J., 1979, Location of rat liver iodothyronine deiodinating enzymes in the endoplasmic reticulum, *Biochim. Biophys. Acta* **587:**12–19.

121. Maciel, R. M. B., Ozawa, Y., and Chopra, I. J., 1979, Subcellular localization

of thyroxine and reverse triiodothyronine outer ring monodeiodinating activities, *Endocrinol.* **104**:365–370.

122. Takaishi, M., Shimizu, T., and Shishiba, Y., 1979, Solubilization of thyroxine-5'-deiodinase activity from rat liver microsome fraction, *Acta Endocrinol. (Copenhagen)* **92**:694–701.

123. Fekkes, D., Overmeeren, E. V., Hennemann, G., and Visser, T. J., 1980, Solubilization and partial characterization of rat liver iodothyronine deiodinases, *Biochim. Biophys. Acta* **613**:41–51.

124. Leonard, J. L., and Rosenberg, I. N., 1980, Iodothyronine 5'-deiodinase from rat kidney: Substrate specificity and the 5'-deiodination of reverse triiodothyronine, *Endocrinology* **107**:1376–1383.

125. Kaplan, M. M., 1980, Thyroxine 5'-monodeiodination in rat anterior pituitary homogenates, *Endocrinology* **106**:567–576.

126. Crantz, F. R., and Larsen, P. R., 1980, Rapid thyroxine to 3,5,3'-triiodothyronine conversion and nuclear 3,5,3'-triiodothyronine binding in rat cerebral cortex and cerebellum, *J. Clin. Invest.* **65**:935–938.

127. Kaplan, M. M., McCann, U. D., Yaskoski, K. A., Larsen, P. R., and Leonard, J. L., 1981, Anatomical distribution of phenolic and tyrosyl ring iodothyronine deiodinases in the nervous system of normal and hypothyroid rats, *Endocrinology* **109**:397–402.

128. Tanaka, K., Inada, M., Ishii, H., Naito, K., Nishikawa, M., Mashio, Y., and Imura, H., 1981, Inner ring monodeiodination of thyroxine and 3,5,3'-L-triiodothyronine in rat brain, *Endocrinology* **109**:1619–1624.

129. Leonard, J. L., Kaplan, M. M., Visser, T. J., Silva, J. E., and Larsen, P. R., 1981, Cerebral cortex responds rapidly to thyroid hormones, *Science* **214**:571–573.

130. Nishikawa, M., Inada, M., Naito, K., Ishii, H., Tanaka, K., Mashio, Y., Nakao, K., Nakai, Y., Udaka, F., and Imura, H., 1981, 3,3',5'-triiodothyronine (reverse T_3) in human cerebrospinal fluid, *J. Clin. Endocrinol. Metab.* **53**:1030–1035.

131. Melmed, S., Nelson, M., Kaplowitz, N., Yamada, T., and Hershman, J. M., 1981, Glutathione-dependent thyroxine 5'-monodeiodination modulates growth hormone production by cultured nonthyrotropic rat pituitary cells, *Endocrinology* **108**:970–976.

132. Roti, E., Fang, S. L., Green, K., Emerson, C. H., and Braverman, L. E., 1981, Human placenta is an active site of thyroxine and 3,3',5-triiodothyronine tyrosyl ring deiodination, *J. Clin. Endocrinol. Metab.* **53**:498–501.

133. Roti, E., Fang, S. L., Braverman, L. E., and Emerson, C. H., 1982, Rat placenta is an active site of inner ring deiodination of thyroxine and 3,3',5-triiodothyronine, *Endocrinology* **110**:34–37.

134. Roti, E., Fang, S. L., Green, K., Braverman, L. E., and Emerson, C. H., 1983, Inner ring deiodination of thyroxine and 3,3',5-triiodothyronine by human fetal membranes, *Am. J. Obstet. Gynecol.* **147**:788–792.

135. El-Zaheri, M., Vagenakis, A. G., Hinerfeld, L., Emerson, C. H., and Braverman, L. E., 1981, Maternal thyroid function is the major determinant of amniotic fluid reverse T_3 in the rat, *J. Clin. Invest.* **67**:1126–1133.

136. Erickson, V. J., Cavalieri, R. R., and Rosenberg, L. L., 1981, Phenolic and

nonphenolic ring iodothyronine deiodinases from rat thyroid gland, *Endocrinology* **108**:1257–1264.

137. Ishii H., Inada, M., Tanaka, K., Mashio, Y., Natto, K., Nishikawa, M., and Imura, H., 1981, Triiodothyronine generation from thyroxine in human thyroid: Enhanced conversion in Graves' thyroid tissue, *J. Clin. Endocrinol. Metab.* **52**:1211–1217.

138. Borges, M., Eisenstein, Z., Burger, A. G., and Ingbar, S. H., 1981, Immunsequestration: A new technique for studying peripheral iodothyronine metabolism in vitro, *Endocrinology* **108**:1665–1671.

139. Pittman, C. S., Shimizu, T., Burger, A., and Chambers, J. B., Jr., 1980, The nondeiodinative pathways of thyroxine metabolism: 3,5,3′,5′-tetraiodothyroacetic acid turnover in normal and fasting human subjects, *J. Clin. Endocrinol. Metab.* **50**:712–716.

140. Gavin, L. A., Bui, F., McMahon, F., and Cavalieri, R. R., 1980, Sequential deiodination of thyroxine to 3,3′-diiodothyronine via 3,5,3′-triiodothyronine and 3,3′,5′-triiodothyronine in rat liver homogenate, *J. Biol. Chem.* **254**:49–53.

141. Gavin, L. A., McMahon, F. A., and Moeller, M., 1981, Dietary modification of thyroxine deiodination in liver is not mediated by hepatic sulfhydryls, *J. Clin. Invest.* **65**:943–946.

142. Harris, A. R., Fang, S. L., Hinerfeld, L., Braverman, L. E., and Vagenakis, A. G., 1979, The role of sulfhydryl groups on the impaired hepatic 3′,3,5-triiodothyronine generation from thyroxine in the hypothyroid, starved, fetal, and neonatal rodent, *J. Clin. Invest.* **63**:516–524.

143. Balsam, A., Ingbar, S. H., and Sexton, F., 1979, Observations on the factors that control the generation of triiodothyronine from thyroxine in rat liver and the nature of the defect induced by fasting, *J. Clin. Invest.* **63**:1145–1156.

144. Kaplan, M. M., 1979, Subcellular alterations causing reduced hepatic thyroxine-5′-monodeiodinase activity in fasted rats, *Endocrinology* **104**:58–64.

145. Chopra, I. J., 1980, Alterations in monodeiodination of iodothyronines in the fasting rat: Effects of reduced nonprotein sulfhydryl groups and hypothyroidism, *Metabolism* **29**:161–167.

146. Gavin, L. A., McMahon, F. A., and Moeller, M., 1981, Carbohydrate in contrast to protein feeding increases the hepatic content of active thyroxine-5′-deiodinase in the rat, *Endocrinology* **109**:530–536.

147. Sato, K., and Robbins, J., 1981, Thyroid hormone metabolism in primary cultured rat hepatocytes, *J. Clin. Invest.* **68**:475–483.

148. Senga, O., Pittman, C. S., Lindsay, R. H., Chambers, J. B., Jr., and Hill, J. B., Jr., 1982, Comparison of the peripheral thyroid hormone metabolism in normal rats and in rats receiving prolonged glucagon infusion, *Endocrinology* **110**:2011–2017.

149. Sorimachi, K., and Robbins, J., 1978, Thyroxine inactivation by starvation in cultured hepatocarcinoma cells: Formation of reverse triiodothyronine, *Horm. Metab. Res.* **10**:459–575.

150. Sato, K., and Robbins, J., 1981, Glutathione deficiency induced by cystine and/or methionine deprivation does not affect thyroid hormone deiodination in cultured rat hepatocytes and monkey hepatocarcinoma cells, *Endocrinology* **109**:844–852.

151. Takai, N. A., Rapoport, B., and Yamamoto, M., 1980, Biliary excretion of iodothyronines in rats as determined by high pressure liquid chromatography: Effect of starvation, *Endocrinology* **107**:176–182.

152. Balsam, A., Sexton, F., and Ingbar, S. H., 1981, The influence of fasting and the thyroid state on the activity of thyroxine 5′-monodeiodinase in rat liver: a kinetic analysis of microsomal formation of triiodothyronine from thyroxine, *Endocrinology* **108**:472–477.

153. Burger, A. G., Weissel, M., and Berger, M., 1980, Starvation induces a partial failure of triiodothyronine to inhibit the thyrotropin response to thyrotropin-releasing hormone, *J. Clin. Endocrinol. Metab.* **51**: 1064–1067.

154. Gardner, D. F., Kaplan, M. M., Stanley, C. A., and Utiger, R. D., 1979, Effect of tri-iodothyronine replacement on the metabolic and pituitary responses to starvation, *N. Engl. J. Med.* **300**:579–584.

155. Schwartz, H. L., Lancer, S. R., and Oppenheimer, J. H., 1980, Thyroid hormones influence starvation-induced hepatic protein loss in the rat: Possible role of thyroid hormones in the generation of labile protein, *Endocrinology* **107**:1684–1692.

156. Oppenheimer, J. H., and Schwartz, H. L., 1980, Factors determining the level of activity of 3,5,3′-triiodothyronine-responsive hepatic enzymes in the starved rat, *Endocrinology* **107**:1460–1468.

157. Mariash, C. N., Kaiser, F. E., Schwartz, H. L., Towle, H. C., and Oppenheimer, J. H., 1980, Synergism of thyroid hormone and high carbohydrate diet in the induction of lipogenic enzymes in the rat, *J. Clin. Invest.* **67**:1126–1134.

158. Forciea, M. A., Schwartz, H. L., Towle, H. C., Mariash, C. N., Kaiser, F. E., and Oppenheimer, J. H., 1981, Thyroid hormone–carbohydrate interaction in the rat, *J. Clin. Invest.* **67**:1739–1747.

159. Mariash, C. N., McSwigan, C. R., Towle, H. C., Schwartz, H. L., and Oppenheimer, J. H., 1981, Glucose and triiodothyronine both induce malic enzyme in the rat hepatocyte culture, *J. Clin. Invest.* **68**:1485–1490.

160. Simat, B. M., Towle, H. C., Schwartz, H. L., and Oppenheimer, J. H., 1980, Difference between thyroidectomized and hypophysectomized animals in their hepatic ribonucleic acid response to thyroid hormone, *Endocrinology* **107**:1338–1344.

161. Walker, P., Weichsel, M. E., Jr., Hoath, S. B., Poland, R. E., and Fisher, D. A., 1981, Effect of thyroxine, testosterone, and corticosterone on nerve growth factor (NGF) and epidermal growth factor (EGF) concentrations in adult female mouse submaxillary gland: Dissociation of NGF and EGF responses, *Endocrinology* **109**:582–587.

162. Gambert, S. R., Ingbar, S. H., and Hagen, T. C., 1981, Interaction of age and thyroid hormone status on Na^+–K^+ ATPase in rat renal cortex and liver, *Endocrinology* **108**:27–30.

163. Dratman, M. B., Futaesaku, Y., Crutchfield, F. L., Berman, N., Payne, B., Sar, M., and Stumpf, W. E., 1982, Iodine-125-labeled triiodothyronine in rat brain: Evidence for localization in discrete neural systems, *Science* **215**:309–312.

164. Kriz, B. M., Fong, B. B., and Goldfine, I. D., 1981, Quantitative electron

microscope autoradiographs of ^{125}I-L-triiodothyronine: Evidence for multiple sites of hormone localization, *Clin. Res.* **29:**506A.

165. Sterling, K., 1979, Thyroid hormone action at the cell level, *N. Engl. J. Med.* **300:**117–124, 173–177.

166. Segal, J., and Ingbar, S. H., 1980, Direct and synergistic interactions of 3,5,3'-triiodothyronine and the adrenergic system in stimulating sugar transport by rat thymocytes, *J. Clin. Invest.* **65:**958–966.

167. Maxfield, F. R., Willingham, M. C., Pastan, I., Dragsten, P., and Cheng, S.-Y., 1981, Binding and mobility of the cell surface receptors for 3,3',5-triiodo-L-thyronine, *Science* **211:**63–64.

168. Young, R. A., Braverman, L. E., and Rajatanavin, R., 1982, Low protein–high carbohydrate diet induces alterations in the serum thyronine binding proteins in the rat, *Endocrinology* **110:**1607–1612.

169. Smallridge, R. C., Glass, A. R., Wartofsky, L., Ward, K. G., and Burman, K. D., 1980, Investigations into the etiology of elevated serum triiodothyronine (T_3) levels in protein malnourished rats, 62nd Annual Meeting of the Endocrine Society, p. 223.

170. Okamura, K., Taurog, A., and Krulich, L., 1981, Elevation of serum 3,5,3'-triiodothyronine and thyroxine levels in rats fed Remington diets: Opposing effects of nutritional deficiency and iodine deficiency, *Endocrinology* **108:**1247–1256.

171. Okamura, K., Taurog, A., and DiStefano, J. J., III, 1981, Elevated serum levels of T_3 without metabolic effect in nutritionally deficient rats, attributable to reduced cellular uptake of T_3, *Endocrinology* **109:**673–675.

172. Hennemann, G., Docter, R., Krenning, E. P., Bos, G., Otten, M., and Visser, T. J., 1979, Raised total thyroxine and free thyroxine index but normal free thyroxine: A serum abnormality due to inherited increased affinity of iodothyronines for serum binding protein, *Lancet* **1:**639–642.

173. Lee, W. N. P., Golden, M. P., van Herle, A. J., Lippe, B. M., and Kaplan, S. A., 1979, Inherited abnormal thyroid hormone-binding protein causing selective increase of total serum thyroxine, *J. Clin. Endocrinol. Metab.* **49:**292–299.

174. Stockigt, J. R., Topliss, D. J., Barlow, J. W., White, E. L., Hurley, D. M., and Taft, P., 1981, Familial euthyroid thyroxine excess: An appropriate response to abnormal thyroxine binding associated with albumin, *J. Clin. Endocrinol. Metab.* **53:**353–359.

175. Ruiz, M., Rajatanavin, R., Young, R. A., Taylor, C., Brown, R., Braverman, L. E., and Ingbar, S. H., 1982, Familial dysalbuminemic hyperthyroxinemia, *N. Engl. J. Med.* **306:**635–639.

176. Moses, A. C., Lawlor, J., Haddow, J., and Jackson, I. M. D., 1982, Familial euthyroid hyperthyroxinemia resulting from increased thyroxine binding to thyroxine-binding prealbumin, *N. Engl. J. Med.* **306:**966–969.

177. Morley, J. E., Shafer, R. B., Elson, M. K., Slag, M. F., Raleigh, M. J., Brammer, G. L., Yuwiler, A., and Hershman, J. M., 1980, Amphetamine-induced hyperthyroxinemia, *Ann. Intern. Med.* **93:**707–709.

178. Geola, F. L., Hershman, J. M., Reed, A. W., and Premachandra, B. N., 1981, Circulating thyroid hormone autoantibodies in a hypothyroid pa-

tient: Effect on thyroxine metabolic clearance rate, *J. Clin. Endocrinol. Metab.* **53**:580–586.

179. Inada, M., Nishikawa, M., Naito, K., Oishi, M., Kurata, S., and Imura, H., 1980, Triiodothyronine-binding immunoglobulin in a patient with Graves' disease and its effect on metabolism and radioimmunoassay of triiodothyronine, *Am. J. Med.* **68**:787–792.

180. Gärtner, R., Henze, R., Horn, K., Pickardt, C. R., and Scriba, P. C., 1981, Thyroxine-binding globulin: Investigation of microheterogeneity, *J. Clin. Endocrinol. Metab.* **52**:657–664.

181. Garnick, M. B., and Larsen, P. R., 1979, Acute deficiency of thyroxine-binding globulin during L-asparaginase therapy, *N. Engl. J. Med.* **301**:252–253.

182. Yabu, Y., Amino, N., Nakatani, K., Ichihara, K., Azukizawa, M., and Miyai, K., 1980, Graves' disease associated with elevated serum thyroxine-binding globulin concentrations, *J. Clin. Endocrinol. Metab.* **51**:325–329.

183. Smals, A. G., Ross, A. H., and Kloppenborg, P. W. C., 1981, Dichotomy between serum free triiodothyronine and free thyroxine concentrations in familial thyroxine-binding globulin deficiency, *J. Clin. Endocrinol. Metab.* **53**:917–922.

184. Fisher, D. A., and Klein, A. H., 1981, Thyroid development and disorders of thyroid function in the newborn, *N. Engl. J. Med.* **304**:702–712.

185. Porterfield, S. P., and Hendrich, C. E., 1981, Alterations of serum thyroxine, triiodothyronine, and thyrotropin in the progeny of hypothyroid rats, *Endocrinology* **108**:1060–1063.

186. Coulombe, P., Ruel, J., and Dussault, J. H., 1980, Effects of neonatal hypo- and hyperthyroidism on pituitary growth hormone content in the rat, *Endocrinology* **107**:2027–2033.

187. Avivi, A., Shemesh, M., and Lindner, H. R., 1981, The ontogeny of the thyrotropin–thyroid axis in early bovine embryos, *Endocrinology* **109**:1611–1618.

188. Oliver, C., Giraud, P., Lissitzky, J. C., Conte-Devolx, B., and Gillioz, P., 1981, Influence of thyrotropin-releasing hormone on the secretion of thyrotropin in neonatal rats, *Endocrinology* **108**:179–182.

189. Theodoropoulos, T., Braverman, L. E., and Vagenakis, A. G., 1979, Thyrotropin-releasing hormone is not required for thyrotropin secretion in the perinatal rat, *J. Clin. Invest.* **63**:588–594.

190. Tonooka, N., and Greer, M. A., 1978, Evidence that control of fetal thyrotropin secretion is independent of both the fetal and maternal hypothalamus, *Endocrinology* **102**:852–858.

191. Frankel, S., and Lange, G., 1980, Maturation of hypothalamic–pituitary–thyroid response in the rat to acute cold, *Am. J. Physiol. Endocrinol. Metab.* **2**:E223–E226.

192. Walker, P., Coulombe, P., and Dussault, J. H., 1980, Effects of triiodothyronine on thyrotropin-releasing hormone-induced thyrotropin release in the neonatal rat, *Endocrinology* **107**:1731–1737.

193. Klein, A. H., and Fisher, D. A., 1980, Thyrotropin-releasing hormone-stimulated pituitary and thyroid gland responsiveness and 3,5,3'-triiodothyronine suppression in fetal and neonatal lambs, *Endocrinology* **106**:697–701.

194. Roti, E., Gnudi, A., Braverman, L. E., Robuschi, G., Emanuele, R., Bandini, P., Benassi, L., Pagliani, A., and Emerson, C. H., 1981, Human cord blood concentrations of thyrotropin, thyroglobulin, and iodothyronines after maternal administrations of thyrotropin-releasing hormone, *J. Clin. Endocrinol. Metab.* **53**:813–817.

195. Pezzino, V., Filetti, S., Belfiore, A., Proto, S., Donzelli, G., and Vigneri, R., 1981, Serum thyroglobulin levels in the newborn, *J. Clin. Endocrinol. Metab.* **52**:364–366.

196. Ket, J. L., de Vijlder, J. J. M., Bikker, H., Gons, M. H., and Tegelaers, W. H. H., 1981, Serum thyroglobulin levels: The physiological decrease in infancy and the absence in athyroidism, *J. Clin. Endocrinol. Metab.* **53**:1301–1303.

197. Tenore, A., Parks, J. S., Gasparo, M., and Koldovsky, O., 1980, Thyroidal response to peroral TSH in suckling and weaned rats, *Am. J. Physiol. Endocrinol. Metab.* **1**:E428–E430.

198. Borges, M., LaBourene, J., and Ingbar, S. H., 1980, Changes in hepatic iodothyronine metabolism during ontogeny of the chick embryo, *Endocrinology* **107**:1751–1761.

199. Galton, V. A., and Munck, K., 1981, Metabolism of thyroxine in *Rana catesbeiana* tadpoles during metamorphic climax, *Endocrinology* **109**:1127–1131.

200. Galton, V. A., 1980, Binding of thyroid hormones in vivo by hepatic nuclei of *Rana catesbeiana* tadpoles at different stages of metamorphosis, *Endocrinology* **107**:1910–1915.

201. Galton, V. A., and Cohen, J. S., 1980, Action of thyroid hormones in premetamorphic tadpoles: An important role of thyroxine?, *Endocrinology* **107**:1820–1826.

202. Gonzales, L. W., and Ballard, P. L., 1981, Identification and characterization of nuclear 3,5,3'-triiodothyronine-binding sites in fetal human lung, *J. Clin. Endocrinol. Metab.* **53**:21–28.

203. Hitchcock, K. R., Harney, J., and Reichlin, S., 1980, Hormones and the lung. III. Thyroid hormone uptake kinetics of perinatal rat lung, *Endocrinology* **107**:294–299.

204. Ballard, P. L., Benson, B. J., Brehier, A., Carter, J. P., Kriz, B. M., and Jorgensen, E. C., 1980, Transplacental stimulation of lung development in the fetal rabbit by 3,5-dimethyl-3'-isopropyl-L-thyroxine, *J. Clin. Invest.* **65**:1407–1417.

205. Matsuura, N., Yamada, Y., Nohara, Y., Konishi, J., Kasagi, K., Endo, K., Kojima, H., and Wataya, K., 1980, Familial neonatal transient hypothyroidism due to maternal TSH-binding inhibitor immunoglobulins, *N. Engl. J. Med.* **303**:738–741.

206. Czernichow, P., Vandalem, J. L., and Hennen, G., 1981, Transient neonatal hyperthyrotropinemia: A factitious syndrome due to the presence of heterophilic antibodies in the plasma of infants and their mothers, *J. Clin. Endocrinol. Metab.* **53**:387–393.

207. Gendrel, D., Feinstein, M.-C., Grenier, J., Roger, M., Ingrand, J., Chaussain, J.-L., Canlorbe, P., and Job, J.-B., 1981, Falsely elevated serum thyrotropin (TSH) in newborn infants: Transfer from mothers to infants of

a factor interfering in the TSH radioimmunoassay, *J. Clin. Endocrinol. Metab.* **52**:62–65.

208. Sugenoya, A., Kidd, A., Row, V. V., and Volpe, R., 1979, Correlation between thyrotropin-displacing activity and human thyroid-stimulating activity by immunoglobulins from patients with Graves' disease and other thyroid disorders, *J. Clin. Endocrinol. Metab.* **48**:398–402.

209. Kuzuya, N., Chiu, S. C., Ikeda, H., Uchimura, H., Ito, K., and Nagataki, S., 1979, Correlation between thyroid stimulators and 3,5,3'-triiodothyronine suppressibility in patients during treatment for hyperthyroidism with thionamide drugs: Comparison of assays by thyroid-stimulating and thyrotropin-displacing activities, *J. Clin. Endocrinol. Metab.* **48**:706–711.

210. Endo, K., Amir, S. M., and Ingbar, S. H., 1981, Development and evaluation of a method for the partial purification of immunoglobulins specific for Graves' disease, *J. Clin. Endocrinol. Metab.* **52**:1113–1123.

211. Kishihara, M., Nakao, Y., Baba, Y., Kobayashi, N., Matsukura, S., Kuma, K., and Fujita, T., 1981, Interaction between thyrotropin (TSH) binding inhibitor immunoglobulins (TBII) and soluble TSH receptors in fat cells, *J. Clin. Endocrinol. Metab.* **52**:665–670.

212. Davies, T. F., 1981, Autoantibodies to the human thyrotropin receptor are not species specific, *J. Clin. Endocrinol. Metab.* **52**:426–430.

213. Ealey, P. A., Marshall, N. J., and Ekins, R. P., 1981, Time-related thyroid stimulation by thyrotropin and thyroid-stimulating antibodies, as measured by the cytochemical section bioassay, *J. Clin. Endocrinol. Metab.* **52**:483–487.

214. Loveridge, N., Zakarija, M., Bitensky, L., and McKenzie, J. M., 1979, The cytochemical bioassay for thyroid-stimulating antibody of Graves' disease: Further experience, *J. Clin. Endocrinol. Metab.* **49**:610–615.

215. Hinds, W. E., Takai, N., Rapoport, B., Filetti, S., and Clark, O. H., 1981, Thyroid-stimulating immunoglobulin bioassay using cultured human thyroid cells, *J. Clin. Endocrinol. Metab.* **52**:1204–1210.

216. Stöcke, G., Wahl, R., and Seif, F. J., 1981, Micromethod of human thyrocyte cultures for detection of thyroid-stimulating antibodies and thyrotropin, *Acta Endocrinol. (Copenhagen)* **97**:369–375.

217. Bidey, S. P., Marshall, N. J., and Ekins, R. P., 1981, Adenylate cyclase activity and the accumulation and release of adenosine 3',5'-monophosphate in normal human thyroid tissue slice preparations: Responses to thyrotropin and thyroid-stimulating antibodies, *J. Clin. Endocrinol. Metab.* **53**:246–253.

218. Atkinson, S., and Kendall-Taylor, P., 1981, The stimulation of thyroid hormone secretion in vitro by thyroid-stimulating antibodies, *J. Clin. Endocrinol. Metab.* **53**:1263–1266.

219. Ozawa, Y., Maciel, R. M. B., Chopra, I. J., Solomon, D. H., and Beall, G. N., 1979, Relationships among immunoglobulin markers in Graves' disease, *J. Clin. Endocrinol. Metab.* **48**:381–387.

220. Kasagi, K., Konishi, J., Endo, K., Mori, T., Nagahara, K., Makimoto, K., Kuma, K., and Torizuka, K., 1980, Adenylate cyclase activity in thyroid tissue from patients with untreated Graves' disease, *J. Clin. Endocrinol. Metab.* **51**:492–499.

221. Kuzuya, N., Uchimura, H., Ikeda, H., Chiu, S. C., Hamada, N., Ito, K.,

and Nagataki, S., 1980, Adenosine 3′,5′-monophosphate concentrations and responsiveness to thyrotropin and thyroid-stimulating immunoglobulins in normal and Graves' thyroids, *J. Clin. Endocrinol. Metab.* **51**:59–63.

222. Drexhage, H. A., Bottazzo, G. F., Doniach, D., Bitensky, L., and Chayen, J., 1980, Evidence for thyroid-growth-stimulating immunoglobulins in some goitrous thyroid diseases, *Lancet* **2**:287–292.

223. Takata, I., Suzuki, Y., Saida, K., and Sato, T., 1980, Human thyroid stimulating activity and clinical state in antithyroid treatment of juvenile Graves' disease, *Acta Endocrinol. (Copenhagen)* **94**:46–52.

224. Fenzi, G., Hashizume, K., Roudebush, C. P., and DeGroot, L. J., 1979, Changes in thyroid-stimulating immunoglobulins during antithyroid therapy, *J. Clin. Endocrinol. Metab.* **48**:572–576.

225. Teng, C. S., and Yeung, R. T. T., 1980, Changes in thyroid-stimulating antibody activity in Graves' disease treated with antithyroid drug and its relationship to relapse: A prospective study, *J. Clin. Endocrinol. Metab.* **50**:144–147.

226. McGregor, A. M., Smith, B. R., Hall, R., Petersen, M. M., Miller, M., and Dewar, P. J., 1980, Prediction of relapse in hyperthyroid Graves' disease, *Lancet* **1**:1101–1103.

227. Zakarija, M., McKenzie, J. M., and Banovac, K., 1980, Clinical significance of assay of thyroid-stimulating antibody in Graves' disease, *Ann. Intern. Med.* **93**:28–32.

228. Karlsson, F. A., and Dahlberg, P. A., 1981, Thyroid stimulating antibodies (TSAb) in patients with Graves' disease undergoing antithyroid drug treatment: Indicators of activity of disease, *Clin. Endocrinol.* **14**:579–585.

229. McGregor, A. M., Petersen, M. M., McLachlan, S. M., Rooke, P., Smith, B. R., and Hall, R., 1980, Carbimazole and the autoimmune response in Graves' disease, *N. Engl. J. Med.* **303**:302–307.

230. McGregor, A. M., Ibbertson, H. K., Smith, B. R., and Hall, R., 1980, Carbimazole and autoantibody synthesis in Hashimoto's thyroiditis, *Br. Med. J.* **281**:968–969.

231. Hallengren, B., Forsgren, A., and Melander, A., 1980, Effects of antithyroid drugs on lymphocyte function in vitro, *J. Clin. Endocrinol. Metab.* **51**:298–301.

232. Weiss, I., and Davies, T. F., 1981, Inhibition of immunoglobulin-secreting cells by antithyroid drugs, *J. Clin. Endocrinol. Metab.* **53**:1223–1228.

233. Fujiwara, H., Torisu, M., Sugisaki, T., and Okano, H., 1981, Immune complex deposits in thyroid glands of patients with Graves' disease, *Clin. Immunol. Immunopathol.* **19**:109–117.

234. Ohtaki, S., Endo, Y., Horinouchi, K., Yoshitake, S., and Ishikawa, E., 1981, Circulating thyroglobulin–antithyroglobulin immune complex in thyroid diseases usig enzyme-linked immunoassays, *J. Clin. Endocrinol. Metab.* **52**:239–246.

235. Van der Heide, D., Bolk, J. H., De Bruin, T. W. A., Van Es, L. A., Daha, M. R., Bussemaker, J. K., Goslings, B. M., and Querido, A., 1980, Circulating immune complexes and thyroid-stimulating immunoglobulins before, during, and after antithyroid drug therapy in patients with Graves' disease, *Lancet* **1**:1376–1379.

236. Jordan, S. C., Johnston, W. H., and Bergstein, J. M., 1978, Immune complex glomerulonephritis mediated by thyroid antigens, *Arch. Pathol. Lab. Med.* **102:**530–533.

237. Horvath, F., Jr., Teague, P., Gaffney, E. F., Mars, D. R., and Fuller, T. J., 1979, Thyroid antigen associated immune complex glomerulonephritis in Graves' disease, *Am. J. Med.* **67:**901–904.

238. Jordan, S. C., Buckingham, B., Sakai, R., and Olson, D., 1981, Studies of immune-complex glomerulonephritis mediated by human thyroglobulin, *N. Engl. J. Med.* **304:**1212–1215.

239. Okita, N., Kidd, A., Row, V. V., and Volpé, R., 1980, Sensitization of T-lymphocytes in Graves' and Hashimoto's disease, *J. Clin. Endocrinol. Metab.* **51:**316–320.

240. Okita, N., Topliss, D., Lewis, M., Row, V. V., and Volpé, R., 1981, T-lymphocyte sensitization in Graves' and Hashimoto's diseases confirmed by an indirect migration inhibition factor test, *J. Clin. Endocrinol. Metab.* **52:**523–527.

241. Okita, N., How, J., Topliss, D., Lewis, M., Row, V. V., and Volpé, R., 1981, Suppressor T lymphocyte dysfunction in Graves' disease: Role of the H-2 histamine receptor-bearing suppressor T lymphocytes, *J. Clin. Endocrinol. Metab.* **53:**1002–1007.

242. Okita, N., Row, V. V., and Volpé, R., 1981, Suppressor T-lymphocyte deficiency in Graves' disease and Hashimoto's thyroiditis, *J. Clin. Endocrinol. Metab.* **52:**528–533.

243. MacLean, D. B., Miller, K. B., Brown, R., and Reichlin, S., 1981, Normal immunoregulation of in vitro antibody secretion in autoimmune thyroid disease, *J. Clin. Endocrinol. Metab.* **53:**801–805.

244. Tanaka, T., Katayama, S., Kuma, K., Tamai, H., Matsuzuka, F., and Hidaka, H., 1980, Clinical and pathological significance of sibling Graves' disease, *Acta Endocrinol. (Copenhagen)* **94:**498–502.

245. Banovac, K., Zakarija, M., McKenzie, J. M., Witte, A., and Sekso, M., 1981, Absence of thyroid-stimulating antibody and long acting thyroid stimulator in relatives of Graves' disease patients, *J. Clin. Endocrinol. Metab.* **53:**651–653.

246. Carey, C., Skosey, C., Pinnamaneni, K. M., Barsano, C. P., and DeGroot, L. J., 1980, Thyroid abnormalities in children of parents who have Graves' disease: Possible pre-Graves' disease, *Metabolism* **29:**369–376.

247. Tamai, H., Ohsako, N., Takeno, K., Fukino, O., Takahashi, H., Kuma, K., Kumagai, L. F., and Nagataki, S., 1980, Changes in thyroid function in euthyroid subjects with a family history of Graves' disease: A follow-up study of 69 patients, *J. Clin. Endocrinol. Metab.* **51:**1123–1127.

248. Mather, B. A., Roberts, D. F., Scanlon, M. F., Mukhtar, E. D., Davies, T. F., Smith, B. R., and Hall, R., 1980, HLA antigens and thyroid autoantibodies in patients with Graves' disease and their first degree relatives, *Clin. Endocrinol.* **12:**155–163.

249. Dallow, R. L., 1978, Reliability of orbital diagnostic tests: Ultrasonography, computerized tomography, and radiography, *Ophthalmology* **85:**1218–1228.

250. Kriss, J. P., and Mehdi, S. Q., 1979, Cell-mediated lysis of lipid vesicles containing eye muscle protein: Implications regarding pathogenesis of Graves' ophthalmopathy, *Proc. Natl. Acad. Sci. USA* **76:**2003–2007.

251. Sergott, R. C., Felberg, N. T., Savino, P. J., Blizzard, J. J., and Schatz, N. J., 1981, Graves' ophthalmopathy-immunologic parameters related to corticosteroid therapy, *Invest. Ophthalmol. Vis. Sci.* **20:**173–182.

252. Teng, C. S., Crombie, A. L., Hall, R., and Ross, W. M., 1980, An evaluation of supervoltage orbital irradiation for Graves' ophthalmopathy, *Clin. Endocrinol.* **13:**545–551.

253. Wall, J. R., Strakosch, C. R., Fang, S. L., Ingbar, S. H., and Braverman, L. E., 1979, Thyroid binding antibodies and other immunological abnormalities in patients with Graves' ophthalmopathy: Effect of treatment with cyclophosphamide, *Clin. Endocrinol.* **10:**79–91.

254. Bigos, S. T., Nisula, B. C., Daniels, G. H., Eastman, R. C., Johnston, H. H., and Kohler, P. O., 1979, Cyclophosphamide in the management of advanced Graves' ophthalmopathy, *Ann. Intern. Med.* **90:**921–923.

255. Amino, N., Yuasa, T., Yabu, Y., Miyai, K., and Kumahara, Y., 1980, Exophthalmos in autoimmune thyroid disease, *J. Clin. Endocrinol. Metab.* **51:**1232–1234.

256. Tamai, H., Nakagawa, T., Ohsako, N., Fukino, O., Takahashi, H., Matsuzuka, F., Kuma, K., and Nagataki, S., 1980, Changes in thyroid functions in patients with euthyroid Graves' disease, *J. Clin. Endocrinol. Metab.* **50:**108–112.

257. Buckingham, B. A., Costin, G., Roe, T. F., Weitzman, J. J., and Kogut, M. D., 1981, Hyperthyroidism in children—A reevaluation of treatment, *Am. J. Dis. Child.* **135:**112–117.

258. Freitas, J. E., Swanson, D. P., Gross, M. D., and Sisson, J. C., 1979, Iodine-131: Optimal therapy for hyperthyroidism in children and adolescents?, *J. Nucl. Med.* **20:**847–850.

259. Zonszein, J., Santangelo, R. P., Mackin, J. F., Lee, T. C., Coffey, R. J.,and Canary, J. J., 1979, Propranolol therapy in thyrotoxicosis—A review of 84 patients undergoing surgery, *Am. J. Med.* **66:**411–416.

260. Rubenfeld, S., Silverman, V. E., Welch, K. M. A., Mallette, L. E., and Kohler, P. O., 1979, Variable plasma propranolol levels in thyrotoxicosis, *Med. Intell.* **300:**353–354.

261. Riddell, J. G., Neill, J. D., Kelly, J. G., and McDevitt, D. G., 1980, Effects of thyroid dysfunction on propranolol kinetics, *Clin. Pharmacol. Ther.* **28:**565–574.

262. Feely, J., Forrest, A., Gunn, A., Hamilton, W., Stevenson, I., and Crooks, J., 1980, Propranolol dosage in thyrotoxicosis, *J. Clin. Endocrinol. Metab.* **51:**658–661.

263. Feek, C. M., Sawers, J. S. A., Irvine, W. J., Beckett, G. J., Ratcliffe, W. A., and Toft, A. D., 1980, Combination of potassium iodide and propranolol in preparation of patients with Graves' disease for thyroid surgery, *N. Engl. J. Med.* **302:**883–885.

264. Emerson, C. H., and El-Zaheri, M. M. S., 1980, Potassium iodide and propranolol in Graves' disease, *N. Engl. J. Med.* **303:**527–528.

265. Feely, J., Crooks, J., Forrest, A. L., Hamilton, W. F. D., Gunn, A., and Browning, M. C. K., 1981, Altered endocrine response to partial thyroidectomy in propranolol-prepared hyperthyroid patients, *Clin. Endocrinol.* **14:**597–604.

266. Nilsson, O. R., Melander, A., and Tegler, L., 1980, Effects and plasma levels of propranolol and metoprolol in hyperthyroid patients, *Eur. J. Clin. Pharmacol.* **18:**315–320.

267. Ross, P. J., Jones, M. K., and John, R., 1980, The effect of propranolol withdrawal on thyroid hormones in normal and hyperthyroid subjects, *Clin. Endocrinol.* **13:**27–31.

268. Rubin, P. C., 1981, Beta-blockers in pregnancy, *N. Engl. J. Med.* **305:**1323–1326.

269. Bradley, E. L., III, DiGirolamo, M., and Tarcan, Y., 1980, Modified subtotal thyroidectomy in management of Graves' disease, *Surgery* **87:**623–629.

270. Rasmusson, B., Borgeskov, S., and Holm-Hansen, B., 1980, Changes in serum calcitonin in patients undergoing thyroid surgery, Surgery **146:** 15–17.

271. Wilkin, T. J., Isles, T. E., Gunn, A., Crooks, J., and Beck, J. S., 1979, Short-term triiodothyronine in prevention of temporary hypothyroidism after subtotal thyroidectomy for Graves' disease, *Lancet* **2:**63–66.

272. Sawers, J. S. A., Toft, A. D., Irvine, W. J., Brown, N. S., and Seth, J., 1980, Transient hypothyroidism after iodine-131 treatment of thyrotoxicosis, *J. Clin. Endocrinol. Metab.* **50:**226–229.

273. Tamai, H., Nakagawa, T., Takahashi, H., Ohsako, N., Fukino, O., Shinzato, R., Suematsu, H., Matsuzuka, F., Kuma, K., and Nagataki, S., 1980, Triiodothyronine suppression tests and TSH-releasing hormone tests before and after I-131 therapy for Graves' disease, *J. Nucl. Med.* **21:**240–245.

274. Vasily, D. B., and Tyler, W. B., 1980, Propylthiouracil-induced cutaneous vasculitis—Case presentation and review of the literature, *J. Am. Med. Assoc.* **243:**458–461.

275. Weiss, M., Hassin, D., and Bank, H., 1980, Propylthiouracil-induced hepatic damage, *Arch. Intern. Med.* **140:**1184–1185.

276. Greer, M. A., Kammer, H., and Bouman, D. J., 1977, Short-term antithyroid therapy for the thyrotoxicosis of Graves' disease, *N. Engl. J. Med.* **297:**173–176.

277. Burr, W. A., Fitzgerald, M. G., and Hoffenberg, R., 1979, Relapse after short-term antithyroid therapy of Graves' disease, *N. Engl. J. Med.* **300:**200.

278. Tamai, H., Nakagawa, T., Fukino, O., Ohsako, N., Shinzato, R., Suematsu, H., Kuma, K., Matsuzuka, F., and Nagataki, S., 1980, Thionamide therapy in Graves' disease: Relation of relapse rate to duration of therapy, *Ann. Intern. Med.* **92:**488–490.

279. Slingerland, D. W., and Burrows, B. A., 1979, Long-term antithyroid treatment in hyperthyroidism, *J. Am. Med. Assoc.* **242:**2408–2410.

280. Wood, L. C., and Ingbar, S. H., 1979, Hypothyroidism as a late sequela in patients with Graves' disease treated with antithyroid agents, *J. Clin. Invest.* **64:**1429–1436.

281. Yamamoto, M., Igarashi, T., Kimura, S., Tsukamoto, S., Togawa, K., and Ogata, E., 1979, Thyroid suppression test and outcome of hyperthyroidism treated with antithyroid drugs and triiodothyronine, *J. Clin. Endocrinol. Metab.* **48:**72–77.

282. Wilkin, T. J., Isles, T. E., Crooks, J., Gunn, A., and Beck, J. S., 1981, Patterns of change in the early (20-minute) radioiodine uptake during

carbimazole treatment for Graves' disease and their relationship to outcome, *J. Clin. Endocrinol. Metab.* **52:**1067–1072.

283. Gardner, D. F., and Utiger, R. D., 1979, The natural history of hyperthyroidism due to Graves' disease in remission: Sequential studies of pituitary–thyroid regulation and various serum parameters, *J. Clin. Endocrinol. Metab.* **49:**417–421.

284. Cooper, D. S., Saxe, V. C., Maloof, F., and Ridgway, E. C., 1981, Studies of propylthiouracil using a newly developed radioimmunoassay, *J. Clin. Endocrinol. Metab.* **52:**204–213.

285. Kampmann, J. P., Mortensen, H. B., Bach, B., Waldorff, S., Kristensen, M. B., and Hansen, J. M., 1979, Kinetics of propylthiouracil in the elderly, *Acta Med. Scand.* **624:**93–98.

286. Skellern, G. G., Knight, B. I., Low, C. K. L., Alexander, W. D., McLarty, D. G., and Kalk, W. J., 1980, The pharmacokinetics of methimazole after oral administration of carbimazole and methimazole, in hyperthyroid patients, *Br. J. Clin. Pharmacol.* **9:**137–143.

287. Dahlberg, P. A., Karlsson, F. A., Lindström, B., and Wide, L., 1981, Studies of thyroid hormone and methimazole levels in patients with Graves' disease on a standardized anti-thyroid drug regimen, *Clin. Endocrinol.* **14:**555–562.

288. Sugrue, D., McEvoy, M., Feely, J., and Drury, M. I., 1980, Hyperthyroidism in the land of Graves: Results of treatment by surgery, radioiodine and carbimazole in 837 cases, *Q. J. Med.* **193:**51–61.

289. Reynolds, L. R., and Kotchen, T. A., 1979, Antithyroid drugs and radioactive iodine—Fifteen years' experience with Graves' disease, *Arch. Intern. Med.* **139:**651–653.

290. Amir, S. M., Sullivan, R., and Ingbar, S. H., 1981, The effect of desialylation on the in vitro interaction of human chorionic gonadotropin with human thyroid plasma membranes, *Endocrinology* **109:**1203–1211.

291. Carayon, P., Amr, S., Nisula, B., and Lissitzky, S., 1981, Effect of carboxypeptidase digestion of the human choriogonadotropin molecule on its thyrotropic activity, *Endocrinology* **108:**1891–1898.

292. Davies, T. F., Taliadouros, G. S., Catt, K. J., and Nisula, B. C., 1979, Assessment of urinary thyrotropin-competing activity in choriocarcinoma and thyroid disease: Further evidence for human chorionic gonadotropin interacting at the thyroid cell membrane, *J. Clin. Endocrinol. Metab.* **49:**353–357.

293. Pekonen, F., and Weintraub, B. D., 1980, Interaction of crude and pure chorionic gonadotropin with the thyrotropin receptor, *J. Clin. Endocrinol. Metab.* **50:**280–285.

294. Carayon, P., Lefort, G., and Nisula, B., 1980, Interaction of human chorionic gonadotropin and human luteinizing hormone with human thyroid membranes, *Endocrinology* **106:**1907–1916.

295. Nikolai, T. F., Coombs, G. J., and McKenzie, A. K., 1981, Lymphocytic thyroiditis with spontaneously resolving hyperthyroidism and subacute thyroiditis, *Arch. Intern. Med.* **141:**1455–1458.

296. Inada, M., Nishikawa, M., Naito, K., Ishii, H., Tanaka, K., and Imura, H., 1981, Reversible changes of the histological abnormalities of the thyroid in patients with painless thyroiditis, *J. Clin. Endocrinol. Metab.* **52:**431–435.

297. Amino, N., Mori, H., Iwatani, Y., Tanizawa, O., Kawashima, M., Tsuge, I., Ibaragi, K., Kumahara, Y., and Miyai, K., 1982, High prevalence of transient post-partum thyrotoxicosis and hypothyroidism, *Med. Intell.* **306:**849–852.

298. Amino, N., Yabu, Y., Miki, T., Morimoto, S., Kumahara, Y., Mori, H., Iwatani, Y., Nishi, K., Nakatani, K., and Miyai, K., 1981, Serum ratio of triiodothyronine to thyroxine, and thyroxine-binding globulin and calcitonin concentrations in Graves' disease and destruction-induced thyrotoxicosis, *J. Clin. Endocrinol. Metab.* **53:**113–116.

299. Weintraub, B. D., Gershengorn, M. C., Kourides, I. A., and Fein, H., 1981, Inappropriate secretion of thyroid-stimulating hormone, *Ann. Intern. Med.* **95:**339–351.

300. Kourides, I. A., Pekonen, F., and Weintraub, B. D., 1980, Absence of thyroid-binding immunoglobulins in patients with thyrotropin-mediated hyperthyroidism, *J. Clin. Endocrinol. Metab.* **51:**271–274.

301. Hamburger, J. I., 1980, Evolution of toxicity in solitary nontoxic autonomously functioning thyroid nodules, *J. Clin. Endocrinol. Metab.* **50:**1089–1093.

302. Mortimer, P. S., Tomlinson, I. W., and Rosenthal, F. D., 1981, Hemiaplasia of the thyroid with thyrotoxicosis, *J. Clin. Endocrinol. Metab.* **52:**152–155.

303. Melnick, J. C., and Stemkowski, P. E., 1981, Thyroid hemiagenesis (hockey stick sign): A review of the world literature and a report of four cases, *J. Clin. Endocrinol. Metab.* **52:**247–251.

304. Sharp, B., Reed, A. W., Tamagna, E. I., Geffner, D. L., and Hershman, J. M., 1981, Treatment of hyperthyroidism with sodium ipodate (Oragrafin) in addition to propylthiouracil and propranolol, *J. Clin. Endocrinol. Metab.* **53:**622–625.

305. Bhasin, S., Wallace, W., Lawrence, J. B., and Lesch, M., 1981, Sudden death associated with thyroid hormone abuse, *Am. J. Med.* **71:**887–890.

306. Nyström, E., Lindstedt, G., and Lundberg, P.-A., 1980, Minor signs and symptoms of toxicity in a young woman in spite of massive thyroxine ingestion, *Acta Med. Scand.* **207:**135–136.

307. Kabadi, U. M., and Eisenstein, A. B., 1980, Glucose intolerance in hyperthyroidism: Role of glucagon, *J. Clin. Endocrinol. Metab.* **50:**392–396.

308. Kabadi, U. M., and Eisenstein, A. B., 1980, Impaired pancreatic α-cell response in hyperthyroidism, *J. Clin. Endocrinol. Metab.* **51:**478–482.

309. Perez, G., Ungaro, B., Covelli, A., Morrone, G., Lombardi, G., Scopacasa, F., and Rossi, R., 1980, Altered glucoregulatory response to physiological infusions of epinephrine and glucagon in hyperthyroidism, *J. Clin. Endocrinol. Metab.* **51:**972–977.

310. Nilsson, O. R., Karlberg, B. E., and Söderberg, A., 1980, Plasma catecholamines and cardiovascular responses to hypoglycemia in hyperthyroidism before and during treatment with metoprolol or propranolol, *J. Clin. Endocrinol. Metab.* **50:**906–911.

311. Tse, J., Wrenn, R. W., and Kuo, J. F., 1980, Thyroxine-induced changes in characteristics and activities of β-adrenergic receptors and adenosine 3',5'-monophosphate and guanosine 3',5'-monophosphate systems in the heart may be related to reputed catecholamine supersensitivity in hyperthyroidism, *Endocrinology* **107:**6–16.

312. Ginsberg, A. M., Clutter, W. E., Shah, S. D., and Cryer, P. E., 1981, Triiodo-thyronine-induced thyrotoxicosis increases mononuclear leukocyte β-adrenergic receptor density in man, *J. Clin. Invest.* **67:**1785–1791.

313. Channick, B. J., Adlin, E. V., Marks, A. D., Dennenberg, B. S., McDonough, M. T., Chakko, C. S., and Spann, J. F., 1981, Hyperthyroidism and mitral-valve prolapse, *N. Engl. J. Med.* **305:**497–500.

314. Marks, A. D., Adlin, E. V., Dennenberg, B. S., and Channick, B. J., 1982, Increased incidence of mitral valve prolapse in chronic lymphocytic thyroiditis, *Clin. Res.* **30:**273A.

315. Bayley, T. A., Harrison, J. E., McNeill, K. G., and Mernagh, J. R., 1980, Effect of thyrotoxicosis and its treatment on bone mineral and muscle mass, *J. Clin. Endocrinol. Metab.* **50:**916–922.

316. Bouillon, R., Muls, E., and De Moor, P., 1980, Influence of thyroid function on the serum concentration of 1,25-dihydroxyvitamin D_3, *J. Clin. Endocrinol. Metab.* **51:**793–797.

317. Haldimann, B., Kaptein, E. M., Singer, F. R., Nicoloff, J. T., and Massry, S. G., 1980, Intestinal calcium absorption in patients with hyperthyroidism, *J. Clin. Endocrinol. Metab.* **51:**995–997.

318. Cooper, D. S., Kaplan, M. M., Ridgway, E. C., Maloof, F., and Daniels, G. H., 1979, Alkaline phosphatase isoenzyme patterns in hyperthyroidism, *Ann. Intern. Med.* **90:**164–168.

319. Wiersinga, W. M., and Touber, J. L., 1980, The relation between gastrin, gastric acid and thyroid function disorders, *Acta Endocrinol. (Copenhagen)* **95:**341–349.

320. Seino, Y., Miyamoto, Y., Moridera, K., Taminato, T., Matsukura, S., and Imura, H., 1980, The role of the β-adrenergic mechanism in the hypergastrinemia of hyperthyroidism, *J. Clin. Endocrinol. Metab.* **50:**368–370.

321. Lipson, A., Tah-Hsiung, H., and Nickoloff, E. L., 1980, Blood gastrin levels in hyperthyroidism, *J. Clin. Endocrinol. Metab.* **50:**176–178.

322. Swanson, J. W., Kelly, J. J., Jr., and McConahey, W. M., 1981, Neurologic aspects of thyroid dysfunction, *Mayo Clin. Proc.* **56:**504–512.

323. Puvanendran, K., Cheah, J. S., Naganathan, N., Yeo, P. P. B., and Wong, P. K., 1979, Neuromuscular transmission in thyrotoxicosis, *J. Neurol. Sci.* **43:**47–57.

324. Rockey, P. H., and Griep, R. J., 1980, Behavioral dysfunction in hyperthyroidism, *Arch. Intern. Med.* **140:**1194–1197.

325. Daneman, D., and Howard, N. J., 1980, Neonatal thyrotoxicosis: Intellectual impairment and craniosynostosis in later years, *J. Pediatr.* **97:**257–259.

326. Hollingsworth, D. R., and Mabry, C. C., 1976, Congenital Graves' disease, *Am. J. Dis. Child.* **130:**148.

327. Kidd, G. S., Glass, A. R., and Vigersky, R. A., 1979, The hypothalamic–pituitary–testicular axis in thyrotoxicosis, *J. Clin. Endocrinol. Metab.* **48:**798–802.

328. Gray, R. S., Borsey, D. Q., Seth, J., Herd, R., Brown, N. S., and Clarke, B. F., 1980, Prevalence of subclinical thyroid failure in insulin-dependent diabetes, *J. Clin. Endocrinol. Metab.* **50:**1034–1037.

329. Crowe, J. P., Christensen, E., Butler, J., Wheeler, P., Doniach, D., Keenan,

J., and Williams, R., 1980, Primary biliary cirrhosis: The prevalence of hypothyroidism and its relationship to thyroid autoantibodies and sicca syndrome, *Gastroenterology* **78:**1437–1441.

330. Gordon, M. B., Klein, I., Dekker, A., Rodnan, G. P., and Medsger, T. A., Jr., 1981, Thyroid disease in progressive systemic sclerosis: Increased frequency of glandular fibrosis and hypothyroidism, *Ann. Intern. Med.* **95:**431–435.

331. Lobo, E. D., Khan, M., and Tew, J., 1980, Community study of hypothyroidism in Down's syndrome, *Br. Med. J.* **280:**1253.

332. Bahn, A. K., Mills, J. L., Snyder, P. J., Gann, P. H., Houten, L., Bialik, O., Hollmann, L., and Utiger, R. D., 1980, Hypothyroidism in workers exposed to polybrominated biphenyls, *N. Engl. J. Med.* **302:**31–33.

333. Smith, R. E., Jr., Adler, R. A., Clark, P., Brinck-Johnsen, T., Tulloh, M. E., and Colton, T., 1981, Thyroid function after mantle irradiation in Hodgkin's disease, *J. Am. Med. Assoc.* **245:**46–49.

334. Schimpff, S. C., Diggs, C. H., Wiswell, J. G., Salvatore, P. C., and Wiernik, P. H., 1980, Radiation-related thyroid dysfunction: Implications for the treatment of Hodgkin's disease, *Ann. Intern. Med.* **92:**91–98.

335. Dussault, J. H., Letarte, J., Guyda, H., and Laberge, C., 1980, Lack of influence of thyroid antibodies on thyroid function in the newborn infant and on a mass screening program for congenital hypothyroidism, *J. Pediatr.* **96:**385–389.

336. Montoro, M., Collea, J. V., Frasier, S. D., and Mestman, J. H., 1981, Successful outcome of pregnancy in women with hypothyroidism, *Ann. Intern. Med.* **94:**31–34.

337. Bastenie, P. A., Bonnyns, M., and Vanhaelst, L., 1980, Grades of subclinical hypothyroidism in asymptomatic autoimmune thyroiditis revealed by the thyrotropin-releasing hormone test, *J. Clin. Endocrinol. Metab.* **51:**163–166.

338. Fisher, D. A., Dussault, J. H., Foley, T. P., Jr., Klein, A. H., LaFranchi, S., Lassen, P. R., Michell, M. L., Murphey, W. H., Walfish, P. G., 1979, Screening for congenital hypothyroidism: Results of screening one million North American infants, *J. Pediatr.* **94:**700–705.

339. Landau, H., Sack, J., Frucht, H., Palti, Z., Hochner-Celnikier, D., Rosenmann, A., 1980, Amniotic fluid 3,3′,5′-triiodothyronine in the detection of congenital hypothyroidism, *J. Clin. Endocrinol. Metab.* **50:**799–801.

340. Santos, A. D., Miller, R. P., Mathew, P. K., Wallace, W. A., Cave, W. T., Jr., Hinojosa, L., 1980, Echocardiographic characterization of the reversible cardiomyopathy of hypothyroidism, *Am. J. Med.* **68:**675–682.

341. Plotnick, G. D., Vassar, D. L., Parisi, A. F., Hamilton, B. P., Carliner, N. H., Fisher, M. L. 1979, Systolic time intervals in hypothyroidism: End organ function as a reflection of clinical status, *Am. J. Med. Sci.* **277:**263–268.

342. Sawin, C. T., Chopra, D., Azizi, F., Mannix, J. E., and Bacharach, P., 1979, The aging thyroid, increased prevalence of elevated serum thyrotropin levels in the elderly, *J. Am. Med. Assoc.* **242:**247–250.

343. Tieche, M., Lupi, G. A., Gutzwiller, F., Grob, P. J., Studer, H., and Bürgi, H., 1981, Borderline low thyroid function and thyroid autoimmunity, risk factors for coronary heart disease?, *Br. Heart J.* **46:**202–206.

344. Hay, I. D., Duick, D. S., Vlietstra, R. E., Maloney, J. D., and Pluth, J. R., 1981, Thyroxine therapy in hypothyroid patients undergoing coronary revascularization: A retrospective analysis, *Ann. Intern. Med.* **95:**456–458.

345. Parving, H.-H., Hansen, J. M., Nielsen, S. L., Rossing, N., Munck, O., and Lassen, N. A., 1979, Mechanisms of edema formation in myxedema— Increased protein extravasation and relatively slow lymphatic drainage, *N. Engl. J. Med.* **301:**460–465.

346. Orr, W. C., Males, J. L., and Imes, N. K., 1981, Myxedema and obstructive sleep apnea, *Am. J. Med.* **70:**1061–1066.

347. Klein, I., Parker, M., Shebert, R., Ayyar, D. R., and Levey, G. S., 1981, Hypothyroidism presenting as muscle stiffness and pseudohypertrophy: Hoffmann's syndrome, *Am. J. Med.* **70:**891–894.

348. Jakubovic, H. R., Salama, S. S. S., and Rosenthal, D., 1982, Multiple cutaneous focal mucinoses with hypothyroidism, *Ann. Intern. Med.* **96:**56–58.

349. Amino, N., Kuro, R., Yabu, Y., Takai, S.-I., Kawashima, M., Morimoto, S., Ichihara, K., Miyai, K., and Kumahara, Y., 1981, Elevated levels of circulating carcinoembryonic antigen in hypothyroidism, *J. Clin. Endocrinol. Metab.* **52:**457–462.

350. Agdeppa, D., Macaron, C., Mallik, T., and Schnuda, N. D., 1979, Plasma high density lipoprotein cholesterol in thyroid disease, *J. Clin. Endocrinol. Metab.* **49:**726–729.

351. Gorman, C. A., Jiang, N.-S., Ellefson, R. D., and Elveback, L. R., 1979, Comparative effectiveness of dextrothyroxine and levothyroxine in correcting hypothyroidism and lowering blood lipid levels in hypothyroid patients, *J. Clin. Endocrinol. Metab.* **49:**1–7.

352. Ingbar, J. C., Borges, M., Iflah, S., Kleinmann, R. E., Braverman, L. E., and Ingbar, S. H., 1982, Elevated serum thyroxine concentration in patients receiving "replacement" doses of levothyroxine, *J. Endocrinol. Invest.* **5:**77–85.

353. Rosenbaum, R. L., and Barzel, U. S., 1982, Levothyroxine replacement dose for primary hypothyroidism decreases with age, *Ann. Intern. Med.* **96:**53–55.

354. LaFranchi, S. H., 1979, Hypothyroidism, *Pediatr. Clin. North Am.* **26:**33–51.

355. Studer, H., and Ramelli, F., 1982, Simple goiter and its variants: Euthyroid and hyperthyroid multinodular goiters, *Endocr. Rev.* **3:**40–61.

356. Van Herle, A. J., Rich, P., Ljung, B.-M. E., Ashcraft, M. W., Solomon, D. H., and Keeler, E. B., 1982, The thyroid nodule, *Ann. Intern. Med.* **96:**221–232.

357. Bolk, J. H., Bussemaker, J. K., Elte, J. W. F., Haak, A., and Van Der Heide, D., 1979, Thyroid-stimulating immunoglobulins do not cause non-autonomous, autonomous, or toxic multinodular goitres, *Lancet* **2:**61–63.

358. Matte, R., Ste-Marie, L. G., Comtois, R., D'Amour, P., Lacroix, A., Chartrand, R., Poisson, R., and Bastomsky, C. H., 1981, The pituitary–thyroid axis after hemithyroidectomy in euthyroid man, *J. Clin. Endocrinol. Metab.* **53:**377–380.

359. Blichert-Toft, M., Egedorf, J., Christiansen, C., and Axelsson, C. K., 1979, Function of pituitary–thyroid axis after surgical treatment of nontoxic nodular goiter, *Acta Med. Scand.* **206:**15–19.

360. McCowen, K. D., Reed, J. W., and Fariss, B. L., 1980, The role of thyroid therapy in patients with thyroid cysts, *Am. J. Med.* **68:**853–855.

361. Rentsch, H., Studer, H., Frauchiger, B., and Siebenhüner, L., 1981, Topographical heterogeneity of basal and thyrotropin-stimulated adenosine 3′,5′-monophosphate in human nodular goiter, *J. Clin. Endocrinol. Metab.* **53:**514–521.

362. Van Sande, J., Mockel, J., Boeynaems, J. M., Dor, P., Andry, G., and Dumont J. E., 1980, Regulation of cyclic nucleotide and prostaglandin formation in normal human thyroid tissue and in autonomous nodules, *J. Clin. Endocrinol. Metab.* **50:**776–785.

363. Nagasaka, A., and Hidaka, H., 1980, Cyclic 3′,5′-nucleotide phosphodiesterase activities in the thyroid glands of patients with various disorders, *J. Clin. Endocrinol. Metab.* **50:**726–733.

364. Saito, K., Yamamota, K., Yoshida, S., Manabe, S., Suzuki, M., Takai, T., Saito, T., Kuzuya, T., and Moriyama, S.-I., 1981, Goitrous hypothyroidism due to iodide-trapping defect, *J. Clin. Endocrinol. Metab.* **53:**1267–1272.

365. Eggo, M. C., Burrow, G. N., Alexander, N. M., and Gordon, J. H., 1980, Iodination and the structure of human thyroglobulin, *J. Clin. Endocrinol. Metab.* **51:**7–11.

366. Cooper, D. S., Axelrod, L., DeGroot, L. J., Vickery, A. L., Jr., and Maloof, F., 1981, Congenital goiter and the development of metastatic follicular carcinoma with evidence for a leak of nonhormonal iodide: Clinical, pathological, kinetic, and biochemical studies and a review of the literature, *J. Clin. Endocrinol. Metab.* **52:**294–306.

367. Gaitan, E., Medina, P., DeRouen, T. A., and Zia, M. S., 1980, Goiter prevalence and bacterial contamination of water supplies, *J. Clin. Endocrinol. Metab.* **51:**957–961.

368. Weiss, M., Kasper, D., and Ingbar, S. H., 1982, A specific, saturable binding site for thyrotropin (TSH) in *Yersinia enterocolitica* and *E. coli, Clin. Res.* **30:**494A.

369. Colacchio, T. A., LoGerfo, P., and Feind, C. R., 1980, Fine needle cytologic diagnosis of thyroid nodules, *Am. J. Surg.* **140:**568–571.

370. Miller, J. M., Hamburger, J. I., and Kini, S., 1979, Diagnosis of thyroid nodules, *J. Am. Med. Assoc.* **241:**481–484.

371. Miller, J. M., Hamburger, J. I., and Kini, S. R., 1981, The needle biopsy diagnosis of papillary thyroid carcinoma, *Cancer* **48:**989–993.

372. Stepanas, A. V., Samaan, N. A., Hill, C. S., Jr., and Hickey, R. C., 1979, Medullary thyroid carcinoma, *Cancer* **43:**825–837.

373. Block, M. A., Jackson, C. E., Greenawald, K. A., and Yott, J. B., 1980, Clinical characteristics distinguishing hereditary from sporadic medullary thyroid carcinoma: Treatment implications, *Arch. Surg. (Chicago)* **115:**142–148.

374. Lamberg, B.-A., Reissel, P., Stenman, S., Koivuniemi, A., Ekblom, M., Mäkinen, J., and Franssila, K., 1981, Concurrent medullary and papillary thyroid carcinoma in the same thyroid lobe and in siblings, *Acta Med. Scand.* **209:**421–424.

375. Deftos, L. J., Bone, H. G., III, Parthemore, J. G., and Burton, D. W., 1980,

Immunohistological studies of medullary thyroid carcinoma and C cell hyperplasia, *J. Clin. Endocrinol. Metab.* **51**:857–862.

376. Schneider, A. B., Bekerman, C., Favus, M., Frohman, L. A., Gonzalez, C., Ryo, U. Y., Sievertsen, G., and Pinsky, S., 1981, Continuing occurrence of thyroid nodules after head and neck irradiation, *Ann. Intern. Med.* **94**:176–180.

377. McDougall, I. R., Coleman, C. N., Burke, J. S., Saunders, W., and Kaplan, H. S., 1980, Thyroid carcinoma after high-dose external radiotherapy for Hodgkin's disease, *Cancer* **45**:2056–2060.

378. Compagno, J., and Oertel, J. E., 1980, Malignant lymphoma and other lymphoproliferative disorders of the thyroid gland, *Am. J. Clin. Pathol.* **74**:1–11.

379. Carayon, P., Morvan, C. T., Castanas, E., and Tubiana, M., 1980, Human thyroid cancer: Membrane thyrotropin binding and adenylate cyclase activity, *J. Clin. Endocrinol. Metab.* **51**:915–920.

380. Schlumberger, M., Charbord, P., Fragu, P., Lumbroso, J., Parmentier, C., and Tubiana, M., 1980, Circulating thyroglobulin and thyroid hormones in patients with metastases of differentiated thyroid carcinoma: Relationship to serum thyrotropin levels, *J. Clin. Endocrinol. Metab.* **51**:513–519.

381. Fui, S. C. N. T., Hoffenberg, R., Maisey, M. N., and Black, E. G., 1979, Serum thyroglobulin concentrations and whole-body radioiodine scan in follow-up of differentiated thyroid cancer after thyroid ablation, *Br. Med. J.* **2**:298–300.

382. Ashcraft, M. W., and van Herle, A. J., 1981, The comparative value of serum thyroglobulin measurements and iodine 131 total body scans in the follow-up study of patients with treated differentiated thyroid cancer, *Am. J. Med.* **71**:806–814.

383. Schneider, A. B., Line, B. R., Goldman, J. M., and Robbins, J., 1981, Sequential serum thyroglobulin determinations, ^{131}I scans, and ^{131}I uptakes after triiodothyronine withdrawal in patients with thyroid cancer, *J. Clin. Endocrinol. Metab.* **53**:1199–1206.

384. Young, R. L., Mazzaferri, E. L., Rahe, A. J., and Dorfman, S. G., 1980, Pure follicular thyroid carcinoma: Impact of therapy in 214 patients, *J. Nucl. Med.* **21**:733–737.

385. Mazzaferri, E. L., and Young, R. L., 1981, Papillary thyroid carcinoma: A 10 year follow-up report of the impact of therapy in 576 patients, *Am. J. Med.* **70**:511–518.

386. DeGroot, L. J., and Reilly, M., 1982, Comparison of 30- and 50-mCi doses of iodine-131 for thyroid ablation, *Ann. Intern. Med.* **96**:51–53.

387. Chung, C. T., Sagerman, R. H., Ryoo, M. C., King, G. A., Yu, W. S., Dalai, P. S., and Emmanuel, I. G., 1980, External irradiation for malignant thyroid tumors, *Radiology* **136**:753–756.

388. Shapiro, S., Slone, D., Kaufman, D. W., Rosenberg, L., Miettinen, O. S., Stolley, P. D., Knapp, R. C., Leavitt, T., Jr., Watring, W. G., Rosenshein, N. B., and Schottenfeld, D., 1980, Use of thyroid supplements in relation to the risk of breast cancer, *J. Am. Med. Assoc.* **244**:1685–1687.

389. Hedley, A. J., Spiegelhalter, D. J., Jones, S. J., Clements, P., Bewsher, P. D., Simpson, J. G., and Weir, R. D., 1981, Breast cancer in thyroid disease: Fact or fallacy?, *Lancet* **1**:131–133.

390. Cerbon, M.-A., Pichon, M.-F., and Milgrom, E., 1981, Thyroid hormone receptors in human breast cancer, *Cancer Res.* **41:**4167–4173.

391. Spitz, I. M., Roith, D. L., Hirsch, H., Carayon, P., Pekonen, F., Liel, Y., Sobel, R., Chorer, Z., and Weintraub, B., 1981, Increased high-molecular-weight thyrotropin with impaired biologic activity in a euthyroid man, *N. Engl. J. Med.* **304:**278–282.

392. Beamer, W. G., Eicher, E. M., Maltais, L. J., and Southard, J. L., 1981, Inherited primary hypothyroidism in mice, *Science* **212:**61–63.

393. Smeds, S., Anderberg, B., Boeryd, B., Ericson, L. E., Gillquist, J., and Persliden, J., 1981, The nude mouse: A possible experimental model for investigation of human thyroid tissue, *J. Endocrinol. Invest.* **4:**11–15.

394. Sternthal, E., Like, A. A., Sarantis, K., and Braverman, L. E., 1981, Lymphocytic thyroiditis and diabetes in the BB/W rat: A new model of autoimmune endocrinopathy, *Diabetes* **3:**1058–1061.

The Testis

Daniel D. Federman

4.1. Introduction

This chapter on the testis follows the outline used in the past. As before, the aim is to present an integrated review rather than an exhaustive compilation of references. Similarly, the emphasis is selective and will, in particular, stress testicular differentiation, puberty and gonadotropin-releasing hormone (LRH), androgen action and resistance, and some new aspects of infertility.

4.2. Intrauterine and Neonatal Function

4.2.1. Embryonic Sex Differentiation

4.2.1.1. Normal Controls

Our current knowledge of the Y chromosome is well reviewed by Bühler.[1] On the basis of almost 20 years' experience, it is clear that:

1. The Y chromosome somehow controls testicular differentiation in the fetus
2. The portion of the Y involved is the pericentric region, particularly on the short arm
3. There is also information (probably regulatory) on the Y that prevents the Turner stigmata in the normal male

DANIEL D. FEDERMAN ● Harvard Medical School, Boston, Massachusetts 02115.

4. No structural gene has been unequivocally assigned to the Y
5. There may be loci on the long arm that influence spermatogenesis
6. There are at least two long stretches of heterochromatin
7. Variation in one of these stretches probably accounts for the heritable variation in length of the Y
8. A segment on the short arm controls linear growth, and duplication leads to excessive growth in XYY men
9. All the above statements must be regarded as tentative

In Fig. 19 of his article, Bühler essays a map of the Y chromosome, but the difficulty entailed is a reminder of the special role of the Y.

The H-Y antigen story is, if anything, murkier than it was a few years ago. The outline seems simple: a locus on the short arm of the Y probably controls expression of a male-specific antigen that is simultaneously a weak histocompatibility factor and the signal for testicular differentiation of the indifferent gonadal anlage of the fetus.[2,3] Wachtel and Koo[4] have marshaled the supporting evidence in man:

1. Presence of H-Y positivity correlates with presence of testis in 46,XX males and 46,XX true hermaphrodites[5]
2. Normal females and 45,X Turner's with gonadal dysgenesis are H-Y negative
3. 46,XY patients with female phenotype (testicular feminization) are H-Y positive and have testes

Some interesting experimental embryology, reported in Volume 1, supports the view outlined above.

But important negative information has begun to accumulate. This includes:

1. 45,X patients who are H-Y positive[6]
2. 46,XX(iso qi) who are H-Y positive
3. 46,XXp patients who have diminished levels of H-Y antigen[7]
4. 46,XY patients with pure gonadal dysgenesis who are H-Y positive, and others who are H-Y negative
5. Reports that some transsexual patients have H-Y results discordant from their karyotype and preoperative phenotype[8]
6. Absence of extensive data about H-Y status of normal males and females

A cautious summary at this time might be that there is a male-specific antigen whose expression is controlled by gene loci on the Y, the long arm of the X, and perhaps an autosome; that this antigen, or a linked substance, is a necessary, but not sufficient, condition for testicular differentiation; that expression of the antigen requires two tissue receptors, one of which is found in all cells, β_2-microglobulin, and one that is found only in gonadal cells[9,10]; and that the evidence is not yet persuasive that the transplantation antigen and the testis-determinant are identical.

There remains some uncertainty about the physiologic control of testosterone (T) secretion *in utero*. Griffin and Wilson[11] suggest that the gonad may be autonomous, although most authors have thought that human chorionic gonadotropin (hCG) is the principal stimulant in the first trimester, and fetal luteinizing hormone (LH) sometime after the 20th week. Huhtaniemi and Lautala[12] have used perifusion of the fetal testis to show a stimulatory effect of hCG in fetuses of 8–18 weeks' gestation. This period overlaps the time when significant difference in clitoral and penile growth has been observed in abortuses by Feldman and Smith.[13] Thus, a small penis, with otherwise normal genitalia, can serve as a clue to intrauterine T deficiency, probably reflecting lack of fetal LH. These interpretations are supported by the consistent finding of differences in amniotic fluid (and often maternal) levels of T throughout mid- and late gestation.[14] Indeed, amniotic fluid T levels remain the best way to distinguish the sex of the fetus.[15] A fine point in hormonal relationships to sex was examined by measuring fetal pituitary LH and follicle-stimulating hormone (FSH) throughout gestation: the female fetus shows a peak in midgestation, with a consistent decline thereafter, whereas the male shows an increase in pituitary LH throughout gestation.[16] This pattern is consistent with the evidence that fetal LH and T, via dihydrotestosterone (DHT), are instrumental in testicular descent during the last trimester.

4.2.1.2. Defects in Fetal Sex Differentiation

As mentioned previously, there is uncertainty about the role of the H-Y antigen in sex differentiation. Nevertheless, some important cases suggesting its role in anomalous development are being reported. Wachtel[17] presents a summary of the influence of H-Y on testicular differentiation, particularly collating reported cases of H-Y defect and testicular deficiency. In 46,XY individuals who lack H-Y antigen, the syndrome of pure gonadal dysgenesis results: normal height, female internal and external genitalia, and streak gonads that sometimes have some testicular-like tubules that serve to differentiate them from the streak gonads of Turner's syndrome. Conversely, 46,XY H-Y positive patients can have gonadal dysgenesis either because of a defect in the H-Y antigen receptor, or because of a defect in the biologically active but not the immunologically reactive portion of the antigen. Similarly, 46,XX males are almost invariably H-Y positive; the accumulating evidence is that the H-Y antigen has been transmitted to an autosome, producing a genetic pattern similar to the autosomal dominant *Sxr* mutation in the mouse. 46,XX true hermaphrodites may be H-Y positive,[18] and at least one article suggests that the translocation is to the X chromosome, with Lyonization leading to intermediate levels of H-Y and, in one of the gonads, to ovarian differentiation. In at least one important case, the testicular portion of an ovotestis was H-Y positive, whereas the remainder was H-Y negative, suggesting an intratissue mosaicism that cytogenetics has rarely demonstrated[19]; this area is not resolved, however, because a secretion of the fetal ovary is capable of blocking the attachment of H-Y antigen to its gonad-specific receptor.

Within the spectrum of sex chromosome errors that produce abnormal sex differentiation, karyotypic mosaicism is an important phenomenon about which several questions exist. Elias *et al.*[20] have addressed two of these uncertainties in a paper that reports repeat studies of three patients with mosaicism for the X chromosome. Simultaneous samplings of blood showed similar frequencies of the various cell lines, and followup over time indicated approximate stability of the proportions. The authors suggest that mosaicism is less variable than has been thought, and that a single blood sample is sufficient for most clinical purposes. (Note, though, that intertissue mosaicism will not be detected with single tissue sampling.)

Undetected mosaicism has been suspected as a factor in XX males, but almost all cases have been H-Y positive. Anomalous H-Y findings have been illuminated by two recent reports. Moreira-Filho *et al.*[21] describe a 46,XX true hermaphrodite with bilateral ovotestes and an ambiguous phenotype; the patient was H-Y positive but with a titer lower than that of his XX/XY father (sic) and lower than that of normal XY controls. The authors suggest that X–Y interchange plus X-chromosome inactivation accounts for the diminished levels, and point out that reduced levels of H-Y in XX males had been seen previously.

More important in a theoretic sense is the report of Bernstein *et al.*[22] regarding a patient and her child, both with normal female gonadal and genital differentiation, but with a curious karyotype interpreted as a duplication of some of the Xq and an apparently normal Y but with an H-Y negative status. The karyotype is important—46,Xdup(X)(p21-pter)—because it is consistent with the existence of regulatory genes on the X that, in excess, suppress H-Y expression. The abnormality was also present in the patient's maternal grandmother and a female sibling, supporting the stability of the karyotype and the interpretation given for it.

Jones *et al.*[23] have raised a dissenting voice regarding the role of H-Y antigen. They report an H-Y positive XX/XY chimera true hermaphrodite, as well as H-Y positive patients without testes and H-Y negative patients with testes, and summarize by saying that the lack of correlation argues strongly against a primary role of H-Y antigen in human sex differentiation.

An intriguing disorder involving macro-orchidism, reported in diverse locales, was summarized by Turner et al.[24] in a paper defining the X-linked nature of the disorder. Although a syndrome of X-linked mental retardation occasionally accompanied by macro-orchidism was known previously, the Australian authors have contributed the insight that the macro-orchidism appears to correlate with the presence of a fragile site on the long arm of the X(Xq27 fra).[25] Patients without the fragile site may have the mental defect but do not have the testicular abnormality, which runs true within affected families.

The endocrine defects contributing to abnormal fetal sex differentiation are being progressively defined. Enzymatic defects in T biosynthesis appear, from the infrequency with which they are reported, to be uncommon. Since three of the diseases involving T deficiency affect cortisol synthesis as well, perhaps their infrequency is accounted for by the extreme disadvantage of the adrenal component.[26]

The syndromes of androgen insensitivity, on the other hand, are accumulating rapidly and may be among the most common of inherited endocrine diorders. In a brilliant series of original contributions and reviews, Wilson et al.[11] have delineated the biochemical defects that underlie this range of phenotypes. The defects in androgen action fall into three categories: impaired conversion of T to DHT in target tissues (steroid 5α-reductase deficiency); defective binding of androgens to the cytosol receptor; or defective stimulation of genetic transcription by the androgen/receptor complex. The disorders are pertinent to both genital differentiation and puberty, and are thus discussed under both headings in this chapter.

Steroid 5α-reductase deficiency, originally described in Dallas and Santo Domingo, has now been reported more widely and with what appears to be a variable degree of enzyme defect. The affected newborn has normal Wolffian development but variable external virilization, and in naive settings more children have been raised as females than as males. Savage et al.[27] reported two Cypriot brothers raised as females who switched to male roles after puberty. Their studies support the interpretation of a defect in the reductase as the mechanism of the disorder. One question that has remained puzzling is why, if T binds to the same cytosol receptor as DHT does, there is a defect in masculinization despite normal or even slightly high T levels. Maes et al.[28] demonstrated that the two hormones do indeed bind to the same receptor, but found that the receptor had a somewhat lower affinity for T and a higher turnover of T than of DHT. Whether these slight differences account for the phenotypic differences is unclear. The finding may, however, illuminate another mystery of the disorder: the excellent masculinization of the patients at puberty. Testosterone may be exerting an effect here as well, with the high plasma levels compensating for the diminished affinity between the ligand and the receptor. Imperato-McGinley et al.[29] have also reported further on the disease, confirming the autosomal recessive inheritance, the impressive masculinization at puberty, and the change in gender identity at that time (vide infra).

4.2.2. Testicular Function in Childhood

The work originally published by Forest et al.[30] that showed a post-natal rise in serum T in males has now been extended. Gendrel et al.[31] have confirmed that this rise is secondary to a rise in LH, which lasts about 4–5 months and subsequently declines to minimal levels until puberty appears. The serum levels of N-acetyl-β-hexosaminidase show a sexual dimorphism during the first 3 months of life, and have been shown to correlate with plasma T levels during that time.[32] Pang et al.[33] showed that DHT and T are both elevated during the first 6 months of life, the values reaching those in the midpubertal range; infants given hCG showed a parallel rise in both hormones. Forest[34] did similar studies, measuring T, androstenedione, and 17-hydroprogesterone (17OH-P) at various times from infancy through the onset of puberty. Her studies indicated that the fall in testicular secretion does not represent testicular hyporesponsiveness but rather a decline in LH secretion (see Gendrel et al. above); that testicular response to hCG can still be elicited during the quiescent period of childhood; and that an increase in testicular responsiveness to gonadotropin is one of the earliest features of puberty. FSH concentrations were slightly higher in female than male infants, and LH values higher in males, in another study.[35] In another report, previously cryptorchid testes descended in males who had a good T rise during early infancy, but did not descend in babies who had little rise in T. This finding correlates with Scorer's much earlier observation that, of those infants cryptorchid at birth, a certain percentage show descent during the first 3 months of life, or not until puberty. Since it appears that DHT is the mediator of testicular descent, the story of a neonatal rise in LH and an accompanying rise in T and DHT fits together nicely.

This background is also useful for understanding and planning for the baby with micropenis. Burstein et al.[36] reported 14 male infants with micropenis, in 9 of whom the condition was a clue to otherwise unsuspected hypopituitarism. This paper reviews the differential diagnosis of micropenis and points to the pitfalls of diagnosis. Evidence of hypopituitarism is provided in nine cases, and hypogonadotropinism cannot be excluded in the other five. T enanthate, 25 or 50 mg monthly for 3 months, was given; the observed penile growth without undue bone maturation is cited by the authors to counter the view of others that patients whose stretched penile length is more than 2 SD below the mean for age should be castrated and raised as girls. This important paper thus proposes an approach to evaluation of the neonate with micropenis and urges a trial of T before considering sex-change surgery. Another paper from the same institution, however, provides a reminder than in some patients microphallus, rather than reflecting an endocrine disorder, is an anomaly requiring surgical repair.[37] The discussion provided in this paper is informative, since it indicates that there is often great difficulty in distinguishing endocrine from nonendocrine causes of microphallus. Finally, Ben-Galim *et al.*[38] report on topical T therapy in older children, with improvement in the condition. However, since topical T is irregularly absorbed, it seems wiser to use the parenteral approach and to monitor the dose administered.

The therapeutic results in micropenis were also studied by Danish *et al.*[39] Of 14 patients with penis 2.5 SD below the mean, 9 were raised as males, and 5 of them received androgen therapy. Of the latter, two achieved penile size within the normal range, but for three penile length remained significantly below normal. The authors point the lesson that, for some patients with a phallus more than 2 SD below the mean, androgen therapy is not necessarily successful. Although they try to suggest a difference between 2.5–3 SD and more than 3 SD below the mean, it is doubtful that this difference can be reliably measured in ordinary clinical work.

Another study based on the neonatal rise in LH and T was reported in seven 45,XY patients with male pseudohermaphroditism.[40] Two patients showed an inadequate rise in T and were found to have adrenal and testicular enzymatic defects in T synthesis. Five patients showed a normal rise, suggesting that they would later have normal T secretion. At the time of the report, none of the patients had demonstrated an abnormally high T, which would predict androgen insensitivity; but it seems likely that this condition will be found, with family studies revealing those patients who are to be studied.

4.3. Puberty

Ojeda *et al.*[41] in the new journal *Endocrine Reviews*, have provided an excellent perspective on human puberty, as well as an interesting comparison with related events in the rat. It would not be wildly off the mark to state that puberty begins about a half-hour after bedtime some evening in late childhood. The heralding event would be a pulse of

LRH, probably not eliciting much of a gonadotropin or T response.[42] But as pulsatile LRH release continues, gonadotropes in the anterior pituitary awake and soon a burst of LH, accompanied by minimal change in FSH, occurs and, about an hour later, elicits a slight rise in plasma T. Over a 4-year period, the plasma T gradually attains the adult level, and the familiar phenotypic changes of puberty appear. Insights into the process have come from a number of sources.

Most authors support the view of Grumbach[43] and his colleagues that puberty is initiated by a reset of the hypothalamic gonadostat, with the result that levels of plasma steroids higher than those present in the child are needed to suppress the secretion of gonadotropin; indeed, the progression of puberty is marked by increasing concentrations of T despite increasing concentrations of LH.[41,43–46] There are, however, several enigmatic features. Plasma levels of adrenal steroids, such as dehydroepiandrosterone (DHEA) and its sulfate (DHEA-S) and androstenedione, rise throughout puberty, and begin to increase before changes in LH or testicular androgens can be found.[47–49] Odell[50] has proposed that the adrenarche is the trigger for puberty, but too many contradictory findings exist to let one adopt that view unmodified. For example, Urban *et al.*[51] (like others before them) have shown that puberty appears on time in male patients with Addison's disease, despite an absence of adrenal androgen production. Nevertheless, there has been a renewed search for a pituitary substance that regulates adrenal androgen secretion, and whose level presumably increases before puberty and decreases in later life; but no viable candidate has as yet been brought forward.[52]

A second puzzle about puberty has been the interrelations between gonadotropin levels and T response on the one hand, and the levels of T secretion and the phenotypic changes on the other.[53] Lucky *et al.*[54] compared gonadotropin bioactivity and immunoreactivity in over 200 samples of plasma from pubertal males, and found that the bioactivity increased eightfold from the beginning to the end of puberty in contrast to a threefold increase in immunoreactivity. Although plasma levels are not the last word—induction of LH receptors by FSH and their downregulation by LH are both potentially important—this study is a reminder of the difference between biological activity and immunoreactivity.

Several longitudinal studies of male puberty have been done, including an important documentation of secondary sex characteristics in American boys aged 12–17.[55,56] While largely corroborative of the Tanner data, these new observations will be useful for clinicians in the United States.[57,58] Interestingly, there were no significant differences in maturation for different geographic regions, or for varied socioeconomic classes. Serum urate, known to be higher in the adult male than female, correlated with bone age and presumably reflects an androgen effect.[59] A potentially important difference between the male and female adolescent has been stressed by Short.[60,61] Whereas most girls go through a 2- to 4-year period of hormone maturation before they ovulate regularly, many boys have spermaturia, and thus may be fertile, before they have much evidence of secondary sexual development. The occasional dramatic case notwithstanding, we remain relatively ignorant of the maturation of fertility in the human pubertal male. Laron[62] has suggested that the age of first conscious ejaculation be used as a milestone in dating male puberty, but he does not indicate in his report how this age was validated, and not every subject in the study could recall a date certain.

Variations in puberty continue to be clinical problems with which even the new refined tests are of limited help. Precocious puberty in the male initially shows modestly elevated FSH values, followed by later rises in LH and T.[63] The phenomenon is usually idiopathic in the female, but careful search for a pathologic cause in the male is indicated. Rosenfeld et al.[64] described a puzzling syndrome of isosexual precocity in a boy, and heterosexual precocity in his sister, both associated with isolated increase of LH; the mechanism was unclear. A new approach to the treatment of idiopathic precocious puberty is the use of long-acting analogs of LRH. Since sustained (rather than pulsatile) LRH administration leads to a fall in LH and T secretion, it was thought that a long-acting analog of LRH might be able to damp down the system.[65]

The distinction between delayed puberty and idiopathic hypogonadotropic hypogonadism remains difficult. Although it was hoped that LRH testing, either alone or after LRH priming, would reveal distinctive patterns, in fact there has been too much overlap in the results obtained.[66] There are, however, some reports of successful induction of puberty by the use of low-dose, pulsatile LRH administration. Some groups have reported disappointment with this approach,[67] but others have been successful in initiating a hormone pattern similar to that of puberty, as well as a clinical response.[68–71]

The psychological disadvantage of delay in male sexual maturation is well known. de Lange et al.[72] report the treatment of eight boys with severely delayed puberty with 6 months of parenteral T. All had a gratifying physical and psychological response, and at follow-up 8–13 months after treatment, all patients had normal plasma T and apparently progressive puberty. The authors raise the venerable question of whether the exogenous androgens may be having a stimulating effect similar to the prepubertal rise in adrenal androgens.

One of the principal achievements of puberty, that of an adult psychosexual identity, is receiving renewed attention. Imperato-McGinley et al.[73] reopened the field by their observations that individuals with steroid 5α-reductase deficiency, although raised as females in childhood, adopted a male-gender identity en route through adolescence. Their observations suggested that this change took 5 years; that it paralleled the other changes of puberty; and specifically, that it was accompanied by marked changes in the external genitalia. Similar findings have been reported in sporadic cases of 5α-reductase deficiency[74] and in at least one case of 17β-hydroxysteroid dehydrogenase deficiency.[75] They therefore propose that gender identity, like other sexually dimorphic attributes, is basically female, and that exposure to T (*in utero,* in infancy, and/or at puberty), in combination with other influences, orients the brain to a male-gender identity. The opposing view, descendant from the classical hypotheses of Money, has suggested that the minimal virilization of the external genitalia of these patients led to a male social sex for these individuals, i.e., that the social signals to the development of gender identity were masculinizing. Although resolution of this interesting and important controversy is not yet possible, the renewed discussion suggests at least two lessons. First, the older views of the development of psychosexual identity were based on rather limited evidence and clearly need reexamination. Second, gender identity is apparently more plastic than had been thought. At least for some individuals, a change from one sex role to the other can be accomplished without the dire consequences formerly predicted. And as a corollary, even if one claims that the children being raised as females were receiving subtle, covert signals of coming masculinity, the ability to sustain one identity until puberty and then switch to the other is remarkable and needs study.

Two additional aspects of this problem should be mentioned. An adult sexuality requires gender identity, object choice, sexual initiative, and sexual arousal. In the past, there has been little evidence of an endocrine determinant of object choice, but Imperato-McGinley et al.[73] have reported that their female-to-male changelings became aware of attraction to female objects at the very beginning of their 5 years of conversion to a male gender identity. These inferences, unfortunately, are derived from retrospective questioning, with all the weakness inherent in that approach. Still they provide a clue to further study and, further, the opportunity to recommend a recent book detailing the erotic life of a French adolescent who changed from a female to a male gender identity during puberty.[76] The autopsy done postsuicide indicates that this person had steroid 5α-reductase deficiency, and puts the issues of gender identity and object choice on center stage of a compelling and haunting story.

A final problem of male puberty, gynecomastia, has received continued attention but remains baffling. In an excellent review, Wilson *et al.*[77] outline the normal production of androgens and estrogens and end in supporting the view, first advanced 30 years ago, that gynecomastia is always the result of a disturbance in the estrogen/androgen ratio. This conclusion means that, in a given patient, the instant cause may be androgen deficiency, estrogen excess, or both. Yet even with this embracing generalization and modern techniques, Wilson avers that only in at most one-quarter of patients with gynecomastia can a particular mechanism be identified. In studies of normal males with moderate gynecomastia and of a few patients with pubertal macromastia, Large and Anderson[78,79] and Marynick et al.[80] could not find consistent abnormalities of circulating androgen or estrogen or prolactin, and in the end Large had to implicate an integrated value of duration of estrogen secretory pulses through the 24-hr period. LeRoith et al.[81] have reported that clomiphene citrate, presumably acting locally as an antiestrogen, can be helpful in the treatment of adolescent gynecomastia.

4.4. Adult Physiology

4.4.1. The Hypothalamus and Pituitary

As in past volumes of this series, the section on neuroendocrinology contains a larger summary of the recent information on the regulation of pituitary–gonadal interrelations than can be provided here. Nevertheless, a few important studies will be cited.

The neuroendocrine control of male reproduction has been the subject of a number of papers, notably one by Bardin.[82] LRH controls the secretion of both gonadotropins, apparently without requiring the mediation of adenylate cyclase.[83] Pulsatile secretion of LRH is critical to its effect; sustained administration or the use of long-acting variants leads to diminished LH secretion and diminished T secretion.[84] It had been assumed that the decrease in T release was secondary to downregulation of LH receptors by a sustained elevation of LH induced by LRH. In fact, however, LH levels fall during prolonged LRH administration and, mirabile dictu, the LRH appears to have a direct effect on the testis.[85-87] If this observation is borne out by further studies in man, the regulation of hormone effect will be shown to have a wholly new dimension: receptor control by a releasing hormone rather than by the primary ligand of the receptor. One suggestion as to how this might occur is provided by Sharpe and Fraser,[88] who describe the induction by hCG of testicular synthesis of an LRH-like activity.

The regulation of LRH and gonadotropin secretion has been studied in several laboratories. Studies cited in previous chapters confirmed that a product of the Sertoli cells, inhibin, has a negative feedback influence on the FSH response of the pituitary to LRH. Estrogen, probably produced intracerebrally from the aromatization of androgen, may also play a small role in this circuit. The negative regulation of LH in man has been much more extensively studied and appears to involve a combination of androgen, androgen metabolites, and estrogen, with perhaps some role for prolactin. A concise but balanced interpretation of this problem was recently provided by Lipsett.[89] Giving primacy to the view of Naftolin et al.[90] that the proximate regulation of LH is exerted by estradiol (E_2), Lipsett reviewed the natural disorders and clinical research in which that explanation does not seem to suffice. T and E_2 given intravenously, each suppress LH, but the androgen has more effect on the excursion of the LH pulses, and the estrogen more effect on their frequency. Nonaromatizable androgens, such as dihydrotestosterone and fluoxymesterone, also suppress LH; conversely, normal or even elevated levels of estrogen, such as occur in testicular feminization, do not suppress LH when androgen is either low or ineffective. An important study was recently done concerning administration of T and Teslac, an inhibitor of peripheral aromatization.[91] In this study, when T was low, LH rose; when T was raised, even though estrogen levels remained low, LH diminished. Lacroix et al.[92] took an interesting approach to this problem by studying the LRH response in normals, androgen-insensitive males, normals given clomiphene to produce estrogen-insensitivity, and androgen-insensitive males given clomiphene to produce combined androgen- and estrogen-insensitivity. The study was marred by having rather few individuals in each cell, and only the basal levels of gonadotropin showed consistent differences: LH was increased in the face of androgen- or estrogen-insensitivity, and further increased when both conditions were present; FSH was partly controlled by estrogen but not by androgen; gonadotropin responsiveness to LRH did not seem to have been consistently affected, perhaps because of the small number of subjects.

There are two additional evidences for a role of androgen: one, the elevation of LH in patients with 5α-reductase deficiency despite increased T and normal E_2[93]; the other, a study by Winters et al.[94] showing that both E_2 and DHT are needed to produce the LH-lowering effect of the equivalent amount of T. The difficulty in the latter type of study, however, is shown by the directly conflicting evidence of Schaison et al.,[95] who administered T and DHT to hypogonadal patients with elevated gonadotropins. In normal men, DHT treatment led to a fall in plasma T and in sex-steroid-binding globulin (SSBG), with LH levels remaining unchanged within the low-normal range. In hypogonadal patients with elevated LH, however, DHT treatment did not lower LH values, whereas T did. In a useful discussion, the authors recognize several alternatives to account for the failure of DHT to lower LH in the hypogonadal patients. These include several possibilities, such as change in levels of free T or E_2 that they did not measure, and that are therefore moot. The fact that T fell during DHT treatment of normal men suggests a decrease in endogenous LH; that LH did not rise when T decreased suggests that DHT may have been a suppressant.

While it may not be possible to come to a final summary of the feedback control of LH secretion, it seems likely that physiological levels of androgen and estrogen are each influential in negative control of LH.

Kinetic aspects of suppressibility have been explored in several papers. Caminos-Torres et al.[96] gave graded doses of androgen for varying periods to normal and hypogonadal men, and used the gonadotropin response to infused LRH as the measure of pituitary suppression. They found that an elevation of serum T must be maintained for at least 1 month in normal men, and 1–2 months or longer in hypogonadal men, to induce pituitary suppression. Similarly, in patients with hypogonadism, there develops a resistance to LH suppression by exogenous T: the amounts and time of administration both have to be longer than in the normal male to show effective central feedback inhibition by the androgen.

Axelrod et al.[97] have described what appears to be a new disorder: a 17-year-old male without signs of puberty had a low plasma T, an elevated immunoassayable plasma LH, and a normal karyotype. The patient's LH was inferred to be biologically inert in him, but when his urinary gonadotropins were assayed in the rodent, the level was high, similar to the level of immunoassayable LH. The authors conclude that the disease is due to a modification in the LH, in which, though immunologically measurable, LH is in fact biologically inactive. The defect appears to be in the LH molecule, since exogenous hCG produced full masculinization in the patient; moreover, the defect appears to be able to distinguish the rodent from the human testis, since the gonadotropin was active in the rat, but not in man. One wonders whether this patient's LH could be used as a probe for differentiating the rodent testicular receptor from that in the human.

The role of positive feedback in the male is unclear. In the preovulatory female, estrogen induces a sudden release of LH-FSH that is responsible for ovulation. Recent beautiful studies by Knobil et al.[98,99] have shown that estrogen-induced cycling can be developed in the sexually immature primate by appropriately timed pulsatile LRH administration. Is this capacity to release a surge of LH in response to high levels of estrogen an intrinsic attribute of the female nervous system? The natural course of human female puberty suggests that the positive feedback is a "learned" response of the CNS secondary to slowly rising estrogen levels; the Knobil experiments support this view. A study by

Barbarino and De Marinis[100] now provides additional evidence: estrogen administration to castrate male humans resulted in acquisition of a positive LH induction after an initial gonadotropin suppression by exogenous estrogen. The authors argue that, in normal man, androgen in fetal and postnatal life suppresses but does not abolish the ability of the CNS to respond to sustained high estrogen levels. This study is potentially relevant to the prior report of Seyler *et al.*[101] that female transsexual patients have a blunted LH response to LRH after estrogen priming.

4.4.2. The Testis

4.4.2.1. Steroidogenesis

At least three major reviews of testicular steroidogenesis have appeared since Volume 1 was published. Preslock[102,103] deals extensively with the biochemistry of T synthesis, whereas Catt *et al.*[104] focus on the influence of gonadotropic hormones and the role of receptor regulation in the response of the testis. Preslock summarizes the extensive comparative literature to conclude that in the rat the Δ^4 pathway (pregnenolone–progesterone– 17OH-progesterone–androstenedione–testosterone) is the preferred pathway; that in subhuman primates there is a greater use of the Δ^5 pathway (17OH-pregnenolone–dehydroepiandrosterone–androstenediol–testosterone), with some use of the Δ^4 pathway; and that in man the preferred pathway is the Δ^5, with minimal use of the Δ^4 unless substrate concentration is artificially controlled. The controlling difference would seem to be the relative activities of the 3β-hydroxysteroid dehydrogenase and isomerase versus the 17-hydroxylase of pregnenolone, but the properties of later enzymes may also be influential.

Two clinical laboratories have been working on aspects of T synthesis. Smals *et al.*[105] reported that, after hCG administration, there occurs a dissociation between 17OH-P and T levels: the first day, there is a greater rise in 17OH-P than in T, and thereafter (for 2–3 days) a continuing rise in T with a fall in 17OH-P. In a later paper, the same group found that tamoxifen, the estrogen antagonist, blunted the temporary block in T synthesis beyond 17OH-P.[106] While the changes were rather small, the study seems important in raising the possibility that intratesticular estrogen levels may have a controlling influence on T synthesis. (In general, hormone synthesis does not seem to be subject to product inhibition in many cases; such a possibility therefore creates special interest.)

Glass and Vigersky[107,108] have looked at the same problem by measuring the Δ^4 versus Δ^5 intermediates 2–4 hr after i.m. hCG before and after 72 hr of hCG treatment. Their observations are important in two ways: first, they find too much overlap between control and hypogonadal subjects to use these tests for differential diagnosis; and, second, they show that 17OH-P metabolism seems to be rate-limiting when hCG sensitivity is declining ("desensitization" is their term), but not when hCG effectiveness is returning ("resensitization"). They postulate an internal shift in the preferred pathway during hCG stimulation. Somewhat puzzling, though, is their finding that the Δ^4 pathway is favored in the early response to hCG, whereas others (see Preslock above) have considered the Δ^5 pathway primary.

Padrón et al.[109] showed a similar biphasic response of plasma T to an injection of hCG. Finding that plasma T was still elevated 6 days after the injection, they suggest that T and hCG therapy be reevaluated. Martikainen et al.[110] used a different protocol, observed less of an immediate response, and found no significant difference between normals given hCG only and those given saline 12 hr before hCG.

Wang et al.[111] similarly studied the response of testicular steroids to varied regimens of hCG administration. They found the early response of androgens less than that of estrogens, and, noting the accumulation of androgen precursors, they suggest that the limiting condition is the shortage of T-synthesizing enzymes. They, too, suggested that androgens and estrogens might be playing a feedback-limiting role.

Davies et al.[112] have used the primate testis (by virtue of its homology with the human) to explore the question of LH-induced decrease in LH receptors. They confirmed that the down-regulation observed in the rat also occurs in the primate and, by inference, in man. In these in vitro studies, they also noted the accumulation of 17OH-P, suggesting that the amount of 17,20-desmolase was rate-limiting in T synthesis after hCG stimulation.

The peripheral fates of testicular hormones are important. Leinonen et al.[113] studied the concentrations of T and its precursors and metabolites in epididymal and proximal ductus deferens fluids. The results suggest that, after being synthesized in the testis, the steroids are transferred to the efferent ducts in testicular lymph or the fluid of the rete, where they may be important in the final steps of spermiogenesis. Another type of peripheral event is the conversion of androgens to estrogens. This step is an important factor in the estrogen milieu of the postmenopausal woman; the percent conversion of androstenedione to estrone inccreases with both age and weight. Prior evidence of an increase in the same step in older men had appeared, and a paper of Kley et al.[114] showed a similar exaggeration of estrogen production in obese males. This aromatization could be a factor in the gynecomastia seen in some obese men.

4.4.2.2. Spermatogenesis

Is the human sperm count declining? This terrible thought, subject of a quiet vendetta during the past several years, was critically reexamined in several recent articles. The paper by MacLeod and Wang[115] is certainly the most important: they assert that, given variations in technique and scoring, there is no significant drift in the human sperm count over the past 40 years. But they do make several important points. First, no count is meaningful without a simultaneous assessment of sperm motility *(vide infra)*. Second, the minimum count consistent with fertility is a shadowy target: the old count of 40 million is certainly too high, and the proposed figure of 10 million may be too low; they are more comfortable with an exception-tolerating 20 million.[116] In this connection, the chapter on assessment of spermatogenesis in the new DeGroot text is valuable.[117]

The correlation between sperm counts and findings on testicular biopsy has been rigorously reexamined by van Dop *et al.*[118] The result is a stereological model of the testis that includes correlation among eight testicular compartments and between the findings in the testis and a semen analysis. Several components of the analysis show an excellent correlation with log total sperm count, but the method seems too complex for clinical use.[119]

Several authors have reassessed the hormonal factors in spermatogenesis, and some consensus can be discerned. Steinberger[120] summarizes the evidence that FSH is required for the initiation of spermatogenesis but that, thereafter, T is sufficient. FSH enters the testis from the arterial blood, attaches to a receptor on the Sertoli cells,[121] and stimulates adenylate cyclase. The resulting cAMP triggers production of an androgen-binding protein (ABP). This compound is a critical intermediary in the process, since it picks up T and DHT produced in the Leydig cells, and transports them to the germ-cell membranes. As the androgen dissociates rapidly from the ABP, a short sequence of pickup–transport–dissociation is established. The androgen then presumably sustains the later steps in spermatogenesis.[122]

Karim and Hillier[123] have summarized the role of prostaglandins in human semen, but there is little agreement on their physiological or clinical significance. As a result, it is impossible to interpret the reports of abnormal levels of prostaglandins in subfertile patients.

4.4.2.3. Effect of Age

At least 10 studies suggest that there is a decline in testicular function with age, although all agree that it is later, less abrupt, less complete, and less universal than the ovarian failure of the menopause. Nuances include: an increase in SSBG rather than a primary change in gonadal secretion as the initial event; an increase in estrogen production from androgen, raising the estrogen/androgen ratio without much fall in basal androgen secretion. Two recent papers state there is no age-related change *if* healthy older males are chosen as subjects.

In one of these papers, Harman and Tsitouras[124] studied 69 male volunteers aged 25–89 years, drawn from the roster of the Baltimore Longitudinal Study on Aging, which is comprised of an exceptionally healthy, employed, middle-class population. This group showed no decline with age in T, DHT, or free T, and no increase in estrone or E_2. There was some increase in LH, and a diminished response of T to exogenous hCG. The authors discuss the philosophical problem of distinguishing a normal aging population and admit the bias probably present in their study. Nevertheless, they make the point that prior studies did not use an identifiably "normal" aged population, either.

Sparrow *et al.*[125] did a similar study, comparing 44 men aged 31–44 with 42 men aged 64–88. Again, subjects were chosen for the absence of known chronic disease, medication, and major surgery within a year; none showed signs of testicular atrophy or significant prostatic hyperplasia. As in the Harman study, there was no evidence of a decline with age in T, free T, or DHT, but there was a slight increase in SSBG, and a definite increase in gonadotropin levels. The authors' conclusions were similar to those of Harman and Tsitouras: that prior aging studies failed to identify a normal aging population and that, when one is identified, there is not the evidence for testicular senescence previously found.

A paper by Sködefors *et al.*[126] comes to the same conclusion, but Serio *et al.*,[127] assaying spermatic venous concentrations of testicular androgens, reported a clear decrease with age. An interesting paper by Kaler and Neaves[128] examined the histology of the testis to assess age-related change. Using a histomorphometric method, they found that the number of Leydig cells decreases with age from a maximum of about 700 million at age 20, with an approximate loss of 80 million per decade. They conclude, however, that there is no certainty of whether the functional capacity of the Leydig cell decreases.

4.5. Adult Pathophysiology

4.5.1. Gonadotropin Deficiencies

The congenital deficiencies of LRH or pituitary gonadotropins continue to receive considerable attention, particularly with tests utilizing LRH or its variants. The importance of chemical modification of the LRH molecule has been reaffirmed by several studies. Smith *et al.*[129]

utilized a long-acting derivative of native LRH to circumvent the need for injections several times each day in treating patients with hypogonadotropic hypogonadism. Using the analog D-Ser(TBU)^6-LH-RH-EA,[10] the authors found that 5μg daily for 1 week produced a progressive rise in the LH response to the test doses of LRH. In the short period of this study, there was no rise in plasma T, but the increasing gonadotropin response suggested that continued treatment would result in some gonadal response. Interestingly, however, in normal patients given the same protocol, plasma LH, its response to LRH, and plasma T all fell; this is presumably another instance of the desensitization of gonadotropin response to long-acting LRH stimulation. In a later report from the same group, longer duration of treatment (27–38 weeks) was associated with a decrease in gonadotropin responses to LRH and a decrease in the transiently raised plasma LH values.[130] This decrease appeared without a significant prior rise in T; thus, the "desensitization" of pituitary response to long-acting LRH analogs cannot be due to negative feedback by T on either the hypothalamus or the pituitary. Another paper[131] suggests that the long duration of action of the analog could be exploited for treatment of hypogonadotropic individuals. The Smith experience, however, contradicts this hope.

Snyder *et al.*[132] reinvestigated the utility of LRH testing in distinguishing hypogonadism of hypothalamic origin from that due to pituitary deficiency. In the past, LRH has been disappointing for this purpose, because some patients with hypothalamic hypogonadism had a deficient response to LRH, suggesting pituitary deficiency and thus making it impossible to differentiate the two sites of disease in undiagnosed patients. Snyder *et al.* studied five patients with presumed hypothalamic disease and five with pituitary disease, all of whom had a deficient LH response to a bolus of LRH. All were given infusions of 500 μg LRH/24 hr for 1 week; a bolus of LRH was administered at the end of that time. The five patients with hypothalamic hypogonadism developed normal LH responses, whereas the five with pituitary disease continued to show a blunted LH response to bolus LRH. Despite the paper's interest, the small numbers studied make it impossible to generalize the significance of this type of attempt to differentiate hypothalamic from hypophyseal deficiency of gonadotropin.

A similar protocol was used by Kletzky *et al.*[133] to locate the site of the gonadotropin deficiency that produced hypogonadism or delayed puberty in thalassemia major. Three female and two male patients were found to be unresponsive to LRH, before and after 1 week of injection of 100 μg LRH. The female patients remained unresponsive after priming with E$_2$ and treatment with gonadotropin, and the males remained unresponsive after treatment with hCG until T was brought into the adult range. Thus, the authors conclude that the defect is secondary to iron deposition in the pituitary, which had earlier been reported at autopsy of a patient.

Patients with hypothalamic hypogonadism have been studied for other traits that might be useful in diagnosis. Smals *et al.*[134] measured the 17OH-P and T responses to a single injection of hCG (studies similar to those reported on p. 170). The normal individual shows a prompt rise in both 17OH-P and T, with a subsequent drop and second rise; during the second phase, 17OH-P increases more than T. Hypogonadal patients, on the other hand, show a minimal initial rise and some later rise, but not the change in the 17OH-P/T ratio found in normals. The authors attribute the lack of early rise to an unprepared steroid biosynthetic machinery (i.e., steroid-producing enzymes were not previously induced), and ascribe the difference in the 17OH-P/T ratio to the possibility in normal man, though not in eunuchoid individuals, that hCG stimulation is followed by a depression in the enzymes required in the pathway between 17OH-P and T.

In another study, patients with hypogonadotropic hypogonadism were compared with patients with primary gonadal deficiency for prolactin values and the response of prolactin to thyrotropin (TSH).[135] The patients with hypogonadotropic eunuchoidism showed low prolactin values that responded poorly to TSH-releasing hormone (TRH). When these patients were treated with androgens, however, the prolactin values rose and responded briskly to TRH. The authors attribute the relative hypoprolactinemia and the poor response to TRH to a lack of sex steroids, treatment with which corrected the prolactin deficiency.

Batrinos *et al.*[136] studied patients with known Kallman's syndrome to try to confirm that there is a gonadal defect as well as a hypothalamic defect. They showed that LRH produced an inadequate LH rise, and that hCG in the same patients produced a blunted T/E_2 response. The authors conclude that there is both a gonadal and a hypothalamic defect in Kallman's syndrome. However, since the protocol was addressed to severely hypogonadal patients whose testes had never been exposed to adequate gonadotropin stimulation, the failure to respond to hCG would appear secondary to the hypogonadotropic state rather than to a separate gonadal defect.

Further phenotypic variation in Kallman's syndrome is suggested by Rogol *et al.*[137] in the first report of HLA tissue-typing in hypogonadal men with progeny. Both patients are interpreted by the authors to show a bridging syndrome between Kallman's (hypogonadotropic hypogonadism with anosmia) and the fertile eunuch (partially eunuchoid, with adequate spermatogenesis on biopsy). The patients each had inadequate secondary sex characteristics, testes smaller than normal, spermatogenesis by biopsy, measurable but not elevated gonadotropins, normal nongonadal pituitary endocrinology, no response to clomiphene, and ultimately responses to hCG. There are some interesting aspects that the authors do not emphasize. One patient is said to have normal testicular tubules on biopsy, yet the clinically measurable sizes were 1.5 cm in longest diameter. The other patient inseminated his wife while being treated with T; this is ordinarily not possible in hypogonadotropic hypogonadal patients, and serves to stress the endogenous gonadotropin function of such patients.[138] It may be a semantic problem to distinguish partial hypogonadotropic hypogonadism (with some spermatogenesis and intratesticular T) from the fertile eunuch, but there are valuable clinical lessons in these patients.

Some useful background for this issue of endogenous gonadotropins affecting the testis without being able to stimulate peripheral hormone levels is provided by an interesting paper from Spain.[139] The authors point out that the Leydig cell is unique among mammalian tissues in that it differentiates twice: during gestation, perhaps under the stimulus of hCG, and again after puberty. Unable to find a prior study of the ultrastructure of the testis at puberty, they report the findings in two males with hypogonadotropic hypogonadism, who had biopsies before and during gonadotropin therapy.

The role of peripheral androgen levels was reexplored in an important paper by Davidson *et al.*[140] Six hypogonadal males were treated with T in varying doses and according to a protocol varied within and among subjects. Daily logs of sexual activity, and interviews conducted by a person unaware of the doses and timing, revealed a good correlation between intensity of sexual activity and plasma T values. This result accords with the view that male sexual potency is androgen-dependent. It is unfortunate that the series was not larger and that it will not be extended.

Another effort to estimate the adequacy of androgen therapy was made by Snyder and Lawrence,[141] who gave varied dosages of T enanthate to 24 hypogonadal males. The doses varied from 100 mg/week–200 mg for 2 weeks, to 300 mg for 3 weeks, to 400 mg for 4 weeks. The plasma T, FSH, and LH were measured. The first three dose schedules suppressed LH effectively. The 400-mg dose schedule did not suppress FSH or LH adequately. Interestingly, the 100 mg/week dose probably achieved higher plasma T levels than are necessary. The authors conclude that the optimum dosage, as judged from these parameters, is either 200 mg for 2 weeks or 300 mg for 3 weeks. They also conclude— an important point—that T in this dose range is able to suppress FSH into the normal range, and that FSH control does not require the postulate of inhibin or another product of the testicular tubule. Whether it is the T itself or the estrogen produced does not, therefore, seem important in the negative argument put forward by Snyder. It is unfortunate that this study did not include measurements of androgenic effects on libido, potency, or other parameters, but if the Davidson data correlating sexuality with T levels and those of this study correlating levels with dosage are combined, a program of 200 mg for 2 weeks, or 300 mg for 3 weeks, should produce adequate androgenization.

Symptoms of androgen deficiency are the most common presenting complaints in patients with pituitary tumors. Recent reports have shown that hyperprolactinemia has an antigonadotropic effect, and that impotence can be associated with prolactinomas, usually with a depressed T level, but sometimes with a normal plasma T. Except for this circumstance, gonadotropin deficiency, signaled by impotence, has most often been the first endocrine difficulty in adults with pituitary tumors. What may be the most surprising recent paper was the report by Snyder *et al.*[142] of the gonadal function of 50 males with untreated pituitary tumors. The unexpected features were: of 14 men able to provide an ejaculate, 4 had normal concentrations of sperm [their T was low, indicating that they were acquired variants of the fertile eunuch syndrome (*vide supra*)], and plasma T and LH responses to LRH did not always correlate. But very remarkable was the fact that 12 of the 50 patients had either a somewhat elevated basal FSH or a hyperresponse to LRH. The authors could find no precedent for these findings in prior reports of pituitary tumors, except for the rare ones associated with primary gonadotropin excess. Similarly, they could not suggest a mechanism for FSH excess in association with hypogonadism and pituitary tumors, but this syndrome must clearly be looked for in the future.

An interesting sidelight of this series was the observation of depressed TSH function in four eugonadal patients. This finding contradicts the usual teaching that gonadotropin failure appears first in patients with progressive pituitary disease. Whether this new lesson is generally applicable or whether it is associated with the particular finding of FSH excess in this series, remains to be seen. In a follow-up report, the patients with pituitary tumors and FSH excess were compared with normals and with pituitary tumor patients without FSH excess, for their responses to TRH.[143] Ten of the patients showed a hyperresponse of LH, and five of the ten an exaggerated response of FSH, when compared to normals or other pituitary tumor patients. The authors recalled the similarity to other pituitary tumors that showed a hyperresponse to a nonspecific stimulation with TRH; on this basis, they suggest that the patients with FSH excess have tumors of gonadotropin-producing cells. In the earlier paper, the authors comment that it is surprising that there was not simultaneous LH excess, because the pituitary gonadotrope is known to produce both FSH and LH.

4.5.2. The Testis

4.5.2.1. Steroidogenesis

A useful report of a patient with 17-ketosteroid reductase deficiency emphasizes early study to avoid confusion with testicular feminization.[144]

Defects in Transport, Binding, or Metabolism. Perhaps the most important paper of the 2-year period was the summary by Griffin and Wilson[11] of the various mechanisms of androgen resistance. They begin with the restatement of the general principle that steroid hormones enter target tissues passively down a concentration gradient and that they attach to cytosol receptors, which then undergo a conformational change, are translocated to the nucleus, and there form a triad of hormone–receptor–chromatin. In the case of T, the situation is modified by the intracellular reduction of T to DHT. Both androgens, however, appear to use the same receptor. As a consequence, androgen insensitivity can occur from one of three causes: failure of androgen binding to the receptor; failure of conversion of T to DHT; or a defect in the postreceptor steps of chromatin binding and genomic activation. Each category may have several abnormalities; thus, the number of disorders is larger than the three-part characterization and allows for considerable genetic heterogeneity.

Failure of conversion of T to DHT has been consistently reported by Imperato-McGinley and sporadically by Wilson and others. At least three defects in the reductase have been identified: one results in failure of attachment of T; a second leads to impaired attachment of the cofactor (NADPH); and a third variant appears to lead to poor attachment of both substrate and cofactor. The phenotypic range is wide, with some patients showing almost normal masculinization at puberty despite severe genital ambiguity at birth (the Santo Domingo group is striking), and others showing much lower degrees of pubertal virilization.

Defects in the androgen receptor comprise the second type of androgen insensitivity. Patients with classic testicular feminization most often have a complete absence of the cytosol receptor. In other families, the hormone attaches to the receptor but binds less well, and the receptor has subtle abnormalities demonstrated by altering the temperature of the reaction. The connection between this defect and the impaired hormonal response is not yet apparent.[145]

Patients with partial deficiency of the receptor show a phenotypic range that stretches from minimal masculinization to—and beyond—almost normal neonatal virilization. The "beyond" is of particular clinical interest, since two variants of minimal androgen insensitivity are of diagnostic importance. At least one family has been seen with gynecomastia as the only abnormality, and confirmation is awaited.[146] Much more important is the suggestion by Griffin and Wilson[11] that T resistance confined to the testicular tubules may underlie 25% of male infertility. These patients are phenotypically normal and do not come to attention until they are investigated for infertility. They are then found to have hypospermatogenesis in association with minimal FSH elevation, but with a diagnostic elevation of T and LH. The diagnostic clue is an (LH × T) product greater than twice the normal level. Confirmation of the frequency of this disorder from other clinics is eagerly awaited.

Finally, some patients with androgen insensitivity have normal binding of ligand to receptor and normal intracellular reduction; by inference they are thought to have a postreceptor defect. The details of this variant remain to be discovered and, when known, will likely reveal more than one mechanism.

The fecundity of Wilson's laboratory is further illustrated by his group's paper on the Seabright bantam syndrome.[147] Many years ago, Albright et al.[148] suggested that the defect leading to absence of the comb in male roosters was a form of end organ resistance, presumably a failure of the androgen to act. Instead, the affected rooster shows an enhanced conversion of T to E_2, and an elevated E_2/T ratio.

4.5.2.2. Tubular Defects

Boisen[149] studied testicular size in XXY, XYY, and XY males ascertained by chromosome pattern rather than by clinical findings. Two insights emerged: the testicular size of 12 XYY individuals was no different from normal; and the testes of 14 XXY males, though smaller than normal, were somewhat larger than has usually been stated for Klinefelter's syndrome.

Several papers on the endocrinology of Klinefelter's syndrome have been published. Smals et al.[150] showed that acute administration of T had little effect on the acute response to LH and LRH infusion (i.e., the readily released LH pool presumed to reflect stored LH). In contrast, chronic administration suppressed the early LH response in three or four patients but had little effect on the delayed LH release (presumed to reflect de novo synthesis). The variability of the results of LH infusion, however, combined with the small number of patients, suggests caution in interpreting this report. A similar caution should be applied to a report by Gabrilove et al.[151] showing a striking decrease in the T/E_2 ratio in the spermatic venous effluent of two patients with Klinefelter's syndrome. However, this observation accords with a number of prior claims that an instrinsic defect of the disorder is the increased conversion of T to E_2 in the testis. Wieland *et al.*[152] found that SSBG was elevated in all of seven patients with Klinefelter's syndrome; this finding was not correlated with an elevated E_2 level. The authors point out, however, that since SSBG is not an important binder of E_2 at physiological temperature, the change in TEBG may result from an increase in effective free E_2/free T.

Barbarino *et al.*[153] investigated the effect of E_2 on LH release in Klinefelter's syndrome (five patients) and in Sertoli-cell-only syndrome (two patients). Observing initially a fall and then a transient rise in LH, they infer that estrogen does have a positive feedback effect on LH release in the human male. This inference, however, is a complex issue on which much more data are needed. The possibility that estrogen-induced positive feedback is genetically determined (i.e., present in XX but absent in XY individuals) seems too simple. But whether the triggering factor is chronic estrogen exposure (as occurs in the pubescent female) or the relationship between estrogen and progesterone (as is suggested by the absence of positive feedback during the luteal phase), or a ratio of T to E_2 is an important issue still to be resolved.

Samaan *et al.*[154] have provided a useful warning that radiologic abnormalities of the pituitary in Klinefelter's and Turner's syndromes may be secondary to the gonadal defect. Two of three patients with Klinefelter's syndrome and two of six with Turner's syndrome had enlarged sellas, but the tomograms of the six other patients showed only minor abnormalities. Caution in interpreting sellar films in patients with end-organ defects seems appropriate. Gabrilove *et al.*[155] studied T/E_2 ratios versus age in Klinefelter's syndrome and showed a progressive decrease in the already low ratio with age, paralleling the change that occurs in the normal individual. They argue that the Klinefelter's testis shows the same age-related progression as that of the normal male, and that the gynecomastia of Klinefelter's patients and of normal older males reflects the abnormal ratio of androgen/estrogen.

Ellison *et al.*[156] reported the first case of breast cancer in a Klinefelter patient in whom estrogen and progesterone receptors were demonstrated in the tumor and a hormonal response was achieved. The paper cites prior studies indicating a 6% incidence of breast cancer in Klinefelter's syndrome, 20-fold higher than in the normal male. Although other cancers are not thought to be any more frequent in patients with Klinefelter's syndrome than in normal males, the recognition of two dysgerminomas in Klinefelter's patients, together with some pathologic findings in the tumors, led Sogge *et al.*[157] to suggest a search for such tumors in chromatin-positive males.

Vaze *et al.*[158] have described a radioimmunoassay for inhibin, and the same laboratory has now reported measurements[159] of this compound in seminal plasma and serum from normal subjects and from patients with a variety of primary gonadal defects. Although the levels of inhibin did not correlate with sperm count or motility, the values in oligospermic and Klinefelter's patients were significantly higher than in normals. A similar report showed that inhibin was almost absent from the semen of azoospermic men, whereas it was readily measured in normals.[160]

A comprehensive review of nonendocrine aspects of male infertility is beyond the scope of this chapter. Varicocele continues to attract much attention, with several reports of large series emphasizing its importance, but with little new of a hormonal nature. Reports of immunologically mediated infertility, sometimes responding to corticosteroid therapy (usually combined with 6 or more months of imposed barrier), have increased, and several thoughtful reviews[161–163] have been published. A number of papers have described defects particularly affecting motility in the sperm. Defects in the cilia, either in the dynein arms or elsewhere, occur in association with bronchiectasis; unfortunately, they are not yet amenable to treatment.[164,165] Defects in spermatogenesis due to cytogenetic abnormalities have been found through meiotic studies and suspected through familial clustering.[166] In all of these studies, however, there is no identifiable endocrine component.

Tubular damage secondary to pesticide exposure has been described by Glass *et al.*[167] Depression of sperm count, elevation of FSH, normal androgen levels, and normal LH were found in pesticide workers with a particular pattern of exposure, though not in other individuals in the same workplace. Epidemiologic observations suggested that a mild early form of damage, sustained on relatively short exposure, could be reversible.

Mention has already been made of the form of minimal androgen insensitivity in which LH and T are both elevated. One practical importance of this finding is the implication that gonadotropin and T values should now be measured in the workup of azoospermic patients and even in oligospermic ones. The LH elevation need not be striking; only its association with an elevated T is important.

What hormonal evaluation, therefore, is appropriate in the investigation of male infertility? Vermeulen *et al.*[168] have summarized their findings in over 500 patients ascertained in a referral practice. They reviewed the results of semen analyses, gonadotropin determinations, T assays, etc., and ended by constructing a flowchart for the endocrine evaluation of the infertile male: one scheme for patients with small testes, and another for those with normal-sized testes. In patients with normal sperm counts and normal-sized testes, they felt that no hormonal tests are useful. Where sperm count is low, FSH should be assayed to determine prognosis and indications for biopsy; if FSH is elevated, LH and T should be measured to discover any T resistance (in fact, they found no such case). When the testes are small, FSH, LH, and T should all be measured. (Rather similar ground is covered by Rosemberg,[169] although from a more theoretical viewpoint.) The stepwise algorithm proposed by Vermeulen et al. appears to be a logical and defensible approach, though perhaps economically questionable. Patients with infertility who seek consultation are usually highly motivated and anxious to reach a diagnosis by any potentially helpful strategy. Even with a normal physical examination, and with a normal or low sperm count, measurement of FSH, LH, T, and perhaps prolactin is advisable as a routine procedure.[170,171] Guides to diagnosis, prognosis, and possible therapy are all provided by this approach and with minimal delay. Some definite inferences can be drawn from endocrine studies; others require further investigation. An elevated FSH eliminates the need for a biopsy and predicts that no therapy will be successful. Normal LH despite T deficiency calls for further workup of the pituitary axis and suggests that gonadotropin therapy may succeed.

Two hormonal agents have been extensively investigated in subfertile but endocrinologically normal patients: bromocryptine and clomiphene. The rationale for bromocryptine derives from the evidence that hyperprolactinemia can cause both T deficiency and hypospermatogenesis, both of which can be reversed by the return of prolactin excess to normal.[172–175] Borrowing this precedent, a number of clinics have treated oligospermic, normoprolactinemic patients with bromocryptine, but the results of several studies show no benefit.[176,177] The story in the case of clomiphene is less clear. In general, doses of 100 mg or higher daily, sometimes with respites, have been used for 3–6 months or even longer. Individual series have claimed good responses or, conversely, denied any benefit.[178] A comprehensive review was therefore welcome. Allag and Alexander's[179] summary of 18 studies, involving a total of 697 patients, suggests on balance that clomiphene is worth trying in the oligospermic, normogonadotropic male. A dosage of 25–50 mg daily, perhaps with a 5-day respite per month, as introduced by Paulson et al.,[180] seems to have the best chance of success without incurring undue side effects.

Schill,[181] in a review of 367 patients from various reports, avers that 55% showed some improvement in sperm counts, but then states that there is as yet no statistical proof of a beneficial effect of clomiphene in male subfertility. This paper, incidentally, provides a broad review of the pharmacologic treatment of male subfertility, with many excellent references.

Treatment with gonadotropin is reviewed by Lunenfeld *et al.*[182] In their experience, retrospective evaluation suggests that patients with low FSH and/or low T, plus low LH, are those likely to respond, i.e., gonadotropin therapy works well for gonadotropin deficiency and much less well in hormonally normal males.[183]

4.6. Effect of Systemic Disease on Gonadal Function

Morley and Melmed[184] have reviewed the literature on the effect of systemic disease on gonadal function, and Federman[185] has edited a volume of *Clinics in Endocrinology and Metabolism* on endocrine manifestations of systemic disease. In the Morley and Melmed review, there are 111 references just in the section on gonadal dysfunction in uremia and cirrhosis; yet for neither disease can a clear pathogenesis or uniform picture be delineated. To consider *uremia* first: there is widespread evidence of hypogonadism in uremic patients. In general, T levels are reduced, estrogen levels are slightly increased, gonadotropins are normal or increased, and prolactin is often elevated. The response to dialysis is rarely satisfactory, and even transplantation is often ineffective in correcting the gonadal dysfunction (steroid therapy and/or immunosuppression may be implicated). Several reports of benefit from bromocryptine have appeared; it would seem that the drug would be worthy of trial in patients not undergoing transplantation.[186] The study by Gómez *et al.*[187] is particularly interesting in this regard, since, in their patients, those who were impotent only seldom had low T values but regularly had elevated prolactin values. This observation was confirmed by Gura *et al.*[188]

The situation in *cirrhosis* is, if possible, even more confused, perhaps because more studies have been done, and because of the additional involvement of a potential chemical toxin, alcohol. A general summary has been given in previous chapters. In broad terms, patients with alcoholic cirrhosis may show gonadal atrophy and gynecomastia on clinical examination, and, on laboratory testing, some combination of low T, elevated plasma estrogens, and normal or low gonadotropins. There is often an increased peripheral conversion of androgen to estrogen, particularly of androstenedione to estrone. But several new papers have dissected the roles of alcohol, malnutrition, and liver disease.

Abel[189] has reviewed the effects of alcohol on sex and reproduction. Using modern quantitative methods to assess both achieved blood level and erectile function, he concludes (with Shakespeare) that acute mild intoxication raises sexual desire but inhibits erectile capacity; chronic alcoholism and in particular high blood alcohol levels appear to inhibit both desire and performance, with reports of impotence varying from 8 to 54%. The effect of alcohol appears to be directly on the spinal reflex arc component of erection. Further, alcohol appears to decrease T formation in the testis and to increase the relative formation of estrogen; it may have central effects as well, since LH levels in hypogonadal alcoholics are not high, as would be expected. Abel's approach is similar to the formulation of van Thiel,[190] who separates the effects of alcohol and of liver disease, and implicates alcohol-induced decreased testicular et al.[187] is particularly interesting in this regard, since, in their patients, those who were impotent only seldom had low T values but regularly had elevated prolactin values. This observation was confirmed by Gura et al.[188]

In *hemochromatosis*, the male gonadal deficiency appears to be primarily due to gonadotropin deficiency, probably secondary to iron deposition in the pituitary rather than to a hypothalamic defect. In *myotonic dystrophy*, the lesion is primarily gonadal and affects spermatogenesis more than steroid synthesis. Gonadotropin levels are usually elevated, and a hyperresponse to LRH, consistent with end organ failure, is common. Patients with *cord damage* and *paraplegia* demonstrate a spermatogenic defect in about a third of cases.[191] Leydig cell function is not usually impaired, but LRH testing shows a hyperresponse of LH in some patients. The tubular dysfunction is attributed to excess warmth of the testis because of the neurogenic defect. Hayes et al.[192] did LRH tests in 15 paraplegic males. FSH was elevated in 8, LH in 9; 14 showed hyperresponse of FSH, and 9 of LH. *Thyrotoxicosis* causes gynecomastia in as many as 5% of patients; the dominant finding is an elevation of unbound E_2/unbound T, thought principally to be due to increased peripheral aromatization of T. Plasma T is elevated in these patients because of the increase in SSBG; this produces the paradoxical finding of impotence, gynecomastia, and elevated T. *Cushing's syndrome* tends to produce hypogonadism through gonadotropin deficiency.[193] The findings are puzzling, however, since gonadotropin levels are not demonstrably low, and yet T is usually low, and impotence common. Some patients with *protein calorie malnutrition* show diminished Leydig cell function, often with an inadequate pituitary reponse (i.e., LH is not high). This combination suggests that there are unknown factors regulating LH and T.

Toone et al.[194] reported an interesting group of 27 male patients with *epilepsy* taking various combinations of phenytoin, phenobarbital, and primidone. There were consistent abnormalities of gonadal tests, with elevation in SSBG, T, LH, FSH, and prolactin. The increases in SSBG, T, and LH were the most striking. The authors are unsure about the mechanism responsible but suggest that the primary event is an effect of the anticonvulsant on the level of SSBG, with elevation in total (but reduction in unbound) T, and secondary changes in LH. Whether there would be enough elevation in estrogen to play a role, and particularly to raise the prolactin, is unclear.

Antitumor therapy is well known to induce damage to the spermatogenic function of the testis. Several papers, however, have suggested Leydig cell damage as well, with diminished T, increased estrogen and LH, and clinical gynecomastia as the result. Sherins *et al.*,[195] Glass and Berenberg,[196] and Friedman and Plymate[197] have come to the same conclusion about the problem.

4.7. Testicular Tumors

The original outline for this chapter made no provision for discussion of testicular tumors, but, in view of the growing literature on the occurrence, diagnosis, staging, and therapy of these neoplasms, a brief survey seems pertinent. There have been several excellent reviews, emphasizing the value of tumor markers (α-fetoprotein and hCG, in particular) in diagnosis, evaluation of therapy, and follow-up.[198,199] One paper reported false-positive elevations of hCG that were really cross-reactions with elevated LH in unilaterally orchiectomized patients; when T therapy was given, the pituitary LH was suppressed, and the false elevations of hCG, thought to represent tumor, disappeared.[200]

It does seem appropriate to call attention to some specifically endocrine aspects of testicular cancer. Lipsett[201] has given an overview of the problem, and several papers have reported functional Leydig cell tumors, and reviewed the literature.[202–204] When functional at all, Leydig cell tumors are usually discovered through feminization rather than supermasculinization. The biochemical explanation is probably an exaggeration of the aromatase step in T to E_2 production, with consequent suppression of endogenous gonadotropin and diminished T production by the uninvolved portions of the testes. If endogenous T production diminishes sufficiently, spermatogenesis would also suffer because of absence of intratesticular delivery of T to the tubules. Just such an endocrine sequence was recently reported by Perez *et al.*[205]; interestingly, the progesterone and prolactin levels were both elevated in this patient before surgery and returned to normal afterwards, as did the preoperative low gonadotropins, low T, and elevated E_2. The case demonstrates the importance of measuring the estrogen level in patients with gynecomastia; without this reading, the picture might have been attributed to hyperprolactinemia.

4.8. Miscellaneous

4.8.1. Gynecomastia

A major review from Wilson's group has delineated the current understanding of pathologic enlargement of the male breast.[77] Using the literature as background, and drawing on their own extensive experience with steroid hormone-turnover studies, they reinforce the view first espoused over 30 years ago that gynecomastia is best explained by an abnormal ratio of T to E_2. This ratio could result from a decrease in T, an increase in E_2, or a combination of the two. Gynecomastia can be seen in all forms of male hypogonadism, but it is more common when the defect is gonadal, since in that circumstance gonadotropins are high and tend to drive the T-to-E_2 step in the testis. Elevated estrogen can occur whenever there is increased estrogen production (liver disease, extreme obesity, old age, thyrotoxicosis, etc.) Both changes can occur in several settings, particularly when increased estrogen both raises SSBG, thus lowering the percent of free T, and suppresses gonadotropin so that testicular androgen synthesis is diminished. Yet Wilson's group finds that, even with the best of techniques, they are able to explain only about 25% of cases of gynecomastia.

Events at the target tissue may also account for gynecomastia. Differential binding of androgen versus estrogen may influence the relative effects of these hormones; the gynecomastia related to cimetidine therapy illustrates this effect. Several authors have shown that there is no measurable difference in androgen/estrogen in the circulating blood, but that cimetidine interferes with androgen binding to cytosol receptors, thus allowing a disproportionate influence of estrogen.[206,207]

The confusion about the gynecomastia induced by spironolactone continues. Prior studies had or had not shown changes in hormone level. Huffman *et al.*,[208] in a study of at least arguable advisability, evaluated the effects of spironolactone in normal males given a low (100 mg daily) or high dose (200 mg daily) for 10 months. None of the placebo group, 30% of the low-dose, and 62% of the high-dose group developed gynecomastia; yet there were no measurable changes in plasma steroid levels or in the clearance rates of labeled androstenedione or T. By inference, the effect of spironolactone may be exerted, at least in part, at the target tissue.

Even when an endocrine causation of gynecomastia is anticipated, the findings are often puzzling. Stepanas *et al.*[209] reported on 45 patients with testicular tumors, 27 of whom had gynecomastia. Measuring PRL, T, E_2 and estrone, and β-hCG, the authors found that, rather than excess of any one hormone, simultaneous elevations of hormones were necessary to account for gynecomastia. E_2/T ratios were particularly abnormal in patients with galactorrhea. Combined gynecomastia and galactorrhea indicated a bad prognosis.

A valuable short report by Jeffreys[210] should be noted. He found that tamoxifen relieved the pain of acute gynecomastia in two patients with gonadotropin-secreting lung tumors and in one with congestive failure being treated with digoxin and spironolactone. (The author has used tamoxifen several times in similar circumstances, with dramatic results.) This approach should, it would seem, have wider notice and use.

4.8.2. Impotence

Erectile dysfunction continues to receive attention in the literature on human sexuality, but good endocrine data are often lacking. Spark *et al.*[211] published an important paper, calling attention to T deficiency and prolactin excess as possible endocrine causes of impotence. Although this series must reflect the bias of their referral practice—37 of 105 patients had endocrine causes of their problem—it was nonetheless extremely valuable in reasserting that even long-standing erectile failure is highly treatable. Cure of hyperprolactinemia in the male, when due to pituitary microadenoma, has been reported by several authors, with consequent recovery of erectile function. An interesting aspect of the syndrome is that, when the T deficiency is corrected by replacement therapy but the hyperprolactinemia is not, impotence persists until the prolactin levels are reduced by surgery or bromocriptine. The lesson from this finding is that, in evaluating patients for endocrine causes of impotence, measurement of the T level alone is not adequate; one should simultaneously measure the prolactin.

The problem of impotence in the diabetic male has been well examined in a supplement to *Annals of Internal Medicine*.[212] Chapters include a review of erectile physiology, investigation of sexual function in male and female diabetics, plethysmographic study of nocturnal tumescence, and approaches to psychological and prosthetic treatment. There is little evidence of a true endocrine defect in the diabetic, but this tragic disorder illustrates the particularly poignant way in which psychological and organic factors interact.

ACKNOWLEDGMENT

The invaluable assistance of Mrs. Margaret Echlin Boorman in preparing this review is gratefully acknowledged.

Submitted January 1981.

References

1. Bühler, E. M., 1980, A synopsis of the human Y chromosome, *Hum. Genet.* **55**:145–175.
2. Short, R. V., 1978, Sex determination and differentiation of the mammalian gonad, *Int. J. Androl. Suppl.* **2**:21–28.
3. Mailhes, J. B., Pittaway, D. E., Rary, J., Chen, H., and Grafton, W. D., 1979, H-Y antigen-positive male pseudohermaphroditism with 45,X/46,XYq-mosaicism, *Hum. Genet.* **53**:57–63.
4. Wachtel, S. S., and Koo, G. C., H-Y antigen in gonadal differentiation, in: *Mechanisms of Sex Differentiation in Animals and Man* (Austin, C.R., and Edwards, U.R., eds.), Academic Press, London.
5. Fraccaro, M., Tiepolo, L., Zuffardi, O., Chiumello, G., Di Natale, B., Gargantini, L., and Wolf, U., 1979, Familial XX true hermaphroditism and the H-Y antigen, *Hum. Genet.* **48**:45–52.
6. Wolf, U., Fraccaro, M., Mayerová, A., Hecht, T., Zuffardi, O., and Hameister, H., 1980, Turner syndrome patients are H-Y positive, *Hum. Genet.* **54**:315–318.
7. Wolf, U., Fraccaro, M., Mayerová A., Hecht, T., Maraschio, P., and Hameister, H., 1980, A gene controlling H-Y antigen on the X chromosome: Tentative assignment by deletion mapping to Xp223, *Hum. Genet.* **54**:149–154.
8. Engel, W., Pfäfflin, F., and Wiedeking, C., 1980, H-Y antigen in transsexuality, and how to explain testis differentiation in H-Y antigen-negative males and ovary differentiation in H-Y antigen-positive females, *Hum. Genet.* **55**:315–319.
9. Müller, U., Aschmoneit, I., Zenzes, M. T., and Wolf, U. W., 1978, Binding studies of H-Y antigen in rat tissues: Indications for a gonad-specific receptor, *Hum. Genet.* **43**:151–157.
10. Schulte, M.-J., 1979, Positive H-Y antigen testing in a case of XY gonadal absence syndrome, *Clin. Genet.* **16**:438–440.
11. Griffin, J. E., and Wilson, J. D., 1980, The syndromes of androgen resistance, *N. Engl. J. Med.* **302**:198–209.
12. Huhtaniemi, I., and Lautala, P., 1979, Stimulation of steroidogenesis in human fetal testes by the placenta during perifusion, *J. Steroid Biochem.* **10**:109–113.
13. Feldman, K. W., and Smith, D. W., 1975, Fetal phallic growth and penile standards for newborn male infants, *J. Pediatr.* **86**:395–398.
14. Naganami, M., McDonough, P. G., Ellegood, J. O., and Mahesh, V. B.,

1979, Maternal and amniotic fluid steroids throughout human pregnancy, *Am. J. Obstet. Gynecol.* **134:**674–680.

15. Lox, C. D., 1978, Amniotic fluid androgens and their relationship to foetal sex, *Int. J. Androl.* **1:**471–476.

16. Siler-Khodr, T. M., and Khodr, G. S., 1980, Studies in human fetal endocrinology. II. LH and FSH content and concentration in the pituitary, *Obstet. Gynecol.* **56:**176–181.

17. Wachtel, S. S., 1980, The dysgenetic gonad: Aberrant testicular differentiation, *Biol. Reprod.* **22:**1–8.

18. Wachtel, S. S., Koo, G. C., Breg, W. R., Thaler, H. T., Dillard, A. M., Rosenthal, I. M., Dosik, H., Gerald, P. S., Saenger, P., New, M., Lieber, E., and Miller, O. J., 1976, Serologic detection of a Y-linked gene in XX males and XX true hermaphrodites, *N. Engl. J. Med.* **295:**750–754.

19. Winters, S. J., Wachtel, S. S., White, B. J., Koo, G. C., Javadpour, N., Loriaux, D. L., and Sherins, R. J., 1979, H-Y antigen mosaicism in the gonad of a 46,XX true hermaphrodite, *N. Engl. J. Med.* **300:**745–749.

20. Elias, S., Martin, A. O., and Simpson, J. L., 1980, Stability of sex chromosome mosaicism, *Am. J. Obstet. Gynecol.* **136:**509–512.

21. Moreira-Filho, C. A., Otto, P. G., Mustacchi, Z., Frota-Pessoa, O., and Otto, P. A., 1980, H-Y antigen expression in a case of XX true hermaphroditism, *Hum. Genet.* **55:**309–314.

22. Bernstein, R., Jenkins, T., Dawson, B., Wagner, J., Dewald, G., Koo, G. C., and Wachtel, S. S., 1980, Female phenotype and multiple abnormalities in sibs with a Y chromosome and partial X chromosome duplication: H-Y antigen and Xg blood group findings, *J. Med. Genet.* **17:**291–300.

23. Jones, H. W., Jr., Rary, J. M., Rock, J. A., and Cummings, D., 1979, The role of the H-Y antigen in human sexual development, *Johns Hopkins Med. J.* **145:**33–43.

24. Turner, G., Daniel, A., and Frost, M., 1980, X-linked mental retardation, macro-orchidism, and the Xq27 fragile site, *J. Pediatr.* **96:**837–841.

25. Sutherland, G. R., and Ashforth, P. L. C., 1979, X-linked mental retardation with macro-orchidism and the fragile site at Xq27 or 28, *Hum. Genet.* **48:**117–120.

26. Forest, M. G., Lecornu, M., and de Peretti, E., 1980, Familial male pseudohermaphroditism due to 17-20-desmolase deficiency. I. *In vivo* endocrine studies, *J. Clin. Endocrinol. Metab.* **50:**826–833.

27. Savage, M. O., Preece, M. A., Jeffcoate, S. L., Ransley, P. G., Rumsby, G., Mansfield, M. D., and Williams, D. I., 1980, Familial male pseudohermaphroditism due to deficiency of 5α-reductase, *Clin. Endocrinol.* **12:**397–406.

28. Maes, M., Sultan, C., Zerhouni, N., Rothwell, S. W., and Migeon, C. J., 1979, Role of testosterone binding to the androgen receptor in male sexual differentiation of patients with 5α-reductase deficiency, *J. Steroid Biochem.* **11:**1385–1390.

29. Imperato-McGinley, J., Peterson, R. E., Gautier, T., and Sturla, E., 1979, Androgens and the evolution of male-gender identity among male pseudohermaphrodites with 5α-reductase deficiency, *N. Engl. J. Med.* **300:**1233–1237.

30. Forest, M. G., Sizonenko, P. C., Cathiard, A. M., and Bertrand, J., 1974, Hypophyso-gonadal function in humans during the first year of life. I. Evidence for testicular activity in early infancy, *J. Clin. Invest.* **53**:819–828.
31. Gendrel, D., Chaussain, J.-L., Roger, M., and Job, J.-C., 1980, Simultaneous postnatal rise of plasma LH and testosterone in male infants, *J. Pediatr.* **97**:600–602.
32. Oberkotter, L. V., Tenore, A., and Koldovsky, O., 1980, Sex differences in serum levels of N-acetyl-β-hexosaminidase in infancy: Correlation of enzyme activity with testosterone levels, *Early Hum. Dev.* **4**:325–332.
33. Pang, S., Levine, L. S., Chow, D., Sagiani, F., Saenger, P., and New, M. I., 1979, Dihydrotestosterone and its relationship to testosterone in infancy and childhood, *J. Clin. Endocrinol. Metab.* **48**:821–826.
34. Forest, M. G., 1979, Pattern of the response of testosterone and its precursors to human chorionic gonadotropin stimulation in relation to age in infants and children, *J. Clin. Endocrinol. Metab.* **49**:132–137.
35. Hammond, G. L., Koivisto, M., Kouvalainen, K., and Vihko, R., 1979, Serum steroids and pituitary hormones in infants with particular reference to testicular activity, *J. Clin. Endocrinol. Metab.* **49**:40–45.
36. Burstein, S., Grumbach, M. M., and Kaplan, S. L., 1979, Early determination of androgen-responsiveness is important in the management of microphallus, *Lancet* **2**:983–986.
37. Hinman, F., Jr., 1980, Microphallus: Distinction between anomalous and endocrine types, *J. Urol.* **123**:412–415.
38. Ben-Galim, E., Hillman, R. E., and Weldon, V. V., 1980, Topically applied testosterone and phallic growth: Its effect on male children with hypopituitarism and microphallus, *Am. J. Dis. Child.* **134**:296–298.
39. Danish, R. K., Lee, P. A., Mazur, T., Amrhein, J. A., and Migeon, C. J., 1980, Micropenis. II. Hypogonadotropic hypogonadism, *Johns Hopkins Med. J.* **146**:177–184.
40. Chaussain, J. L., Gendrel, D., Roger, M., Boudailliez, B., and Job, J. C., 1979, Longitudinal study of plasma testosterone in male pseudohermaphrodites during early infancy, *J. Clin. Endocrinol. Metab.* **49**:305–306.
41. Ojeda, S. R., Andrews, W. W., Advis, J. P., and White, S. S., 1980, Recent advances in the endocrinology of puberty, *Endocr. Rev.* **1**:228–257.
42. Beck, W., and Wuttke, W., 1980, Diurnal variations of plasma luteinizing hormone, follicle-stimulating hormone, and prolactin in boys and girls from birth to puberty, *J. Clin. Endocrinol. Metab.* **50**:635–639.
43. Grumbach, M. M., 1980, The neuroendocrinology of puberty, *Hosp. Pract.* **15**(3):51–60.
44. Lee, P. A., and Gisriel, D. L., 1980, Correlation of gonadotropins with unbound testosterone during puberty in males, *Horm. Res.* **12**:130–136.
45. Styne, D. M., Kaplan, S. L., and Grumbach, M. M., 1980, Plasma glycoprotein hormone α-subunit in the neonate and in prepubertal and pubertal children: Effects of luteinizing hormone-releasing hormone, *J. Clin. Endocrinol. Metab.* **50**:450–455.
46. Conte, F. A., Grumbach, M. M., Kaplan, S. L., and Reiter, E. O., 1980, Correlation of luteinizing hormone-releasing factor-induced luteinizing

hormone and follicle-stimulating hormone release from infancy to 19 years with the changing pattern of gonadotropin secretion in agonadal patients: Relation to the restraint of puberty, *J. Clin. Endocrinol. Metab.* **50**:163–168.

47. Ducharme, J. R., Catin-Savoie, S., Taché, Y., Bourel, B., and Collu, R., 1979, Sequential hormonal changes and activation of the hypothalamic–pituitary–gonadal axis, *J. Steroid Biochem.* **11**:563–569.

48. Herrera-Justiniano, E., Galvez, M. D., Aznar, A. M., Gomez, S. M. M., Sendon, P. A., Zurita, A. R., Malagon, C. M., and Aznar, R. A., 1979, Changes in the plasma levels of androstenedione, dehydroepiandrosterone and cortisol after stimulation with ACTH and hCG and suppression with dexamethasone during male puberty, *Acta Endocrinol. (Copenhagen)* **90**:113–121.

49. Pakarinen, A., Hammond, G. L., and Vihko, R., 1979, Serum pregnenolone, progesterone, 17α-hydroxyprogesterone, androstenedione, testosterone, 5α-dihydrotestosterone and androsterone during puberty in boys, *Clin. Endocrinol.* **11**:465–474.

50. Odell, W. D., 1979, The physiology of puberty: Disorders of the pubertal process, in: *Endocrinology*, Volume 3 (L. J. DeGroot, G. F. Cahill, Jr., L. Martini, D. H. Nelson, W. D. Odell, J. T. Potts, Jr., E. Steinberger, and A. I. Winegrad, eds.), pp. 1363–1379, Grune & Stratton, New York.

51. Urban, M. D., Lee, P. A., Gutai, J. P., and Migeon, C. J., 1980, Androgens in pubertal males with Addison's disease, *J. Clin. Endocrinol. Metab.* **51**:925–929.

52. Sklar, C. A., Kaplan, S. L., and Grumbach, M. M., 1980, Evidence for dissociation between adrenarche and gonadarche: Studies in patients with idiopathic precocious puberty, gonadal dysgenesis, isolated gonadotropin deficiency, and constitutionally delayed growth and adolescence, *J. Clin. Endocrinol. Metab.* **51**:548–566.

53. Olweus, D., Mattsson, ÅA., Schalling, D., and Löw, H., 1980, Testosterone, aggression, physical, and personality dimensions in normal adolescent males, *Psychosom. Med.* **42**:253–269.

54. Lucky, A. W., Rich, B. H., Rosenfield, R. L., Fang, V. S., and Roche-Bender, N., 1980, LH bioactivity increases more than immunoreactivity during puberty, *J. Pediatr.* **97**:205–213.

55. Lee, P. A., 1980, Normal ages of pubertal events among American males and females, *J. Adolesc. Health Care* **1**:26–29.

56. Root, A. W., 1980, Hormonal changes in puberty, *Pediatr. Ann.* **9**(10): 11–27.

57. Harlan, W. R., Grillo, G. P., Cornoni-Huntley, J., and Leaverton, P. E., 1979, Secondary sex characteristics of boys 12 to 17 years of age: The U. S. Health Examination Survey, *J. Pediatr.* **95**:293–297.

58. Daniel, W. A., Jr., 1979, Sex maturity ratings, *J. Pediatr.* **95**:255–256.

59. Round, J. M., 1980, Changes in plasma urate, creatinine, alkaline phosphatase and the 24 hour excretion of hydroxyproline during sexual maturation in adolescents, *Ann. Hum. Biol.* **7**:83–88.

60. Short, R. V., 1976, The evolution of human reproduction, *Proc. R. Soc. London Ser. B* **195**:3–24.

61. 1979, Adolescent sexuality and adolescent fertility (editorial), *Lancet* **2:**129–130.

62. Laron, Z., Arad, J., Gurewitz, R., Grunebaum, M., and Dickerman, Z., 1980, Age at first conscious ejaculation: A milestone in male puberty, *Helv. Paediatr. Acta* **35:**13–20.

63. Raiti, S., Maclaren, N. K., and Akesode, F. A., 1980, Precocious and delayed puberty: Studies of FSH and LH production and metabolism, *Acta Endocrinol. (Copenhagen)* **94:**475–479.

64. Rosenfeld, R. G., Reitz, R. E., King, A. B., and Hintz, R. L., 1980, Familial precocious puberty associated with isolated elevation of luteinizing hormone, *N. Engl. J. Med.* **303:**859–862.

65. Crowley, W. F., Jr., Comite, F., Vale, W., Rivier, J., Loriaux, D. L., and Cutler, G. B., Jr., 1981, Therapeutic use of pituitary desensitization with a long-acting LHRH agonist: A potential new treatment for idiopathic precocious puberty, *J. Clin. Endocrinol. Metab.* **52:**370–372.

66. Kelch, R. P., Hopwood, N. J., and Marshall, J. C., 1980, Diagnosis of gonadotropin deficiency in adolescents: Limited usefulness of a standard gonadotropin-releasing hormone test in obese boys, *J. Pediatr.* **97:**820–824.

67. Brook, C. G. D., and Dombey, S., 1979, Induction of puberty: Long-term treatment with high-dose LHRH, *Clin. Endocrinol.* **11:**81–87.

68. Jacobson, R. I., Seyler, L. E., Jr., Tamborlane, W. V., Jr., Gertner, J. M., and Genel, M., 1979, Pulsatile subcutaneous nocturnal administration of GnRH by portable infusion pump in hypogonadotropic hypogonadism: Initiation of gonadotropin responsiveness, *J. Clin. Endocrinol. Metab.* **49:**652–654.

69. Valk, T. W., Corley, K. P., Kelch, R. P., and Marshall, J. C., 1980, Hypogonadotropic hypogonadism: Hormonal responses to low dose pulsatile administration of gonadotropin-releasing hormone, *J. Clin. Endocrinol.* **51:**730–738.

70. Crowley, W. F., and McArthur, J. W., 1980, Simulation of the normal menstrual cycle in Kallman's syndrome by pulsatile administration of luteinizing hormone-releasing hormone (LHRH), *J. Clin. Endocrinol. Metab.* **51:**173–175.

71. McArthur, J. W., 1980, Induction of puberty in hypogonadotropic males: Use of low dose pulsatile luteinizing hormone releasing hormone (LHRH) administration, Abstract No. 743, 62nd Annual Meeting of the Endocrine Society.

72. de Lange, W. E., Snoep, M. C., and Doorenbos, H., 1979, The effect of short-term testosterone treatment in boys with delayed puberty, *Acta Endocrinol. (Copenhagen)* **91:**177–183.

73. Imperato-McGinley, J., Peterson, R. E., Gautier, T., and Sturla, E., 1979, Male pseudohermaphroditism secondary to 5α-reductase deficiency—A model for the role of androgens in both the development of the male phenotype and the evolution of a male gender identity, *J. Steroid Biochem.* **11:**637–645.

74. Imperato-McGinley, J., Peterson, R. E., Leshin, M., Griffin, J. E., Cooper, G., Draghi, S., Berenyi, M., and Wilson, J. D., 1980, Steroid 5α-reductase

deficiency in a 65-year-old male pseudohermaphrodite: The natural history, ultrastructure of the testes, and evidence for inherited enzyme heterogeneity, *J. Clin. Endocrinol. Metab.* **50**:15–22.

75. Imperato-McGinley, J., Peterson, R. E., Stoller, R., and Goodwin, W. E., 1979, Male pseudohermaphroditism secondary to 17β-hydroxysteroid dehydrogenase deficiency: Gender role change with puberty, *J. Clin. Endocrinol. Metab.* **49**:391–395.

76. Foucault, M. (ed.), 1980, *Herculine Barbin: The Recently Discovered Memoirs of a Nineteenth-Century French Hermaphrodite*, Pantheon Books, New York.

77. Wilson, J. D., Aiman, J., and MacDonald, P. C., 1980, The pathogenesis of gynecomastia, *Adv. Intern. Med.* **25**:1–32.

78. Large, D. M., and Anderson, D. C., 1979, Twenty-four hour profiles of circulating androgens and oestrogens in male puberty with and without gynaecomastia, *Clin. Endocrinol.* **11**:505–521.

79. Large, D. M., Anderson, D. C., and Laing, I., 1980, Twenty-four hour profiles of serum prolactin during male puberty with and without gynaecomastia, *Clin. Endocrinol.* **12**:293–302.

80. Marynick, S. P., Nisula, B. C., Pita, J. C., Jr., and Loriaux, D. L., 1980, Persistent pubertal macromastia, *J. Clin. Endocrinol. Metab.* **50**:128–130.

81. LeRoith, D., Sobel, R., and Glick, S. M., 1980, The effect of clomiphene citrate on pubertal gynaecomastia, *Acta Endocrinol. (Copenhagen)* **95**:177–180.

82. Bardin, C. W., 1979, The neuroendocrinology of male reproduction, *Hosp. Pract.* **14**(12):65–75.

83. Pinto, H., Wajchenberg, B. L., Lima, F. B., Goldman, J., Comaru-Schally, A. M., and Schally, A. V., 1979, Evaluation of the gonadotrophic responsiveness of the pituitary to acute and prolonged administration of LH/FH-releasing hormone (LH-RH) in normal females and males, *Acta Endocrinol. (Copenhagen)* **91**:1–13.

84. Bergquist, C., Nillius, S. J., Bergh, T., Skarin, G., and Wide, L., 1979, Inhibitory effects on gonadotrophin secretion and gonadal function in men during chronic treatment with a potent stimulatory luteinizing hormone-releasing hormone analogue, *Acta Endocrinol. (Copenhagen)* **91**:601–608.

85. Catt, K. J., Baukal, A. J., Davies, T. F., and Dafau, M. L., 1979, Luteinizing hormone-releasing hormone-induced regulation of gonadotropin and prolactin receptors in the rat testis, *Endocrinology* **104**:17–25.

86. Clayton, R. N., Katikineni, M., Chan, V., Dufau, M. L., and Catt, K. J., 1980, Direct inhibition of testicular function by gonadotropin-releasing hormone: Mediation by specific gonadotropin-releasing hormone receptors in interstitial cells, *Proc. Natl. Acad. Sci. USA* **77**:4459–4463.

87. Bourne, G. A., Regiani, S., Payne, A. H., and Marshall, J. C., 1980, Testicular GnRH receptors—Characterization and localization on interstitial tissue, *J. Clin. Endocrinol. Metab.* **51**:407–409.

88. Sharpe, R. M., and Fraser, H. M., 1980, HCG stimulation of testicular LHRH-like activity, *Nature (London)* **287**:642–643.

89. Lipsett, M. B., 1979, The role of testosterone and other hormones in regulation of LH, *J. Steroid Biochem.* **11**:659–661.

90. Naftolin, F., Ryan, K. J., Davies, I. J., Reddy, I. I., Flores, F., Petro, Z.,

Kulin, M., White, R. J., Takaoka, Y., and Wolin, L., 1975, The formation of estrogens by central neuroendocrine tissues, *Recent Prog. Horm. Res.* **31:**295–315.

91. Marynick, S. P., Loriaux, D. L., Sherins, R. J., Pita, J. C., Jr., and Lipsett, M. B., 1979, Evidence that testosterone can suppress pituitary gonadotropin secretion independently of peripheral aromatization, *J. Clin. Endocrinol. Metab.* **49:**396–398.

92. Lacroix, A., McKenna, T. J., and Rabinowitz, D., 1979, Sex steroid modulation of gonadotropins in normal men and in androgen insensitivity syndrome, *J. Clin. Endocrinol. Metab.* **48:**235–240.

93. Martini, L., Celotti, F., and Serio, M., 1979, 5α-reductase deficiency in humans: Support to the theory that 5α-reduction of testosterone is an essential step in the control of LH secretion [letter], *J. Endocrinol. Invest.* **2:**463.

94. Winters, S. J., Janick, J. J., Loriaux, D. L., and Sherins, R. J., 1979, Studies on the role of sex steroids in the feedback control of gonadotropin concentrations in men. II. Use of the estrogen antagonist, clomiphene citrate, *J. Clin. Endocrinol. Metab.* **48:**222–227.

95. Schaison, G., Renoir, M., Lagoguey, M., and Mowszowicz, I., 1980, On the role of dihydrotestosterone in regulating luteinizing hormone secretion in man, *J. Clin. Endocrinol. Metab.* **51:**1133–1137.

96. Caminos-Torres, R., Ma, L., and Snyder, P. J., 1977, Testosterone-induced inhibition of the LH and FSH responses to gonadotropin-releasing hormone occurs slowly, *J. Clin. Endocrinol. Metab.* **44:**1142–1153.

97. Axelrod, L., Neer, R. M., and Kliman, B., 1979, Hypogonadism in a male with immunologically active, biologically inactive luteinizing hormone: An exception to a venerable rule, *J. Clin. Endocrinol. Metab.* **48:**279–287.

98. Knobil, E., Plant, T. M., Wildt, L., Belchetz, P. E., and Marshall, G., 1980, Control of the rhesus monkey menstrual cycle: Permissive role of hypothalamic gonadotropin-releasing hormone, *Science* **207:**1371–1373.

99. Wildt, L., Marshall, G., and Knobil, E., 1980, Experimental induction of puberty in the infantile female rhesus monkey, *Science* **207:**1373–1375.

100. Barbarino, A., and De Marinis, L., 1980, Estrogen induction of luteinizing hormone release in castrated adult human males, *J. Clin. Endocrinol. Metab.* **51:**280–286.

101. Seyler, L. E., Jr., Canalis, E., Spare, S., and Reichlin, S., 1978, Abnormal gonadotropin secretory responses to LRH in transsexual women after diethylstilbestrol priming, *J. Clin. Endocrinol. Metab.* **47:**176–183.

102. Preslock, J. P., 1980, A review of *in vitro* testicular steroidogenesis in rodents, monkeys and humans, *J. Steroid Biochem.* **13:**965–975.

103. Preslock, J. P., 1980, Steroidogenesis in the mammalian testis, *Endocr. Rev.* **1:**132–139.

104. Catt, K. J., Harwood, J. P., Clayton, R. N., Davies, T. F., Chan, V., Katikineni, M., Nozu, K., and Dufau, M. L., 1980, Regulation of peptide hormone receptors and gonadal steroidogenesis, *Recent Prog. Horm. Res.* **36:**557–622.

105. Smals, A. G. H., Pieters, G. F. F. M., Lozekoot, D. C., Benraad, T. J., and

Kloppenborg, P. W. C., 1980, Dissociated responses of plasma testosterone and 17-hydroxyprogesterone to single or repeated human chorionic gonadotropin administration in normal men, *J. Clin. Endocrinol. Metab.* **50:**190–193.

106. Smals, A. G. H., Pieters, G. F. F. M., Drayer, J. I. M., Boers, G. H. J., Benraad, T. J., and Kloppenborg, P. W. C., 1980, Tamoxifen suppresses gonadotropin-induced 17α-hydroxyprogesterone accumulation in normal men, *J. Clin. Endocrinol. Metab.* **51:**1026–1029.

107. Glass, A. R., and Vigersky, R. A., 1980, Correlation of acute and chronic increases in serum gonadal steroid levels after administration of human chorionic gonadotropin, *Fertil. Steril.* **34:**41–45.

108. Glass, A. R., and Vigersky, R. A., 1980, Resensitization of testosterone production in men after human chorionic gonadotropin-induced desensitization, *J. Clin. Endocrinol. Metab.* **51:**1395–1400.

109. Padrón, R. S., Wischusen, J., Hudson, B., Burger, H. G., and de Kretser, D. M., 1980, Prolonged biphasic response of plasma testosterone to single intramuscular injections of human chorionic gonadotropin, *J. Clin. Endocrinol. Metab.* **50:**1100–1104.

110. Martikainen, H., Huhtaniemi, I., and Vihko, R., 1980, Response of peripheral serum sex steroids and some of their precursors to a single injection of hCG in adult men, *Clin. Endocrinol.* **13:**157–166.

111. Wang, C., Rebar, R. W., Hopper, B. R., and Yen, S. S. C., 1980, Functional studies of the luteinizing hormone–Leydig cell–androgen axis: Exaggerated response in C-18 and C-21 testicular steroids to various modes of luteinizing hormone stimulation, *J. Clin. Endocrinol. Metab.* **51:**201–208.

112. Davies, T. F., Hodgen, G. D., Dufau, M. L., and Catt, K. J., 1979, Regulation of primate testicular luteinizing hormone receptors and steroidogenesis, *J. Clin. Invest.* **64:**1070–1073.

113. Leinonen, P., Hammond, G. L., and Vihko, R., 1980, Testosterone and some its precursors and metabolites in the human epididymis, *J. Clin. Endocrinol. Metab.* **51:**423–428.

114. Kley, H. K., Deselaers, T., Peerenboom, H., and Krüskemper, H. L., 1980, Enhanced conversion of androstenedione to estrogens in obese males, *J. Clin. Endocrinol. Metab.* **51:**1128–1132.

115. MacLeod, J., and Wang, Y., 1979, Male fertility potential in terms of semen quality: A review of the past, a study of the present, *Fertil. Steril.* **31:**103–116.

116. David, G., Jouannet, P., Martin-Boyce, A., Spira, A., and Schwartz, D., 1979, Sperm counts in fertile and infertile men, *Fertil. Steril.* **31:**453–455.

117. Smith, K. D., and Rodriguez-Rigau, L. J., 1979, Laboratory evaluation of testicular function, in: *Endocrinology*, Volume 3 (L. J. DeGroot, G. F. Cahill, Jr., L. Martini, D. H. Nelson, W. D. Odell, J. T. Potts, Jr., E. Steinberger, and A. I. Winegrad, eds.), pp. 1539–1547, Grune & Stratton, New York.

118. van Dop, P. A., Scholtmeijer, R. J., Kruver, P. H. J., Baak, J. P. A., Oort, J., and Stolte, L. A. M., 1980, A quantitative structural model of the testis of fertile males with normal sperm counts, *Int. J. Androl.* **3:**153–169.

119. van Dop, P. A., Kruver, P. H. J., Scholtmeijer, R. J., Baak, J. P. A., Oort, J., and Stolte, L. A. M., 1980, Correlations between the quantitative mor-

phology of the human testis and sperm production: The testis of healthy men with normal sperm counts, *Int. J. Androl.* **3:**170–176.

120. Steinberger, E., 1979, Hormonal control of spermatogenesis, in: *Endocrinology*, Volume 3 (L. J. DeGroot, G. F. Cahill, Jr., L. Martini, D. H. Nelson, W. D. Odell, J. T. Potts, Jr., E. Steinberger, and A. I. Winegrad, eds.), pp. 1535–1538, Grune & Stratton, New York.

121. Means, A. R., Dedman, J. R., Tindall, D. J., and Welsh, M. J., 1978, Hormonal regulation of Sertoli cells, *Int. J. Androl. Suppl.* **2:**403–423.

122. Ritzén, E. M., Hansson, V., and French, F. S., 1978, Androgen action on spermatogenesis, *Int. J. Androl. Suppl.* **1:**108–115.

123. Karim, S. M. M., and Hillier, K., 1979, Prostaglandins in the control of animal and human reproduction, *Br. Med. Bull.* **35:**173–180.

124. Harman, S. M., and Tsitouras, P. D., 1980, Reproductive hormones in aging men. I. Measurement of sex steroids, basal luteinizing hormone, and Leydig cell response to human chorionic gonadotropin, *J. Clin. Endocrinol. Metab.* **51:**35–40.

125. Sparrow, D., Bosse, R., and Rowe, J. W., 1980, The influence of age, alcohol consumption, and body build on gonadal function in men, *J. Clin. Endocrinol. Metab.* **51:**508–519.

126. Sköldefors, H., Carlström, K., and Eneroth, P., 1978, Influence of aging upon the serum hormone levels in the male, *Int. J. Androl.* **1:**306–316.

127. Serio, M., Gonnelli, P., Borrelli, D., Pampaloni, A., Fiorelli, G., Calabresi, E., Forti, G., Pazzagli, M., Mannelli, M., Baroni, A., Giannotti, P., and Giusti, G., 1978, Human testicular secretion with increasing age, *J. Steroid Biochem.* **11:**893–897.

128. Kaler, L. W., and Neaves, W. B., 1978, Attrition of the human Leydig cell population with advancing age, *Anat. Rec.* **192:**513–518.

129. Smith, R., Donald, R. A., Espiner, E. A., Stronach, S. G., and Edwards, I. A., 1979, Normal adults and subjects with hypogonadotropic hypogonadism respond differently to D-Ser(TBU)[6]-LH-RH-EA[10], *J. Clin. Endocrinol. Metab.* **48:**167–170.

130. Smith, R., Donald, R. A., Espiner, E. A., and Stronach, S., 1979, The effects of prolonged administration of D-Ser(TBU)[6]-LH-RH-EA[10] (HOE 766) in subjects with hypogonadotrophic hypogonadism, *Clin. Endocrinol.* **11:**553–559.

131. Heath, M., Scanlon, M. F., Mora, B., Snow, M. H., Gomez-Pan, A., Watson, M. J., Mulligan, F., and Hall, R., 1979, The pituitary–gonadal response to the gonadotrophin releasing hormone analogue D-Ser(TBU)[6]-des Gly[10]-LHRH-ethylamide in normal men, *Clin. Endocrinol.* **10:**297–303.

132. Snyder, P. J., Rudenstein, R. S., Gardner, D. F., and Rothman, J. G., 1979, Repetitive infusion of gonadotropin-releasing hormone distinguishes hypothalamic from pituitary hypogonadism, *J. Clin. Endocrinol. Metab.* **48:**864–868.

133. Kletzky, O. A., Costin, G., Marrs, R. P., Bernstein, G., March, C. M., and Mishell, D. R., Jr., 1979, Gonadotropin insufficiency in patients with thalassemia major, *J. Clin. Endocrinol. Metab.* **48:**901–905.

134. Smals, A. G. H., Pieters, G. F. F. M., Kloppenborg, P. W. C., Lozekoot, D.

C., and Benraad, T. J., 1980, Lack of a biphasic steroid response to single human chorionic gonadotropin administration in patients with isolated gonadotropin deficiency, *J. Clin. Endocrinol. Metab.* **50:**879–881.

135. Spitz, I. M., Zylber, E., Cohen, H., Almaliach, U., and Leroith, D., 1979, Impaired prolactin response to thyrotropin-releasing hormone in isolated gonadotropin deficiency and exaggerated response in primary testicular failure, *J. Clin. Endocrinol. Metab.* **48:**941–945.

136. Bartrinos, M. L., Panitsa-Faflia, C., Pitoulis, S., and Petraki, N., 1980, Pituitary–gonadal function in three relatives presenting with Kallmann's syndrome, *Horm. Res.* **12:**79–86.

137. Rogol, A. D., Mittal, K. K., White, B. J., McGinness, M. H., Lieblich, J. M., and Rosen, S. W., 1980, HLA-compatible paternity in two "fertile eunuchs" with congenital hypogonadotropic hypogonadism and anosmia (the Kallmann syndrome), *J. Clin. Endocrinol. Metab.* **51:**275–279.

138. Barenetsky, N. G., and Carolson, H. E., 1980, Persistence of spermatogenesis in hypogonadotropic hypogonadism treated with testosterone, *Fertil. Steril.* **34:**477–482.

139. Nistal, M., and Paniagua, R., 1979, Leydig cell differentiation induced by stimulation with HCG and HMG in two patients affected with hypogonadotropic hypogonadism, *Andrologia* **11:**211–222.

140. Davidson, J. M., Camargo, C. A., and Smith, E. R., 1979, Effects of androgen on sexual behavior in hypogonadal men, *J. Clin. Endocrinol. Metab.* **48:**955–958.

141. Snyder, P. J., and Lawrence, D. A., 1980, Treatment of male hypogonadism with testosterone enanthate, *J. Clin. Endocrinol. Metab.* **51:**1335–1339.

142. Snyder, P. J., Bigdeli, H., Gardner, D. F., Mihailovic, V., Rudenstein, R. S., Sterling, F. H., and Utiger, R. D., 1979, Gonadal function in fifty men with untreated pituitary adenomas, *J. Clin. Endocrinol. Metab.* **48:**309–314.

143. Snyder, P. J., Muzyka, R., Johnson, J., and Utiger, R. D., 1980, Thyrotropin-releasing hormone provokes abnormal follicle-stimulating hormone (FSH) and luteinizing hormone responses in men who have pituitary adenomas and FSH hypersecretion, *J. Clin. Endocrinol. Metab.* **51:**744–749.

144. Schnakenburg, K. v., Bidlingmaier, F., Engelhardt, D., Butenandt, O., and Knorr, D., 1980, 17-Ketosteroid reductase deficiency—Plasma steroids and incubation studies with testicular tissue, *Acta Endocrinol. (Copenhagen)* **94:**397–403.

145. Maes, M., Lee, P. A., Jeffs, R. D., Sultan, C., and Migeon, C. J., 1980, Phenotypic variation in a family with partial androgen insensitivity syndrome, *Am. J. Dis. Child.* **134:**470–473.

146. Larrea, F., Benavides, G., Scaglia, H., Kofman-Alfaro, S., Ferrusca, E., Medina, M., and Pérez-Palactios, G., 1978, Gynecomastia as a familial incomplete male pseudohermaphroditism type 1: A limited androgen resistance syndrome, *J. Clin. Endocrinol. Metab.* **46:**961–970.

147. George, F. W., and Wilson, J. D., 1980, Pathogenesis of the henny feathering trait in the Sebright bantam chicken: Increased conversion of androgen to estrogen, *J. Clin. Invest.* **66:**57–65.

148. Albright, F., Burnett, C. H., Smith, P. H., and Parson, W., 1942, Pseu-

dohypoparathyroidism—An example of 'Seabright–Bantam syndrome,' *Endocrinology* **30:**922–932.

149. Boisen, E., 1979, Testicular size and shape of 47,XYY and 47,XXY men in a double-blind, double-matched population survey, *Am. J. Hum. Genet.* **31:**697–703.

150. Smals, A. G. H., Kloppenborg, P. W. C., Pieters, G. F. F. M., Hoefnagels, W. H. L., Lequin, R. M., and Benraad, T. J., 1979, Modulation of the gonadotropin response to constant luteinizing hormone-releasing hormone infusion by acute and chronic testosterone administration in Klinefelter's syndrome, *J. Clin. Endocrinol. Metab.* **48:**148–152.

151. Gabrilove, J. L., Freiberg, E. K., and Nicolis, G. L., 1980, Testicular function in Klinefelter's syndrome, *J. Urol.* **124:**825–826.

152. Wieland, R. G., Zorn, E. M., and Johnson, M. W., 1980, Elevated testosterone-binding globulin in Klinefelter's syndrome, *J. Clin. Endocrinol. Metab.* **51:**1199–1200.

153. Barbarino, A., De Marinis, L., LaFuenti, G., Muscatello, P., and Matteucci, B. R., 1979, Presence of positive feedback between oestrogen and LH in patients with Klinefelter's syndrome, and Sertoli-cell-only syndrome, *Clin. Endocrinol.* **10:**235–242.

154. Samaan, N. A., Stepanas, A. V., Danziger, J., and Trujillo, J., 1979, Reactive pituitary abnormalities in patients with Klinefelter's and Turner's syndromes, *Arch. Intern. Med.* **139:**198–201.

155. Gabrilove, J. L., Freiberg, E. K., Thornton, J. C., and Nicolis, G. L., 1979, Effect of age on testicular function in patients with Klinefelter's syndrome, *Clin. Endocrinol.* **11:**343–347.

156. Ellison, H. S., Scheuer, S. A., and Eichner, E. R., 1980, Metastatic breast carcinoma with positive estrogen and progesterone receptors in a man with Klinefelter's syndrome, *South. Med. J.* **73:**1393–1396.

157. Sogge, M. R., McDonald, S. D., and Cofold, P. B., 1979, The malignant potential of the dysgenetic germ cell in Klinefelter's syndrome, *Am. J. Med.* **66:**515–518.

158. Vaze, A. Y., Thakur, A. N., and Sheth, A. R., 1979, Development of radioimmunoassay for human seminal plasma inhibin, *J. Reprod. Fertil. Suppl.* **26:**135–146.

159. Asch, R. H., Vaze, A. Y., Thakur, A. N., and Sheth, A. R., 1980, Concentrations of immunoreactive inhibin in seminal plasma and serum from normospermic, oligospermic, vasectomized, Klinefelter's syndrome, and Sertoli-cell-only syndrome subjects, *J. Androl.* **1:**252–254.

160. Scott, R. S., and Burger, H. G., 1980, Inhibin is absent from azoospermic semen of infertile men, *Nature (London)* **285:**246–247.

161. Editorial, 1979, Recognisable patterns of male infertility, *Br. Med. J.* **2:**1169–1170.

162. Haas, G. G., Jr., Cines, D. B., and Schreiber, A. D., 1980, Immunologic infertility: Identification of patients with antisperm antibody, *N. Engl. J. Med.* **303:**722–727.

163. Troen, P., and Oshima, H., 1980, The male factor [editorial], *N. Engl. J. Med.* **303:**751–752.

164. Sturgess, J. M., Chao, J., Wong, J., Aspin, N., and Turner, J. A. P., 1979, Cilia with defective radial spokes: A cause of human respiratory disease, *N. Engl. J. Med.* **300:**53–56.
165. Editorial, 1980, Flagellating cilia, *Lancet* **1:**346–347.
166. Marmor, D., Taillemite, J.-L., Van den Akker, J., Portnoi, M.-F., Le Porrier, N., Joye, N., Delafontaine, D., and Roux, C., 1980, Semen analysis in subfertile balanced-translocation carriers, *Fertil. Steril.* **34:**496–502.
167. Glass, R. I., Lyness, R. N., Mengle, D. C., Powell, K. E., and Kahn, E., 1979, Sperm count depression in pesticide applicators exposed to dibromochloropropane, *Am. J. Epidemiol.* **109:**346–351.
168. Vermeulen, A., Comhaire, F., and Vendeweghe, M., 1979, Hormonal exploration of male infertility, *Acta Eur. Fertil.* **10:**105–112.
169. Rosemberg, E., 1978, Importance of endocrine evaluation in the diagnosis and treatment of disorders of the male reproductive tract, *Int. J. Androl. Suppl.* **1:**21–35.
170. Glass, A. R., and Vigersky, R. A., 1980, Leydig cell function in idiopathic oligospermia, *Fertil. Steril.* **34:**144–148.
171. Rodriguez-Raigau, L. J., Smith, K. D., and Steinberger, E., 1980, A possible relation between elevated FSH levels and Leydig cell dysfunction in azoospermic and oligospermic men, *J. Androl.* **1:**127–132.
172. Segal, S., Yaffe, H., Laufer, N., and Ben-David, M., 1979, Male hyperprolactinemia: Effects on fertility, *Fertil. Steril.* **32:**556–561.
173. Pont, A., Shelton, R., Odell, W. D., and Wilson, C. B., 1979, Prolactinsecreting tumors in men: Surgical care, *Ann. Intern. Med.* **91:**211–213.
174. Jequier, A. M., Crich, J. C., and Ansell, I. D., 1979, Clinical findings and testicular histology in three hyperprolactinemic infertile men, *Fertil. Steril.* **31:**525–530.
175. Spark, R. F., and Dickstein, G., 1979, Bromocriptine and endocrine disorders, *Ann. Intern. Med.* **90:**949–956.
176. Hovatta, O., Koskimies, A. I., Ranta, T., Stenman, U.-H., and Seppälä, M., 1979, Bromocriptine treatment of oligospermia: A double blind study, *Clin. Endocrinol.* **11:**377–382.
177. Glatthaar, C., Donald, R. A., Smith, R., and McRae, C. U., 1980, Pituitary function in normoprolactinaemic infertile men receiving bromocriptine, *Clin. Endocrinol.* **13:**455–459.
178. Charny, C. W., 1979, Clomiphene therapy in male infertility: A negative report, *Fertil. Steril.* **32:**551–555.
179. Allag, I. S., and Alexander, N. J., 1979, Clomiphene citrate therapy for male infertility, *Urology* **14:**500–503.
180. Paulson, D. F., Hammond, C. B., White, R., d., and Wiebe, R. H., 1977, Clomiphene citrate: Pharmacologic treatment of hypofertile male, *Urology* **9:**419–421.
181. Schill, W.-B., 1979, Recent progress in pharmacological therapy of male subfertility—A review, *Andrologia* **112:**77–107.
182. Lunenfeld, B., Olchovsky, D., Tadir, Y., and Glezerman, M., 1979, Treatment of male infertility with human gonadotrophins: Selection of cases, management and results, *Andrologia* **11:**331–336.

183. Chehval, M. J., and Mehan, D. J., 1979, Chorionic gonadotropins in the treatment of the subfertile male, *Fertil. Steril.* **31:**666–668.
184. Morley, J. E., and Melmed, S., 1979, Gonadal dysfunction in systemic disorders, *Metabolism* **28:**1051–1073.
185. Federman, D. D. (ed.), 1980, *Endocrine Manifestations of Systemic Disease, Clin. Endocrinol. Metab.* **8.**
186. Bommer, J., del Pozo, E., Ritz, E., and Bommer, G., 1979, Improved sexual function in male haemodialysis patients on bromocriptine, *Lancet* **2:**496–497.
187. Gómez, F., De La Cueva, R., Wauters, J.-P., and Lemarchand-Béraud, T., 1980, Endocrine abnormalities in patients undergoing long-term hemodialysis: The role of prolactin, *Am. J. Med.* **68:**522–530.
188. Gura, V., Weizman, A., Maoz, B., Zevin, D., and Ben-David, M., 1980, Hyperprolactinemia: A possible cause of sexual impotence in male patients undergoing chronic hemodialysis, *Nephron* **26:**53–54.
189. Abel, E. L., 1980, A review of alcohol's effects on sex and reproduction, *Drug Alcohol Depend.* **5:**321–332.
190. van Thiel, D. H., 1979, Feminization of chronic alcoholic men: A formulation, *Yale J. Biol. Med.* **52:**219–225.
191. Morley, J. E., Distiller, L. A., Lissoos, I., Lipschitz, R., Kay, G., Searle, D. L., and Katz, M., 1979, Testicular function in patients with spinal cord damage, *Horm. Metab. Res.* **11:**679–682.
192. Hayes, P. J., Krishnan, K. R., Diver, M. J., Hipkin, L. J., and Davis, J. C., 1979, Testicular endocrine function in paraplegic men, *Clin. Endocrinol.* **11:**549–552.
193. McKenna, T. J., Lorber, D., Lacroix, A., and Rabin, D., 1979, Testicular activity in Cushing's disease, *Acta Endocrinol. (Copenhagen)* **91:**501–510.
194. Toone, B. K., Wheeler, M., and Fenwick, P. B. C., 1980, Sex hormone changes in male epileptics, *Clin. Endocrinol.* **12:**391–395.
195. Sherins, R. J., Olweny, C. L. M., and Ziegler, J. L., 1978, Gynecomastia and gonadal dysfunction in adolescent boys treated with combination chemotherapy for Hodgkin's disease, *N. Engl. J. Med.* **299:**12–16.
196. Glass, A. R., and Berenberg, J., 1979, Gynecomastia after chemotherapy for lymphoma, *Arch. Intern. Med.* **139:**1048–1049.
197. Friedman, N. M., and Plymate, S. R., 1980, Leydig cell dysfunction and gynaecomastia in adult males treated with alkylating agents, *Clin. Endocrinol.* **12:**553–556.
198. Fraley, E. E., Lange, P. H., and Kennedy, B. J., 1979, Germ-cell testicular cancer in adults, *N. Engl. J. Med.* **301:**1370–1377, 1420–1426.
199. National Institutes of Health Conference, 1979, Testicular germ-cell neoplasms: Recent advances in diagnosis and therapy, *Ann. Intern. Med.* **90:**373–385.
200. Catalona, W. J., Vaitukaitis, J. L., and Fair, W. R., 1979, Falsely positive specific human chorionic gonadotropin assays in patients with testicular tumors: Conversion to negative with testosterone administration, *J. Urol.* **122:**126–128.
201. Lipsett, M. B., 1979, Functional tumors of the testis, in: *Endocrinology,* Volume 3 (L.J. DeGroot, G.F. Cahill, Jr., L. Martini, D.H. Nelson, W.D. Odell, J.T. Potts, Jr., E. Steinberger, and A.I. Winegrad, eds.), pp. 1573–1576, Grune & Stratton, New York.

202. Damjanov, I., Katz, S. M., and Jewett, M. A. S., 1979, Leydig cell tumors of the testis, *Ann. Clin. Lab. Sci.* **9**:157–163.
203. Caldamone, A. A., Altebarmakian, V., Frank, I. N., and Linke, C. A., 1979, Leydig cell tumor of testis, *Urology* **14**:39–43.
204. Klippel, K. F., Jonas, U., Hohenfellner, R., and Walther, D., 1979, Interstitial cell tumor of testis: A delicate problem, *Urology* **14**:79–82.
205. Perez, C., Novoa, J., Alcañiz, J., Salto, L., and Barcelo, B., 1980, Leydig cell tumour of the testis with gynaecomastia and elevated oestrogen, progesterone and prolactin levels: Case report, *Clin. Endocrinol.* **13**:409–412.
206. van Thiel, D. H., Gavaler, J. S., Smith, W. I., Jr., and Paul, G., 1979, Hypothalamic–pituitary–gonadal dysfunction in men using cimetidine, *N. Engl. J. Med.* **300**:1012–1015.
207. Temple, R. J., Jones, J. K., and Crout, J. R., 1979, Adverse effects of newly marketed drugs [editorial], *N. Engl. J. Med.* **300**:1046–1047.
208. Huffman, D. H., Kampmann, J. P., Hignite, C. E., and Azarnoff, D. L., 1978, Gynecomastia induced in normal males by spironolactone, *Clin. Pharmacol. Ther.* **24**:465–473.
209. Stepanas, A. V., Samaan, N. A., Schultz, P. N., and Holoye, P. Y., 1978, Endocrine studies in testicular tumor patients with and without gynecomastia: A report of 45 cases, *Cancer* **41**:369–376.
210. Jeffreys, D. B., 1979, Painful gynaecomastia treated with tamoxifen, *Br. Med. J.* **1**:1119–1120.
211. Spark, R. F., White, R. A., and Connolly, P. B., 1980, Impotence is not always psychogenic: Newer insights into hypothalamic–pituitary–gonadal dysfunction, *J. Am. Med. Assoc.* **243**:750–755.
212. Bradley, W. E., 1980, Aspects of diabetic autonomic neuropathy, *Ann. Intern. Med.* **2**(Suppl., Part 2):289–342.

5

Aldosterone and Renin

Edward G. Biglieri

5.1. A Reexamination and Further Definition of Congenital Adrenal Hyperplasia through the Examination of Steroids in the Mineralocorticoid Hormone Pathways

To appreciate the origins of the steroids produced in the zona glomerulosa (ZG) and zona fasciculata (ZF), the reader is referred to Fig. 1. The unique steroids from the ZG are 18-hydroxycorticosterone (18OH-B) and aldosterone. The contribution of ZG corticosterone (B) and deoxycorticosterone (DOC) to peripheral blood levels must be minimal because current evidence suggests that they are primarily ACTH-dependent and of ZF origin. Only in the 17α-hydroxylase deficiency type of congenital adrenal hyperplasia (CAH) does 18OH-B originate from the ZF. Angiotensin II is the principal regulator of this zone, but acute or short-term administration of ACTH stimulates 18OH-B and aldosterone.

The ZF contains two major pathways: a glucocorticoid hormone pathway leading to the formation of 17-hydroxylated steroids, 17-hydroxyprogesterone (17OH-P), 11-deoxycortisol (S), and cortisol (F), and a mineralocorticoid hormone (MCH) pathway leading to the formation of the 17-deoxysteroids, DOC, 18-hydroxy-DOC (18OH-DOC), and B.

EDWARD G. BIGLIERI ● Endocrinology Service of the Medical Services, and Clinical Study Center, San Francisco General Hospital Medical Center, and Department of Medicine, University of California School of Medicine, San Francisco, California 94120.

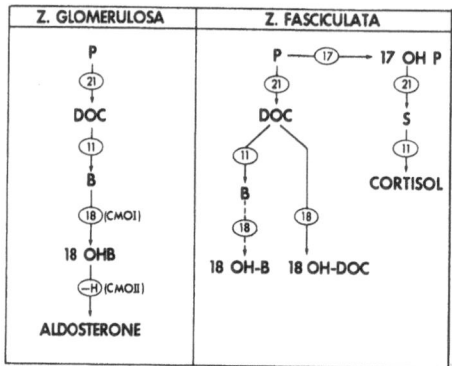

Fig. 1. The steroid pathways in the zona glomerulosa and fasciculata. P, progesterone; DOC, deoxycortico-sterone; B, corticosterone; 18 OH-B, 18-hydroxycorticosterone; 18OH-DOC, 18-hydroxydeoxycorticosterone; 17OH, 17-hydroxyprogesterone; S, 11-deoxycortisol. Circled numbers indicate hydroxylation steps. CMO, corticosterone methyl oxidase type I or II. −H, dehydrogenation.

The peripheral concentrations of DOC, B, 18OH-DOC, 17OH-P, S, and F are due primarily to ZF production and are regulated by ACTH. There is no evidence that angiotensin II or III stimulates ZF steroids.

5.1.1. 21-Hydroxylase Deficiency [Simple Virilizing (SV), Nonsalt-Losing, and Salt-Losing (SL) Types]

Aldosterone production has been documented to be increased in the SV form and decreased in the SL form. Recently, there has been additional documentation that plasma aldosterone concentrations are increased in the SV form.[1-4] Renin levels, usually measured as plasma renin activity (PRA), are elevated in this type regardless of whether or not salt loss is present, presumably due to the degree of hypovolemia, and is in part the reason for the elevated aldosterone levels observed. Several mechanisms for the elevated renin levels have been proposed. The elevated levels of ACTH stimulate the secretion of aldosterone antagonists, which act as inhibitors of the action of aldosterone in the renal tubule and neutralize its effect. These events activate homeostatic mechanisms. The renin–angiotensin system increases aldosterone production to establish a compensated state that does not lead to sodium wasting. Sodium wasting occurs only if this compensation is inadequate, i.e., sufficient increases of aldosterone are not possible.[5] This could in part explain the great range in values for plasma aldosterone concentration in the SL. In addition, angiotensin II may directly stimulate the ZF to increase ACTH-dependent aldosterone antagonists, increase the sensitivity of the ZF to ACTH, or increase ACTH levels. In fact, inadequate suppression of ACTH with glucocorticoid therapy may well be a consequence of an increased renin–angiotensin system.

The documentation of elevated aldosterone levels in 21-hydroxylase deficiency SV has suggested that the steroids produced in the ZG were essentially normal and 21-hydroxylation was not impaired.[1] However, further examination of the steroids in the MCH pathways introduced new insights into other events that were occurring in both the ZF and the ZG.

In the presence of low and fixed levels of F and increased levels of ACTH and 17OH-P, normal levels of B and 18OH-DOC and usually elevated levels of DOC are observed. Attention was directed to the MCH pathway (17-deoxy pathway in the ZF). Steroids distal to the 21 block, B and 18OH-DOC, were normal and failed to increase under ACTH stimulation. However, the elevated DOC levels although high showed a limited increase. Because DOC is the immediate precursor of B and 18OH-DOC, ZF DOC, by inference, should at least be normal and not elevated. Thus, this strongly suggests that the DOC measured was of ZG origin.[2]

The ZG at first appears to be operating normally. Aldosterone and 18OH-B levels are increased above normal ranges, presumably due to elevated renin levels. B secretion from the ZG is difficult to assess, but it must be minimal. It is further complicated by the fact that levels of B are normally much higher than all the other components of the MCH pathway of the ZG. The elevated level of DOC is presumably of ZG origin and must be primarily under ACTH control. DOC is not stimulated by angiotensin II nor in other disorders in which activation of the renin system occurs. A good example of normal DOC in the presence of high PRA occurs in the salt-losing disorder due to corticosterone methyl oxidase deficiency type II in which renin levels are extremely high with elevated levels of 18OH-B but decreased aldosterone production.

Aldosterone, DOC, and 18OH-B increase with acute ACTH infusions, but the increases are quantitatively small and the percentage increases are less than normal. This suggests that although basal values are increased, further increments are restricted and may represent limited 21-hydroxylation in the ZG. The continued administration of superphysiologic doses of ACTH achieves much greater levels of DOC than achieved with ACTH in the 21-hydroxylase deficiency SV. With similar treatment in normal subjects, aldosterone and 18OH-B return to control levels after initial increases (up to 30 hr). This "turn off" of aldosterone and 18OH-B requires normal adrenal steroid production. Several mechanisms have been suggested.[6] In rat experiments, suppression of PRA and angiotensin II receptors in the adrenal gland are offered as an explanation for the decrease.[7] In man the turn off occurs even without changes in renin (in patients with an aldosterone-producing adenoma) and, in addition, there is a reduction of initially elevated levels of 18OH-DOC and B (ZF steroids). Thus, reduced 11β- and 18-hydroxylating activity is not just confined to the ZG and a decrease in PRA and angiotensin II receptors. These studies are important because patients with 21-hydroxylase deficiency do not show the early turn off of aldosterone[3] and 18OH-B with continued ACTH treatment. The limited increases in aldosterone and DOC combined with blocked F production may prevent suppression of the elevated PRA and permit the maintenance of the elevated aldosterone and 18OH-B levels. DOC levels are maintained by increases in ACTH.

A single enzymatic defect in the ZG and ZF of the adrenal gland is supported by these observations. Although the numbers are limited in the SL form, plasma aldosterone, 18OH-B, and even DOC appear to be lower and are less responsive to ACTH. They also appear to have a greater degree of 21-hydroxylase deficiency by lower basal levels of B, 18OH-DOC, and F than in the SV form.

An intriguing observation has been made in 21-hydroxylase deficiency and suggests that a possible aldosterone biosynthetic defect may also be present in both SL and SV forms. This would imply that in the 21-hydroxylation defect the SL and SV forms differ only in degree and are not of different genotypes. The ratio of the urinary metabolite of 18OH-B to the tetrahydro metabolite of aldosterone was always elevated in SL and most SV. The levels of the ratios in the SL were similar to those observed in the corticosterone methyl oxidase type II defect.[8] These findings strongly suggest a limitation of aldosterone-secreting reserve in both forms of 21-hydroxylase deficiency regardless of the level of aldosterone.

In summary, the SV has elevations of steroids produced in the ZG: DOC, 18OH-B, and aldosterone. They are elevated by ACTH (DOC) and angiotensin II (18OH-B and aldosterone). Because of the production of ACTH-dependent aldosterone antagonists, renin is increased. There appears to be a limited capacity to increase 21-hydroxylation in the ZG normally. A biosynthetic defect in the conversion of 18OH-B to aldosterone may be present, thus limiting aldosterone secretory reserve. Activation of the renin system increases the glucocorticoid requirement for ACTH-suppressive therapy. The MCH pathway in the ZF (17-deoxysteroids) is also involved. B, 18OH-DOC, and ZF DOC are normal and not responsive to ACTH. A high 18OH-B level and normal or low 18OH-DOC level are characteristics of the SV.

5.1.2. 11β-Hydroxylase Deficiency

There is now *in vivo* evidence that the 11β-hydroxylase and 18-hydroxylase functions may well appear on the same enzyme protein or be the same enzyme.[6,9] In this disorder, elevated DOC and 11-deoxycortisol are associated with reduced and limited increases of 18OH-DOC, 18OH-B, and aldosterone production after administration of ACTH.[9] One may argue that the reduced 18OH-B and aldosterone production were due to an inhibition of ZG 11β-hydroxylation and/or suppression of PRA by DOC. That 18-hydroxylation was also involved in this reduction is suggested by the low levels of 18OH-DOC, which does not undergo 11-hydroxylation. A case for the suppression of possibly a normal ZG is presented by the observation (in four patients) that suppression of ACTH by dexamethasone followed by the challenge of sodium restriction results in a rise in PRA, 18OH-B, and aldosterone[10]; the ZG appears normal. 18OH-DOC remains low, because the defect in the ZF persists. Thus, this disorder might be considered to have normal 11β- and 18-hydroxylation in the ZG but deficient hydroxylation in the ZF. However, clinical experience has shown that caution must be exercised when treatment is initiated in this type of CAH because hypovolemic crises due to inadequate aldosterone production may occur and persist. As observed in the 21-hydroxylase deficiency type, there is most likely a spectrum of disorders with varying degrees of 11β- and 18-hydroxylase deficiency in both the ZF and the ZG.

5.1.3. 17α-Hydroxylase Deficiency

The zonal origins of the MCHs of this type of CAH are somewhat easier to define because 17α-hydroxylation is absent in the ZG but present in other zones. This is uniquely a disorder of the MCH pathway in the ZF (17-deoxysteroid pathway). DOC, B, 18OH-DOC, and 18OH-B are elevated, leading to renin suppression and subsequent reduction of ZG aldosterone to very low levels.[11] The discrepancy between the levels of aldosterone and 18OH-B is characteristic for this type of nonvirilizing hypertension with hypokalemia, suppressed PRA, and virtual absence of aldosterone. The mechanism of the production of 18OH-B from the ZF is almost unique for this disorder. It is most likely due to the large amounts of B produced in the substrate for 18OH-B.[8,12] The elevated 18OH-B is easily suppressed by dexamethasone, in contrast to the slight decrease seen in normal subjects in whom 18OH-B is of ZG origin. It responds to ACTH and has an ACTH-dependent circadian rhythm.[11-13] The ZG returns to normal when adequate suppression of ACTH by glucocorticoid hormone treatment is achieved.

5.2. The Hypokalemic and Hypertensive Syndromes with Suppressed Renin and Aldosterone Production

The index disorders with the hypertension associated with suppressed renin and aldosterone and hypokalemia are the 11β- and 17α-hydroxylase-deficient types of CAH and Liddle's syndrome (a renal tubular defect in sodium–potassium transport). Two recently described disorders have additional biochemical findings that identify unusual mechanisms for the clinical findings—defects in terminal steroid metabolism and glucocorticoid insensitivity.

5.2.1. Defect in Terminal (or Peripheral) Steroid Metabolism

This disorder was first described in 1977.[14] New cases have now been reported.[15,16] The defect in metabolism has been observed only in children. It is clinically recognizable by hypertension, hypokalemia, suppressed PRA and aldosterone levels, correction of biochemical abnormalities and elevated blood pressure by spironolactone, and a reduced tetrahydrocortisone/tetrahydrocortisol ratio.

The conversion of F to cortisone is the major route of inactivation and metabolism of F. 11β-Hydroxyoxidoreductase normally oxidizes at least half of the secreted F and the reverse, (reduction) cortisone to F, returns steroid to the F pool. The conversion of F to cortisone is impaired but the reverse is not in this disorder. Normally, the excretory ratios of cortisone to F and their metabolites are at least 2 : 1. In this disorder the ratio is extremely low at about one-tenth of the normal value.

The characteristic abnormality is a reduced production of tetrahydrocortisone, indicating reduced activity of the 11β-hydroxyoxidoreductase. There is also greatly increased excretion of free steroids containing the 3-keto[4] group, another marker of greatly reduced metabolism. 5α-Dihydrocortisol (a weak MCH) is increased, but its contribution to the apparent MCH excess must be limited because it disappears with time, whereas the defect persists. In one study, the hepatic and renal oxidoreductive activity was able to handle reduced steroid loads when F levels were reduced by dexamethasone, but the defect was magnified by ACTH-induced increases in F.[16] However, in other studies the defect persisted whether exogenous F or ACTH was given. These variations of the steroid loads to the 11β-hydroxysteroid oxidoreductase system need further documentation in more of these unusual patients.

Other abnormalities in F metabolism characterize this disorder. The F half-disappearance time is prolonged, resulting in reduced secretion and excretion with a normal blood level. At present, there is no direct evidence that the disturbance in F metabolism is involved with the MCH excess-like abnormality. The tetrahydrocortisone/tetrahydrocortisol ratio is the marker of this syndrome.

The existence of an unknown MCH, rather than a renal tubular defect as in Liddle's syndrome, is supported by clinical improvement with spironolactone. However, bioassay of urine extract for sodium-retaining activity has been inconsistent, and an MCH receptor assay showed normal activity. That an adrenal steroid is involved is further suggested by occasional improvement when treated with dexamethasone for short periods of time, clinical features aggravated by ACTH, and improvement with sodium restriction.

5.2.2. Glucocorticoid Insensitivity

In 1976, a patient was reported[17] who had hypertension, hypokalemia, and normal-to-low aldosterone production rates with normal-to-reduced PRA. However, plasma F levels were markedly elevated (>61.1 μg/dl) on three occasions. Corticosterone-binding globulin was normal, but free plasma F and its urinary metabolites were elevated. There were no clinical findings of Cushing's syndrome. To suppress the elevated F levels, 5 mg of dexamethasone per day was required and the patient has been maintained on 3 mg of dexamethasone to reduce F levels and correct the hypokalemia. This sustained large daily dose of dexamethasone effected no signs of glucocorticoid excess. A primary insensitivity to glucocorticoid is postulated without a major insensitivity to the MCH action of F. The insensitivity to glucocorticoids must be fairly generalized because the high levels of F do not suppress ACTH (which was elevated) sufficiently to reduce adrenal gland production to a normal level. F alone could explain the hypertension and hypokalemia by its sitll intact MCH action.

The ZG appeared to function normally as PRA and aldosterone secretion increased during sodium restriction and was suppressed with sodium loading. The question of whether other MCHs were present was not clear at that time. However, the elevated urinary excretion of the metabolites and of B, while consistent with patterns seen in Cushing's disease, could have suggested increased activity of the MCH pathway of the ZF. The investigators believed that tetrahydrodeoxycorticosterone levels were normal (without documentation). At the 33rd annual meeting of the Endocrine Society, restudy of the patient and son showed tissue insensitivity to F and, most important, elevation of both plasma B and DOC.[18] Thus, the increase of these two MCHs provides the mechanism for the hypertension and hypokalemia. The patterns are similar to the increased secretion of the steroids of the ZF MCH pathway in the 17α-hydroxylase deficiency. The normal values and dynamics of the renin–aldosterone system may in part be due to the inhibitory effects of ACTH on 11β- and 18-hydroxylation in the ZG. The normal renin values could also in part be due to the effect of F on renin substrate.

5.3. Primary Hyperaldosteronism

5.3.1. Primary Aldosteronism

Primary aldosteronism due to a unilateral adrenocortical adenoma (APA) can be precisely identified by measuring the precursor steroids of the MCH pathway of the ZG. The simultaneous measurements of these steroids (DOC, B, 18OH-DOC, aldosterone) at 0800 hr after overnight recumbency reveal that frequent elevations of plasma DOC and B and constant elevations of plasma 18OH-B concentrations occur only in patients with APA.[19] Plasma DOC, B, and 18OH-B are usually normal in hyperplastic disorders. Of greater importance is that the elevated 18OH-B levels (usually >85 ng/dl) in patients with APA show no overlap with, at times, the slightly increased levels seen in idiopathic hyperaldosteronism (hyperplasia).[19] At lower serum potassium concentrations (2.0 mEQ/liter), the 18OH-B/aldosterone ratio increases. This suggests that potassium may retard conversion of 18OH-B to aldosterone, the last step of aldosterone synthesis, or that some 18OH-B is of ZF origin and not influenced by potassium depletion as is aldosterone production in the ZG. 18OH-B declines like aldosterone with upright posture, which provides additional evidence that both originate in the ZG. 18OH-B may prove to be a more useful marker of an APA because it is less potassium dependent.

The anomalous fall or lack of change of the 0800 hr overnight recumbent plasma aldosterone level after 2 hr in the upright posture in over 90% of the patients continues to be an almost constant characteristic of patients with an APA. In fact, when rises do occur, they are always less than the total percentage increase seen in normal subjects.[20] Success with this maneuver varies with different laboratories[21,22]; patient preparation is crucial. Equilibration or fixing salt intake for 3–4 days is required as well as recumbency for at least 6–8 hr before the 0800 hr sample is obtained. F or preferably steroids such as B and 18OH-DOC should be measured at the same time, e.g., at 0800 and 1000 hr. These steroids respond more vigorously to ACTH and provide a more sensitive marker than F for an ACTH discharge that might occur during the test period, which invalidates the postural maneuver. Greater accuracy can be achieved by suppressing what little renin is produced by high salt intake or fluorocortisone before the postural response is examined.[23]

A secure biochemical diagnosis is followed by computed axial tomography for lateralization or identification of hyperplastic glands. This procedure has added a new dimension to adrenal gland visualization. Its accuracy in locating an adenoma is greater than 80%.[24]

5.3.2. Idiopathic Hyperaldosteronism (IHA, Adrenal Hyperplasia)

As keenness in identifying patients with an APA increases, the diagnosis of IHA is made more frequently. Patients with this type of hyperaldosteronism also show greater variation in their responses to factors that control aldosterone production and most likely represent a heterogeneous group. The well-documented increased sensitivity of plasma aldosterone concentration to graded infusions of angiotensin II and ACTH reveals a unique response in both patients with IHA and low-renin essential hypertension.[25,26] This presumably persistent abnormality may in part be responsible for the inappropriate secretion of aldosterone relative to the renin levels in these two low-renin states. Such sensitivity may also be operating in response to other extraadrenal factors (e.g., prostaglandins, kallikreins, catecholamines, potassium). Perhaps blood pressure *per se* and adrenal function may be more closely interdependent than can currently be demonstrated even though adrenalectomy rarely cures the hypertension in patients with IHA. Secretory products of the adrenergic nervous system, norepinephrine, epinephrine, and isoproterenol, can increase both blood pressure and aldosterone production but through the stimulation of renin. It is of great interest that dopamine receptors exist in the adrenal gland. Can abnormalities of secretion by the dopaminergic system and its inhibitors manipulate adrenocortical biosynthetic pathways to cause hyperplasia and hyperaldosteronism? Acute increases in plasma aldosterone concentration by a dopamine inhibitor (metoclopramide) have been observed in normal subjects.[27] However, the chronic administration of this inhibitor does not sustain the hypersecretion of aldosterone.[28] In patients with an APA, the levels of dopamine may influence the plasma aldosterone concentration: diminishing the dopamine levels results in episodic surges of plasma aldosterone concentration and increasing dopamine levels augments its reduction produced by ACTH suppression.[29] Transient interruption of a serotonin transmitter pathway in the CNS leads to the interesting decrease in plasma aldosterone concentration in patients with IHA but not APA.

Secretagogues of CNS origin warrant close attention because they may play an active role in adrenal hyperplasia and hypertension. Newly observed, presumably pituitary, regulators appear to be specific aldosterone stimulators *in vitro*. These secretagogues are melanocyte-stimulating hormone,[30] β-lipotropin,[31] and the N-terminal 16K peptide of pro-opiomelanotropin.[32] An aldosterone stimulatory hormone, isolated from human urine, of pituitary origin has been identified.[33] A link with IHA has not been established.

Although these observations are novel and important, is the chronic excessive secretion of aldosterone the major factor in the elevated blood pressure in IHA? Adrenalectomy rarely cures the hypertension in patients with IHA. The role of aldosterone in the IHA syndrome may not be as critical for elevated blood pressure by the time patients present with the abnormality. The interdependence between adrenal function and blood pressure is not clearly established in this disorder. Perhaps IHA is merely a variant of essential hypertension—part of a broad spectrum of a disorder with varying hormonal contributions.[34]

5.3.3. Glucocorticoid-Remediable Hyperaldosteronism (GRHA)

This rare autosomal dominant form of MCH hypertension continues to be a most unusual form of adrenal hyperplasia. The hypertension, hypokalemia, and suppressed renin with hyperaldosteronism are all corrected by the administration of ACTH-suppressive doses of glucocorticoid hormones. It also is a type of adrenal hyperplasia in which adrenal overactivity and hypertension are intimately linked. That aldosterone alone is the effector of hypertension is not unequivocally established.[35] Aldosterone levels in this disorder are clearly ACTH dependent.[35,36] Aminoglutethemide reduces aldosterone levels and corrects hypertension. However, administration of aldosterone or DOC alone to these patients does not increase blood pressure, but administration of ACTH does increase it. These observations have led to speculation that an additional ACTH-dependent MCH may be a factor in the clinical manifestations of MCH excess. Increases in both 18OH-DOC and DOC production have been seen in some of these patients. In one patient, the elevated radioreceptor assay of plasma MCH activity could not be explained entirely by the levels of F, aldosterone, or DOC as is usually the case. This additional unexplained activity appeared to be ACTH dependent.[37] Thus, the possibility of another ACTH-dependent MCH still remains a possibility. With continued treatment with glucocorticoid hormones, the reduced levels of aldosterone rise in response to the renin increase effected by sodium restriction. The ZG functions normally when ACTH is suppressed.[35,38]

The confirmation, from two laboratories, that the continued administration of excessive amounts of ACTH for 5–7 days fails to turn off aldosterone production appears characteristic of this disorder.[35,36] This failure of continued ACTH administration to restore the initial elevations of aldosterone levels to normal is an unusual occurrence and is seen only in patients with CAH with limited F production. F and DOC production showed normal and sustained increases with ACTH. The suppressed renin system, normal urinary levels of 18OH-DOC and plasma corticosterone concentration, and usually normal plasma DOC levels

suggest that ACTH has a unique effect only on the ZG steroids.[38] 11β-
and 18-hydroxylation appear normal in the ZF, but the expected inhibition of these hydroxylations does not occur with ACTH in the ZF. The
mechanism for the sustained elevations of aldosterone production with
ACTH is not known.

References

1. Kuhnle, U., Chow, D., Rapaport, R., Pang, S., Levine, L. S., and New, M.
   I., 1981, The 21-hydroxylase activity in the glomerulosa and fasciculata of
   the adrenal cortex in congenital adrenal hyperplasia, *J. Clin. Endocrinol.
   Metab.* **52:**534–544.
2. Biglieri, E. G., Wajchenberg, B. L., Malerbi, D. A., Okada, H., Lemme, C.
   E., and Kater, C. E., 1981, The zonal origins of the mineralocorticoid hormones in the 21-hydroxylation, deficiency of congenital adrenal hyperplasia,
   J. Clin. Endocrinol. Metab. **53:**964–969.
3. Beitins, I. Z., Bayard, F., Kowarski, A., and Migeon, C. J., 1972, The effect
   of ACTH administration on aldosterone production in nonsalt-losing congenital adrenal hyperplasia, *J. Clin. Endocrinol. Metab.* **35:**595–603.
4. Horner, J. M., Hintz, R. L., and Luetscher, J. A., 1979, The role of renin
   and angiotensin in salt-losing, 21-hydroxylase deficient congenital adrenal
   hyperplasia, *J. Clin. Endocrinol. Metab.* **48:**776–783.
5. Lemal, J. M., Rapaport, R., and Bayard, F., 1976, Plasma aldosterone, renin
   activity, and 17α-hydroxyprogesterone in salt-losing congenital adrenal hyperplasia. I. Response to ACTH on hydrocortisone treated patients and
   effect of 9α-fluorocortisol, *J. Clin. Endocrinol. Metab.* **45:**551–559.
6. Biglieri, E. G., Chang, B., Hirai, J., Brust, N., Rost, C. R., and Schambelan,
   M., 1979, Adrenocorticotropin inhibition of mineralocorticoid hormone
   production, *Clin. Sci.* **56:**307–311.
7. Aquilera, G., Fujita, K., and Catt, K. J., 1981, Mechanisms of inhibition of
   aldosterone secretion by adrenocorticotropin, *Endocrinology* **108:**522–526.
8. Ulick, S., Eberlein, W. R., Bliffeld, A. R., Chu, M. D., and Bongioanini, A.
   F., 1980, Evidence for an aldosterone biosynthetic defect in congenital adrenal hyperplasia, *J. Clin. Endocrinol. Metab.* **51:**1346–1353.
9. Sonino, N., Levine, L. S., Vecsei, P., and New, M. I., 1980, Parallelism of
   11β and 18-hydroxylation demonstrated in urinary free hormones in man,
   J. Clin. Endocrinol. Metab. **51:**557–560.
10. Levine, L. S., Rauh, W., Gottesdiener, K., Chow, D., Gunczler, P., Rapaport,
    R., Pang, S., Schneider, B., and New, M.I., 1980, New studies of the 11β-
    hydroxylase and 18-hydroxylase enzymes in the hypertensive form of con-
    genital adrenal hyperplasia, *J. Clin. Endocrinol. Metab.* **50:**258–265.
11. Biglieri, E. G., 1979, Mechanisms establishing the mineralocorticoid hor-
    mone patterns in the 17α-hydroxylase deficiency syndrome, *J. Steroid Biochem.*
    11:653–658.
12. Kater, C. E., Biglieri, E. G., and Brust, N., 1981, An explanation for the

sequential variation leading to the unique zona fasciculata mineralocorticoid levels in the 17α-hydroxylase deficiency, Program of Endocrinology of Hypertension Symposium, Serano, Italy, P. 34.

13. Ulick, S., 1976, Adrenocortical factors in hypertension. I. Significance of 18-hydroxy-11-deoxycorticosterone, *Am. J. Cardiol.* **38**:814–824.

14. New, M. I., Levine, L. S., Biglieri, E. G., Pareira, J., and Ulick, S., 1977, Evidence for an unidentified steroid in a child with an apparent mineralocorticoid hypertension, *J. Clin. Endocrinol. Metab.* **44**:924–933.

15. Ulick, S., Levine, L. S., Gunczler, P., Zanconato, G., Ramirez, L. C., Rauh, W., Rosler, A., Bradow, H. L., and New, M. I., 1979, A syndrome of apparent mineralocorticoid excess associated with defects in the peripheral metabolism of cortisol, *J. Clin. Endocrinol. Metab.* **49**:757–764.

16. Shackleton, C. H. L., Honour, J. W., Dillon, M. J., Chansler, C., and Jones, R. W. A., 1980, Hypertension in a four year old child: Gas chromatographic and mass spectrometric evidence for deficient hepatic metabolism of steroids, *J. Clin. Endocrinol. Metab.* **50**:786–792.

17. Vingerhoeds, A. C. M., Thijssen, J. H. H., and Schwartz, F., 1976, Spontaneous, hypercortisolism without Cushing's syndrome, *J. Clin. Endocrinol. Metab.* **43**:1128–1133.

18. Chrousos, C. P., Vingerhoeds, A., Brandon, D., de Regt, J., Pugeat, M., Eli, C., Loriaux, D. L., and Lipsett, M. B., 1981, Primary cortisol resistance: A glucocorticoid receptor-mediated disease, 33rd Annual Meeting of the Endocrine Society, p. 276.

19. Biglieri, E. G., and Schambelan, M., 1979, Significance of elevated levels of plasma hydroxycorticosterone in patients with primary aldosteronism, *J. Clin. Endocrinol. Metab.* **49**:87–91.

20. Biglieri, E. G., and Baxter, J. D., 1981, The endocrinology of hypertension, in: *Endocrinology and Metabolism* (B. Felig, J. D. Baxter, A. Broadus, and L. Frohman, eds.), p. 551.

21. Vetter, H., Siebenschein, R., Stude, A., Witassek, F., Furrer, J., Glanzer, L., Siegenthaler, W., and Vetter, W., 1979, Primary aldosteronism: Inability to differentiate unilateral from bilateral adrenal type lesions by various routine clinical and laboratory data and by peripheral plasma aldosterone, *Acta Endocrinol. (Copenhagen)* **89**:710–725.

22. Weinberger, N. H., Grim, C. E., Hollifield, J. M., Kem, D. C., Ganguly, A., Kramer, N. J., Yume, N. H., Wellman, H., and Donohue, J. P., 1979, Primary aldosteronism: Diagnosis, localization and treatment, *Ann. Intern. Med.* **90**:386–395.

23. Vaughan, N. J. A., Slater, J. D. H., Lightman, S., Jowett, T. P., Wiggins, R. C., Ma, J. T. C., and Payne, N. N., 1981, The diagnosis of primary hyperaldosteronism, *Lancet* **1**:120–125.

24. White, E. A., Schambelan, M., Sigala, J. F., Glynn, R. D., and Biglieri, E. G., 1980, Use of computed tomography in diagnosing the cause of primary aldosteronism, *N. Engl. J. Med.* **303**:1503–1507.

25. Wisgerhoff, M., Carpenter, P. C., and Brown, R. D., 1978, Increased adrenal sensitivity to angiotensin II in idiopathic hyperaldosteronism, *J. Clin. Endocrinol. Metab.* **47**:938–943.

26. Kem, D. C., Weinberger, M. H., Higgins, J. R., Kramer, N. J., Gomez-Sanchez, C., and Holland, O. B., 1978, Plasma aldosterone response to ACTH in primary aldosteronism and patients with low renin hypertension, *J. Clin. Endocrinol. Metab.* **46:**552–560.

27. Carey, R. M., Thorner, M. O., and Ortt, E. M., 1980, Dopaminergic inhibition of metoclopramide-induced aldosterone secretion in man, *J. Clin. Invest.* **66:**10–18.

28. Noth, R. H., McCallum, R. W., Contino, C., and Havelick, J., 1980, Tonic dopaminergic suppression of plasma aldosterone, *J. Clin. Endocrinol. Metab.* **51:**64–69.

29. Kuchel, O., Buu, N. T., Vescei, P., Bourque, M., Hamet, P., and Genest, J., 1980, Are plasma aldosterone surges in primary aldosteronism due to a loss of an inhibiting dopaminergic control?, *J. Clin. Endocrinol. Metab.* **51:**337–343.

30. Vinson, G. P., Whitehouse, B. J., Dell, A., Etienne, T., and Morris, H. R., 1980, Characterization of an adrenal zona glomerulosa-stimulating component of posterior pituitary extracts as α-MSH, *Nature (London)* **284:**464–467.

31. Matsuoka, H., Mulrow, P.J., and Li, C. H., 1980, Beta-lipotropin: A new aldosterone-stimulating factor, *Science* **209:**307–308.

32. Lis, M., Hamet, P., Gutkowska, J., Maurice, G., Seidah, N. G., Larivere, N., Chretien, M., and Genest, J. 1981, Pro-opiomelanocortin in aldosterone release by human adrenal adenoma in vitro, *J. Clin. Endocrinol. Metab.* **52:**1053–1056.

33. Sen, S., Valenzuela, R., Smeby, R., Bravo, E., and Bumpus, F. M., 1981, Localization, purification and biological activity of a new aldosterone stimulating factor, *Hypertension* **3**(Suppl. I):I-81–I-89.

34. Brown, J. J., Lever, A. F., Robertson, J. I. S., Beeveb, D. G., Cumming, A. M., Davies, D. L., Fraser, R., Mason, P., Morton, J. S., Tree, M., 1979, Are idiopathic hyperaldosteronism and low-renin hypertension variants of essential hypertension?, *Ann. Clin. Biochem.* **16:**380–388.

35. Gill, J. R., Jr., and Bartter, F. C., 1981, Overproduction of sodium retaining steroids by the zona glomerulosa is adrenocorticotropin-dependent and mediates hypertension in dexamethasone-suppressible aldosteronism, *J. Clin. Endocrinol. Metab.* **53:**335–337.

36. Rauh, W., Levine, L. S., Gottesdiener, K., and New, M. I., 1978, Mineralocorticoids, salt balance and blood pressure after prolonged ACTH administration in juvenile hypertension, *Klin. Wochenschr.* **56**(Suppl. I):161–167.

37. Lau, N. C., Matulich, D. T., Stockigt, J. R., Biglieri, E. G., New, M. I., Wenter, J. S. D., McKenzie, J. K., and Baxter, J. D., 1980, Radioreceptor assay of plasma mineralocorticoid activity: Role of aldosterone, cortisol, deoxycorticosterone in various mineralocorticoid excess states, *Circ. Res.* **46**(Suppl. I):I-94–I-100.

38. Oberfield, S. E., Levine, L. S., Stoner, E., Chow, D., Rauh, W., Greig, F., Lee, S. M., Lightner, E., Witte, M., New, M. I., 1981, Adrenal glomerulosa function in patients with dexamethasone-suppressible hyperaldosteronism, *J. Clin. Endocrinol. Metab.* **53:**158–164.

6

Sympathoadrenal System

L. Landsberg and J. B. Young

6.1. Introduction

Previous chapters in this series (*The Year in Endocrinology 1975-76, The Year in Endocrinology 1977,* and *Contemporary Endocrinology,* Volume 1) have considered in depth a variety of topics related to the sympathoadrenal system. Among the topics explored have been the assessment of sympathetic nervous system activity, familial pheochromocytoma, catecholamines and essential hypertension, the sympathoadrenal system and the regulation of hormone secretion, and the role of the sympathoadrenal system in the regulation of metabolism. In recent years, increasing interest has developed in the sympathetic nervous system regulation of thermogenesis, and some of the current literature will be reviewed here. The sympathetic response to acute and chronic cold exposure provides an excellent example of the manner in which sympathetic regulation of metabolism, the vasculature, and hormone secretion may be integrated into a comprehensive physiological response. In addition, the potential role of the sympathetic nervous system in the regulation of dietary thermogenesis will be reviewed, along with implications for obesity, therapeutic dieting, and weight loss. The final section will briefly review some of the recent literature dealing with the diagnosis and localization of pheochromocytoma.

L. LANDSBERG AND J. B. YOUNG • Departments of Medicine, Beth Israel Hospital, Charles A. Dana Research Institute, and Thorndike Laboratories, Harvard Medical School, Boston, Massachusetts 02115.

6.2. Sympathetic Responses during Cold Exposure: Regulation of Nonshivering Thermogenesis

6.2.1. Role of the Sympathetic Nervous System in Temperature Maintenance during Cold Exposure

Experiments from the laboratory of L. D. Carlson over 25 years ago clearly demonstrated the important role of the sympathetic nervous system in the mammalian defense against exposure to a cold environment.[1] In these studies it was conclusively demonstrated that cold-acclimated curarized rats failed to increase oxygen consumption and to maintain body temperature when treated with ganglionic blocking agents. In contradistinction to ganglionic blockade, parasympathetic blockade with atropine did not impair the cold response. The administration of norepinephrine (NE), however, along with ganglionic blocking agents, restored oxygen consumption and temperature maintenance to normal. Epinephrine (E) was much less effective than NE in this regard. These results implied that the sympathetic nervous system plays a major role in the mammalian defense of body temperature during cold exposure. The various components of the sympathetic response, as they relate to maintenance of body temperature, as well as the biochemical and physiological mechanisms involved, have been studied in detail over the last 25 years; much has been learned about the role of the sympathetic nervous system in the mammalian defense against cold exposure and in the regulation of thermogenesis.

6.2.2. Sympathetic Activation in the Cold

Both acute and chronic cold exposure are associated with marked stimulation of the sympathetic nervous system. Sympathetic stimulation has been convincingly demonstrated in a variety of mammalian species, including man, by many diverse techniques, including assessment of urinary NE excretion[2] and plasma NE levels,[3,4] as well as by measurements of NE turnover rate in sympathetically innervated organs,[5-10] and direct recording of sympathetic nervous activity from implanted microelectrodes in cutaneous nerves.[11,12] In chronic cold exposure, the degree of sympathetic stimulation tends to diminish slowly, although evidence of increased activity persists for long periods of time.[2] The increase in sympathetic nervous system activity, moreover, appears to be discriminating rather than generalized. Studies of NE turnover and biosynthesis suggest increased sympathetic activity in heart, spleen, and skeletal muscles, with negligible increases in salivary gland, liver, intestine, and kidney.[5,6,9,13] Nerve recordings from implanted microelectrodes, similarly, demonstrate increased sympathetic activity in cutaneous sympathetic efferents, with diminished impulse traffic in visceral splanchnic nerves.[12]

6.2.2.1. Adrenal Medulla

Many studies demonstrate activation of the adrenal medulla as well as the sympathetic nervous system during cold exposure.[2,4,14] The increase in adrenal medullary secretion, however, is less marked than the stimulation of the sympathetic nervous system, and of brief duration despite the sustained increase in sympathetic nervous system activity.[2] In some studies[15,16] adrenal medullary stimulation has not been demonstrated during cold exposure. The adrenal medullary response to cold exposure, therefore, is less pronounced and less reproducible than activation of the sympathetic nervous system is. Stimulation of the adrenal medulla is most marked when cold exposure is very severe, in warm-adapted as compared with cold-adapted animals, and in situations in which the function of the sympathetic nervous system is impaired.[15]

6.2.2.2. Central Regulation

Temperature is sensed by specialized neurons in the skin, spinal cord, and hypothalamus.[17,18] Afferent information related to temperature regulation is integrated in the anterior hypothalamus and preoptic area; the posterior hypothalamus contains the efferent centers that regulate the increase in sympathetic outflow during cold exposure. Many different neurotransmitters appear to be involved in the central regulation of thermoregulatory responses, including acetylcholine, the biogenic amines, prostaglandins, amino acids, and a variety of neuropeptides[19,20]; the role played by the various transmitters is not yet established.

6.2.3. Components of the Sympathetic Response

Sympathetic stimulation contributes to the mammalian defense against cold in several different important ways. First and foremost, sympathetic stimulation increases the metabolic rate, with resultant increase in oxygen consumption and heat production. Second, the sympathetic nervous system regulates changes in cardiac output and in the distribution of blood flow so that metabolizing tissues receive an adequate supply of oxygen and substrate. Third, the sympathetic nervous system and the adrenal medulla are importantly involved in the mobilization of substrate from fuel depots to provide an energy source for the increase in metabolic rate. In addition, the sympathetic nervous system is involved in heat conservation. Changes in blood flow distribution and pilo-erection, both mediated by the sympathetic nervous system, limit dissipation of body heat by increasing insulation. And finally, the sympathetic nervous system is intimately involved in the process of cold acclimation, whereby the production of metabolic heat in response to cold exposure is markedly increased in animals chronically exposed to a cold environment.

Stimulation of metabolic rate or thermogenesis by the sympathetic nervous system is referred to as nonshivering thermogenesis; it is distinct from shivering thermogenesis, in which heat production is consequent to muscle contraction. Shivering thermogenesis is under the control of the somatic motor system, although it is probable that the sympathetic nervous system facilitates shivering thermogenesis,[21–23] at least by the maintenance of adequate blood flow to shivering muscle and by provision of substrate as an energy source.

6.2.4. Nonshivering Thermogenesis

6.2.4.1. "Adaptive" or "Regulatory" Thermogenesis

Mammalian thermogenesis has both an obligatory and a facultative component. Obligatory thermogenesis, which encompasses the basal metabolic rate, is derived from the chemical friction inherent in the metabolic processes required to maintain homeostasis under basal conditions. Facultative thermogenesis, on the other hand, depends upon heat production secondary to those physiological and biochemical processes that are necessary for maintenance of the organism at a functional level above basal requirements.[24] A portion of facultative thermogenesis is "regulatory" or "adaptive" in that it subserves a homeostatic need for heat production. The capability of regulating heat production is an important characteristic of mammalian homeotherms and contributes a critical component in the maintenance of the internal milieu. Although heat production may be a by-product of a variety of physiological and biochemical processes, the term adaptive thermogenesis is reserved for those processes in which production of heat is the primary goal. Adaptive thermogenesis, therefore, encompasses those processes in which heat production may be specifically increased in fulfillment of a homeostatic need. Increased heat production in response to cold exposure (nonshivering thermogenesis) is the best studied example of adaptive thermogenesis in mammals.

6.2.4.2. Thermogenic Effects of Catecholamines

Although the suggestion that changes in heat production might result from alterations in metabolic rate has been attributed to German physiologists, particularly Rubner, at the end of the 19th century, it was W. B. Cannon, in 1926, who first proposed that catecholamines of adrenal medullary origin stimulate "chemical" thermogenesis by mechanisms independent of shivering. Subsequent studies clearly demonstrated that catecholamines increased metabolic rate when shivering was inhibited[25,26] and identified NE as a more potent thermogenic hormone than E. It is now generally recognized that the sympathetic nervous system regulates nonshivering thermogenesis and that NE is the principal thermogenic mediator. In small mammals the effects of both cold exposure[23] and NE on heat production are mediated by the β-adrenergic receptor[27–29] since they are elicited by β-adrenergic agonists and blocked by β-adrenergic antagonists.

6.2.4.2a. Cold Acclimation. Chronic exposure to a cold environment enhances the thermogenic response to a subsequent cold exposure in a variety of laboratory animals, a phenomenon known as cold acclimation. Cold-acclimated animals also demonstrate a marked increase in thermogenesis in response to catecholamines.[25,26] Enhancement of the thermogenic effects of catecholamines appears, therefore, to contribute importantly to the cold-acclimation process.[30] An even more intimate association of the sympathetic nervous system with cold acclimation is suggested by the fact that chronic daily infusions of NE, in the warm-acclimated rat, are associated with an enhanced thermogenic response to NE.[31] The chronic administration of NE, therefore, appears to reproduce some of the elements of the cold-acclimated state; NE administration by itself, however, does not mimic all the features of cold acclimation.[31]

6.2.4.2b. Nonshivering Thermogenesis and Cold Acclimation in Man. Although formerly a point of some controversy, it has been clearly established that larger mammals, including man, demonstrate both nonshivering thermogenesis and cold acclimation. A brief period of cold exposure during curarization has been shown to increase metabolic rate in noncold-acclimated man, an increase associated with a rise in plasma NE level.[16] NE infusions in noncold-acclimated humans have also been shown to increase oxygen consumption.[32] Evidence of cold acclimation has been produced in man as well.[33–36] As in rodents, cold acclimation in man is associated with enhancement of the thermogenic effects of NE, although the magnitude of the enhancement is considerably less than in rodents.[37]

6.2.4.3. Role of Brown Adipose Tissue In Nonshivering Thermogenesis

How does sympathetic stimulation result in increased heat production? A small amount of the total metabolic heat produced during cold exposure undoubtedly arises as a result of sympathetic stimulation of the cardiovascular system and of the metabolic pathways that result in substrate mobilization, as described below. Participation of the splanchnic viscera in nonshivering thermogenesis seems unlikely as judged from measurements of oxygen consumption[16,38] and from studies in the rat indicating reasonable preservation of the thermogenic response to cold exposure and to NE infusions following functional evisceration of the liver and the gut.[39–41] Skeletal muscle, by virtue of its large mass, has been considered a potentially important site of nonshivering thermogenesis, and some evidence has appeared consistent with participation of skeletal muscle in increased heat production during cold exposure and cold acclimation.[42–48] The available evidence, however, does not support a major role for skeletal muscle in nonshivering thermogenesis.[42,49]

Nonshivering thermogenesis has been best studied in the rat. In this species it is reasonably clear that brown adipose tissue (BAT) is the major site of metabolic heat production in response to cold exposure.[49]

6.2.4.3a. BAT. BAT, unlike white adipose tissue, is not involved primarily in fuel storage; it is an organ highly specialized for the production of metabolic heat. The importance of BAT in temperature regulation in neonates of many mammalian species, in arousal from hibernation, and in temperature regulation in cold-acclimated rodents is well recognized.[50] In these situations the importance of BAT as a heat-producing organ is clearly established. The role of BAT in the regulation of thermogenesis in adult, warm-acclimated mammals, particularly larger species including man, has, in contrast, not been established. The possibility that BAT plays a significant role in thermogenesis in these other situations has, however, stirred considerable interest.

BAT is localized in the interscapular and paraspinal regions and within the thoracic and abdominal cavities. Because of its anatomical location, interscapular BAT has been studied most extensively. Although BAT accounts for only a small percent of the total body weight of the rat, evidence has been produced indicating that over 60% of NE-induced thermogenesis in cold-acclimated rats may be attributed to BAT.[49] The heat-producing capacity of BAT is regulated by the sympathetic nervous system in all species studied.

6.2.4.3b. Sympathetic Regulation of BAT. BAT receives a dense sympathetic innervation.[50–52] During cold acclimation the density of sympathetic innervation increases,[51] as does the NE content of BAT.[52] Electrical stimulation of the nerves supplying BAT increases heat production within the BAT *in situ.*[50,53] Both acute and chronic cold exposure markedly increase sympathetic activity in interscapular BAT *in vivo.*[52,54] BAT denervation, on the other hand, adversely affects BAT metabolism,[53,55] and chemical sympathectomy has been shown to diminish nonshivering thermogenesis.[56]

NE locally released from sympathetic nerve endings increases the metabolic rate within BAT and markedly increases BAT blood flow. The increase in metabolic rate results in local warming of the tissue and export of heat to other regions of the body, both by a local effect on contiguous structures, and by increasing the temperature of the blood perfusing BAT, which is then distributed to other organs.[50] The concentration of NE required to induce these changes within BAT markedly exceeds the circulating level of NE under most circumstances, thereby providing further evidence for the primary role of the sympathetic nervous system, as compared with circulating catecholamines from the adrenal medulla, in the regulation of thermogenesis.[57]

6.2.4.3c. Effect of NE on BAT Blood Flow, Metabolism, and Hypertrophy. Both cold exposure and NE infusion markedly increase BAT blood flow. Foster and Frydman have shown that NE administration results in an approximately 16-fold increase in interscapular BAT blood flow in warm-acclimated rats and in a 25-fold increase in cold-acclimated rats.[49] The mechanisms involved in this prodigious increase in blood flow have not been established.

The metabolic response to NE in the brown adipocyte begins with depolarization of the cell membrane. Although both α- and β-adrenergic receptor agonists cause depolarization,[58] the subsequent thermogenic response to NE depends, at physiologic concentrations, on stimulation of the β receptor of the β_1 subtype.[59] Propranolol completely blocks NE-stimulated oxygen consumption in isolated brown adipocytes.[59]

The development of the thermogenic response within the brown adipocyte is complex, and the mechanisms involved are controversial. Evidence in support of two distinct mechanisms has been produced. One involves NE-stimulated changes in membrane permeability, with resultant increase in sodium influx and potassium efflux from the brown adipocyte.[54] The subsequent change in intracellular ionic concentration obligates increased ion pumping by the Na^+-K^+ ATPase system in order to maintain ionic equilibrium. The increased ion pumping utilizes ATP and, according to this model, the thermogenic response is secondary to the hydrolysis of ATP,[54,60] and to mitochondrial substrate oxidation that results from the increase in intracellular ADP. In support of such a mechanism, catecholamines have been shown to increase Na^+-K^+ ATPase activity in brown adipocytes.[54] Another possible mechanism involves uncoupling of mitochondrial respiration. BAT mitochondria may be uncoupled by the activation of a specific proton conductance pathway[61] stimulated by NE. Uncoupling would increase oxygen consumption within the cell by dissociating substrate oxidation and ATP generation, so that the major portion of the energy released during oxidation is dissipated as heat. NE-stimulated lipolysis, mediated via the adenylate cyclase–cAMP system, provides free fatty acids as an internal substrate for oxidation within the brown adipocyte.[60,62,63]

NE may also contribute to the hypertrophy of BAT that occurs during cold acclimation. Chronic administration of NE or isoproterenol induces hypertrophy of BAT in the rat,[29,61,64] although factors other than NE may be involved in cold-induced BAT hypertrophy.[65]

6.2.5. Substrate Mobilization

The energy requirements for both shivering and nonshivering thermogenesis are met by dissolution of fuel reserves in white adipose tissue, liver, and skeletal muscle.[66] Under the influence of catecholamines, free fatty acids, glucose, ketone bodies, and lactate are released into the circulation and transported to metabolizing tissues. The sympathetic nervous system appears to have the major role in the regulation of lipolysis within white adipose tissue, while the adrenal medulla may be more important in the enhancement of hepatic glucose output.[67,68]

6.2.5.1. Lipid Metabolism

Fat is the major substrate utilized during cold exposure. The respiratory quotient falls during both cold exposure[69] and NE infusion,[70] indicating increased utilization of fat as substrate. Free fatty acid turnover is increased by NE infusions to a greater extent in cold-acclimated than in warm-acclimated animals.[70] NE also increases ketone body turnover in cold-acclimated rats,[71] an effect that reflects increased free fatty acid delivery to the liver. Plasma triglyceride levels are reduced during chronic and acute cold exposure in the rat, along with a fall in the very-low-density lipoprotein fraction,[66,72] changes that reflect increased lipid utilization. During cold exposure, both body composition studies and carcass analysis in experimental animals and man indicate that cold exposure diminishes body fat even if feeding is maintained *ad lib*.[73–75] A significant portion of the caloric deficit induced by cold exposure is, therefore, derived from fat stores. As cold exposure progresses, increased caloric intake makes up a major portion of the energy deficit induced by increased thermogenesis, although the carcass analysis and body composition studies cited above imply that mobilization of fat stores continues to play an important role in substrate supply throughout the period of cold exposure.

The sympathetic nervous system is generally considered to play the critical role in the regulation of lipolysis within white adipose tissue[76] during cold exposure,[68] despite the fact that the adrenergic innervation is sparse in comparison with that of BAT. NE activates hormone-sensitive lipase within white fat by a mechanism that involves the β_1 adrenergic receptor and the adenylate cyclase–cAMP system. Ganglionic blockade or chemical sympathectomy both diminish the rise in free fatty acids that occurs during acute cold exposure in the rat, while adrenal demedullation is without effect on either plasma free fatty acid level or the activity of hormone-sensitive lipase,[77] findings consistent with a crucial role for the sympathetic nervous system.

6.2.5.2. Carbohydrate Metabolism

Although quantitatively less important than mobilization of free fatty acids from adipose tissue, increased hepatic glucose output, as determined by glucose turnover studies,[69] occurs during cold exposure and is enhanced in cold-acclimated rats.[69] Hepatic glycogen stores are known to decrease during cold exposure,[69] and if mobilization of free fatty acids from adipose tissue is impaired, metabolism of carbohydrates may compensate for this deficiency.[66]

Although the liver receives a parenchymal sympathetic innervation, sympathetic activity in the liver is only marginally increased during cold exposure.[5] Noncold-acclimated rats develop a substantial increase in plasma glucose level when exposed to cold[67]; following adrenal demedullation, however, the plasma glucose level fails to rise. The adrenal medulla, therefore, may play a significant role in stimulating hepatic glucose output,[21] especially in warm-acclimated animals.

6.2.5.3. Role of Insulin and Effects on Lipoprotein Lipase

Suppression of insulin release during cold exposure may contribute to substrate mobilization, since the effects of insulin of fuel stores are generally antagonistic to those of catecholamines. Insulin diminishes the activity of hormone-sensitive lipase, thereby diminishing free fatty acid release from white adipose tissue; insulin also inhibits hepatic glycogenolysis and gluconeogenesis, thereby reducing glucose release from the liver. During chronic cold exposure in the rat, insulin levels are diminished,[78] a change that would favor substrate mobilization. It is possible that catecholamines contribute to the suppressed insulin level since, in at least one study, α-adrenergic blockade was shown to increase insulin release during cold-induced hypothermia.[79]

Changes in lipoprotein lipase activity may also affect substrate mobilization and utilization in the cold. Lipoprotein lipase activity, which is importantly involved in the uptake and utilization of plasma triglycerides by extra hepatic tissues, is diminished in rat white adipose tissue and increased in heart and BAT.[72] Both the sympathetic nervous system and insulin may be involved in these alterations in lipoprotein lipase activity since they are partially reversed by insulin, and NE administration promotes changes in lipoprotein lipase activity in warm animals that resemble those that occur in cold.[72] The changes in lipoprotein lipase activity that occur during cold exposure would favor fat utilization in BAT and heart and suppress storage of fat in white adipose tissue.

6.2.6. Cardiovascular System

Cardiovascular responses during cold exposure conserve heat and enhance the delivery of oxygen and substrates to actively metabolizing tissues. The changes in blood flow distribution and cardiac output that occur during cold exposure are consistent with the changes in sympathetic nervous system activity that have been demonstrated during cold exposure, as described above (Section 6.2.2). Subcutaneous vasoconstriction diverts blood from the skin, thereby enhancing the insulating capacity of the subcutaneous tissues and inhibiting heat loss. In addition, cardiac output increases markedly; in noncold-acclimated man, a brief period of cold exposure has been shown to double cardiac output.[80] The correlation between increased oxygen uptake and cardiac output during cold exposure suggests that the increased metabolic rate is the stimulus for the increase in cardiac output.[80] Peripheral resistance falls during cold exposure, reflecting increased blood flow to both shivering muscles and tissues involved in nonshivering thermogenesis. The fact that cold exposure increases pulse pressure and cross product (pulse rate times systolic blood pressure) in noncold-acclimated subjects suggests that these cardiovascular responses are secondary to increased sympathetic activity.

6.2.6.1. Vascular Responsiveness to NE

A number of studies demonstrate that environmental temperature itself alters vascular responsiveness to NE. The contractile response to NE is enhanced in superficial cutaneous veins and arteries,[81–83] thereby diminishing subcutaneous blood flow at a given level of sympathetic activity and diminishing heat loss to the environment. One aspect of heat conservation fostered by this mechanism appears to be an enhancement of countercurrent heat exchange within limb vessels; by shifting venous drainage from the superficial subcutaneous veins to the deeper venae comitantes, heat is returned from the arteries perfusing the extremities to the central venous pool.

6.2.6.2. Cold Acclimation

In addition to the direct effect of environmental temperature, cold acclimation alters the vascular response to sympathetic stimulation. In noncold-acclimated animals, including man,[80,84,85] acute cold exposure increases blood pressure approximately 20%; after cold acclimation, however, the blood pressure response both to a cold stimulus[84,86] and to infused NE[37] is diminished. Enhancement of vagal parasympathetic tone during cold exposure may contribute to this change in cardiovascular response.[86] Additionally, changes involving adrenergic receptors may be involved as well, since alterations in receptor sensitivity to adrenergic agonists have been demonstrated in cold-acclimated rats.[87,88] The cold-acclimation process is associated with diminution in α-adrenergic responses and enhancement of those mediated by the β receptor,[87] changes that may contribute to the differential patterns of cardiovascular response noted in warm- and cold-acclimated mammals.

6.2.7. Summary: The Role of the Sympathetic Nervous System and the Adrenal Medulla in the Mammalian Defense against Cold Exposure

Cold exposure, therefore, is associated with stimulation of the sympathetic nervous system. Sympathetic stimulation increases metabolic heat production (nonshivering thermogenesis), alters the cardiovascular system so that heat is conserved and adequate supplies of oxygen and substrate are delivered to metabolizing tissues, and increases the mobilization of substrate, particularly free fatty acids from fuel stores in adipose tissue. Cold acclimation, in which metabolic heat production in response to cold exposure is enhanced following prolonged exposure to a cold environment, is associated with enhancement of the thermogenic effects of catecholamines as well as with alterations in the vascular sensitivity to NE.

The role of the adrenal medulla is less clearly defined. Stimulation of the adrenal medulla is less marked during cold exposure than stimulation of the sympathetic nervous system. If the sympathetic nervous system is impaired, stimulation of the adrenal medulla is more marked, and circulating E can compensate, at least in part, for the deficient nervous system responses. While stimulation of nonshivering thermogenesis and cardiovascular regulation are clearly within the province of the sympathetic nervous system, the adrenal medulla may play an important role in substrate mobilization during cold exposure, particularly in the regulation of hepatic glucose output.

6.3. Dietary Thermogenesis

6.3.1. Luxusconsumption: Adaptive Changes in Thermogenesis in Relation to Changes in Dietary Intake

The possibility of a regulatory change in thermogenesis in response to alterations in caloric intake was first proposed at the end of the 19th century by German physiologists, including Rubner and Neumann.[89] Simply stated, these workers suggested that changes in energy production in response to alterations in dietary intake modify metabolic efficiency so that body mass remains relatively unchanged on diets of different caloric value. The increase in metabolic rate secondary to increased intake was referred to as luxusconsumption. This concept has been the subject of considerable controversy over the last century. It has been recognized for some time that oxygen consumption changes in response to semistarvation or overfeeding; the point of issue has been whether these changes in thermogenesis are adaptive in nature or whether they reflect either changes in the mass of metabolizing tissue caused by alterations in body size or composition, or the energy required to assimilate ingested nutrients. Although the controversy over adaptive thermogenesis in response to changes in dietaty intake has not been conclusively settled, the continued development of data consistent with adaptive dietary thermogenesis,[89] particularly in the rat,[90] supports the notion of a functionally significant "luxusconsumption."

Further evidence in support of adaptive dietary thermogenesis is provided by evidence demonstrating diet-induced changes in sympathetic nervous system activity. Since the sympathetic nervous system plays such an important role in the regulation of nonshivering thermogenesis, it is not an unreasonable hypothesis that diet-induced changes in sympathetic nervous system activity may be related to thermogenesis as well. The demonstration of an essential similarity between diet-induced thermogenesis and nonshivering thermogenesis, in both physiological and biochemical terms, also supports such a hypothesis.

6.3.2. Effect of Dietary Intake on Sympathoadrenal Activity

6.3.2.1. Suppression of Sympathetic Activity during Fasting and Caloric Restriction

NE turnover techniques have clearly indicated that sympathetic nervous system activity is diminished during fasting in a variety of organs of the experimental animal[91-93] including interscapular BAT.[94] In the rat, suppressed sympathetic activity can be demonstrated during the first day of fasting.[95]

6.3.2.1a. Human Studies. Although data in humans are less complete, the available evidence indicates that suppression of sympathetic activity occurs in human subjects during fasting or caloric restriction. Plasma NE levels are reduced in obese subjects during semistarvation[96,97] and in starved patients with anorexia nervosa.[98] Refeeding elevates plasma NE levels to control values.[98] In human subjects of normal weight, a 3-day fast is associated with a fall in urinary NE excretion (R. Rosa, J. B. Young, and L. Landsberg, unpublished observation). In all of these studies, a fall in blood pressure and pulse rate during caloric restriction has been noted, thereby providing physiological evidence of sympathetic suppression.

6.3.2.1b. The Adrenal Medullary Response to Caloric Restriction. Preliminary studies of human subjects of normal weight show an increase in E excretion during a 3-day fast (R. Rosa, J. B. Young, and L. Landsberg, unpublished observation) consistent with stimulation of adrenal medullary secretion. Since glucose lowering in normal and diabetic human subjects from 95 to 60 mg/dl has been shown to increase plasma E levels,[99] the possibility arises that lowered plasma glucose concentrations during fasting may stimulate the adrenal medulla. The adrenal medullary response to caloric restriction warrants further study; it should be noted that the increase in E excretion or plasma E levels in the studies cited above is a small fraction of the adrenal medullary response to frank hypoglycemia such as occurs when the plasma glucose level is reduced below a value in the range of 50 mg/dl. As noted below, however, even a small increase in adrenal medullary secretion during fasting may have physiologically significant consequences.

6.3.2.1c. Physiological Role of the Sympathetic Nervous System and the Adrenal Medulla during Caloric Restriction. It is a reasonable hypothesis that suppression of sympathetic nervous system activity during caloric restriction contributes to the decrease in metabolic rate observed when caloric intake is limited. Suppression of sympathetic activity during fasting in rat BAT,[94] the major thermogenic organ in this species, is consistent with such an interpretation. The decrease in metabolic rate associated with fasting cannot be ascribed to functional hypothyroidism, since it is demonstrable even in thyroid-deficient animals.[100] Furthermore, the administration of L-dopa, which has a sympathomimetic effect, blocks the fall in oxygen consumption that normally occurs when obese human subjects undergo semistarvation,[101] without increasing the lowered triiodothyronine level. Thus, available evidence is consistent with an important role for the sympathetic nervous system in the mediation of depressed thermogenesis during diminished caloric intake.

During cold exposure the sympathoadrenal system plays an important role in the substrate mobilization that occurs along with the increase in metabolic rate. The role of the sympathoadrenal system in the regulation of substrate mobilization during fasting or caloric restriction is more complex. Since sympathetic activity is suppressd, it is unlikely that substrate mobilization is mediated by the sympathetic nervous system. It is possible, however, that a small increase in adrenal medullary E secretion, in conjunction with a low circulating level of insulin, may be involved. Lipolysis is extremely sensitive to small changes in plasma E level within the physiological range.[102] Recent studies also demonstrate that, in human subjects *in vivo*, fasting enhances sensitivity to the lipolytic effect of catecholamines.[103] Since small increments of E would be unlikely to increase thermogenesis, the pattern of sympathetic nervous system suppression coupled with adrenal medullary activation may contribute to both the diminished thermogenesis and the substrate mobilization that occurs when caloric intake is restricted.

6.3.2.2. Stimulation of Sympathetic Nervous System Activity and Thermogenesis during Feeding and Excessive Caloric Intake

The relationships between feeding, overfeeding, sympathetic activity, and thermogenesis are complex. The sympathetic nervous system is stimulated acutely during discrete episodes of food intake, and chronically, in response to a sustained increase in dietary intake. The thermogenic response to feeding also has two components: an acute, short-lived, meal-related thermogenic response, and a sustained increase in resting metabolic rate that reflects antecedent diet. The former, previously referred to as specific dynamic action and now more frequently called the thermic effect of food, appears to reflect, at least in part, the energy cost of digestion, assimilation, and metabolism of the ingested nutrients. The latter, often referred to as dietary-induced thermogenesis, may represent an adaptive change in energy balance and is subject to significant regulation by the sympathetic nervous system.

6.3.2.2a. Acute Sympathetic Responses to Feeding. In normal man, glucose ingestion raises plasma NE levels.[104,105] Isocaloric meals of protein or fat, by contrast, are devoid of effect on plasma NE level.[106] All three nutrients, however, when administered singly, increase oxygen consumption, an effect that is greatest after protein.[106] Thus, fat and protein meals increase thermogenesis in the absence of definitive evidence of sympathetic stimulation. Furthermore, the increase in oxygen consumption seen after glucose administration, despite the rise in plasma NE level, is not antagonized by prior β blockade.[107] Evidence in human subjects thus suggests that the thermic effect of feeding may be independent of sympathetic stimulation and not, predominantly, an adaptive form of thermogenesis. With glucose administration, the possibility still remains, however, that part of the acute thermic response may be mediated by the sympathetic nervous system.

6.3.2.2b. Overfeeding.   In the rat, chronic overfeeding increases both sympathetic nervous system activity and oxygen consumption. Overfeeding of sucrose in the rat, utilizing a regimen that increases caloric intake approximately 30%, increases sympathetic nervous system activity in a variety of organs.[92,93,108,109] The effects of sucrose overfeeding on sympathetic activity are sustained through at least 8 days and are restored to control levels by 1 day of normal feeding.[109] Preliminary experiments in the rat indicate that supplemental rations of fat increase sympathetic nervous system activity as well. When added to rat chow, lard increases sympathetic activity in heart, the magnitude of the effect resembling or possibly exceeding that of sucrose.[110] Overfeeding a mixed, highly palatable ("cafeteria") diet, which increases caloric intake between 50 and 100%, for 10 days or longer also increases sympathetic nervous system activity in heart and interscapular BAT.[94] On this regimen, oxygen consumption is markedly increased and the increase is antagonized by β-adrenergic blockade.[90] This form of overfeeding also potentiates the thermogenic effects of NE in the rat,[90] an effect resembling that of cold acclimation. The fact that overfeeding increases sympathetic activity in interscapular BAT, and that the increase in oxygen consumption associated with overfeeding is blocked by propranolol, suggests an important role for the sympathetic nervous system in the regulation of dietary thermogenesis in the rat.

In human subjects, chronic overfeeding increases resting metabolic rate[111] although the thermogenic effects of NE infusions are not enhanced,[111] in contradistinction to what occurs in the rat. The effect of chronic overfeeding on sympathetic activity in man, and the effect of β-adrenergic blockade on the increase in metabolic rate associated with overfeeding, have not been clearly established.

6.3.2.2c. Nonshivering Thermogenesis and Diet-Induced Thermogenesis.   Thus, at least in the rat, sympathetic responses to cold exposure and increased dietary intake are similar. Both cold and diet stimulate NE turnover in interscapular BAT,[94] and the thermogenic effect of NE is potentiated by both chronic cold exposure or chronic ingestion of a high-calorie diet.[90] Other evidence, in the rat, supports the essential similarity between nonshivering thermogenesis and diet-induced thermogenesis. With regard to BAT, overfeeding has been shown to stimulate hypertrophy,[90] increase NE-stimulated oxygen consumption,[112] and increase interscapular BAT blood flow; these changes are all similar to those noted during cold acclimation. Chronic overfeeding has also been shown to increase the proton conductance pathway in isolated mitochondria from BAT[113] and to increase BAT Na^+-K^+ ATPase activity,[114] changes similar to those seen in cold acclimation. Thus, BAT, the major thermogenic organ of the rat, undergoes similar structural and functional changes during chronic overfeeding and cold exposure.

Overfeeding has also been shown to diminish shivering in warm-acclimated animals acutely exposed to cold.[65] The effects of overfeeding and cold-acclimation on the thermogenic response to NE appear to be additive and are greater than those obtained with either overfeeding or cold acclimation alone.[65] Activation of the sympathetic nervous system during cold exposure is significantly reduced by fasting.[115] These additional data also support the similarity of thermogenic mechanisms induced by cold, on the one hand, and dietary intake on the other.

6.3.2.2d. Physiological Role of the Sympathetic Nervous System during Overfeeding. The survival value of increased sympathetic activity with overfeeding is less clear than that of sympathetic suppression during caloric restriction. Increased sympathetic activity with overfeeding might result in an increase in oxygen consumption and dissipation of calories taken in excess of need. The ability to expend excess calories would be of particular benefit to organisms on a subsistence diet with, for example, a low nitrogen content. The capacity for diet-induced thermogenesis under these circumstances might permit such organisms to satisfy the basic requirement for nitrogen by increasing dietary intake of foodstuffs low in protein. Stimulation of sympathetic nervous system activity with consequent increase in dietary thermogenesis would prevent undue accumulation of fat while assuring adequate nutrition.

The efficiency of utilization of calories is not the same in different individuals.[89] Individuals displaying decreased dietary thermogenesis might be considered to have a thrifty metabolic trait; increased efficiency of fuel utilization would favor survival during periods of famine, but might predispose to obesity in the face of abundant food supply. It is conceivable that alterations in either the extent of activation of the sympathetic nervous system,[116] or alterations in thermogenic effects of NE,[32] may be involved in the different patterns of metabolic efficiency noted in different individuals. Both sympathetic nervous system function and the thermogenic effects of NE warrant further study in obese and formerly obese subjects.

6.3.3. CNS Assessment of Nutritional Status: The Signal That Couples Changes in Dietary Intake with Changes in Sympathetic Activity

The mechanisms involved in the stimulation of the sympathetic nervous system during cold exposure are straightforward; cold-sensitive neurons in the periphery and in the CNS change their firing rate in response to a fall in temperature, and the information is relayed to the hypothalamic centers that integrate sympathetic activity. The coupling of sympathetic activity with dietary intake is more complex and requires a virtually continuous assessment of the nutritional status by the CNS. Changes in body mass or body composition cannot explain diet-induced changes in sympathetic activity since the latter are demonstrable long before appreciable changes in the former could occur.[109] Mechanisms whereby the CNS assesses body mass or body composition, moreover, have not been clearly defined. Although different mechanisms are probably involved with different nutrients, the relationship of carbohydrate metabolism to changes in sympathetic nervous system activity has been best studied.

6.3.3.1. Possible Role of Glucose and Insulin

A reasonable hypothesis can be developed in support of a mechanism whereby insulin-mediated glucose metabolism within the CNS is involved in the coupling of carbohydrate intake and sympathetic nervous system activity. In contrast to a stimulatory effect on the adrenal medulla, both hypoglycemia[117,118] and 2-deoxyglucose,[95] which disrupts intracellular glucose metabolism, suppress sympathetic nervous system activity. Thus, diminished intracellular glucose metabolism may be linked to suppression of sympathetic activity. It seems unlikely, however, that plasma glucose level *per se* is a sufficient determinant of intracellular glucose metabolism to function as the sole signal that couples changes in sympathetic activity with changes in diet or even changes in carbohydrate intake. Although the decrements in plasma glucose levels that occur during fasting may contribute to decreased glucose availability, changes in plasma glucose level during sucrose feeding cannot adequately explain the increase in sympathetic activity under these circumstances.

It is possible, however, that insulin-mediated glucose metabolism may be involved. In contradistinction to glucose, plasma insulin level varies widely and reflects, in a general sense, the intake of carbohydrates. Moreover, insulin is the major signal to tissues throughout the body that calories have been assimilated and it is, therefore, logical that insulin serve the same function for the CNS. Furthermore, insulin is known to affect specifically certain regions of the brain, particularly the hypothalamus,[119,120] and a direct stimulatory effect of insulin on sympathetic nervous system activity has been demonstrated.[121]

Central Neuronal Integration. The portion of the brain responsive to changes in glucose and insulin concentration may be located in the ventromedial portion of the hypothalamus.[120,122–125] This region of the brain is known to be responsive to glucose and insulin and is involved, as well, in the regulation of satiety and food intake. Treatment with gold thioglucose, an agent that destroys glucose-sensitive neurons in the region of the ventromedial nucleus, has been shown to block diet-induced changes in sympathetic nervous system activity in the mouse.[125] In the rat, stimulation of this portion of the hypothalamus increases BAT thermogenesis.[123] Although an entirely coherent and internally consistent model of ventromedial hypothalamic regulation of diet-induced changes in sympathetic activity cannot be constructed at the present time, the data accumulated thus far suggest an important role for this region of the brain in the integration of diet with sympathetic activity. Available evidence is consistent with the hypothesis that glucose metabolism (facilitated by insulin) within glucose-sensitive cells in the ventromedial portion of the hypothalamus influences central sympathetic outflow so that diminished glucose utilization is associated with suppression, and increased glucose utilization with stimulation, of sympathetic activity.

6.3.3.2. Visceral Afferents

Since mixed diets and high-fat diets also stimulate sympathetic nervous system activity, it is obvious that signals other than glucose and insulin must be involved in the coupling of sympathetic activity with dietary intake. Although studies of the role of visceral afferents in the regulation of metabolism are in their infancy, available evidence does suggest that receptors for substrates and hormones in visceral organs, particularly liver, may initiate afferent neural discharges that convey information to the CNS about the nutritional state of the organism.[126] Glucose administration has been shown to diminish the discharge rate of hepatic vagal afferents while 2-deoxyglucose has been shown to have a stimulatory effect.[126] Cholecystokinin (CCK), when given by intravenous infusion, decreases hepatic vagal afferent discharge.[126] These results suggest a resemblance to the venous and arterial baroreceptor systems that regulate sympathetic activity in accord with the needs of the circulation. Changes in hormone and substrate levels in association with feeding (increased glucose level, increased CCK), for example, might result in enhanced sympathetic nervous system activity by diminishing inhibitory input into the centers that regulate sympathetic outflow, analogous to the increase in sympathetic outflow that results from diminished baroreceptor impulses from the aorta, carotid sinus, and great veins when arterial or venous blood pressure is lowered. Possible effects of CCK and other gut hormones, particularly gastric inhibitory polypeptide, on the CNS need to be explored as well.

6.3.4. Summary: Adaptive Thermogenesis

Thus, the sympathetic nervous system has a critical role in the regulation of adaptive thermogenesis in response to changes in environmental temperature and changes in caloric intake. These changes help the mammalian organism to defend not only body temperature, but also energy balance, and may contribute in an important way to the regulation of body mass. It seems likely, moreover, that the sympathetic nervous system is involved in a variety of other situations in which thermogenesis is altered. Thus, hibernation, fever, malignant hyperpyrexia, tetanus, traumatic injury, and shock, among others, are all situations in which alterations in thermogenesis are well characterized, and a relationship to alterations in sympathetic nevous system activity seems likely. At present, evidence for participation of the sympathetic nervous system in these other situations is only fragmentary, but investigation of the role played by the sympathetic nervous system in these various physiological and pathophysiological states may be important in understanding the physiologic mechanisms that underlie the characteristic changes in thermogenesis associated with these disorders.

6.4. Pheochromocytoma

6.4.1. Usefulness of Plasma Cathecholamine Measurements in the Diagnosis of Pheochromocytoma

6.4.1.1. Diagnostic Considerations

Measurement of catecholamines or catecholamine metabolites in a 24-hr urine sample remains the standard test in the diagnosis of pheochromocytoma. The diagnosis can be confirmed in the great majority of patients by the proper analysis of a single 24-hr urine sample, providing the patient is hypersensitive or symptomatic at the time the collection is made. The commonly employed assays include unconjugated or "free" catecholamines, VMA, and the metanephrines. Although opinions differ about the relative usefulness of these assays, the different measurements are probably equivalent if properly performed. Diagnostic accuracy is improved when two of the three determinations are employed, although it is not usually necessary to obtain more than one as a screening procedure. The determination selected as the basic screening test should depend on the expertise of the laboratory available to the physician.

The following general considerations apply to all the urinary determinations. (1) In patients with paroxysmal hypertension, the yield of the 24-hr collection is enhanced if the urine collection is initiated when the patient experiences a crisis. (2) Although claims have been made for the adequacy of measurements made on random urine samples and expressed per milligram of creatinine, the correlation of random samples with 24-hr urine collections is not perfect, and analysis of a full 24-hr urine sample is clearly preferable. Creatinine should always be determined as well to ensure the adequacy of collection. (3) The urine collection should be properly acidified and kept cold during the collection and prior to analysis. (4) Where possible, the collection should be obtained when the patient is at rest, on no medication, and without recent exposure to radiographic contrast media, which may alter the renal catecholamine secretion. Where it is not feasible to discontinue antihypertensive medications, those drugs known specifically to interfere in the assays should be avoided. Thiazide diuretics, propranolol, and hydralazine usually cause no interference; catecholamines, in any form, particularly α-methyldopa, interfere with urine catecholamine determinations for periods of up to 2 weeks. With high-quality assays, dietary restrictions are usually not necessary. The physician should consult his reference laboratory for their instructions with regard to diet and interfering drugs.

Although pheochromocytoma will be diagnosed in most cases on the first urine collection, an occasional case with borderline values and a compelling clinical picture will need to be investigated further. The first step generally will be to repeat the urine collection at a time when the patient is symptomatic. It is customary to do this by initiating the urine collection at the beginning of a crisis or paroxysm. In the rare case, where repeated urinary determinations are not decisive, measurements of plasma catecholamines may be of value.

6.4.1.2. Plasma Catecholamines

It is important to emphasize that plasma catecholamines should not be used as a screening test for pheochromocytoma. These measurements should be reserved for difficult cases where the diagnosis cannot be established or excluded with reasonable certainty by the urinary methods. It is also important to note that the blood obtained for catecholamine measurements must be obtained under basal conditions. By convention, basal conditions consist of 30 min supine in a relaxed environment with an intravenous line in place for blood withdrawal. The test should be performed after an overnight fast or at least 3 hr after the last meal. Casually obtained plasma catecholamine levels are uninterpretable, since normal individuals in an upright position have plasma levels as high or higher than those seen in some patients with pheochromocytoma. Basal levels of total catecholamines over 2000 pg/ml support the diagnosis of pheochromocytoma. Patients who have essential hypertension with "hyperadrenergic" features generally have levels in the range 400–600 pg/ml.[127]

Stimulation and Suppression of Plasma Catecholamines in Patients with Pheochromocytoma. Preliminary studies indicate that the usefulness of plasma catecholamine measurements in the diagnosis of pheochromocytoma may be improved by the application of suppression and stimulation tests. Both clonidine[128] and pentolinium[129] decrease plasma catecholamine levels in patients with essential hypertension, but are without effect on circulating catecholamine concentrations in patients with pheochromocytoma. The rationale for the use of the suppression test is based on the fact that pheochromocytomas are not innervated. Both clonidine and pentolinium diminish central sympathetic activity, clonidine at the level of the sympathetic centers in the brain stem, pentolinium at the level of the autonomic ganglia, and therefore diminish sympathoadrenal activity with resultant fall in circulating catecholamines. Pheochromocytomas, in contrast, are not affected, and plasma catecholamines are unaltered.

Although provocative tests have largely been replaced in the diagnosis of pheochromocytoma by the measurement of catecholamines and catecholamine metabolites, in an exceptional patient in whom the clinical features are highly suggestive, and the diagnosis cannot be excluded by the other techniques, a glucagon stimulation test coupled with plasma catecholamine measurements may be of value.[127] Glucagon is without effect on plasma catecholamines in subjects without pheochromocytoma; in patients with pheochromocytoma, marked increases in plasma catecholamine concentrations have been documented. It must be emphasized, however, that glucagon may induce severe and life-threatening paroxysms. This test should never be done casually, therefore, and must be carried out only under close supervision, with phentolamine readily at hand and adequate intravenous access. Although the percentage of false-negative tests is not known, in the study by Bravo *et al.* from the Cleveland Clinic,[127] all of six patients with pheochromocytoma had positive plasma catecholamine responses (threefold increase and achievement of a value greater than 2000 pg/ml), criteria not filled by any of 40 similarly studied controls.

It must be emphasized once again, however, that it is an unusual patient who requires these specialized tests for diagnosis. These tests will be most useful in excluding the diagnosis in patients with suggestive clinical futures and borderline urinary catecholamine values.

6.4.2. Localization of Pheochromocytoma

6.4.2.1. CT-Scan

CT-scan has become the method of choice for the localization of intraadrenal pheochromocytomas. The efficacy of CT has been clearly demonstrated in a number of recent studies.[130–133] Angiography is rarely necessary for the localization of intraadrenal tumors, providing the adrenals can be clearly demonstrated on the CT-scan. Angiography continues to play a role, however, in the demonstration of extraadrenal pheochromocytomas, which frequently have a large aberrant artery readily demonstrable on abdominal aortogram. Although some centers have had reasonable experience with ultrasonic demonstration of adrenal tumors, in general this technique is substantially inferior to CT-scan.

6.4.2.2. Venous Sampling and Scintographic Localization

Venous sampling at different levels of the inferior vena cava may be of value in localizing extraadrenal pheochromocytomas.[134] Although claims have been made for the usefulness of venous sampling in the localization of intraadrenal pheochromocytoma,[135] this technique is of limited usefulness, since the normal adrenal may secrete large amounts of E in response to instrumentation and catheter placement. The demonstration of a large amount of NE coming from an adrenal vein, in comparison with the opposite side may be useful on some occasions, but in general probably adds little to localization by the CT-scan.

Radionuclide scintiscanning using labeled (^{131}I) *meta*-iodobenzylguanidine has also been described.[136,137] This compound, which is a guanidine congener of NE, is a substrate for the neuronal uptake and storage systems, and is, therefore, incorporated in the catecholamine store of adrenergic tissues, including pheochromocytoma. Preliminary studies indicate reasonable demonstration of intra- and extraadrenal tumors.[136,137] The general usefulness of this technique, however, remains to be established.

References

1. Hsieh, A. C. L., Carlson, L. D., and Gray, G., 1957, Role of the sympathetic nervous system in the control of chemical regulation of heat production, *Am. J. Physiol.* **190:**247–251.
2. Leduc, J., 1961, Catecholamine production and release in exposure and acclimation to cold, *Acta Physiol. Scand.* **53:**1–101.
3. Bergh, U., Harley, H., Landsberg, L., and Ekblom, B., 1979, Plasma norepinephrine concentrations during submaximal and maximal exercise at lowered skin and core temperatures, *Acta Physiol. Scand.* **106:**383–384.
4. Therminarias, A., Chirpaz, M. F., and Tanche, M., 1979, Catecholamines in dogs during cold adaptation by repeated immersions, *J. Appl. Physiol.* **46:**662–668.
5. Young, J. B., and Landsberg, L., 1976, Effect of diet and cold exposure on norepinephrine turnover in pancreas and liver, *Am. J. Physiol.* **236:**E524–E533.

6. Jones, S. B., and Musacchia, X. J., 1976, Norephinephrine turnover in heart and spleen of 7-, 22-, and 34 C-acclimated hamsters, *Am. J. Physiol.* **230:**564–568.

7. Oliverio, A., and Stjarne, L., 1965, Acceleration of noradrenaline turnover in the mouse heart by cold exposure, *Life Sci.* **4:**2339–2343.

8. Bralet, J., Beley, A., and Lallemant, A. M., 1972, Alterations in norepinephrine turnover in various peripheral organs of the rat during exposure and acclimation to cold, *Pfluegers Arch.* **335:**186–197.

9. Tedesco, J. L., Flattery, K. V., and Sellers, E. A., 1977, Effects of thyroid hormones and cold exposure on turnover of norepinephrine in cardiac and skeletal muscle, *Can. J. Physiol. Pharmacol.* **55:**515–522.

10. Johnson, T. S., Young, J. B., and Landsberg, L., 1981, Norepinephrine turnover in lung: Effect of cold exposure and chronic hypoxia, *J. Appl. Physiol.* **51:**614–620.

11. Iriki, M., Riedel, W., and Simon, E., 1971, Regional differentiation of sympathetic activity during hypothalamic heating and cooling in anesthetized rabbits, *Pfluegers Arch.* **328:**320–331.

12. Walther, O. E., Iriki, M., and Simon, E., 1970, Antagonistic changes of blood flow and sympathetic activity in different vascular beds following central thermal stimulation. II. Cutaneous and visceral sympathetic activity during spinal cord heating and cooling in anesthetized rabbits and cats, *Pfluegers Arch.* **319:**162–184.

13. Beley, A., Beley, P., Rochette, L., and Bralet, J., 1976, Evolution in vivo of the synthesis rate of catecholamines in various peripheral organs of the rat during cold exposure, *Pfluegers Arch.* **366:**259–264.

14. Cannon, W. B., Querido, A., Britton, S. W., and Bright, E. M., 1979, Studies on the conditions of activity in endocrine glands. XXI. The role of adrenal secretion in the chemical control of body temperature, *Am. J. Physiol.* **79:**466–507.

15. Young, J. B., and Landsberg, L., 1981, Effect of concomitant fasting and cold exposure on sympathoadrenal activity in rats, *Am. J. Physiol.* **240:**E314–E319.

16. Jessen, K., Rabol, A., and Winkler, K., 1980, Total body and splanchnic thermogenesis in curarized man during a short exposure to cold, *Acta. Anaesthesiol. Scand.* **24:**339–344.

17. Thompson, G. E., 1977, Physiological effects of cold exposure, in: *International Review of Physiology: Environmental Physiology II* (D. Robertshaw, ed.), pp. 29–69, University Park Press, Baltimore.

18. Gale, C. C., 1973, Neuroendocrine aspects of thermoregulation, *Annu. Rev. Physiol.* **35:**391–430.

19. Hellon, R. F., 1975, Monoamines, pyrogens and cations: Their actions on central control of body temperature, *Pharmacol Rev.* **26:**289–321.

20. Blatteis, C. M., 1981, The newer putative central neurotransmitters: Roles in thermoregulation. Hypothalamic substances in the control of body temperature: General characteristics, *Fed. Proc.* **40:**2735–2740.

21. Himms-Hagen, J., 1975, Role of the adrenal medulla in adaptation to cold, in: *Handbook of Physiology*, Section VII, *Endocrinology* (R. O. Greep and E.

B. Astwood, eds.), pp. 637–665, American Physiology Society, Washington, D.C.

22. Feist, D. D., and Feist, C. F., 1978, Catecholamine-synthesizing enzymes in adrenals of seasonally acclimatized voles, *J. Appl. Physiol.* **44:**59–62.

23. Banet, M., Hensel, H., and Liebermann, H., 1978, The central control of shivering and non-shivering thermogenesis in the rat, *J. Physiol. (London)* **283:**569–584.

24. Horwitz, B. A., 1979, Metabolic aspects of thermogenesis: Neuronal and hormonal control, *Fed. Proc.* **38:**2147–2149.

25. Hsieh, A. C. L., and Carlson, L. D., 1957, Role of adrenaline and noradrenaline in chemical regulation of heat production, *Am. J. Physiol.* **190:**243–246.

26. Hemingway, A., Price, W. M., and Stuart, D., 1964, The calorigenic action of catecholamines in warm acclimated and cold acclimated non-shivering cats, *Int. J. Neuropharmacol.* **3:**495–503.

27. Komaromi, I., 1977, Effects of alpha- and beta-adrenergic blockers on the actions of noradrenaline on body temperature in the newborn guinea-pig, *Experientia* **33:**1083–1084.

28. Schonbaum, E., Johnson, G. E., Sellers, E. A., and Gill, M. J., 1966, Adrenergic beta-receptors and non-shivering thermogenesis, *Nature (London)* **210:**426.

29. LeBlanc, J., Vallieres, J., and Vachon, C., 1972, Beta-receptor sensitization by repeated injections of isoproterenol and by cold adaptation, *Am. J. Physiol.* **222:**1043–1046.

30. Sellers, E. A., and Schonbaum, E., 1963, Catecholamines in acclimation to cold: Historical survey, *Fed. Proc.* **22:**909–910.

31. Hsieh, A. C. L., and Wang, J. C. C., 1971, Calorigenic responses to cold of rats after prolonged infusion of norepinephrine, *Am. J. Physiol.* **221:**335–337.

32. Jung, R. T., Shetty, P. S., James, W. P. T., Barrand, M. A., and Callingham, B. A., 1979, Reduced thermogenesis in obesity, *Nature (London)* **279:**322–323.

33. Davis, T. R. A., and Johnston, D. R., 1961, Seasonal acclimatization to cold in man, *J. Appl. Physiol.* **16:**231–234.

34. Scholander, P. F., Hammel, H. T., Lange Anderson, K., and Loyning, Y., 1958, Metabolic acclimatization to cold in man, *J. Appl. Physiol.* **12:**1–8.

35. Budd, G. M., and Warhaft, N., 1966, Cardiovascular and metabolic responses to noradrenaline in man, before and after acclimatization to cold in Artarctica, *J. Physiol. (London)* **186:**233–242.

36. Davis, T. R. A., 1961, Chamber cold acclimatization in man, *J. Appl. Physiol.* **16:**1011–1015.

37. Joy, R. J. T., 1963, Responses of cold-acclimated men to infused norepinephrine, *J. Appl. Physiol.* **18:**1209–1212.

38. Mejsnar, J., and Jansky, L., 1976, Mode of catecholamine action during organ regulation of nonshivering thermogenesis, in: *Regulation of Depressed Metabolism and Thermogenesis* (L. Jansky and X. J. Musacchia, eds.), pp. 225–242, Thomas, Springfield, Ill.

39. Depocas, F., 1958, Chemical thermogenesis in the functionally eviscerated cold-acclimated rat, *Can. J. Biochem. Physiol.* **36:**691–699.

40. Depocas, F., 1960, The calorigenic response to cold-acclimated white rats to infused noradrenaline, *Can. J. Biochem. Physiol.* **38:**107–114.

41. Depocas, F., 1960, Calorigenesis from various organ systems in the whole animal, *Fed. Proc.* **5:**19–24.

42. Davis, T. R. A., 1967, Contribution of skeletal muscle to nonshivering thermogenesis in the dog, *Am. J. Physiol.* **213:**1423–1426.

43. Jansky, L., and Hart, J. S., 1963, Participation of skeletal muscle and kidney during nonshivering thermogenesis in cold-acclimated rats, *Can. J. Biochem. Physiol.* **41:**953–964.

44. Guernsey, D. L., and Stevens, E. D., 1977, The cell membrane sodium pump as a mechanism for increasing thermogenesis during cold acclimation in rats, *Science* **196:**908–910.

45. Horwitz, B. A., and Eaton, M., 1977, Ouabain-sensitive liver and diaphragm respiration in cold-acclimated hamster, *J. Appl. Physiol.* **42:**150–153.

46. Greenway, D. C., and Himms-Hagen, J., 1978, Increased calcium uptake by muscle mitochondria of cold-acclimated rats, *Am. J. Physiol.* **234:**C7–C13.

47. Himms-Hagen, J., Behren, W., Hbous, A., and Greenway, D., 1976, Altered mitochondria in skeletal muscle of cold acclimated rats and the adaptation for nonshivering thermogenesis, in: *Regulation of Depressed Metabolism and Thermogenesis* (L. Jansky and X. J. Musacchia, eds.), pp. 243–260, Thomas, Springfield, Ill.

48. Kurahashi, M., and Kuroshima, A., 1978, Creatine metabolism in skeletal muscle of cold-acclimated rats, *J. Appl. Physiol.* **44:**12–16.

49. Foster, D. O., and Frydman, M. L., 1978, Nonshivering thermogenesis in the rat. II. Measurements of blood flow with microspheres point to brown adipose tissue as the dominant site of the calorigenesis induced by noradrenaline, *Can. J. Physiol. Pharmacol.* **56:**110–122.

50. Smith, R. E., and Horwitz, B. A., 1969, Brown fat and thermogenesis, *Physiol. Rev.* **49:**330–425.

51. Cottle, M. K. W., and Cottle, W. H., 1970, Adrenergic fibers in brown fat of cold-acclimated rats, *J. Histochem. Cytochem.* **18:**116–119.

52. Young, J. B., Saville, E., Rothwell, N. J., Stock, M. J., and Landsberg, L., 1982, Effect of diet and cold exposure on norepinephrine turnover in brown adipose tissue of the rat, *J. Clin. Invest.* **69:**1061–1071.

53. Hull, D., and Segall, M. M., 1965, Sympathetic nervous control of brown adipose tissue and heat production in the new-born rabbit, *J. Physiol. (London)* **181:**458–467.

54. Horwitz, B. A., 1979, Cellular events underlying catecholamine-induced thermogenesis: Cation transport in brown adipocytes, *Fed. Proc.* **38:**2170–2176.

55. Slavin, B. G., and Bernick, S., 1974, Morphological studies on denervated brown adipose tissue, *Anat. Rec.* **179:**497–506.

56. Alexander, G., and Stevens, D., 1980, Sympathetic innervation and the development of structure and function of brown adipose tissue: Studies on lambs chemically sympathectomized *in utero* with 6-hydroxydopamine, *J. Dev. Physiol.* **2:**119–137.

57. Foster, D. O., Depocas, F., and Frydman, M. L., 1980, Noradrenaline-induced calorigenesis in warm- and cold-acclimated rats: Relations between

concentration of noradrenaline in arterial plasma, blood flow to differently located masses of brown adipose tissue, and calorigenic response, *Can. J. Physiol. Pharmacol.* **58:**915–924.

58. Fink, S. A., and Williams, J. A., 1976, Adrenergic receptors mediating depolarization in brown adipose tissue, *Am. J. Physiol.* **231:**700–706.

59. Bukowiecki, L., Follea, N., Paradis, A., and Collet, A., 1980, Stereospecific stimulation of brown adipocyte respiration by catecholamines via beta-1-adrenoreceptors, *Am. J. Physiol.* **238:**E552–E563.

60. Himms-Hagen, J., 1976, Cellular thermogenesis, *Annu. Rev. Physiol.* **38:**315–351.

61. Desautels, M., and Himms-Hagen, J., 1979, Roles of noradrenaline and protein synthesis in the cold-induced increase in purine nucleotide binding by rat brown adipose tissue mitochondria, *Can. J. Biochem.* **57:**968–976.

62. Rabbi, T., Cassuto, Y., and Gutman, A., 1977, Lipolysis in brown adipose tissue of cold- and heat-acclimated hamsters, *J. Appl. Physiol.* **43:**1007–1011.

63. Lindberg, O., Bieber, L. L., and Houstek, J., 1976, Brown adipose tissue metabolism: An attempt to apply results from *in vitro* experiments on tissue *in vivo*, in: *Regulation of Depressed Metabolism and Thermogenesis* (L. Jansky and X. J. Musacchia, eds.), pp. 117–136, Thomas, Springfield, Ill.

64. Leblanc, J., and Villemaire, A., 1970, Thyroxine and noradrenaline on noradrenaline sensitivity, cold resistance, and brown fat, *Am. J. Physiol.* **218:**1742–1745.

65. Rothwell, N. J., and Stock, M. J., 1980, Similarities between cold- and diet-induced thermogenesis in the rat, *Can. J. Physiol. Pharmacol.* **58:**842–848.

66. Himms-Hagen, J., 1972, Lipid metabolism during cold-exposure and during cold-acclimation, *Lipids* **7:**310–323.

67. Maickel, R. P., Matussek, N., Stern, D. N., and Brodie, B. B., 1967, The sympathetic nervous system as a homeostatic mechanism. I. Absolute need for sympathetic nervous function in body temperature maintenance of cold-exposed rats, *J. Pharmacol. Exp. Ther.* **157:**103–110.

68. Gilgen, A., Maickel, R. P., Nikodijevic, O., and Brodie, B. B., 1962, Essential role of catecholamines in the mobilization of free fatty acids and glucose after exposure to cold, *Life Sci.* **12:**709–715.

69. Depocas, F., 1961, Biochemical changes in exposure and acclimation to cold environments, *Br. Med Bull.* **17:**25–31.

70. LaFrance, L., Lagace, G., and Routhier, D., 1980, Free fatty acid turnover and oxygen consumption: Effects of noradrenaline in nonfasted and non-anesthetized cold-adapted rats, *Can. J. Physiol. Pharmacol.* **58:**797–804.

71. Maekubo, H., Moriya, K., and Hiroshige, T., 1977, Role of ketone bodies in nonshivering thermogenesis in cold-acclimated rats, *J. Appl. Physiol.* **42:**159–165.

72. Radomski, M. W., and Orme, T., 1971, Response of lipoprotein lipase in various tissues to cold exposure, *Am. J. Physiol.* **220:**1852–1856.

73. Sugahara, M., Baker, D. H., Harmon, B. G., and Jensen, A. H., 1969, Effect of ambient temperature and dietary amino acids on carcass fat deposition in rats, *J. Nutr.* **98:**344–350.

74. Kodama, A. M., and Pace, N., 1964, Effect of environmental temperature on hamster body fat composition, *J. Appl. Physiol.* **19:**863–867.

75. O'Hara, W. J., Allen, C., Shephard, R. J., and Allen, G., 1979, Fat loss in the cold—A controlled study, *J. Appl. Physiol. Respir. Environ. Exercise Physiol.* **46:**872–877.
76. Rosell, S., and Belfrage, E., 1979, Blood circulation in adipose tissue, *Physiol. Rev.* **59:**1078–1104.
77. Maickel, R., Sussman, H., Yamada, K., and Brodie, B., 1963, Control of adipose tissue lipase activity by the sympathetic nervous system, *Life Sci.* **3:**210–214.
78. Beck. L. V., Zaharko, D. S., and Kalser, S. C., 1967, Variation in serum insulin and glucose of rats with chronic cold exposure, *Life Sci.* **6:**1501–1506.
79. Baum, D., and Porte, D., 1971, Alpha-adrenergic inhibition of immunoreactive insulin release during deep hypothermia, *Am. J. Physiol.* **221:**303–311.
80. Raven, P. B., Niki, I., Dahms, T. E., and Horvath, S. M., 1970, Compensatory cardiovascular responses during an environmental cold stress, 5°C, *J. Appl. Physiol.* **29:**417–421.
81. Janssens, W. J., and Vanhoutte, P. M., 1979, Instantaneous changes of alpha-adrenoceptor affinity caused by moderate cooling in canine cutaneous veins, *Am. J. Physiol.* **234:**H330–H337.
82. Webb-Peploe, M. M., and Shepard, J. T., 1968, Responses of the superficial limb veins of the dog to changes in temperature, *Circ. Res.* **22:**737–746.
83. Millard, R. W., and Reite, O. B., 1975, Peripheral vascular response to norepinephrine at temperatures from 2 to 40°C, *J. Appl. Physiol.* **38:**26–30.
84. Budd, G. M., and Warhaft, N., 1966, Body temperature, shivering blood pressure and heart rate during a standard cold stress in Australia and Antarctica, *J. Physiol. (London)* **186:**216–232.
85. Wasserstrum, N., and Herd, J. A., 1977, Elevation of arterial blood pressure in the squirrel monkey at 10°C, *Am. J. Physiol.* **232:**H459–H463.
86. LeBlanc, J., Dulac, S., Cote, J., and Girard, B., 1975, Autonomic nervous system and adaptation to cold and man, *J. Appl. Physiol.* **39:**181–186.
87. Fregly, M. J., Field, F. P., Nelson, E. L., Tyler, P. E., and Dasler, R., 1977, Effect of chronic exposure to cold on some responses to catecholamines, *J. Appl. Physiol.* **42:**149–154.
88. Koo, A., and Liang, I. Y. S., 1978, Microvascular responses to norepinephrine in skeletal muscle of cold-acclimated rats, *J. Appl. Physiol.* **44:**190–194.
89. Landsberg, L., and Young, J. B., 1981, Diet-induced changes in sympathoadrenal activity: Implications for thermogenesis and obesity, *Obesity Metab.* **1:**5–33.
90. Rothwell, N. J., and Stock, M. J., 1979, A role for brown adipose tissue in diet-induced thermogenesis, *Nature (London)* **281:**31–35.
91. Young, J. B., and Landsberg, L., 1977, Suppression of sympathetic nervous system during fasting, *Science* **196:**1473–1475.
92. Young, J. B., and Landsberg, L., 1979, Effect of diet and cold exposure on norepinephrine turnover in pancreas and liver, *Am. J. Physiol.* **236:**E524–E533.
93. Rappaport, E. B., Young, J. B., and Landsberg, L., 1981, Impact of age on basal and diet-induced changes in sympathetic nervous system activity of Fischer rats, *J. Gerontol.* **36:**152–157.

94. Young, J. B., Saville, E., Rothwell, N. J., Stock, M. J., and Landsberg, L., 1982, Effect of diet and cold exposure on norepinephrine turnover in brown adipose tissue in the rat, *J. Clin. Invest.* **69:**1061–1071.

95. Rappaport, E. B., Young, J. B., and Landsberg, L., 1982, Effects of 2-deoxy-D-glucose on the cardiac sympathetic nerves and the adrenal medulla in the rat: Further evidence for a dissociation of sympathetic nervous system and adrenal medullary responses, *Endocrinology* **110:**650–656.

96. Jung, R. T., Shetty, P. S., Berrand, M., Callingham, B. A., and James, W. P. T., 1979, Role of catecholamines in hypotensive response to dieting, *Br. Med. J.* **1:**12–13.

97. DeHaven, J., Sherwin, R., Hendler, R., and Felig, P., 1980, Nitrogen and sodium balance and sympathetic-nervous-system activity in obese subjects treated with a low-calorie protein or mixed diet, *N. Engl. J. Med.* **302:**477–482.

98. Gross, H. A., Lake, C. R., Ebert, M. H., Ziegler, M. G., and Kopin, I. J., 1979, Catecholamine metabolism in primary anorexia nervosa, *J. Clin. Endocrinol. Metab.* **49:**805–809.

99. Santiago, J. A., Clarke, W. L., Shah, S. D., and Cryer, P. E., 1980, Epinephrine, norepinephrine, glucagon, and growth hormone release in association with physiological decrements in the plasma glucose concentration in normal and diabetic man, *J. Clin. Endocrinol. Metab.* **51:**877–883.

100. Wimpfheimer, C., Saville, E., Voirol, M. J., Danforth, E., Jr., and Burger, A. G., 1979, Starvation-induced decreased sensitivity of resting metabolic rate to triiodothyronine, *Science* **205:**1272–1273.

101. Shetty, P. S., Jung, R. T., and James, W. P., 1979, Effect of catecholamine replacement with levodopa on the metabolic response to semistarvation, *Lancet* **1:**77–79.

102. Burke, D., Sundlof, G., and Wallin, G., 1977, Postural effects on muscle nerve sympathetic activity in man, *J. Physiol. (London)* **272:**399–414.

103. Arner, P., Engfeldt, P., and Nowak, J., 1981, *In vivo* observations on the lipolytic effect of noradrenaline during therapeutic fasting, *J. Clin. Endocrinol. Metab.* **53:**1207–1212.

104. Young, J. B., Rowe, J. W., Pallotta, J. A., Sparrow, D., and Landsberg, L., 1980, Enhanced plasma norepinephrine response to upright posture and glucose administration in elderly human subjects, *Metabolism* **29:**532–539.

105. Welle, S., Lilavivathana, U., and Campbell, R. G., 1980, Increased plasma norepinephrine concentrations and metabolic rates following glucose ingestion in man, *Metabolism* **29:**806–809.

106. Welle, S., Lilivivat, U., and Campbell, R. G., 1981, Thermic effect of feeding in man: Increased plasma norepinephrine levels following glucose but not protein or fat consumption, *Metabolism* **30:**953–958.

107. Zwillich, C., Martin, B., Hofeldt, F., Charles, A., Subryan, V., and Burman, K., 1981, Lack of effects of beta sympathetic blockade on the metabolic and respiratory responses to carbohydrate feeding, *Metabolism.* **30:**451–456.

108. Young, J. B., and Landsberg, L., 1977, Stimulation of the sympathetic nervous system during sucrose feeding, *Nature* **269:**615–617.

109. Rappaport, E. B., Young, J. B., and Landsberg, L., 1982, Initiation, duration, and dissipation of diet-induced changes in sympathetic nervous system activity in the rat, *Metabolism* **31:**143–146.

110. Schwartz, J., Young, J. B., and Landsberg, L., 1982, Increased cardiac sympathetic nervous system (SNS) activity with fat (lard) feeding: A more potent stimulus than sucrose, *Clin. Res.* **30:**247A.

111. Katzeff, H. L., and Danforth, E., Jr., 1981, The thermogenic response to norepinephrine, food and exercise in lean man during overfeeding, *Clin. Res.* **29:**663A.

112. Rothwell, N. J., and Stock, M. J., 1981, Influence of noradrenaline on blood flow to brown adipose tissue in rats exhibiting diet-induced thermogenesis, *Pfluegers Arch.* **389:**237–242.

113. Brooks, S. L., Rothwell, N. J., Stock, M. J., Goodbody, A. E., and Trayhurn, P., 1980, Increased proton conductance pathway in brown adipose tissue mitochondria of rats exhibiting diet-induced thermogenesis, *Nature (London)* **286:**274–276.

114. Rothwell, N. J., Saville, M. E., Stock, M. J., and Wyllie, M. G., 1982, Catecholamine and thyroid hormone influence on brown fat Na^+K^+-ATPase activity and thermogenesis in the rat, *Horm. Metab. Res.* **14:**261–265.

115. Young, J. B., and Landsberg, L., 1981, Effect of concomitant fasting and cold exposure on sympathoadrenal activity in rats, *Am. J. Physiol.* **240:**E314–E319.

116. Landsberg, L., and Young, J. B., 1981, Diet-induced changes in sympathoadrenal activity: Implications for thermogenesis, *Life Sci.* **28:**1801–1817.

117. Young, J. B., and Landsberg, L., 1979, Sympathoadrenal activity in fasting pregnant rats: Dissociation of adrenal medullary and sympathetic nervous system responses, *J. Clin. Invest.* **64:**109–116.

118. Landsberg, L., Greff, L., Gunn, S., and Young, J. B., 1980, Adrenergic mechanisms in the metabolic adaptation to fasting and feeding: Effects of phlorizin on diet-induced changes in sympathoadrenal activity in the rat, *Metabolism* **29:**1128–1137.

119. Van Houten, M., and Posner, B. I., 1981, Cellular basis of direct insulin action in the central nervous system, *Diabetologia* **20:**255–267.

120. Oomura, Y., and Kita, H., 1981, Insulin acting as a modulator of feeding through the hypothalamus, *Diabetologia* **20:**290–298.

121. Rowe, J. W., Young, J. B., Minaker, K. L., Stevens, A. L., Pallotta, J., and Landsberg, L., 1981, Effect of insulin and glucose infusions on sympathetic nervous system activity in normal man, *Diabetes* **30:**219–225.

122. Shimazu, T., and Takahashi, A., 1980, Stimulation of hypothalamic nuclei has differential effects on lipid synthesis in brown and white adipose tissue, *Nature (London)* **284:**62–63.

123. Perkins, M. N., Rothwell, N. J., Stock, M. J., and Stone, T. W., 1981, Activation of brown adipose tissue thermogenesis by the ventromedial hypothalamus, *Nature (London)* **289:**401–402.

124. Shimazu, T., 1981, Central nervous system regulation of liver and adipose tissue metabolism, *Diabetologia* **20:**343–356.

125. Young, J. B., and Landsberg, L., 1980, Impaired suppression of sympathetic activity during fasting in the gold thioglucose-treated mouse, *J. Clin. Invest.* **65:**1086–1094.

126. Niijima, A., 1981, Visceral afferents and metabolic function, *Diabetologia* **20:**325–330.

127. Bravo, E. L., Tarazi, R. C., Gifford, R. W., and Stewart, B. H., 1979, Circulating and urinary catecholamines in pheochromocytoma: Diagnostic and pathophysiologic implication, *N. Engl. J. Med.* **301:**682–686.

128. Bravo, E. L., Tarazi, R. C., Fouad, F. M., Vidt, D. G., and Gifford, R. W., Jr., 1981, Clonidine-suppression test: A useful aid in the diagnosis of pheochromocytoma, *N. Engl. J. Med.* **305:**623–626.

129. Brown, M. J., Jenner, D. A., Allison, D. J., Lewis, P. J., and Dollery, C. T., 1981, Increased sensitivity and accuracy of phaeochromocytoma diagnosis achieved by use of plasma-adrenaline estimations and a pentolinium-suppression test, *Lancet* **1:**174–177.

130. Laursen, K., and Damgaard-Pedersen, K., 1980, CT for pheochromocytoma diagnosis, *Am. J. Roentgenol.* **134:**277–280.

131. Thomas, J. L., Bernardino, M. E., Samaan, N. A., and Hickey, R. C., 1980, CT of pheochromocytoma, *Am. J. Roentgenol.* **135:**477–482.

132. Thomas, J. L., and Bernardino, M. E., 1981, Pheochromocytoma in multiple endocrine adenomatosis: Efficacy of computed tomography, *J.A.M.A.* **245:**1467–1469.

133. Ganguly, A., Henry, D. P., Yune, H. Y., Pratt, J. H., Grim, C. E., Donohue, J. P., and Weinberger, M. H., 1979, Diagnosis and localization of pheochromocytoma: Detection by measurement of urinary norepinephrine excretion during sleep, plasma norepinephrine concentration and computerized axial tomography (CT-scan), *Am. J. Med.* **67:**21–26.

134. Paulubinskas, A. J., Roizen, M. F., and Conte, F. A., 1980, Localization of functioning pheochromocytomas by venous sampling and radioenzymatic analysis, *Radiology* **136:**495–496.

135. Jones, D. H., Reid, J. L., Hamilton, C. A., Allison, D. J., Welbourn, R. B., and Dollery, C. T., 1980, The biochemical diagnosis, localization and follow up of phaeochromocytoma: The role of plasma and urinary catecholamine measurements, *Q. J. Med.* **49:**341–361.

136. Sisson, J. C., Frager, M. S., Valk, T. W., Gross, M. D., Swanson, D. P., Wieland, D. M., Tobes, M. C., Beierwaltes, W. H., and Thompson, N. W., 1981, Scintigraphic localization of pheochromocytoma, *N. Engl. J. Med.* **305:**12–17.

137. Valk, T. W., Frager, M. S., Gross, M. D., Sisson, J. C., Wieland, D. M., Swanson, D. P., Mangner, T. J., and Beierwaltes, W. H., 1981, Spectrum of pheochromocytoma in multiple endocrine neoplasia: A scintigraphic portrayal using ^{131}I-metaiodobenzylguanidine, *Ann. Intern. Med.* **94:**762–767.

Parathyroid Hormone and Calcitonin

Karen E. Kleeman and Charles R. Kleeman

7.1. Introduction

In the course of reading and thinking a great deal about parathyroid hormone (PTH)—its purpose, its evolution, the effects of its excess and its deficiency—we have been led into speculation about the role of calcium in cellular economy. Increasingly we appreciate calcium's critical role as a regulator in all kinds of cells and in organisms of all levels of complexity. Even the simplest organisms appear to employ calcium; it regulates chemotactic behavior[1] and sporulation[2] in bacteria; and it has been adapted to more and more uses in multicellular organisms. Cell aggregation, cell–cell communication, membrane integrity and permeability, microtubular assembly, cell division and growth, blood coagulation, hormone–response coupling, and electrical stimulus–response coupling, including muscle contraction and neurotransmitter release, all require calcium and are to some degree regulated by it.[3]

Life evolved in a high-calcium environment, the ocean. One assumes that the evolving organism would have found the most effective and efficient way to make its peace with the calcium ion. It almost seems

KAREN E. KLEEMAN ● Department of Psychiatry and Biobehavioral Science, UCLA Neuropsychiatric Institute and School of Medicine, Los Angeles, California 90024. CHARLES R. KLEEMAN ● Division of Nephrology, Department of Medicine, UCLA Center for the Health Sciences and School of Medicine, Los Angeles, California 90024.

paradoxical, therefore, that living things have evolved in such a way that calcium, unless tightly controlled, is poisonous to them. Even unicellular organisms have ways of keeping their cytosolic calcium low, though it costs them energy to dispose of the calcium that is always diffusing in from the environment. On the other hand, its very availability might be said to make calcium a logical choice for a regulator; if energy must be expended to maintain control over it, at least no energy was required to find it and hoard it—not, that is, as long as life remained in the ocean. PTH, incidentally, first appeared with the move to land.

Kretsinger[4] has suggested that the initial "choice" made by the cell was not the choice of calcium as a regulator, but the choice of phosphate as an energy source. Phosphate having been so chosen, it would then become necessary to find a way to keep intracellular free calcium very low, so that it would not precipitate with phosphate and render the latter useless to the cell. Kretsinger suggests that the unicellular organism, first having found a way to keep calcium concentration down, made a virtue of necessity by adapting the resultant extracellular-to-intracellular calcium gradient for use in information transfer and cell regulation.

As techniques for measuring cytosolic free calcium have improved, our estimate of this value has fallen, and free calcium concentration is now felt to be between 10^{-7} and 10^{-8}M in most resting cells.[4] This means that the extracellular free calcium level is *10,000 to 100,000 times* the intracellular free calcium level. No remotely comparable gradient exists for any other ion or molecule in the circulation. This fantastically large gradient makes calcium an ideal regulator or "second messenger": because of the large gradient, the slightest alteration in the cell membrane that increases its permeability to calcium permits a relatively large increase in the amount of calcium entering the cell at the alteration site. Calcium-regulated processes near the alteration site are switched on; then, the excess calcium is rapidly taken up and the gradient reestablished. The calcium-regulated processes may thereby be switched off, or they may be perpetuated by calcium-activated agents, such as cyclic nucleotides.

It is evident that if this system is to be maintained, the excess calcium that enters the cell must be rapidly sequestered by intracellular organelles, until it can eventually be pumped out of the cell. This ultimate disposition is the responsibility of a ubiquitous calcium pump located in the cell membrane, supplied with energy by a calcium-dependent ATPase. The pump prevents the cell from becoming completely loaded with calcium and therefore nonfunctional, but it does not, at least in most cell types, appear to have the capacity to bring down cytosolic calcium quickly. Mitochondria and reticular membranes share this responsibility. They are able not only to lower cytosolic calcium quickly, but also to prevent its free diffusion from its point of entry throughout the cytoplasm. When calcium is delivered into a cell with a micropipette, there is a short-lived rise in cytosolic calcium only in the vicinity of the micropipette; the calcium does not spread far before being sequestered.[5] Rapid sequestration increases the effectiveness and versatility of calcium as a second messenger, since it permits different processes in different parts of the cell to be regulated independently by changes in cytosolic calcium.

The importance of mitochondria versus that of reticular membranes in the rapid sequestration of calcium is still being debated and almost certainly varies from cell type to cell type. There is evidence to suggest that in nerve terminals[6] and skeletal and cardiac muscle cells[7] rapid calcium uptake is primarily accomplished by calcium pumps in reticular membranes, mitochondria acting as a backup system to deal with particularly heavy calcium loads. That calcium-transport ATPase represents *70 to 80%* of the total protein content of cardiac sarcoplasmic reticulum, and 60 to 90% of total protein in sarcoplasmic reticulum from various other muscles[7], gives us some indication of how important a function calcium transport is for these membranes. For most cell types, however, mitochondria probably carry most of the burden of intracellular calcium uptake.[8] Mitochondria from virtually all vertebrate and some invertebrate tissues can transport calcium inward with high affinity in an energy-dependent process, coupled to respiration and ATP production, and requiring virtually simultaneous uptake of an appropriate anion (usually phosphate) so that the calcium taken up can be stored in a bound, electroneutral form.[9,10] Calcium uptake is such an important function of animal mitochondria that it takes precedence over the production of ATP for other purposes.[9] By the time ambient calcium concentration rises above a few micromolar, mitochondria are using most of the energy derived from electron transport to sequester calcium.[9] The need for this kind of priority is readily understandable when we consider that critical calcium-regulated processes may be activated at a calcium level of 10^{-6} M and inhibited at a cytosolic calcium level of 10^{-5}.[11,12]

Hypocalcemia will, of course, decrease the extracellular-to-intracellular calcium gradient and so can be expected to interfere with all manner of basic cellular processes. The body clearly has some capacity to adapt to chronic hypocalcemia, although complete adaptation does not occur. The evolving organism, having become dependent on calcium, did not change course when it found itself no longer literally surrounded by an abundance of this element, but found ways, first to increase its absorption, and next to exploit a store of it in the form of the calcified skeleton. It seems undeniable to us that PTH evolved to meet the need to maintain the serum calcium in the face of a scarcity of environmental calcium. In keeping with this function, PTH exerts its regulatory effect only at low to normal calcium levels; above a serum calcium of about 11 mg/dl (2.75 mM/liter), PTH no longer effectively regulates calcium metabolism. Compared with our ability to defend against hypocalcemia, we are ill-equipped in general to defend against hypercalcemia. We have, in fact, a somewhat ironic situation in which individual cells, whose function still reflects a high-calcium environment, are more equipped to deal with high calcium than are whole land animals, which have "learned" to adapt to a scarcity of calcium.

7.2. Chemistry, Synthesis, and Secretion

PTH is a single polypeptide chain of 84 amino acids. The complete amino acid sequence of the human hormone has been published by Keutmann et al.[13] It differs from that of the bovine hormone at 11 positions, 10 of which represent single-step mutations in a triplet-base codon. Six of these substitutions occur in the region 40–47, or midportion of the hormone, three occur in the N-terminal segment (residues 1, 7, and 16), and two in the C-terminal segment (residues 79 and 83). The substitutions may suffice to produce significant conformational changes in the PTH molecule; this would explain the incomplete immunologic cross-reactivity between human hormone and hormone from other species, particularly with antisera directed at the middle portion of the molecule.

PTH has no cysteine residues, so it has no disulfide bridges, but it does appear to have a secondary and tertiary structure.[14,15] Presumably this structure affects hormone binding, metabolism, and activity, but very little is known of this aspect of PTH chemistry. Habener and Potts[16] showed that an antiserum raised against synthetic fragment 1–12 of bovine PTH reacted very weakly with bPTH 1–26, bPTH 1–28, bPTH 1–34, bPTH 2–34, and bPTH 3–34. They interpret these results to mean that the biologically active N-terminal peptide normally exists in a three-dimensional conformation that shields residues 1–12 from interaction with antibody. The folding of the PTH molecule might serve to bring the receptor-binding region, which probably lies in the neighborhood of residues 20–25,[17] into proximity with the N-terminal residues 1–3, which are required to activate adenylate cyclase.[18]

Quite a lot of attention has been focused on the precursor forms of PTH, their definition and their roles. The 84-amino-acid PTH molecule is originally synthesized in a larger form, the 115-amino-acid peptide preproPTH, which has a 31-amino-acid N-terminal sequence that is absent from the final PTH molecule. The 25 N-terminal amino acids are cleaved from preproPTH, leaving the 90-amino-acid proPTH, which is then cleaved to PTH. Nothing longer than the 115-amino-acid preproPTH can be shown to be synthesized, either on preproPTH mRNA or on DNA prepared from mRNA by reverse transcriptase, so it seems established that preproPTH is, in fact, the first and longest form of the hormone and the "authentic and complete representation of the gene for PTH."[19]

Our knowledge of the details of the PTH synthetic process has grown enormously. Habener and Kronenberg[20] have developed the most complete model. The painstaking work of many investigators has identified numerous possible loci of control of synthesis, and eventually we should know exactly where calcium acts to regulate the amount of PTH released into the circulation. The work has applications that extend beyond the parathyroid gland, however: the process of PTH synthesis is felt to be analogous to that of "exportable" proteins in general, including insulin, immunoglobulins, albumin, and pancreatic enzymes.[20]

Proteins destined for export from secretory cells are believed to be synthesized on polyribosomes attached to the endoplasmic reticulum, while proteins that are to remain inside the cell are synthesized on free ribosomes.[21] Many of these export proteins are first synthesized in precursor forms that have highly hydrophobic N-terminal precursor sequences. Blobel and Sabatini[22] proposed in 1971 that these hydrophobic sequences bind to the reticular membrane and function to direct the new protein, as it is synthesized, into the endoplasmic reticulum, where it is sequestered from the proteins that are to remain in the cell[20] and somehow guided to the Golgi complex for packaging and eventual secretion (the "signal hypothesis").

What is the evidence that this sequence occurs in the parathyroid cell? The 25-amino-acid precursor sequence of preproPTH contains 20 hydrophobic amino acids.[23] Habener et al. have synthesized this sequence and shown that it binds to the microsomal fraction of parathyroid gland homogenates.[23] Similarly, both preproPTH and proPTH, when added to subcellular fractions of parathyroid gland, tend to associate with membranes.[23,24] PreproPTH can be synthesized in a cell-free system, but no proPTH is formed unless microsomes are added (indicating that the as yet uncharacterized enzyme that cleaves preproPTH must be associated with these membranes); however, to obtain proPTH, these membranes must be added during, not after, preproPTH synthesis.[25] Since the preproPTH molecule will bind to the membrane either during or after synthesis, the cleavage enzyme is probably not present on the outer reticular membrane. Habener and Potts[24] added trypsin and chymotrypsin to particulate fractions of bovine parathyroid gland and showed that endogenous preproPTH was almost completely degraded, while

40–50% of endogenous PTH and proPTH remained intact; however, all but 2–8% of *added* PTH and proPTH was degraded, and when membranes were dispersed with detergent, endogenous hormone became similarly susceptible to proteolysis. Thus, it seems likely that most of the proPTH and PTH inside the cell is enclosed and protected in membranes.

ProPTH is transported within the endoplasmic reticulum, by a process requiring energy and probably microtubules, to the Golgi apparatus, where cleavage to PTH occurs simply by removal of the 6-amino-acid N-terminal sequence.[26] The entire process, from initiation to secretion of PTH, takes 15 to 20 min, so that synthesis of new hormone obviously cannot be relied upon to correct acute hypocalcemia rapidly.

There are several points along the course of hormone synthesis where control might be effected, but there is surprisingly little evidence with regard to any of them. The amount of hormone stored within the parathyroid gland is small compared to stores in other endocrine glands; Mayer and Hurst have estimated that bovine glands contain enough hormone for 5–6 hr of basal secretion or 1–1½ hr of maximal secretion.[27] It is obvious, therefore, that although hypocalcemic stress may first be met by increased secretion of PTH, this increase must somehow be coupled to an increase in the synthetic rate; how or where this is accomplished is unknown. As we stated in an earlier volume of this series,[28] cleavage of hormone precursors does not appear to be regulated. Habener *et al.*[23] found in preliminary studies that the association of prepro PTH with microsomal membranes appeared to be enhanced by the calcium chelator EDTA; however, since Smith and Boime[29] observed the same effect of EDTA, and the opposite effect of calcium, on the processing of human placental lactogen—a hormone whose synthesis is not stimulated by hypocalcemia—it is hard to conclude that Habener *et al.* have uncovered a step at which calcium regulates PTH synthesis. *In vitro*, it takes hours for the rate of proPTH synthesis to change in response to a change in the extracellular calcium concentration[30]; given this time course, it is most likely that regulation occurs at the transcriptional level,[31] although there is no direct proof of this. However, as pointed out by Habener and Potts,[31] now that the DNA for preproPTH has been synthesized,[19] it could be used as a probe to measure change in RNA levels in response to changes in the ambient calcium concentration.

In 1975, Habener *et al.*[32] described the apparent intracellular degradation of a large fraction of newly synthesized PTH in parathyroid slices exposed to high calcium. Although they failed to find any quantity of PTH fragments in medium or tissue, their work takes on new interest in the light of recent recognition that the parathyroid gland secretes C-terminal PTH fragments. Until lately, there was general agreement that only intact PTH 1–84, and no smaller peptides, were secreted by the parathyroid gland. However, more and more evidence is accumulating that this may not be the case. Silverman and Yalow[33] identified in crude parathyroid extracts hormone fragments identical to those circulating in plasma. Flueck et al.[34] found C-terminal hormone fragments in large quantity in the venous effluent of parathyroid tumors. Di Bella et al.[35] found abundant C-terminal fragments in an extract of parathyroid tumors. An obvious question is whether these C-terminal fragments reflect the activity of a regulated degradation process that controls the amount of biologically active PTH secreted by the parathyroid gland; two groups have reported supporting evidence for this hypothesis. Dambacher et al.[36] took serum samples from normal volunteers, patients with primary hyperparathyroidism, patients with pseudohypoparathyroidism, and patients with secondary hyperparathyroidism of vitamin D deficiency. They then separated hormone and hormone fragments using gel filtration, and analyzed the different peaks with a sensitive C-terminal assay. C-terminal fragments predominated in patients with primary and both kinds of secondary hyperparathyroidism; however, the ratio of C-terminal to intact hormone was many times greater in the *hyper*calcemic patients with primary hyperparathyroidism than in the *hypo*calcemic patients with secondary hyperparathyroidism, suggesting that the quantity of C-terminal fragments was somehow controlled by the level of serum calcium (though this work does not fix the locus of control in the parathyroid gland rather than in the peripheral sites of hormone metabolism; see below). In a more direct study, Mayer et al.[37] collected samples of parathyroid venous blood from anesthetized calves during normocalcemia, hypocalcemia, and hypercalcemia, separated hormone and fragments with gel filtration, and analyzed the fragments with N-terminal and C-terminal assays. They found two peaks of immunoreactivity, one recognized by both N- and C-terminal assays (presumably intact hormone) and one recognized only by the C-terminal assay (presumably C-terminal fragments) in all samples; however, in the hypocalcemic samples there was almost no fragment peak, in the normocalcemic samples the two peaks were approximately equal, and in the hypercalcemic samples almost nothing but presumed C-terminal fragments was detected. We should point out, however, that in contrast, Morrissey and Cohn,[38] studying dispersed parathyroid cells, detected secretion of C-terminal fragments but found no change in the ratio of fragments to intact hormone with change in ambient calcium concentration.

It is unlikely that these fragments are synthesized *de novo;* the weight of the evidence suggests that they are a by-product of calcium-regulated intracellular degradation of hormone. Since fragments have been detected even in low calcium, when the quantity of fragments produced is very small, it seems likely that the gland cannot further degrade them but simply secretes all that are produced. It is unclear, however, why Habener et al.[32] were unable to find hormone fragments in their original experiments with parathyroid slices.

7.3. Control of Secretion

Unquestionably, PTH secretion is controlled primarily by the plasma concentration of free calcium ion. In all likelihood, calcium, the first recognized regulator of PTH secretion, is the only one of any physiologic importance. However, there are other agents that have been found to stimulate or inhibit PTH release, and these have been the focus of quite a lot of study lately, despite the fact that there is no evidence to suggest that their role is of much significance.

In our minds, the most interesting question that remains to be answered is: what does calcium do to the parathyroid cell, and how does it do it? Or, in more specific terms: at what points in the sequence of synthesis and secretion does calcium act? What, if any, are the mediators of its effects? And why does the parathyroid cell react differently from all other cells? For, as we and others have pointed out, other secretory cells are activated, not inactivated, by calcium entry and are little, if at all, affected by changes in serum calcium within the normal range, while parathyroid cells are exquisitely sensitive to such changes.[27] We will report some progress that has been made toward finding answers to these questions, and we will add some speculations as well.

As an aside, we would mention a technical advance that has made it possible to study some aspects of the process of PTH secretion with much greater exactness. This is the dispersed cell preparation. Brown et al.[39] first described in 1976 a method of preparing viable bovine parathyroid cells free of their connective tissue stroma; more recently they have applied the same method to the preparation of dispersed cells from human glands removed at surgery.[40] Use of these cell preparations, rather than whole glands or gland slices, ensures that any control agent being tested reaches all cells more or less equally. Also, since in this preparation the extracellular space and the incubation medium are the same, it is easy to distinguish the intracellular from the extracellular. This separation has made it possible to define more clearly the time course of the parathyroid cell's response to various stimuli (see below).

7.3.1. Control by Calcium

The basic pattern of the parathyroid response to changes in ambient calcium has been defined: a sigmoidal, rather than a linear relationship

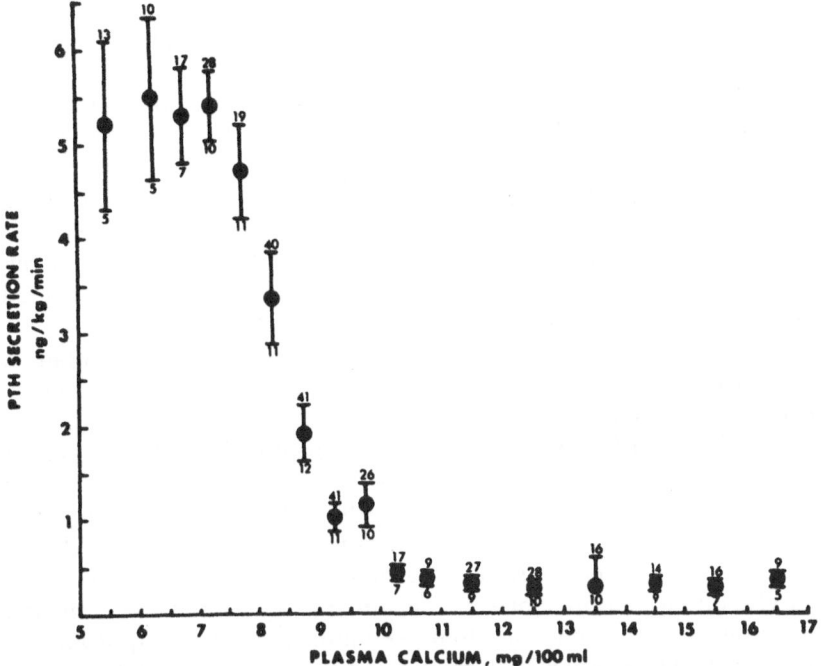

Fig. 1. Secretory response of bovine parathyroid glands to induced alterations of plasma calcium concentration. The symbols and vertical bars indicate the secretory rate (mean ± SE) in calcium concentration ranges of 1.0 or 0.5 mg/100 ml. The number of calves and samples are indicated, respectively, by numbers below and above the bars. From Ref. 27.

exists between calcium concentration and hormone secretion. This relationship was first demonstrated by Blum et al.[41] who measured peripheral plasma PTH in cows, and has more recently been confirmed by Mayer and Hurst,[27] who measured PTH in parathyroid venous effluent in calves. As can be seen in Fig. 1, Mayer and Hurst found that PTH secretion rate increased very little as long as serum calcium, though falling, remained within the normal range. As soon as serum calcium fell below 9 mg/dl, however, hormone secretion increased very rapidly. Maximum secretion was reached at a serum calcium of about 7.5 mg/dl, and a further fall in calcium did not elicit any greater secretion. The figure also confirms previous reports[42] that some degree of secretion continues, albeit at a very low level, even during marked hypercalcemia (so-called "nonsuppressible" secretion). In light of the work that has demonstrated secretion of hormone fragments by the parathyroid gland, the obvious question arises as to whether the measured "nonsuppressible" secretion might consist only of fragments, not of active hormone. However, in demonstrating fragment secretion with specific N-terminal and C-terminal assays, Mayer et al.[37] incidentally showed that the immunoreactive material secreted by the gland during hypercalcemia definitely contains at least some intact hormone (i.e., material that was recognized by both N- and C-terminal assays). Brown *et al.* obtained similar results using N- and C-terminal assays to study the secretory product of dispersed human parathyroid cells at high calcium.[40] There are, in addition, older observations on the handling of excess calcium by normal and hypoparathyroid subjects that suggested that a basal level of nonsuppressible PTH secretion must exist: when hypercalcemia is experimentally induced in normal and hypoparathyroid subjects, urinary calcium excretion in the normal subjects never reaches the level attained by the hypoparathyroid subjects.[43] From these old and new data, we can confidently conclude that a basal level of PTH secretion is maintained irrespective of the plasma calcium, at least during acute hypercalcemia. Parfitt[3] has stressed the observation that, even during prolonged hypercalcemia, parathyroid glands do not atrophy, as do other glands whose secretion can be completely suppressed.

Although it responds most vigorously to frank hypocalcemia, the parathyroid gland does not permit serum calcium to fluctuate freely within the normocalcemic range. Mayer and Hurst were able to show, by careful manipulation of plasma calcium, that small changes in calcium, even within the normal range, do indeed induce small, but appropriate, changes in PTH secretion.[27] Dispersed human parathyroid cells are also very sensitive to changes in ambient calcium within the normocalcemic range, responding with obvious changes in hormone secretion rate.[40] Finally, in studies on normal human subjects, Broadus *et al.* found that nephrogenous cAMP, the production of which has been shown to correlate very well with the PTH secretion rate,[44] was as fully suppressed by low-dose calcium infusion, which did not raise serum calcium to hypercalcemic levels, as by high-dose calcium infusion, which produced frank hypercalcemia.[45] All this should not be taken to mean that in any given individual, serum ionized calcium will always be the same from hour to hour and day to day; as we will discuss below, there are other influences on PTH secretion and on calcium homeostasis that can affect the serum calcium level. However, the fact that PTH secretion rate and serum calcium are indeed related within the normocalcemic range does mean that adequately refined measurements of circulating PTH and nephrogenous cAMP, plotted against serum calcium, should be able to distinguish a patient with high-normal serum calcium who truly is hyperparathyroid from one who is not. The close relationship between PTH secretion and ambient calcium must also be taken into account by any theorist who tries to explain how the calcium ion manipulates the parathyroid cell. This question, though of less immediate interest to clinicians than the accurate diagnosis of hyperparathyroidism, takes us into intriguing realms of cellular physiology.

Before we address this question, we will consider what we know about where, as opposed to how, calcium acts in the parathyroid cell to alter secretion of hormone. Since increased PTH is released from dispersed bovine parathyroid cells less than 5 min after exposure to low calcium,[46] while new hormone synthesis takes at least 15 to 20 min, a decrease in serum calcium must affect *secretion* directly. We do not know whether there is a necessary coupling between these two processes, such that any change in secretion rate somehow triggers a corresponding change in synthetic rate, or whether the two are regulated independently; in the first case, calcium might need to act at only one point, while in the second case it would need to act at at least two. We also do not know whether calcium acts directly on the secretory process—which has, itself, not been well described—or whether it simply inhibits degradation of the intact hormone present in the cell, with available hormone then being automatically secreted, as Habener *et al.* have suggested.[32]

We believe it likely that calcium will eventually be found to act at several points. Morrissey and Cohn[38] found evidence of two hormone pools in parathyroid cells, an older "storage" pool and a pool of newly synthesized hormone, which could contain the PTH subject to calcium-dependent degradation. Low calcium stimulated secretion of hormone from both pools. Their experiments also showed that the two pools are regulated independently, which would suggest that calcium must act directly on both of them.

Parfitt[3] has prepared a timetable of the various stages in parathyroid gland response to the stimulus of low calcium (Table I).

We will discuss three tentative answers to the question of how calcium manipulates the parathyroid cell: through cAMP, through pros-

Table I. Parathyroid Cell Response to Hypocalcemia[a]

Mechanism	Time scale
1. Release of preformed hormone ↑	Seconds to minutes
2. Intracellular degradation ↓	Minutes to hours
3. Hormone synthesis ↑	Hours to days
4. Quiescent interval ↓	Days to weeks
5. Hyperplasia	Weeks to months

[a] Reproduced with permission from Parfitt and Kleerekoper.[3]

taglandins, and through modification or abandonment of the mechanisms that other cells use to maintain intracellular calcium homeostasis.

Because there is good evidence that cAMP mediates the effect of sympathomimetics, among other agents, on PTH release (see below), it has seemed natural to postulate that calcium, also, might act through cAMP. Human parathyroid gland, like that of the horse,[47] contains a calcium-inhibitable adenylate cyclase that is very sensitive to low concentrations of calcium.[48] Brown et al.[46] found that in dispersed bovine parathyroid cells, increasing ambient calcium from 0.1mM to over 1mM produced a parallel and proportionate decrease of intracellular cAMP concentration and PTH release (Fig. 2). Increasing calcium, even within the normocalcemic range, also inhibited both cAMP accumulation and PTH release in response to various agonists.

Nonetheless, although there is reason to believe that cAMP is involved in the response of the parathyroid cell to changes in ambient calcium, there are many reasons to think it unlikely that cAMP is the sole mediator. The calcium-inhibitable adenylate cyclase described by Rodriguez et al.[48] showed maximum activity in zero calcium; in contrast,

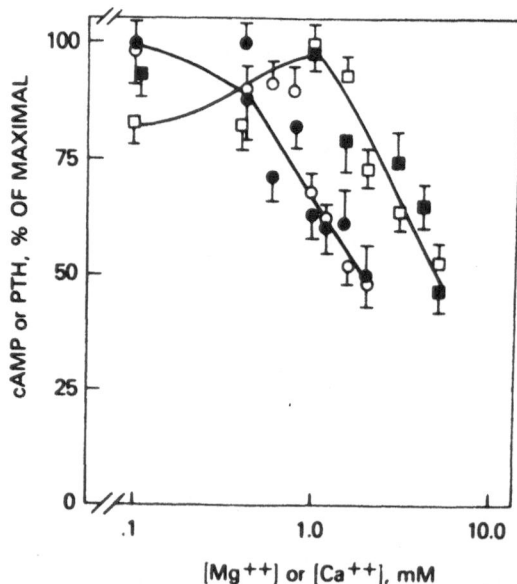

Fig. 2. Inhibition of cAMP accumulation and PTH release by divalent cations. Dispersed cells were incubated for 15 min at 37°C in standard medium with either 0.5 mM $MgSO_4$ or 0.5 mM $CaCl_2$ and increasing concentrations of $CaCl_2$ (●, ○) or $MgSO_4$ (■, □), respectively. Intracellular cAMP (●, ■) and PTH (○, □) were determined on separate sets of incubation vials. From Ref. 46.

Ramp et al.[49] found that parathyroid glands incubated in calcium-free medium released *no* detectable PTH (thereby incidentally demonstrating that parathyroid cells do share with all other secretory cells a requirement for at least *some* calcium to permit secretion.) The calcium-inhibitable adenylate cyclase was also 75% inhibited by only 0.5 mM calcium, a concentration at which PTH secretion is maximal; thus, it would appear that the range of calcium concentrations within which modulation of PTH secretion occurs and that within which adenylate cyclase is progressively inhibited are not very well matched. High calcium alters the relationship between isoproterenol-stimulated cAMP accumulation and PTH secretion, such that at any given level of cAMP less PTH is released[32]; one would not expect this to be the case if calcium regulated PTH release only by changing the intracellular concentration of cAMP. Finally, Morrissey and Cohn[38] found that the effects of dibutyryl cAMP and low calcium on PTH secretion were not identical: low calcium appeared to stimulate release of hormone from two different pools, dibutyryl cAMP from only one. We think it likely that cAMP mediates some, but not all, of the stimulatory effects of low calcium on the parathyroid cell. For instance, it may be that release of PTH from the "storage pool" of hormone described by Morrissey and Cohn[38] is effected via cAMP, while the calcium-dependent degradation process described by Habener and co-workers,[19] and perhaps some steps in the synthesis of hormone, are controlled by intracellular calcium independent of cAMP. Since adenylate cyclase appears to be located only at the surface of the parathyroid cell,[50] cAMP is unlikely to be involved in any process, such as hormone synthesis, which takes place far from the cell membranes.

Prostaglandins have been examined as possible mediators of PTH release, as they have been found to inhibit hormone-stimulated cAMP accumulation in several systems. Gardner et al. found that $PGF_{2\alpha}$ markedly inhibited PTH release from dispersed bovine parathyroid cells at low to normal ambient calcium. Secretion at high calcium levels—i.e., the "nonsuppressible" secretion—was not affected. $PGF_{2\alpha}$, by an apparently intracellular mechanism, also inhibited cAMP accumulation and PTH release induced by isoproterenol, dopamine, and methylisobutylxanthine (a phosphodiesterase inhibitor).[51] The same group reported PGE_2 stimulation of both cAMP and PTH release; however, PGE_2-mediated release could be suppressed by high calcium.[52] Moreover, Licata et al.[53] found an *inhibitory* effect of PGE_2 as well as PGE_1 on secretion. Though all this work is interesting, the various findings are hard to reconcile, and the possible role of endogenous prostaglandins in modulating PTH release must be considered speculative.

It would seem intuitively evident that the parathyroid cell must do something with calcium that other kinds of cells do not. Although the amount of calcium entering any kind of cell will fluctuate somewhat as the serum calcium fluctuates, it must be the aim of all but the parathyroid cell to prevent this fluctuation from affecting either the cytosolic free calcium level or any cell function. It would clearly not do to leave delicately balanced calcium-regulated processes at the mercy of transient and unrelated changes in the serum calcium. In the parathyroid cell, however, this is precisely what *must* happen. Given our knowledge of the elements of cellular calcium regulation, discussed in Section 7.1, we can think of several possible alterations in the system that would confer upon it calcium sensitivity:

1. The parathyroid cell might handle calcium exactly as other cells do, with rapid uptake by mitochondria and/or smooth endoplasmic reticulum, outward pumping, and maintenance of a constant cytosolic free calcium; but either the mitochondria, reticular membrane, or cell membrane pump would be linked to some kind of sensing element that would detect changes in calcium influx and link these to the processes of hormone synthesis and secretion. There is at present no evidence for such a sensor.

2. As compared to other cell types, mitochondria in parathyroid cells might be either very few in number, or have relatively little capacity for rapid uptake or storage of calcium. Thus, if serum calcium were to rise, cytosolic calcium would also rise, because a rapid, high-capacity calcium "buffering" system would not be available. Over time, of course, if the cell were not to be overcome and killed by continuous influx of calcium, either the cell membrane pump would have to adapt to pumping more calcium outward, or mitochondria would have to multiply. The fact that oxyphil cells, which are nonsecretory and therefore have relatively low metabolic demands, not only increase in number during hypercalcemia[54] but are packed with mitochondria (despite their lesser need for ATP production) as compared with the actively secreting chief cell suggests that hypercalcemia does indeed lead to mitochondrial multiplication. There have been, to our knowledge, no studies of the kinetics of calcium influx and efflux in parathyroid mitochondria, although the appropriate methodology exists and has been applied in numerous studies on mitochondria from other tissues (Refs. 55–57, and others). The latter studies have revealed, however, that there are considerable differences in mitochondrial calcium transport in different tissues. For instance, mitochondria from cerebral cortex take up calcium more rapidly, and much more efficiently at very low calcium concentrations, than do heart or liver mitochondria[58]; mitochondria in calcifying cartilage can store 200 times as much calcium as mitochondria from most other tissues.[59] It is certainly conceivable, therefore, that parathyroid cell mitochondria could lie at the low end of a spectrum with regard to capacity

for calcium uptake, and that the parathyroid cell could thus be rendered sensitive to calcium.

3. The plasma membrane pump, which pumps calcium out of the cell, might be incapable of responding to changes in intracellular calcium with an increase or decrease in outward pumping. Then, if storage by intracellular organelles did not change, a change in ambient calcium would result in a new steady-state cytosolic free calcium level. Glick and Mockel[60] have recently studied ^{45}Ca kinetics in parathyroid tissue and come to the conclusion that the parathyroid cell behaves as if it had such a nonadapting calcium pump. Uptake of ^{45}Ca by parathyroid gland slices was rapid and avid over a wide range of medium calcium concentration, from 0.5 to 2.5 mM; however, the rate of ^{45}Ca *efflux* from the tissue was constant and independent of the rate of influx, so that the tissue calcium content steadily increased as the medium calcium was raised.

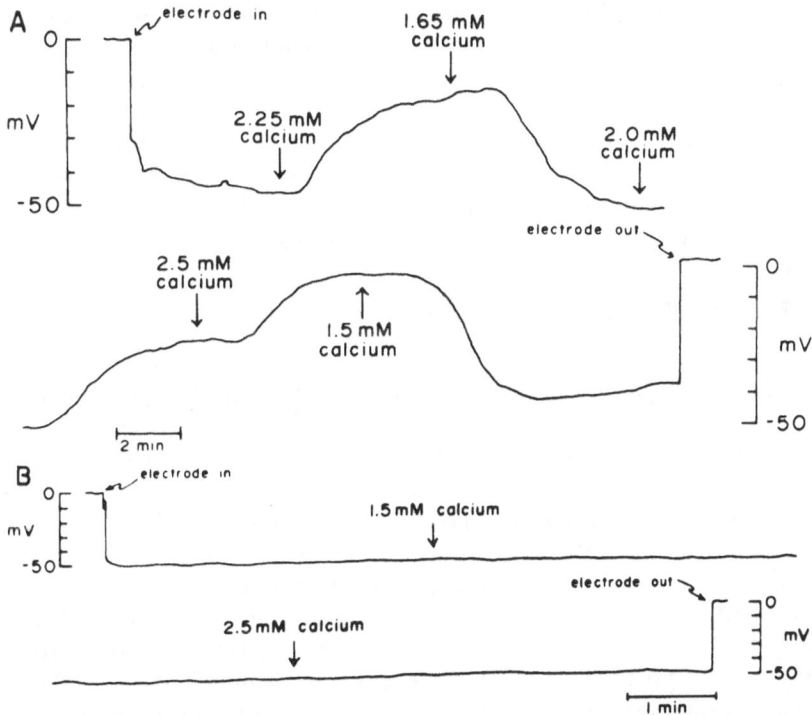

Fig. 3. (A) Continuous intracellular record from mouse parathyroid cell showing response to alterations in calcium concentration (1.5, 1.65, 1.8, 2.0, 2.25, and 2.5 mM Ca). Cell was impaled in 1.8 mM Ca. (B) Continuous intracellular record from mouse thyroid cell showing response to alterations in calcium concentration (1.5 and 2.5 mM Ca). Cell was impaled in 2.5 mM Ca. Arrows corresponding with solution changes in both A and B indicate introductions of a new solution to superfusion reservoir. From Ref. 61.

Bruce and Anderson[61] have published an important study of the response of the parathyroid cell membrane potential to changes in calcium. The study of the electrophysiology of glands has attracted substantial interest only in the last 10 years or so, but enough has been discovered to make it seem clear that all secretory cells respond to secretagogues with changes in membrane potential; that these changes result from changes in membrane permeability to one or another ion, with increased flow of the ion along its concentration gradient; and that the permeability and potential changes are linked to the secretory response.[62] Bruce and Anderson found the resting membrane potential of the parathyroid cell to be responsive to external calcium concentration, with an abrupt depolarization occurring at higher concentrations, between 1.5 and 2.5 mM (Fig. 3). This response was quite unlike that seen in other kinds of secretory cells tested, which do not show this dependence of resting potential on external calcium. We can only speculate as to the possible significance of this effect, but it is interesting that the change in potential occurs at approximately the level of external calcium at which calcium-suppressible hormone secretion is completely suppressed and only "nonsuppressible" secretion continues.

The work of Bruce and Anderson, like that of Glick and Mockel,[60] supports what we have postulated must be true, that the parathyroid cell handles calcium in its own unique way. It will be of great interest to discover, in future studies, what this way may be.

7.3.2. Control by Catecholamines

It has been more than amply demonstrated over the past few years that adrenergic agonists can affect PTH secretion. A highly detailed review of this literature has been recently published.[63] In brief, it is clear that β-adrenergic agonists stimulate both cAMP accumulation in and PTH release from parathyroid glands. The original observations made on minced and sliced parathyroid tissue[64] have recently been confirmed in studies of dispersed cells from normal bovine[65] and abnormal human parathyroid tissue.[40] cAMP is presumed to mediate the secretory response, although for unclear reasons far more cAMP is produced than is required for maximal stimulation of hormone release,[46] and Brown *et al.*[66] have reported studies on some abnormal human parathyroid cells in which β-agonists stimulated normal cAMP accumulation but no hormone release at all. β-Receptors have been directly demonstrated on dispersed human cells through their binding of [125I]hydroxypindolol.[66] Whether these receptors are of β_1 or β_2 type is debated, and at least in abnormal human parathyroid glands seems to be variable, some glands having more receptors of the β_1 type and some having more receptors of the β_2 type.[66] Both cAMP accumulation and PTH release can be blocked by propranolol *in vitro*.[46,64]

Hormone release is stimulated by both isoproterenol and epinephrine, both *in vitro* and *in vivo*, within 2 to 5 min, indicating that secretion of preformed hormone, rather than hormone synthesis, must be at least the initial process affected.[46,67] There is evidence that the only effect of adrenergic stimulation is to release hormone from a storage pool, not to stimulate further synthesis; the secretory effect is transient, lasting about 1 hr.[67,68] Unlike changes in calcium concentration, infusion of epinephrine did not alter the ratio of intact hormone to fragments secreted in the studies of Mayer *et al.*,[67] further suggesting that the processes affected by β-agonists and by low calcium are not the same. Kukreja *et al.*[69] have suggested that the calcium-nonsuppressible component of PTH secretion might be sustained by β-adrenergic activity; they infused propranolol into normal volunteers made hypercalcemic by calcium infusion and found PTH levels fell significantly. However, Hanley *et al.* could not demonstrate any effect of β-blockade on calcium-nonsuppressible secretion in bovine glands.[68]

α-Agonists inhibit both cAMP accumulation and PTH release from dispersed bovine parathyroid cells,[46] and the mixed α- and β-agonist properties of epinephrine and norepinephrine may account for the fact that these agents stimulate PTH release less effectively than does the pure β-agonist isoproterenol,[63] since the α-blocker phentolamine has been shown to enhance epinephrine- and norepinephrine-induced secretion from dispersed bovine cells.[70] Overall, one would have to say, however, that the effect of α-adrenergic activity on PTH secretion is neither so clear-cut nor nearly so marked as the effect of β-adrenergic activity.[71]

The implications of all these findings have not yet become perfectly clear; however, we can say with assurance that they will prove less than immense. Studies in experimental animals do not provide evidence of a consistent effect of endogenous catecholamines on PTH release. In the rat, an animal whose calcium metabolism is in many ways very different from that of the human, Harney *et al.*[72] were able to show a long-term, persistent, and quite marked effect of both propranolol and epinephrine on PTH secretion; however, even in this animal, Heath[73] could demonstrate no effect of adrenalectomy or chemical sympathectomy on calcium homeostasis, and concluded that endogenous catecholamines played no part in calcium control. Blum *et al.*[74] reported stress-related increases in PTH, but *not* in serum calcium, in cattle. A quick mental review of one's experience with patients under stress, patients receiving sympathomimetic drugs, and patients receiving β-blocking drugs reassures one that hyper- and hypocalcemia do not ordinarily develop in these patients. Pheochromocytoma (without associated primary hyper-parathyroidism) is occasionally accompanied by hypercalcemia that disappears with removal of the tumor, but only rarely is this hypercalcemia referable to increased PTH secretion.[63]

Based on the limited evidence of adrenergic control of PTH secretion, attempts have been made to treat primary and secondary hyperparathyroidism with propranolol. The results and implications of these studies are discussed in Section 7.4.

7.3.3. CNS Control

The enormous current interest in neuroendocrine connections prompts us to comment on studies suggesting that the CNS influences calcium homeostasis. A diurnal variation in serum PTH in normal subjects was demonstrated by Arnaud *et al.*[76] in 1971. Sinha *et al.*[77] confirmed this finding, reporting that an increase in PTH occurs after 8 p.m. They observed this pattern not only in normal subjects, but also in 14 patients with primary hyperparathyroidism and two with pseudohypoparathyroidism. Hypercalcemia, induced by calcium infusion between 8 p.m. and midnight, inhibited the rise in PTH in all three groups. Kripke *et al.*[78] studied serum PTH and calcium in normal volunteers in relation to sleep stage cycles and found a pattern of PTH peaks and troughs with a periodicity of about 100 min throughout the day and night. At night, a significant phase relationship was observed between PTH and sleep stages 3 and 4. The PTH pattern appeared to be independent of fluctuations in serum calcium.

These PTH fluctuations cannot be said to be of any evident physiologic importance. It is very possible that they are vestigial. CNS involvement in calcium regulation seems most likely to be significant in fish, which do not have parathyroid glands but still support their serum calcium effectively. Euryhaline fish, which move between the sea and freshwater rivers, thereby transfer from an ambient calcium of 10 mM to one as low as 0.2 mM without becoming hypocalcemic.[79] This remarkable adaptation depends on the pituitary gland and has been ascribed to the hypercalcemic action of fish prolactin,[80,81] a hormone whose composition lies somewhere between mammalian GH and prolactin [both of which, interestingly, stimulate $1,25\text{-}(OH)_2D_3$ production in rats[82]; prolactin can even induce hypercalcemia[83]]. PTH itself has no hypercalcemic effect in fish, which presumably have evolved no receptors for this hormone. However, Parsons *et al.*[84] have extracted from eel and cod pituitaries a substance (not prolactin) that induces hypercalcemia in trout within 2 hr and that, unlike prolactin, exerts an effect in nonhypophysectomized fish. It is fascinating that this substance showed significant immunologic cross-reactivity with human PTH 1–34. Moreover, although a similar substance could not be extracted from human pituitary, both rat and guinea pig pituitary extracts were found to contain "considerable PTH-like reactivity."[84] It is certainly conceivable that there might be a hypothalamic factor, comparable to TRH, LHRH, etc., that would regulate secretion of this hypercalcemic substance and in turn be subject to circadian rhythms or other periodic regulation. If parathyroid cells are indeed descended from cells that once made part of the pituitary, they might still carry receptors for hypothalamic regulatory substances, even if this "regulation" were no longer of any importance. Lee et al.[85] have reported isolation of two fractions from bovine hypothalamus that induce hypocalcemia in intact, but not in thyroparathyroidectomized, rats. It would be interesting to see whether these extracts could affect hormone secretion from human parathyroid cells.

7.3.4. Vitamin D

As we discussed in the last volume of this series,[86] there is good evidence that $1,25\text{-}(OH)_2D_3$ is taken up by parathyroid cells. A cytoplasmic receptor for this form of vitamin D in chicken parathyroid cells was described in 1977 by Wecksler et al.[87] Hughes and Haussler[88] have since identified the cytoplasmic receptor in chick, bovine, and adenomatous human parathyroid glands, have shown that binding of $1,25\text{-}(OH)_2D_3$ to this receptor occurs at low concentration and with high affinity, and have demonstrated a time-dependent movement of the vitamin to the cell nucleus. Stumpf et al.[89] found that labeled $1,25(OH)_2D_3$ given to vitamin D-deficient rats became concentrated in the nuclei of parathyroid cells (as well as in the nuclei of small and large intestinal epithelial cells, renal distal tubular cells, epidermal cells, stomach, and pituitary cells).

There is no consensus, however, on the effect or the significance of $1,25\text{-}(OH)_2D_3$ binding. The evidence for and against a meaningful direct effect on PTH secretion of this or any other form of vitamin D [cholecalciferol, $25\text{-}OH\text{-}D_3$, 24,25- and $25,26\text{-}(OH)_2D_3$ have been studied as well[90–93]] was summarized in 1979 by Golden et al.[94] Several studies have suggested that $1,25\text{-}(OH)_2D_3$ binding inhibits PTH secretion, closing a negative feedback loop, but just as many others have failed to confirm this inhibition. Golden et al. concluded that the issue "remains confusing." In general, in vitro studies have found an inhibitory effect, while in vivo studies have not. In 1979, Dietel et al.[93] reported that at physiologic concentrations $1,25\text{-}(OH)_2D_3$ markedly inhibited both PTH secretion and cAMP release from porcine and human glands in culture and even produced clear ultrastructural changes in the cells indicative of decreased activity. Oldham et al.,[95] however, could find no direct inhibitory effect of 1,25-$(OH)_2D_3$ in the intact dog, although they suggested it might increase parathyroid sensitivity to calcium suppression. We should point out, however, lest the problem seem to come down to an *in vitro* versus *in vivo* issue, that at least one recent *in vitro* study was completely negative[94] and one *in vivo* study positive, though for a *stimulatory* effect of 1,25-$(OH)_2D_3$ and a suppressive effect of 24,25-$(OH)_2D_3$.[92]

Oldham *et al.*[96] in 1974 isolated from porcine parathyroid gland a calcium-binding protein resembling vitamin D-dependent intestinal calcium-binding protein; they also reported that parathyroid gland calcium-binding activity increased when vitamin D-deficient dogs were repleted with vitamin D.[97] More recently, however, they have better characterized this calcium-binding protein and concluded that it is not vitamin-D dependent.[98]

While falling short of throwing up our hands at all this, we do conclude that the evidence for any significant direct feedback effect of vitamin D on parathyroid secretion is lacking and is unlikely to be forthcoming, although the various contradictory findings will no doubt be reconciled in time.

7.3.5. Miscellaneous Effectors and Integrative Speculation

Numerous biogenic amines and hormones will stimulate PTH secretion in various experimental preparations. *Dopamine* has been shown by Brown *et al.* to produce short-lived increases in cAMP and PTH secretion from dispersed bovine cells, a process that is not affected by adrenergic antagonists[99] but is inhibited by calcium.[46] The same group reported more recently, however, finding no effect of dopamine on dispersed human parathyroid cells from adenomatous and hyperplastic tissue.[66] We also know of no evidence of an effect of phenothiazines (dopaminergic blocking agents) on human calcium metabolism, although these drugs block the dopamine effect on bovine cells.[99]

Histamine has been reported to increase PTH release from bovine parathyroid gland slices, an effect blocked by cimetidine,[100] and to increase cAMP and PTH release from dispersed abnormal human parathyroid cells.[66] We will have more to say about cimetidine in Section 7.4. As Heath[63] points out, hypercalcemia is not seen in the histamine-excess disorder systemic mastocytosis, although osteopenia is. *Glucagon*, in contrast to dopamine, did not affect PTH secretion from dispersed bovine cells in one study,[101] but has been found to increase cAMP and PTH secretion from abnormal human cells[66] and to stimulate the adenylate cyclase of human parathyroid gland.[48] *Secretin* increased cAMP and PTH release from dispersed bovine cells in one study[101]; the process was not affected by α-, β-, or dopaminergic blockade. The effect of *somatostatin* has been studied in two laboratories. Deftos et al.[102] and Metz et al.[103] found no effect of somatostatin infusions on PTH levels in normal human volunteers and in one hyperparathyroid patient. Hargis et al.,[104] on the other hand, produced with somatostatin infusion a 50–60% decrease in the levels of both PTH and calcitonin (CT) with minimal change in calcium, in rats and monkeys. One might suggest that the primary effect of somatostatin here was on CT secretion, the effect on PTH being secondary; however, the authors also demonstrated significant inhibition of PTH secretion from bovine parathyroid slices at low, normal, and high calcium. In a rather ingenious experiment aimed at demonstrating that endogenous somatostatin helps regulate hormone secretion, Williams et al.[105] gave antisomatostatin antiserum to intact rats and produced a 150% increase in circulating PTH and CT. PTH secretion was also increased in bovine parathyroid slices incubated with antiserum.

What are we to make of all this work, this appearance on the scene of myriad new "regulators" of a hormone whose purpose is, after all, to maintain calcium homeostasis—something with which all of these substances, as far as we know, have little or nothing to do? We see two possible interpretations. The one that we prefer, and believe that clinical experience supports, is that the responses to all agents other than calcium are vestigial—remnants of earlier stages of either evolutionary or embryologic development. Some of these agents may exert meaningful control over the secretion of PTH or other hypercalcemic factors in species lower than man; some of them may bind to receptors "left over" from less differentiated stem cells that have developed, by birth or later, into fully differentiated parathyroid cells. In any case, their effect on mature parathyroid cells would be minimal, of no physiologic significance, and easily overridden by the effect of calcium.

Another possibility, which appeals because it suggests a control system similar to that that regulates secretion of ADH, insulin, and various other hormones, is that PTH secretion is regulated by the integration, within the parathyroid cell, of a number of "signals," that of calcium being by far the loudest. The obvious site for this integration would be the cAMP system (adenylate cyclase, cAMP phosphodiesterase, or both), through which virtually every agent, other than calcium, seems to exert its effect, and which seems to be involved in calcium-mediated secretion to at least some degree. Gardner et al.[52] found that PGE_2 stimulates cAMP accumulation and PTH release from dispersed bovine cells; the effect was greatest at low calcium and completely suppressed by high calcium (2.0 mM). The stimulatory effect of epinephrine on PTH release in calves was either greatly or completely suppressed by hypercalcemia in the study of Mayer et al.[67] Secretin-stimulated cAMP accumulation and PTH release were suppressed 50% by mild hypercalcemia in the study of Windeck *et al.*[101] High calcium inhibited isoproterenol-stimulated cAMP accumulation and PTH release and also altered the relationship between the two, decreasing the apparent sensitivity of hormone release, to cAMP in the study of Brown *et al.*[46] And Brown *et al.*[106] recently showed that the calcium ionophore A23187, which raises intracytoplasmic calcium in parathyroid cells, similarly suppresses dopamine-stimulated cAMP accumulation and PTH release and partially dissociates the two.

The link between calcium and the cAMP system, and very possibly a critical element in the control of PTH secretion generally, may be the calcium-dependent regulator protein, calmodulin. This fascinating protein is attracting enormous and rapidly increasing interest from investigators in many fields.[107] It probably occurs in virtually every cell type; it has been found in Protozoa.[108] It belongs to a small group of related calcium-binding proteins that includes troponin and vitamin D-dependent intestinal calcium-binding protein. Calmodulin binds to and confers calcium sensitivity on adenylate cyclase, cyclic nucleotide phosphodiesterase, myosin light-chain kinase and other kinases, and probably numerous other enzymes. It has also been linked to the control of neurotransmitter release, platelet aggregation, calcium pumping in sarcoplasmic reticulum and plasma membranes, axonal transport, and hormone secretion[107]; it may well in time be linked to all calcium-regulated processes. Oldham *et al.*[109] have now isolated calmodulin from the parathyroid gland, and we expect that further work along this line will go far toward explaining the control of PTH secretion.

7.4. Metabolism

Despite a great deal of productive work, this remains a confusing area. Many results that at present appear irreconcilable have entered the literature. The scheme that seemed straightforward several years ago—secretion of intact hormone, binding to receptors in the recognized target organs with cleavage to N- and C-terminal peptides, and release of C-terminal peptide to the circulation for eventual disposal—has been extensively modified. We will try to summarize the questions being asked and to condense, without oversimplification, the answers offered.

1. What are the plasma kinetics of intact hormone and its fragments? Attention has shifted away from this area of late. There is a consensus that intact hormone is rapidly cleared from the circulation in all mammalian species, with a half-life of 10 min or less.[110] The metabolically inactive C-terminal fragment is generally held to circulate for a somewhat

longer period, although estimates of its half-life have been variable.[110] Its longer half-life is not universally accepted; Neuman *et al.*[111] recently published a study of continuous hormone infusion in dogs in which the steady-state levels of intact hormone and of fragments were reached at the same time, apparently indicating equal clearance rates for hormone and fragments. These results are consistent with those of single-injection studies from the same group,[112] but are difficult for us to reconcile with those of other groups, including Papapoulos *et al.*,[113] who used a similar experimental design, i.e., lengthy hormone infusion, in humans and showed N-terminal reactivity (representing intact hormone) peaking by 30 min, while C-terminal reactivity (intact hormone plus C-terminal fragments) did not peak for 80 min and also declined at a much slower rate when the infusion was discontinued. The weight of evidence still would have to be said to support the slower clearance of the C-terminal fragment.

2. What is the source of the heterogeneity of circulating PTH? As is well known, circulating PTH, as measured by most immunoassays, comprises mostly inactive C-terminal fragments, produced in the periphery by splitting of intact hormone between positions 33 and 34 or 36 and 37,[114] some intact hormone, and probably a very small quantity of biologically active N-terminal peptide, PTH 1–34 or 1–36.[115] We have discussed above (Section 7.2) evidence that circulating C-terminal fragments are secreted directly by the parathyroid gland. Segre *et al.* have shown, however, that at least some of the fragments in circulation must be derived from peripheral metabolism of the hormone[116]: they found that the level of circulating C-terminal fragments was decreased by 75% in animals infused with a synthetic PTH fragment containing residues 28–48, which acts as a competitive inhibitor of intact hormone cleavage.[117] C-terminal fragments in the circulation have been thought to derive primarily from cleavage of intact hormone in the kidney and in the liver, with return of fragments to the circulation (see review by Martin *et al.*[110]), but there is debate about the relative roles of these organs. D'Amour *et al.*[114] injected iodinated PTH into rats and studied the fragments generated in liver and kidney by microsequence analysis. They found that the C-terminal fragment generated in the kidney was not the same as that in the circulation, having amino acid 39 as its N-terminal peptide. They also mentioned having found markedly decreased levels of C-terminal fragments in hepatectomized rats injected with intact PTH. They believe their studies show that the liver, rather than the kidney, is primarily responsible for generating C-terminal fragments from circulating intact hormone. The question cannot be considered settled.

Freitag *et al.*[118] have demonstrated that fetal rat bone and isolated bone cells metabolize intact PTH, with release of C-terminal fragments but apparent complete degradation of N-terminal fragments. Their findings suggest that skeletal PTH metabolism contributes to the heterogeneity of circulating immunoreactive PTH.

3. What is the ultimate fate of intact hormone and its fragments? Surprisingly, given the fact that it has not been thought to be a target organ for PTH, it seems that a large fraction of circulating intact hormone is actually taken up by the liver. Uptake has been demonstrated in dog, chick, and rat liver *in vivo* and *in vitro*.[110] In the study of D'Amour et al.,[114] 32% of a single injected dose of PTH was taken up by the liver. Oldham et al.[119] have now demonstrated hepatic uptake in humans. They obtained blood samples from femoral artery and hepatic veins in patients undergoing catheterization prior to parathyroid surgery and found a 44% A-V difference in intact hormone levels across the liver. Hepatic uptake is specific for biologically active intact hormone; N- and C-terminal fragments are rejected.[110,120] Exactly what the liver does with the hormone it extracts is less clear. The hormone is cleaved,[120] and C-terminal fragments are released into the circulation. However, it has not been shown that N-terminal fragments are released, although Canterbury et al.[121] did report hepatic release of a fragment active in the renal cortical adenylate cyclase assay.

After the liver, it appears that the largest fraction of intact hormone is taken up by the kidney: 28% in the study of D'Amour et al.[114] and 34% extraction in the patients studied by Oldham et al.[119] D'Amour et al. found 9% of injected hormone taken up by muscle and 6.4% by bone. Oldham et al. were able to show a 16% A-V difference in intact PTH across the leg (femoral artery to femoral vein) in man, something not previously demonstrated.

C-terminal fragments appear to be cleared solely by the kidney. Unlike active forms of the hormone, they are not bound to receptors but simply filtered and probably catabolized in tubules.[122] Therefore, the rate of disappearance of C-terminal PTH from the circulation after parathyroidectomy, a measurement that has frequently been used to assess PTH kinetics, will be directly proportional to the glomerular filtration rate. It has been clearly shown that the enormous plasma PTH values obtained with common C-terminal assays in patients with chronic renal failure reflect the large quantities of retained, inactive, C-terminal fragments in these patients.[123]

4. What is the purpose of PTH cleavage in the liver? No answer has emerged since we last wrote.[86] There are three possibilities. First, the hormone might simply be degraded and inactivated; the degradation process could be specific and purposefully regulated, or it could be incidental. Second, the hormone might be activated, i.e., "active" N-terminal fragments would be released into the circulation; to accept this

explanation, one must believe that there are target organs for PTH that do not respond fully to intact hormone and for which PTH would need to be "activated" elsewhere (see below). Third, the liver may be an un-appreciated end organ for PTH. The liver clearly has several responses to PTH: various effects on carbohydrate metabolism in mitochondria, uptake of calcium, adenylate cyclase activation, release of phosphate and glucose, uptake of lactate and amino acids, and production of urea have all been reported.[120] In addition, regeneration after partial hepatectomy is delayed in parathyroidectomized animals. We have seen no evidence, however, that hepatic function is in any way abnormal in hypoparathy-roid patients.

5. Is PTH metabolism a control point in the calcium homeostatic system? In 1979 we mentioned the possibility that concepts of calcium regulation might have to expand to encompass not just the source of PTH, but the sites of its metabolism; there was evidence that the deg-radative processes in both liver and kidney were responsive to the serum calcium level.[86] This possibility has received little attention since our last writing. Oldham et al.,[119] who studied PTH extraction by liver, kidney, and leg in nine hyperparathyroid patients, found a weak direct corre-lation between extraction by the kidney and the serum calcium but no correlation between serum calcium and extraction by the liver or leg.

6. What is the nature of active PTH? There is an ongoing debate (active, though short of being heated) over whether intact PTH itself activates its receptor cells or must first be split, either at its end-organ receptor site or elsewhere, into inactive C-terminal peptide and active 1–34 PTH. It is unquestionable that in a wide variety of *in vitro* test systems, from both kidney and bone, no difference has been detected between the effects of 1–84 and 1–34 PTH. Most recently, Goltzman *et al.*, who showed in 1976 that intact PTH normally stimulated renal cor-tical adenylate cyclase,[124] have shown that it also activates adenylate cy-clase in fetal rabbit bone.[125] Feitag *et al.*[118] showed that fetal rat bone and isolated bone cells both respond to intact PTH with cAMP produc-tion. Rosenblatt *et al.*[117] found that their synthetically produced PTH fragment 28–48, an effective competitive inhibitor of PTH cleavage, did not inhibit renal cortical adenylate cyclase activation by intact hormone.

Against all this evidence must be ranged certain solid and currently inexplicable findings. Martin *et al.*[126] infused both intact PTH and syn-thetic 1–34 PTH into blood perfusing the isolated dog tibia. They found 36% extraction of 1–34 PTH but *no* extraction of intact hormone, despite repeated perfusion. cAMP production was stimulated, as expected, dur-ing perfusion with 1–34 PTH but very little stimulation occurred during perfusion with intact hormone. Their results are consistent with those of Parsons and Robinson,[127] who in 1968 reported finding no mobilization of calcium from the isolated cat limb perfused with PTH; Mueller *et al.*,[128] who failed similarly with perfused hen femur in 1973; and the author's (C.R.K.) unpublished results with the isolated perfused kidney, on which parathyroid gland extract had no effect. They conflict with the results of Oldham *et al.*,[119] discussed above, who measured 16% PTH extraction across the leg with an immunoassay detecting *only* intact hormone. Although differences between species, age of test subjects, and experimental design can be raised as possible explanations for these apparently irreconcilable findings, none is very satisfactory, and explication will have to await further work or more insightful thinking.

7.5. Physiology of PTH And Its Evolution

We will not attempt to provide an integrated overview of human calcium metabolism. The reviews of Neer[43] and Parfitt and Kleerekoper[3] contain clear and useful formulations.

Although PTH can be shown to have some effect on a variety of cells not usually considered its targets, such as hepatocytes and leukocytes, its only effects of demonstrated physiologic significance are those involved in calcium and phosphate homeostasis. We believe that the primary function of PTH is to maintain a normal calcium level in extracellular fluid, and that it does this primarily by drawing upon skeletal calcium. This might seem a completely obvious statement, but it has been challenged in the recent past. Some of the first investigators to try to study the effects of truly physiologic, rather than pharmacologic, doses of PTH in animals concluded that PTH could produce hypercalcemia and hypocalciuria without, apparently, drawing calcium from the skeleton. Parsons[129] has suggested that in the physiologic state, PTH produces skeletal *anabolism*, while serum calcium is controlled by renal calcium reabsorption. As Neer[43] points out, however, renal calcium turnover is normally so low that even if calcium excretion drops abruptly to zero, serum calcium will increase by only 0.2 mg/dl in 6 hr; therefore, he states, "it is necessary to conclude that renal and intestinal calcium clearance can affect serum calcium homeostasis in a major fashion only over a long time interval (weeks)." We suggest that Parsons' conclusions were made possible by the fact that the store of calcium in the skeleton is so large, and the amount that must leave the skeleton to produce hypercalcemia, given avid renal calcium reabsorption, is so small, that the fairly insensitive methods that were available to study the skeleton simply could not detect the PTH effect. New techniques (see below) that show that bone-resorbing cells are just as responsive as kidney cells to PTH, support the conclusion to which such calculations as Neer describes lead us: that short-term calcium homeostasis must depend, first, on the release of skeletal calcium, and second, on the reabsorption of this calcium by the kidney. Skeletal primacy in the hierarchy of PTH targets is supported by studies of the earliest animals to produce PTH, the urodele amphibians; results suggest that PTH affects bone but not kidney in the most primitive of these animals.[130]

The evolution of PTH makes an intriguing study. The evidence suggests to us that in the course of evolution the combination of the move from water to land with development of the calcified skeleton made a PTH-like substance necessary: the land animal needed a hormone that could draw on an *endogenous* calcium store to meet acute demands on the serum calcium. While fish moving from sea to freshwater face an acute challenge to their serum calcium, they still can meet it simply by increasing calcium absorption, as a source of calcium is continuously available in the water surrounding them. With the move to land, this is no longer the case; food cannot be considered a reliable source of calcium to meet immediate needs.

The move to land also required the support of the calcified skeleton. Paradoxically, the existence of the calcified skeleton simultaneously solves and complicates the problem of calcium homeostasis on land. The skeleton represents a calcium reservoir, true. However, when it is *growing* it represents the single greatest challenge to calcium homeostasis that the organism is required to meet. Growth, pregnancy, and lactation are periods during which the skeleton, either of the organism or of its offspring, is absorbing calcium voraciously in a process that, were it not for the moderating influence of PTH, would be wholly autonomous.

Nowhere is the challenge of skeletal growth better demonstrated than in the rat. It has become clear over the years that this animal's calcium metabolism differs quite markedly from ours and that results of rat studies cannot be automatically extrapolated to man; however, the force exerted by the growing skeleton, although stronger in the rat, can be seen in human children as well.

Radar *et al.*[131] have recently published a fascinating study of calcium homeostasis in weanling rats, in whom bone growth is tremendously rapid. Serum calcium in these animals is strongly dependent on dietary calcium. Weanling rats fed a low-calcium diet developed mild hypocalcemia after 6 days and severe hypocalcemia by 3 weeks, serum calcium reaching a stable level of 5.5 mg/dl (normal, about 11) after 5 weeks. Hypocalcemia developed in spite of 13-fold increases in PTH and 10-fold increases in $1,25$-$(OH)_2D_3$ levels, but without PTH, hypocalcemia would have been even more severe. It is not because weanling bone is insensitive to PTH that the hypocalcemia develops; *in vitro,* weanling bone is more responsive than adult bone. Rather, skeletal growth behaves as an almost autonomous process that, in the rat, takes clear precedence over maintaining the serum calcium. Skeletal growth can be slowed, perhaps even stopped, but not reversed. The slow-growing adult rat, in contrast, can by increasing PTH secretion keep serum calcium near normal during dietary calcium deficiency.[132] Although humans defend the serum calcium much more effectively than rats do, mild hypocalcemia (to about 8 mg/dl) will still develop in rapidly growing infants and young children when their diet is low in calcium, while adults will never become hypocalcemic on the basis of dietary calcium deficiency alone.

Calcium metabolism during pregnancy has been well reviewed by Pitkin.[133] During pregnancy, calcium is transferred against a concentration gradient from mother to fetus. During most of gestation, maternal PTH levels increase progressively, and ionic calcium declines only very slightly, despite the fetal drain on maternal calcium.[134] $1,25\text{-}(OH)_2D$ levels also increase progressively,[135] and this increase may be ascribed to an increase in PTH-stimulated 1α-hydroxylation, since circulating 25-OH-D levels do not increase.[133] Under normal circumstances, fetal calcium needs are ultimately met through increased maternal calcium absorption, as a normal pregnancy does not decrease maternal bone density,[133] but since the fetal calcium drain is continuous and maternal calcium absorption is not, intermittent maternal hypocalcemia would be inevitable were it not for PTH.

During lactation, the calcium drain trom mother to baby continues. Lactating rats have more parathyroid tissue by weight than nonlactating rats,[136] and parathyroidectomy in lactating animals results in a rapid fall in serum calcium that is not observed in nonlactating rats.[137] Although we have not seen data on PTH levels in lactating women, Kumar et al.[135] found that $1,25\text{-}(OH)_2D$ levels remained elevated postpartum in lactating women, presumably reflecting elevated PTH.

We suggest that when PTH first appeared in the course of evolution, it served to support the serum calcium only in times of hypocalcemic stress. Humans, however, have become much more dependent on it than lower animals are and, unlike many of them, cannot adapt to its absence without pharmacologic help. The functions served by human PTH have been well characterized by Parfitt and Kleerekoper[3]:

1. To set the steady-state level of plasma calcium; this requires a coordinated effect on the skeleton, where the level of blood–bone calcium exchange is set, and the kidney, where calcium reabsorption is adjusted to maintain the desired ECF calcium level without unnecessary calcium wasting. Calcium absorption from the gut is adjusted appropriately via regulation of the supply of 1,25-dihydroxycholecalciferol, but the steady-state calcium level is not dependent on the calcium available from the diet.

2. To detect and correct deviations in plasma calcium from the normal. As we have said, it is hypo- rather than hypercalcemic deviations that PTH corrects; since its secretion is suppressed to baseline by barely supranormal calcium levels, it can play no regulatory role if calcium goes higher. Acute hypocalcemia *must* be met by withdrawal of calcium from the skeleton, though avid renal conservation of this calcium increases the rate and improves the efficiency of the response. This calcium can be withdrawn without irretrievable skeletal mineral loss; the structure of the skeleton is not affected, and the calcium can be replaced once the hypocalcemic stress is gone. (The situation changes, of course, when the hypocalcemic stress becomes chronic.) The rapid hypercalcemic response requires the presence of normal amounts of 1,25-dihydroxycholecalciferol and is impeded by hyperphosphatemia, which will tend to cause the calcium mobilized from the skeleton to be redeposited in the form of calcium phosphate crystals. Since increased intestinal calcium absorption can only occur in response to an increase in 1,25-dihydroxycholecalciferol production, which takes hours, intestinal calcium absorption does not play any part in the rapid hypercalcemic response.

3. To determine the rate of bone remodeling. Parfitt and Kleerekoper make the very important point that this "skeletal homeostasis" can be considered for clinical purposes to be *completely independent* of the calcium homeostatic process, each being able to proceed normally in the face of severe derangement of the other, each being for the most part accomplished by its own types of cells. Skeletal remodeling does not require 1,25-dihydroxycholecalciferol; in fact, in vitamin D deficiency, skeletal remodeling is accelerated.

It is useful to keep these three distinct functions of PTH in mind while sifting the data on PTH effects on the skeleton.

7.5.1. PTH and the Skeleton

The overall intestinal and renal effects of PTH have been generally agreed upon for some time, with only the exact mechanisms and cellular loci remaining to be elucidated. In contrast, the skeletal effects of PTH are still debated. There are four main reasons for this continued controversy. One is the complexity of bone tissue: not only does it contain a variety of cell types, all of which respond to PTH differently, but travecular bone differs from cortical bone, woven bone differs from Haversian bone, growing bone differs from nongrowing bone, and bone from one species differs from that of another. Advances in the technique of enzymatic dispersion have made it possible to isolate populations of bone cells,[138] but it is by no means clear how far we can extrapolate responses of isolated cells to the overall response of the tissue. We do not know enough about the effect on these bone cells of their complex microenvironment. A second reason is the extreme difficulty of studying the skeleton *in vivo*, a process that in humans has had to depend solely on radiolabeled calcium studies, whose limitations we are increasingly coming to appreciate, and on bone biopsy, whose practical limitations are obvious (not to mention sampling error, related to the complexity of bone described above). A third is the fact that the effect of PTH on the skeleton is far from independent, but depends at the very least on the availability of calcium, phosphate, 1,25-dihydroxycholecalciferol, estrogen, thyroid hormone, and, as Wong[139] has recently confirmed, glucocorticoids. And finally, there is the increasingly appreciated fact—unfortunately, not taken into account in many experimental studies—that the observed effect of PTH on the skeleton varies markedly with the dose of hormone used (as well as, in all likelihood, the duration of the study). As Parsons[129] points out, the classic descriptions of PTH as an agent of pure bone destruction were derived from the results of studies performed by injecting massive amounts of hormone, as well as the study of patients with very severe hyperparathyroidism. Patients with mild hyperparathyroidism, in contrast, "may not show any reduction in bone density over several years of continuous observation."[129]

Calcium turnover in the skeleton can be studied in two ways: through kinetic studies of skeletal uptake and release of radiolabeled calcium, and histologically. Of course, histological studies do not examine mineral turnover directly, but rather infer it from microscopic observations of bone loss and deposition. The electron microscope, which can in addition detect the signs of cell activation, has made it possible to correlate turnover rates with the activity of various cell types, but we should remember that an exact correlation, though it might satisfy our desire for a neat model, does not exist in fact. Kinetic and histologic studies do, however, agree fully on one point: every turnover rate is controlled, and every bone cell type affected, by PTH. The greatest recent advances in our knowledge of PTH effects on the skeleton have come from the application of electron microscopy and scanning electron microscopy to the study of bone. These methods have permitted clear demonstration of PTH-stimulated periosteocytic mini-remodeling[140] and of the rapid responsiveness of bone-lining cells[141] and osteoclasts[142,143] to PTH.

Calcium kinetic studies prove that skeletal mineral is in constant flux. In a young adult, skeletal calcium turnover amounts to 30 to 40 g of calcium per day, or a more than complete replacement of plasma calcium every hour; and this measured turnover does not include min-

Table II. Blood–Bone Calcium Exchanges in Hypoparathyroid, Normal, Primary Hyperparathyroid Humans[a]

Component	Effective equilibration time[b]	Magnitude[c]		
		Hypo	Normal	Hyper
Fast	1.1 hr	(11.2)	16.6	17.3
Slow	18 hr	(2.0)	3.7	3.1
Slower	8 days	(0.40)	0.66	0.90
Slowest	40+ days	(0.19)	0.24	(0.55)

[a] Reproduced with permission from Neer.[43]
[b] Four half-lives.
[c] Mean value for grams of calcium/day per square meter body surface. Parentheses indicate values significantly different from normal.

eral that may be mobilized and redeposited within the skeleton without ever reaching the systemic ECF. The abundance of the skeletal blood supply—up to 25% of the cardiac output, much more than is needed to meet skeletal metabolic demands—attests to the importance to the organism of blood–bone calcium turnover.

Table II summarizes the results of many calcium kinetic studies. The division into four components is a heuristic device, as turnover rates actually distribute themselves along a continuum, but it has been useful to envision turnover as occurring between the blood and a series of compartments in bone. As can be seen, while a small fraction of calcium turnover is extremely slow, most is quite rapid. A large part of the rapid turnover occurs between the blood and the "surface compartment," i.e., calcium in bone-lining cells, calcium in bone ECF, and calcium ions in solution in the "hydration shell" that surrounds loose surface bone mineral crystals; all this calcium behaves kinetically as one compartment. Calcium exchange between the blood and the surface compartment is so rapid that the two are functionally one pool[43]; if this exchange slows, then serum calcium will fall. Blood–bone exchange is felt to be the process that maintains the steady-state serum calcium and buffers small transient fluctuations in the serum calcium. Blood–bone exchange is probably mediated by the bone-lining cells, which form a syncytium that covers all bone surfaces and appear, somehow, to maintain a calcium concentration gradient between the plasma and the bone ECF. They are presumably involved in mobilizing calcium from the surface compartment, the most readily accessible calcium in the skeleton, to meet acute hypocalcemic challenges. Because PTH can stimulate calcium release from the skeleton within minutes[43] and because it somehow "sets" bone to maintain a certain level of calcium flux and thereby an appropriate serum calcium,[3] it has been assumed that PTH must have an effect on bone-lining cells. Norimatsu et al.[141] and Vander Wiel et al.[144] have now shown directly, using electron and scanning electron microscopy, that PTH does in fact stimulate calcium uptake and morphologic changes (an increase in distended endoplasmic reticulum, swelling of the Golgi complex, and roughening of the cell surface, suggesting increased membrane activity) in the bone-lining cells. Moreover, these changes were produced within 5 min, showing that the skeletal response to PTH is as rapid and sensitive as the renal response—rapid enough to meet minute-to-minute challenges to the serum calcium.

In experimental human hypocalcemia (a 25% fall in serum calcium produced by a 2-hr EDTA infusion), preinfusion serum calcium is fully restored in about 12 hr. Parfitt and Kleerekoper[3] estimate that from one-half to two-thirds of this calcium deficit could be met from the surface compartment, but the rest of the repair would require resorption of bone mineral. Osteocytes can rapidly resorb mineral without matrix from the perilacunar bone, which they keep loose-packed and accessible through the process of periosteocytic mini-remodeling. Osteocytes, like bone-lining cells, show structural changes within a few minutes of exposure to PTH,[145] which are followed by periosteocytic osteolysis.[146] The effects of PTH on osteocytes and the perilacunar wall have been fully reviewed recently by Baud and Boivin.[146]

Osteoclasts are the only bone cells that resorb both matrix and mineral. Although they certainly contribute to calcium homeostasis when there is a chronic drain on ECF calcium, it is not clear that they are involved in the acute regulation of calcium homeostasis. Even though Miller,[143] and Holtrop et al.,[142] using sophisticated electron microscopic techniques, have now shown that large doses of PTH in vivo can affect osteoclast structure within 30 min, and Burger et al.[147] have shown PTH to increase osteoclast calcium transport within 1 hr, we still incline to the view of Parfitt and Kleerekoper[3] that osteoclasts are, under normal circumstances, responsible for skeletal homeostasis rather than for calcium turnover.

Schulz et al.,[148] Krempien et al.,[149] and Bonucci et al.[150] have used the electron microscope to study bone in patients with hyperparathyroidism, confirming the findings in experimental animals and the inferences drawn from light microscopy in human patients: periosteocytic and osteoclastic resorption and osteoblastic remodeling activity are all increased.[150] Bonucci et al. found ultrastructural evidence of delayed and incomplete calcification,[150] but Meunier et al., who used light microscopy and tetracycline labeling to study bone histology in hyperparathyroid patients, did not find any evidence for a PTH-induced mineralization defect[151]; thus, the effect of PTH on mineralization is still unclear.

Acute and chronic metabolic acid loads exceeding the capacity of extracellular buffers are thought to be buffered primarily by bone. A role for PTH in the buffering process was suggested in 1970.[152] Fraley and Adler[153] showed recently that PTH was required for rats and dogs to buffer large metabolic acid loads. Intact rats and dogs buffered 39 and 50% of administered acid extracellularly, while thyroparathyroidectomized animals buffered 97 and 78% extracellularly and did not survive the acid loading. Thyroparathyroidectomized animals given PTH 2 hr before acid infusion did survive. Although the authors did not demonstrate directly that PTH was exerting its effect on the skeleton, they ruled out a renal effect by nephrectomy and could not find an effect on skeletal muscle.

7.5.2. PTH and the Kidney

In the kidney, PTH increases phosphate and bicarbonate clearance and decreases calcium clearance. These effects were observed "black-box" fashion many years ago, and subsequent efforts have been directed toward localizing the effects more exactly within the kidney and toward establishing the mechanisms by which they are accomplished. These efforts have been advanced by the development of progressively sophisticated techniques for studying the renal tubule, both *in situ* and after dissection from the kidney. Two useful new techniques have recently been applied to studies of renal PTH effects: electron probe microanalysis[154] and the isolation of membrane vesicles.[155–158] The first technique permits the chemical analysis of very tiny fluid and tissue samples, including tubular fluid drawn from extremely small segments of the nephron. The second technique makes it possible to study brush border and basal lateral renal tubular cell membranes in isolation from other segments of these cells, in a system in which these membranes appear to function just as they do in intact cells.

7.5.2.1. Calcium Clearance

Calcium transport in the various segments of the nephron has recently been reviewed by Suki.[159] As he points out, we are increasingly coming to appreciate the heterogeneity, not only of the total nephron population, but of the various segments of the nephron, both along their length and between different parts of the kidney, specifically between the cortical and the juxtamedullary or "deep" nephrons. While our new knowledge permits sophisticated investigators to clarify the nature of ion transport throughout the kidney, it also must lead us to question the validity and utility of the results of many older studies that were done before this heterogeneity was appreciated.[159]

Active reabsorption of calcium occurs throughout the nephron, even in the proximal tubule (as studies with membrane vesicles[156] have shown), where calcium absorption was once thought to be wholly passive. More than 95% of filtered calcium is ordinarily reabsorbed. Approximately 60% of calcium reabsorption occurs in the proximal tubule, mostly in the convoluted segment, although the straight tubule also appears to be capable of active transport[160]; 20% occurs in the loop of Henle, 10% in the distal convoluted tubule, and 5% in the collecting duct. Although maximum calcium reabsorption is decreased by many factors, including PTH, it appears that the actual regulation of calcium clearance takes place in the distal convoluted tubule and collecting duct.[159] Shareghi and Stoner,[161] using microperfusion, and Greger et al.,[162] using microinjection of ^{45}Ca into the tubule, have both shown that PTH increases calcium transport in the distal convoluted tubule. The same two groups of investigators also reported PTH-enhanced calcium absorption in the collecting duct, supporting the report of Agus et al.[163] that parathyroidectomy abolished calcium absorption beyond the distal tubule.

The details of calcium transport from the tubular lumen, across the cell, and out into the blood are poorly understood. Gmaj et al.[156] have produced basal lateral and brush border membrane vesicles from the rat proximal tubule and have shown that the basal lateral vesicles contain both a calcium-stimulated ATPase and a Na^+–Ca^{2+} exchange system, while the brush border membrane vesicles do not transport calcium. This work would seem to indicate that the driving force for calcium transport, at least in the proximal tubule, is at the basal lateral membrane, calcium entry at the brush border being passive. If calcium transport systems are similarly constituted in other segments of the nephron, we might hypothesize that PTH would be most likely to act at the basal lateral membrane to influence calcium transport; since PTH binds to this side of the tubular cell, it would seem most efficient for it to act at a nearby site. However, we do not know how the calcium transport process may vary from segment to segment along the nephron or how it is affected by PTH at any site. Although we have learned a bit more about the cAMP response of the renal cell to PTH, PTH-stimulated calcium entry, and the relationship between calcium, cAMP, and cGMP in the PTH-stimulated cell, there remains a huge gap in our knowledge: we know nothing of the steps between this activation process and its observable ultimate result, i.e., absorption of calcium and rejection of bicarbonate and phosphate.

Phosphate depletion or dietary phosphate deficiency results in hypercalciuria, comprising that calcium released into the circulation as bone is broken down for its phosphate content. Grabic et al.[164] have recently shown that this hypercalciuria is moderated by PTH, even though PTH secretion may be suppressed to baseline in this state, and that the hypercalciuria is more severe in parathyroidectomized animals than in their intact counterparts.

The mechanism of thiazide-induced hypocalciuria has recently been clarified by Costanzo and Windhager,[165] who directly demonstrated by microperfusion and micropuncture that these diuretics enhance calcium reabsorption in the distal convoluted tubule (as has previously been suspected). Thiazide hypocalciuria is partly PTH-dependent and is most apparent in the presence of high circulating PTH.[3] Thiazide hypocalciuria can be observed in any patient given thiazides, but thiazide-induced hypercalcemia has been considered relatively rare. In our last review we reported the finding of Christenson et al.[166] that 14 of 70 patients with supposed thiazide-induced hypercalcemia remained hypercalcemic when taken off thiazides and were subsequently found to be hyperparathyroid. In contrast, Mohamadi et al.[167] have now reported that 8 of 22 thiazide-treated patients studied retrospectively developed transient (2–4 weeks), self-limited episodes of hypercalcemia at various times during their treatment. Total protein, albumin, and globulin also increased during these episodes. The authors then prospectively studied 11 patients and observed the same phenomenon of transient hypercalcemia in all of them, in addition to a constant elevation in mean serum calcium that was due to increased protein-bound, *not* increased free calcium, and that was ascribed to volume depletion. They concluded that mild, transient thiazide-induced hypercalcemia is common and need not be presumed to be pathological. We infer from their results that in any patient with thiazide-induced hypercalcemia, free rather than total calcium measurements are essential; if the *free* calcium concentration is high, the patient's bone turnover rate can be assumed to be accelerated, either because of hyperparathyroidism or some other process, such as hyperthyroidism or vitamin D intoxication.

7.5.2.2. Phosphate Clearance

We would like to stress again, as in our last review, the enormous superiority of the measurement of the renal phosphate threshold, TmP/GFR, over all other measures of phosphate clearance. The TmP/GFR is a simple and extremely accurate measure of renal phosphate handling in any physiologic or pathologic situation. Its measurement and use are well described by Parfitt and Kleerekoper.[3]

Studies using electron probe microanalysis have confirmed and extended previous findings on the sites at which PTH inhibits phosphate reabsorption. Lechene et al.[168] and Pastoriza-Munoz et al.[169] have confirmed a direct effect of PTH on phosphate transport in the distal convoluted tubule and proximal tubule and have shown that PTH also inhibits phosphate reabsorption in the loop of Henle. Evers *et al.*,[155] using isolated brush border (luminal) membrane vesicles, have shown that although PTH binds to the contraluminal membrane, it appears to exert its effect on phosphate clearance (at least in the proximal tubule) on the luminal side: vesicles isolated from PTH-treated rats took up 30% less phosphate than vesicles isolated from untreated rats.

Two groups of investigators have used membrane vesicles to study the phenomenon of renal tubular adaptation to phosphate depletion, showing that the increased phosphate reabsorption is mediated at the luminal membrane and confirming that it is independent of the presence of PTH.[157,158]

7.5.2.3. Glomerular Filtration

Sraer *et al.*,[170] using binding of labeled PTH and labeled anti-PTH antibodies, have demonstrated glomerular receptors for PTH. This demonstration supports the same group's finding of PTH-sensitive adenylate cyclase in rabbit glomeruli[171] and Dousa and colleagues' demonstration by immunocytochemical methods of an increase in cAMP in glomerular epithelial cells in response to PTH.[172] Humes *et al.* have shown that PTH decreases the single-nephron GFR in the rat by reducing the glomerular capillary ultrafiltration coefficient[173] and that acute hypercalcemia has a similar, PTH-dependent, effect, not on just the single nephron but on the whole kidney GFR.[174] Do these interesting findings have any clinical relevance? Lins[175] has studied GFR and renal plasma flow in eight patients with hyperparathyroid and ten with nonhyperparathyroid hypercalcemia, and his findings are exactly the *opposite* of those that we might predict from the experimental results of Humes, Ichikawa, and colleagues: GFR and filtration fraction were significantly *higher* in the patients with primary hyperparathyroidism than in the others. Mean serum calcium was the same in both groups. In the hyperparathyroid patients, parathyroidectomy with correction of hypercalcemia had no effect on GFR or on renal plasma flow. The only finding that agrees with the experimental results of Humes, Ichikawa, and colleagues is that correction of hypercalcemia in the nonhyperparathyroid patients was followed by a significant increase in GFR. Whether the discrepancy between Lins' findings and those of Humes, Ichikawa, and colleagues reflects a difference between the effects of acute and chronic hypercalcemia, or between the response of human and rat glomerular cells to calcium and PTH, cannot be inferred from the available evidence, but we expect future studies will lead to a reconciliation.

7.5.3. PTH and Vitamin D

Studies published in the last few years have not changed our previous conceptions, hazy as they are, of the respective roles and interaction of PTH and vitamin D.[28,86]

Of the major targets of PTH action, the kidney is the one least affected by vitamin D, even though it is the site of PTH-stimulated 1α-hydroxylation of this hormone. Levine et al.[176] have thoroughly reviewed the evidence for an effect of vitamin D on the renal handling of calcium and phosphorus, concluding that "the verdict indicates that vitamin D sterols *can* affect the renal tubular handling of Ca and P; however, the question 'what is the physiologic significance of this?' leads to a vague, uncertain answer." We would agree that although an effect of vitamin D can be demonstrated in certain experimental settings, its physiologic significance is open to grave doubt. In hypoparathyroid subjects, vitamin D will increase urinary calcium, but Bernstein et al.[177] observed in 1959 that this calciuria was due solely to an increase in the filtered load of calcium. Hugi et al.[178] have recently made similar observations in rats. In both intact and thyroparathyroidectomized animals, $1,25-(OH)_2D_3$ changed urinary calcium excretion only in proportion to the change in filtered calcium; only PTH was capable of changing the renal threshold for calcium excretion.

Vitamin D-deficient rats show a blunted phosphaturic response to PTH, which Forte et al.[179] showed to be associated with decreased responsiveness of renal adenylate cyclase to PTH. Kakuta et al.[180] have more recently confirmed the finding that in the vitamin D-deficient rat the response of renal adenylate cyclase to PTH is blunted, although the vitamin D-deficient animals start from a higher renal cAMP level, presumably because of their secondary hyperparathyroidism. Kakuta et al. further showed, however, that the hyporesponsiveness of the renal adenylate cyclase was not related to vitamin D deficiency per se, but rather to hypocalcemia, since vitamin D-deficient rats made normocalcemic with dietary calcium alone recovered their adenylate cyclase response. The fact that the adenylate cyclase response *in vitro* has been found to be not blunted by low calcium, but instead enhanced, only illustrates again the complexity and confusion of this field and underscores the necessity for clinicians to draw their conclusions from observations on whole, human subjects.

In the intestine, PTH does not appear to act directly, but adjusts calcium absorption indirectly, as dictated by the serum calcium, by altering the production of $1,25-(OH)_2D$ from 25-OH-D in the kidney. The sequence of the human response to an excess or deficiency of dietary calcium has been beautifully delineated in experiments by Adams et al.[181] High calcium intake in 32 healthy volunteers produced a rise in serum calcium within 6 hr, hypercalciuria, a fall in plasma PTH and urinary cAMP, and a subsequent sustained and marked fall in plasma 1,25-$(OH)_2D$ within 18–24 hr. An extreme reduction in dietary calcium produced exactly the opposite effects, a sustained rise in plasma 1,25-$(OH)_2D$ being produced within 48 hr. Since injected 1,25-$(OH)_2D_3$ is metabolized very rapidly,[182] Adams et al. inferred that the observed changes in plasma 1,25-$(OH)_2D$ reflected changes in the renal synthesis of this hormone, presumably under the control of PTH. Although no one has attempted to discover whether 1,25-$(OH)_2D$ synthesis is in any way affected by changes in dietary calcium in hypoparathyroid human subjects, it seems safe to assume that any effect would be slight and that PTH, in the human as in other species, is the critical factor in adaptation to changes in dietary calcium. Hughes et al.[183] showed that 1,25-$(OH)_2D_3$ levels in parathyroidectomized rats are minimally responsive to dietary calcium deprivation, and Ribovich and DeLuca[184] have more recently confirmed that thyroparathyroidectomy in rats eliminates the adaptation of 1,25-$(OH)_2D$ production to changes in dietary calcium.

Hyperparathyroidism is a state of "hypervitaminosis D." The increased intestinal calcium absorption observed in primary hyperparathyroidism has been attributed to the increase in plasma 1,25-$(OH)_2D$, which correlates positively with the increased absorption.[185] Bone et al.[186] have recently reported the interesting observation that in 5 of 11 hyperparathyroid patients with elevated 1,25-$(OH)_2D$ levels preoperatively, intestinal calcium absorption was still abnormally avid several months after surgery had returned both serum calcium and 1,25-$(OH)_2D$ levels to normal. Their findings suggest that something besides high 1,25-$(OH)_2D$ contributes to calcium hyperabsorption in primary hyperparathyroidism. Further light will no doubt be shed on this point in the future.

It is an old clinical observation that severe bone disease and renal stones tend to occur in different groups of patients, those with severe bone disease also having more severe hypercalcemia and those with stones greater hypercalciuria (Table III). A few years ago, studies began to suggest that differences in 1,25-$(OH)_2D$ production might account for this stratification. Current studies appear to confirm this theory. Figure 4, taken from the study of Adams et al.[181] on human adaptation to changes in dietary calcium, shows that the correlation between a change in serum PTH and a change in plasma 1,25-$(OH)_2D$, though clearly positive and direct, is far from uniform from person to person. Peacock et al.[187] studied a group of patients with primary hyperparathyroidism and found that after an overnight fast, plasma 1,25-$(OH)_2D$ could be low, normal, or high and that it behaved as if regulated by both PTH

Table III. Comparison of Two Types of Primary Hyperparathyroidism[a]

	Type 1	Type 2
Number of cases	44	88
Mean tumor weight (g)	5.90	1.05
Range	0.70–26.0	0.15–3.5
Length of history (years)	3.56 ± 4.8	6.66 ± 7.2
Doublings (from 50 mg)	6.9	4.3
Doubling time (months)	6.2	18.6
Linear growth rate (g/year)	1.64	0.15
Plasma Ca (mmoles/liter)	3.34 ± 0.60	2.91 ± 0.2
Plasma P (mmoles/liter), BUN 7.5	0.70 ± 0.13 (32)	0.76 ± 0.15
Plasma P (mmoles/liter), BUN 7.5	1.43 ± 0.43 (12)	1.05 ± 0.02
BUN (mmoles/liter)	9.3	5.5
Urinary Ca (mmoles/24 hr)	8.42	10.20
Nephrolithiasis	5%	100%
Nephrocalcinosis	30%	25%
AP (K.A.U.)	40.1 ± 23.2	8.1 ± 3.0
Bone disease	Osteitis fibrosa	Osteoporosis

[a] Reproduced with permission from Parfitt and Kleerekoper.[3]

and plasma calcium: the higher the plasma calcium, the *lower* the 1,25-$(OH)_2D$ level relative to the plasma PTH. Broadus *et al.*[188] have recently published a very important study implicating 1,25-$(OH)_2D$ in the pathogenesis of hyperparathyroid hypercalciuria and renal stone formation. They found that 50 unselected patients with primary hyperparathy-

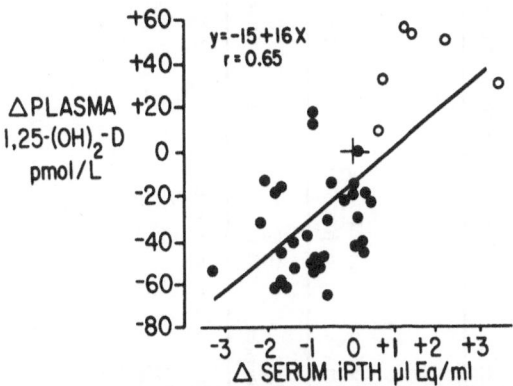

Fig. 4. The individual changes from baseline of plasma 1,25(OH)₂D concentrations as a function of the individual changes from baseline of serum PTH concentrations at the end of four days of CaCO₃ loading (●) or dietary Ca deprivation (○). From Ref. 181.

Table IV. Features of Absorptive and Nonabsorptive Patients with Primary Hyperparathyroidism[a]

Category of patient	No. of patients	Serum 25-OH-D (ng/ml)	Serum calcium (mg/dl)	Serum phosphorus (mg/dl)	Renal tubular phosphorus threshold (mg/dl)	Glomerular filtration rate (ml/min)	Serum iPTH (µl-Eq/ml)	Nephrogenous cAMP (nmoles/dl glomerular filtrate)	Age (years)	Sex (M/F)
Absorptive	20	20 ± 9	11.0 ± 0.5	2.6 ± 0.5	2.3 ± 0.5	91 ± 18	129 ± 58	4.13 ± 1.14	49 ± 12	8/22
Nonabsorptive	30	22 ± 10	11.3 ± 1.2	2.7 ± 0.5	2.3 ± 0.3	100 ± 27	123 ± 44	3.60 ± 1.01	55 ± 14	8/22

[a] Reproduced with permission from Broadus et al.[188]

roidism separated readily into two populations along a continuum: 30 patients with hyperabsorption of dietary calcium, marked hypercalciuria, very high plasma levels of $1,25-(OH)_2D$, and a high incidence of stones (19 of 30 patients) and 20 patients with normal calcium absorption, normocalciuria, normal or high-normal $1,25-(OH)_2D$, and a low incidence of stones (3 of 20 patients). As can be seen in Table IV, these two groups of patients could not be distinguished by any of the more conventional measurements of parathyroid function. From the standpoint of the pathogenesis of primary hyperparathyroidism and its manifestations, two fascinating findings emerge from this study. One, as the authors point out, is that nothing that we now know about the control of $1,25-(OH)_2D$ production can explain the very marked differences seen in this production. The other finding is that the patients with high $1,25-(OH)_2D$ levels, who showed greater postprandial hypercalcemia than the patients in the low-$1,25-(OH)_2D$ group, also showed more marked dietary suppression of nephrogenous cAMP. The authors postulate that in the hyperabsorptive population, postprandial hypercalcemia leads to a high filtered load of calcium, as well as both a suppression of PTH secretion and a PTH-stimulated renal calcium reabsorption in the distal nephron, where urinary concentration predisposes to stone formation. As we will discuss in Section 7.1, both *in vitro* and *in vivo* studies show that the responsiveness of abnormal parathyroid glands to suppression by calcium varies widely. It is tempting to speculate that the patients in the hyperabsorptive group might also have more readily suppressible glands, which could account for their tendency to more benign illness and lower serum calcium. In the small series of patients reported by Brown *et al.*,[40] those whose glands showed calcium-suppressible secretion *in vitro* tended to have lower serum calcium preoperatively than those whose glands proved to be nonsuppressible. Adequate data to confirm or refute our speculation are not yet available, however.

It is on bone that PTH and vitamin D truly act in concert. In vitamin D deficiency, serum calcium always falls (though not always to frankly hypocalcemic levels), despite severe secondary hyperparathyroidism. As we stated in our last review,[28] normal mineral homeostasis or calcium turnover requires both vitamin D and PTH, while normal skeletal homeostasis or bone turnover can probably be maintained by either. Certainly, active bone turnover can continue in the face of severe deficiency of vitamin D, as the occurrence of osteitis fibrosa (highly accelerated and poorly controlled bone turnover) in chronic renal failure attests. Patients with another kind of renal disease, nephrotic syndrome, may have vitamin D deficiency even when GFR is normal, probably because of loss of vitamin D and its binding protein into the urine. Malluche *et al.*[189] studied six such patients, all with low blood 25-OH-D, low total and free calcium, and elevated PTH; bone biopsy showed evidence of increased bone resorption in all six, in addition to the usual histologic changes of osteomalacia.

Weisbrode et al.[190] performed electron microscopy on bone taken from thyroparathyroidectomized rats treated with 1,25-$(OH)_2$D. Consistent with the clinical evidence that vitamin D can maintain bone turnover but not mineral homeostasis, electron microscopy showed evidence of marked activation of osteoclasts, some activation of osteoblasts, but little or no activation of osteocytes.

We know no more than we did a few years ago of the reason why PTH-supported calcium homeostasis requires vitamin D. We hold to our opinion that vitamin D may be required solely to make adequate ECF calcium available to enter and activate the PTH-stimulated cell (Section 7.6).

7.6. Cellular Response to PTH

Our knowledge of the cellular response to PTH is still rudimentary, and recent work has added relatively little to the picture. We will briefly outline the present "working model" of PTH action and point out additions and clarifications that recent studies have supplied.

PTH is assumed to initiate its effect by binding to a specific receptor on its target cells. The receptor has not been isolated, and its exact composition is unknown. Nissenson and Arnaud,[191] using binding of labeled hormone, demonstrated the presence of a specific PTH-binding site in chicken renal plasma membranes; the sites appeared to be of one class and to bind PTH with high affinity; stimulation of adenylate cyclase and hormone binding occurred in parallel in their system. Segre et al.[192] have also used hormone binding to identify the PTH-binding site in canine renal cortical plasma membranes and have shown that binding is specific for biologically active PTH. They also found a close correlation between the relative binding affinity of intact hormone and several synthetic analogs and their ability to stimulate adenylate cyclase in the same membranes. However, using synthetic inactive PTH analogs, Segre et al.[192] and Mahaffey et al.[17] showed that hormone binding can be dissociated from adenylate cyclase activation. Mohr and Hesch,[193] working with basal lateral membranes of bovine renal cortex, were able to separate three components of the receptor complex: a PTH-binding site, PTH-sensitive adenylate cyclase, and a "PTHase" or PTH-degrading activity.

After binding to its receptor, PTH activates adenylate cyclase and alters plasma membrane permeability to calcium, so that calcium enters the target cell down its concentration gradient. It is an old observation that PTH administration is followed by transient hypocalcemia, which has been assumed to reflect PTH-stimulated entry of calcium into a variety of cells. Mazzuoli et al.[194] have provided indirect support for this assumption in an ingenious study of the change in serum calcium that occurs immediately following parathyroidectomy. In 12 patients, surgical removal of parathyroid adenomas was followed within 2 hr by a short-lived *increase* in plasma calcium, preceding the usual decrease. Presumably, the acute drop in PTH following surgery permitted efflux of the intracellular calcium that had accumulated under the influence of PTH. Comparable results in a very different system, cultured kidney cells, were obtained by Borle and Uchikawa.[195] They showed that PTH increased total cell calcium content, calcium content in all cellular exchangeable pools, and all calcium exchange rates, the greatest effect being on the mitochondrial calcium pool; when PTH was removed, calcium efflux from these cells occurred. Results such as these support the contention that in hyperparathyroidism, intracellular calcium load and possibly cytoplasmic calcium levels increase in a variety of cells. Many of the symptoms of hyperparathyroidism may be ascribable to the toxic effects of this increase (Section 7.2).

There has been disagreement as to whether PTH stimulates cAMP production and calcium transport independently or whether one effect is primary and the other secondary. Borle and Uchikawa[196] claim that cAMP and dibutyryl cAMP have the same effect on renal cell calcium uptake and exchange that PTH does; however, high concentrations of nucleotide were needed to produce these effects. The weight of evidence indicates that PTH-stimulated calcium uptake and cAMP production are independent, but that target cell response requires both. Dziak and Stern[197] reported that PTH-stimulated calcium uptake in bone cells continued even when cAMP production was blocked. Nagata et al.[198] reported that cholera toxin, which increases cAMP production in bone, actually inhibited calcium mobilization from bone. Kakuta et al.[199] reported that PTH-stimulated bone adenylate cyclase activation was normal in hypocalcemic vitamin D-deficient rats, but bone calcium mobilization did not occur. Some studies do suggest that the cAMP response sometimes depends on available calcium: Carnes et al.[200] and Kakuta et al.[180] both found the cAMP response to PTH in renal cortex blunted by vitamin D deficiency, and Kakuta et al. showed that the blunted response was due to hypocalcemia rather than to vitamin D deficiency per se.

The steps that intervene in the target cells between calcium entry and cAMP production and the grossly observable effects of PTH are still not clear. One of the early steps may be a change in cell membrane potential. Mears[201] observed several years ago that PTH rapidly depolarized osteoclasts, presumably by increasing their calcium permeability;

calcitonin (CT), in contrast, polarized osteoclasts. More recently, Dietrich et al.[202] reported that drugs that inhibit cell depolarization—propranolol, lidocaine, tetracaine, and quinidine—also inhibited the demineralization of bone induced by PTH, 1,25-dihydroxycholecalciferol, cAMP, prostaglandin E_2, and osteoclast-activating factor. The ability of PTH to release calcium from fetal rat bone was completely abolished by simultaneous treatment with propranolol.

Studies on a variety of hormones that stimulate adenylate cyclase indicate that hormone binding is linked to cyclase activation by a protein called guanine nucleotide regulatory protein (GNRP). Hormone binding appears to cause this protein to bind GTP, and the complex then stimulates adenylate cyclase. The action of PTH probably involves this process.[203] Goltzman et al.[204] found that in the renal cortical membrane adenylate cyclase assay, GTP and its analogs increased the activity of all partially active synthetic PTH analogs. More recently, Drezner and Burch[205] and Levine et al.[206] have suggested that a deficiency of GNRP may be the cause of the defective cAMP response to PTH in pseudo-hypoparathyroidism type I. Levine et al. hypothesized that a generalized deficiency in GNRP might be present in these patients, and found low GNRP activity, as predicted, in erythrocyte membranes of all of their patients but one. cGMP, also, is almost certainly involved in the response to PTH. Walling et al.[207] have shown that PTH stimulates guanylate cyclase in fetal bone osteogenic cells, and Wrenn et al.[208] that PTH increases cGMP concentration in renal tubules; the rise in cGMP depends on the PTH-stimulated increase in intracellular calcium. Despite the continued work of many investigators, however, we do not seem to be appreciably closer than we were at the time of our last review to an adequate model linking calcium, cAMP, and cGMP in the PTH target cell.

Prostaglandins have been studied as possible mediators of the cellular response to PTH. The results of several studies in both kidney and bone strongly indicate that the responses of these cell types to PTH and to prostaglandins are independent of each other.[209–213] Indomethacin does not appear to affect the cAMP response to PTH. [211–213]

7.7. Hyperparathyroidism

7.7.1. Nature of Hyperparathyroidism

Further studies in hyperparathyroid patients,[214,215] on whole adenomatous and hyperplastic glands removed at surgery,[216] and on dispersed cells prepared from such glands[40,66,214] have confirmed that most of these pathologic glands are not totally autonomous, but respond both to changes in serum calcium and to other regulators. Brown et al.[214] found that preoperative in vivo suppressibility, assessed by the effect of calcium infusion on nephrogenous cAMP, and postoperative in vitro gland suppressibility, assessed by the effect of medium calcium on PTH release, correlated very well in 12 patients.

All studied have demonstrated a large range of responsiveness among pathologic glands, some glands showing near-normal calcium suppressibility and some very little. There seems to be no clear-cut qualitative distinction in response between normal and abnormal cells. Some have found that adenomatous glands tend to be less responsive than hyperplastic glands,[40,214] but the difference is by no means clear-cut or significant enough to make suppressibility useful as a preoperative diagnostic test. Responsiveness to β-adrenergic stimuli, glucagon, histamine, and prostaglandin E_2 also seems to vary enormously from gland to gland.[66]

This variability may account for the discrepant reports of the effects of propranolol and cimetidine on hyperparathyroidism. Caro and Besarab[217] reported a patient with probable primary hyperparathyroidism who was treated with propranolol for angina; serum calcium and PTH levels were incidentally noted to fall to near normal during this treatment. Fournier et al.[218] then reported that infusion of propranolol decreased PTH levels in nine patients with hyperparathyroidism secondary to uremia, an effect that was later reported to occur consistently in normal subjects.[69] Caro et al.[219] reported that PTH and alkaline phosphatase levels were lower, and evidence of renal osteodystrophy less, in uremic patients taking propranolol for hypertension or angina than in patients not taking propranolol. Examination of their data shows that the effect was not universal, however, and varied greatly from patient to patient. The same group also studied the effect of 5 months' treatment with high doses of propranolol (320 mg/day) in eight patients with primary hyperparathyroidism.[220] In four patients, serum calcium and PTH fell to normal; the other four subjects showed no significant improvement.

Similarly variable results have been reported for cimetidine. Sherwood et al.[221] reported a patient with primary hyperparathyroidism whose neck exploration was deferred for cimetidine treatment of a bleeding peptic ulcer. After 1 month of treatment she no longer had symptoms of hyperparathyroidism, and her serum calcium and PTH had fallen to normal. The patient was tested for full cycles on and off cimetidine therapy, and the results of each cycle of treatment were the same. Palmer et al.[222] then briefly reported on 14 hyperparathyroid patients treated for 4 weeks with cimetidine, 1200 mg/day. They found no effect on serum calcium, even though PTH was said to have fallen to normal or near normal in eight. Jacob et al.[223] reported 74% suppression of PTH levels in seven uremic patients by cimetidine treatment for 10 weeks. Serum ionized calcium fell slightly but not significantly.

All these reports are open to criticism. In no case have pharmacokinetic studies been done to see whether individual differences in drug metabolism might account for some of the observed variability in response. There have been no studies comparing *in vivo* and *in vitro* (postoperative) gland response. In the patients reported by Palmer et al., it is impossible that biologically active PTH could have fallen to normal without any change in serum calcium.

We would suggest, however, that the observed variable responses could well reflect differences in the nature of the pathologic parathyroid cells themselves. If, as we suggested in Section 7.3.5, normal parathyroid cells evolve from cells of greater potential, and may sometimes retain receptors for a variety of hormones and transmitters that have no significant effect on the normal mature parathyroid cell, it seems reasonable that pathologic cells might have dedifferentiated to a variable degree, becoming responsive once again to some of these secretagogues. Since the process would almost certainly be different in different individuals, some pathologic glands might become extra-responsive to β-adrenergic agonists and antagonists, some to histamine and cimetidine, and so forth.

7.7.2. Clinical Characteristics

We will not try to do justice to the polymorphous nature of hyperparathyroidism, but there are a few aspects of its presentation and character that have received attention recently.

The connection between previous radiotherapy to the head and neck and the development decades later (mean, 30 years) of hyperparathyroidism can be considered well established. In three recent series of patients with hyperparathyroidism, the number with a history of neck irradiation varied from 8 of 58[224] to 10 of 16,[225] in all cases significantly greater than control. Russ et al.[226] found 25% of 74 consecutive patients with hyperparathyroidism to have a history of neck irradiation; almost half of these patients also had developed a malignancy in the radiation field, of either thyroid, skin, parotid gland, or breast. One interesting report described a patient who had had unilateral neck irradiation for tuberculous nodes 61 years before and developed two hyperplastic parathyroid glands, a neuroma, and a nodular goiter all on the irradiated side.[227]

Two of the commonly accepted associations between primary hyperparathyroidism and other disorders have recently been questioned.

Christensson and Einarsson[228] could not confirm an increased frequency of cholelithiasis in hyperparathyroid patients; 82 such patients had the same incidence of cholelithiasis as a group of matched controls. Linos et al.[229] studied the association between hyperparathyroidism and peptic ulcer disease and concluded that the association is probably no more than coincidental. On the other hand, McCarthy et al.[230] reported a patient with a gastrinoma successfully treated with cimetidine in whom acid secretion became cimetidine-resistant when hyperparathyroidism developed. Surgical treatment of the hyperparathyroidism restored the response to cimetidine. It may well be that hyperparathyroidism stimulates acid secretion but not the development of ulcer disease per se.

Serum urate is often elevated in hyperparathyroidism. Christensson[231] studied this phenomenon in patients with hyperparathyroid and nonhyperparathyroid hypercalcemia and found that hyperparathyroidism, rather than hypercalcemia, seems to produce the hyperuricemia; although the elevations in serum urate and serum calcium were correlated in hyperparathyroid patients, there was no correlation between serum calcium and serum urate in the nonhyperparathyroid patients. We believe that a decrease in renal urate clearance is responsible for the hyperuricemia of hyperparathyroidism, but cannot explain why this should occur.

Akgun and Ertel[232] reported on two diabetic patients in whom hyperparathyroidism was diagnosed. In the first, removal of a parathyroid adenoma resulted in frequent hypoglycemic attacks, requiring a decrease in insulin dose from 45 to 20 U/day; in the second, surgery produced a marked improvement in glucose tolerance.

7.7.2.1. Familial Hypocalciuric Hypercalcemia

Marx et al. have published three studies of patients with what has been called familial hypocalciuric hypercalcemia (FHH).[233-235] This familial disorder is distinct from multiple endocrine neoplasia and closely resembles primary hyperparathyroidism. The differential diagnosis is important, because parathyroid surgery will not cure patients with FHH. These patients have normal PTH levels, but both their urinary calcium excretion and calcium clearance rate are *lower* than those of hyperparathyroid patients with comparable serum calcium levels. The primary pathologic defect could be a renal supersensitivity to the anticalciuretic effect of PTH; why PTH is not fully suppressed by the hypercalcemia is not clear, however. Although Marx et al.[235] reported significant differences in serum PTH and urinary cAMP between primary hyperparathyroidism and FHH (both were higher in primary hyperparathyroidism), it is very important for purposes of differential diagnosis to note that these authors found that after corrections for age, creatinine clearance, and serum calcium, *only* the TmP/GFR measurement (the renal phosphate threshold) still distinguished FHH from primary hyperparathyroidism.

7.7.2.2. PTH as the "Uremic Toxin"

Poorly understood breakdowns in many organ systems may make the lives of even patients with "well-controlled" renal failure miserable. Because various metabolic by-products accumulate in renal failure, and because uremic serum has toxic effects on many cells *in vitro*, the "uremic syndrome" has been ascribed to the effect of some metabolic toxin or toxins. Many candidates have been proposed, but none has been satisfactorily proven.

Some believe that PTH is the major, if not the sole, uremic toxin. Massry and Goldstein[236] reviewed those uremic concomitants in whose pathogenesis PTH has been implicated: CNS disorders, soft tissue calcification and necrosis, itching, bone disease, anemia, hyperlipidemia, and impotence. For some of these the evidence for the involvement of PTH is much better than for others.

Primary hyperparathyroidism is well known to be associated with a range of neuropsychiatric aberrations from depression, subtle personality change and decreased clarity of thought to psychosis. Cogan *et al.*[237] performed EEGs and tests of intellect on seven patients with primary and six with secondary hyperparathyroidism before and after parathyroidectomy. Before surgery, all patients showed an increase in the percentage of EEG slow-wave activity, about twice normal in primary and four times normal in secondary hyperparathyroidism. After surgery, the EEG returned to normal in the former group and to much nearer normal in the latter; in addition, the performance of the latter group on tests of intellect was much improved by surgery.

Guisado *et al.*[238] reported that brain calcium was increased in animals with acute renal failure and that their EEG abnormalities could be largely prevented by parathyroidectomy. Goldstein and Massry[239] have confirmed that brain calcium and EEG slow-wave activity are markedly increased in dogs by both acute uremia and treatment with parathyroid extract for only 3 days. The effects of parathyroid extract were reversible, disappearing 5 days after treatment was discontinued. Cooper *et al.*[240] studied patients with acute renal failure of less than 48 hr duration; despite only modest increases in urea and creatinine, their EEGs were strikingly abnormal, with *20 times* the normal percentage of slow-wave and one-third the normal percentage of high-frequency activity. These changes correlated with a twofold increase in plasma PTH. In a group of patients with acute renal failure who died, brain calcium was twice normal. The authors concluded that the increased brain calcium and EEG changes were attributable to the effect of PTH.

Some recent studies have suggested that PTH may be responsible for another common concomitant of chronic renal failure, peripheral neuropathy. Goldstein *et al.*[241] studied peripheral nerve calcium and motor nerve conduction velocity (MNCV) in dogs given PTH, dogs with acute renal failure and intact parathyroid glands, and parathyroidectomized dogs with acute renal failure. In the first two groups, peripheral nerve calcium was much increased and MNCV markedly slower; neither of these changes was observed in the animals parathyroidectomized before the induction of acute renal failure, and both returned to normal in the supplemented dogs after withdrawal of PTH. Avram *et al.*[242] measured MNCV and parathormone level in 42 uremic patients and found a roughly inverse relationship between PTH level and MNCV. Although objections can and have been raised to their attribution of decreased MNCV to high PTH—that the PTH measured in uremic patients is mostly inactive, and that it might just be a marker for severity of uremia[243]—the report of Avram *et al.*, coupled with the experimental findings of Goldstein *et al.*, must be considered suggestive. Avram *et al.*[244] also reported two patients with chronic renal failure whose MNCV increased significantly after parathyroidectomy. Others have not found a consistent effect of parathyroidectomy on MNCV, though some patients do seem to have improved.[245,246] Massry *et al.* have suggested that PTH may produce uremic impotence,[247] which would certainly be possible if PTH is, in fact, a neurotoxin.

We must point out that despite all these suggestive studies, there are no good data in humans substantiating that parathyroidectomy positively affects the length or long-term quality of life in azotemic patients or has any effect on the course of their disease, except in regard to itching and metastatic calcification, both of which are decreased. It is not possible at this time to conclude that PTH is the only, or even the most important, uremic toxin. The results we have described do, however, add to the growing evidence that PTH is able to affect many, if not most, body tissues. How it does this—whether through specific receptor binding or some other route—and what the physiologic significance of its effect may be, are unanswered questions. However, studies in uremic subjects do indicate, as have *in vitro* studies, that it is PTH itself and not simply PTH-induced hypercalcemia that affects these tissues.

7.7.3. Diagnosis

Although the diagnosis of hyperparathyroidism is usually not difficult, new techniques for diagnosis and for locating pathologic glands continue to be introduced and refined.

The marked superiority of ionized calcium measurements for detecting true hypercalcemia has been reconfirmed by Ladenson et al.[248] and by Conceicao et al.[249] Ladenson et al. measured total and ionized calcium and also calculated ionized calcium (using formulas to correct total calcium for albumin and pH) in 691 patients with suspected hypercalcemia. In almost 20%, the ionized calcium measurement revealed hypercalcemia when the total calcium was normal. The ionized calcium measurement proved particularly useful in patients with suspected hyperparathyroidism and in patients with hypoalbuminemia, mostly those with malignancies or renal transplants. The formulas for calculating ionized calcium proved inadequate substitutes for the ionized calcium measurement. Conceicao et al. similarly measured and calculated ionized calcium in 104 patients with chronic renal failure and 83 transplant recipients; of 129 samples in which ionized calcium was *measurably* high, ionized calcium was *calculated* as normal in over 70%. With presently available methods, ionized calcium can be measured with remarkable accuracy and reproducibility.[250]

Although numerous PTH radioimmunoassays are available, the literature consistently confirms that any of the commonly used assays will detect PTH excess very reliably. Although the C-terminal assays detect mostly C-terminal fragments rather than newly secreted intact PTH, Parthemore et al.[251] showed that a C-terminal assay can nevertheless sensitively detect acute and chronic changes in PTH secretion. The fine points of the various assays need not concern us, but the interested reader is referred to a recent comprehensive review by Christensen.[253]

The nephrogenous cAMP measurement reflects the activity of circulating PTH very accurately. Broadus et al.[254] have shown that nephrogenous cAMP is remarkably sensitive, even to very small changes in the serum calcium. Figure 5 shows the effect of low-dose infusion, which does not even produce hypercalcemia, on serum iPTH, urinary cAMP, and nephrogenous cAMP in eight normal subjects. As can be seen, the immediate response in all normal subjects was a marked fall in urinary and nephrogenous AMP. Both indices also declined in patients with hyperparathyroidism, but to a lesser extent, so that postinfusion values for both clearly separated normal subjects from those with hyperparathyroidism. Although most physicians still turn first to the PTH immunoassay to diagnose hyperparathyroidism, the nephrogenous cAMP measurement is as sensitive a test as any PTH radioimmunoassay currently in use.

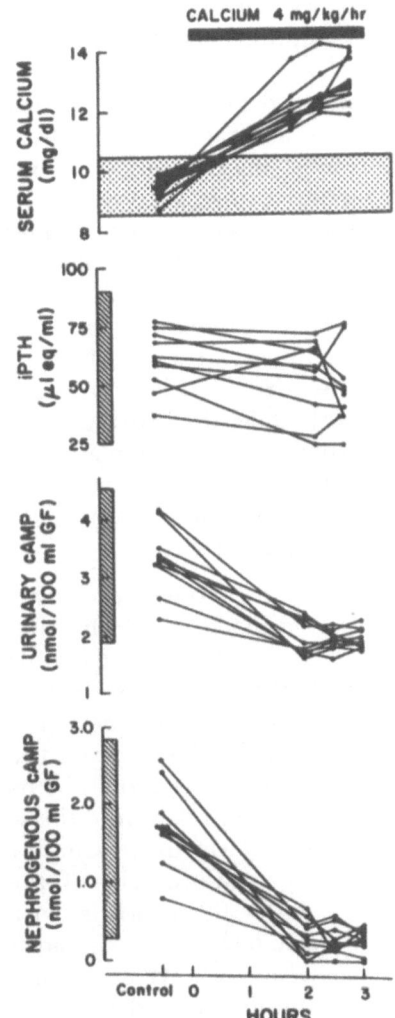

Fig. 5. The results of calcium injection in eight normal subjects. From Ref. 254.

In a sense, the nephrogenous cAMP measurement is a PTH bioassay. Unfortunately, it is of no use in precisely the patients in whom a measurement of biologically active rather than immunoreactive PTH is needed: patients with chronic renal failure and hypercalcemia. Many bioassays for PTH have been used experimentally, but they have been too insensitive to be useful diagnostically. However, some extremely sensitive bioassays have recently been developed.[255-257] If such assays can be made generally available, they will not only be applicable to patients with chronic renal failure but may completely replace the PTH radioimmunoassays now in use.

Various imaging techniques have been used to try to locate enlarged parathyroid glands prior to surgery. These include ultrasound,[258] ultrasound and radionuclide subtraction,[259] computed tomography,[260] and, of course, angiography.[261] Brote et al.[262] have confirmed that the combination of angiography and venous sampling can provide accurate preoperative localization in most cases. Wang[263] has suggested that a conventional barium swallow should be done in all patients before "second-look" parathyroid surgery, since an enlarged gland can sometimes be seen indenting the esophagus. Sofianides et al.[264] have studied the usefulness of a modified form of cervical esophagography, using rapid sequential filming of the maximally distended esophagus. Using this technique, they correctly localized parathyroid adenomas in 19 of 20 patients; five of these adenomas measured 1.5 cm or less.

Given the current state of diagnostic testing, we would recommend the following evaluation procedure for a patient with suspected hyperparathyroidism:

1. At least three blood samples for total calcium and phosphorus; the blood should be free-flowing and should be separated immediately, so that erythrocyte phosphate will not leak into the plasma.
2. If there is any question whether serum calcium is high-normal or in fact high, ionized calcium should be measured.
3. Serum PTH should be measured with any good assay and evaluated in relation to the serum calcium.
4. Two 24-hr urine samples should be obtained on a random diet for measurement of the rate of calcium excretion and the TmP/GFR, which is perhaps our most sensitive currently available test of parathyroid function.[4]
5. Urinary cAMP can be measured if the preceding tests leave any question as to diagnosis.

As good as current assays are, we think the PTH assay result should always be corroborated by another test of parathyroid function such as the TmP/GFR or urinary cAMP; a patient should not be taken to surgery on the basis of an elevated PTH measurement alone.

The results obtained by Sofianides et al. with their modified esophagography are so impressive that we feel this study should be part of every patient's preoperative evaluation. Routine use of other imaging techniques before neck exploration is not warranted, however: the noninvasive techniques are insensitive and costly, and angiography and venous sampling involve significant risk as well as expense. Before second-look surgery, use of the various noninvasive techniques may be justified, but we still believe that angiography and venous sampling should be done only if the first operation was a meticulous exploration by an experienced parathyroid surgeon. Van Vroonhoven and Muller[265] have reaffirmed Wang's conclusion[263] that most failures in parathyroid surgery are preventable: they have been the result of "inadequate anatomical knowledge [or] inadequate surgical technique."[265]

7.7.4. Treatment

Hyperparathyroidism should be treated, for two reasons: one, that the patient will feel better (we believe that "asymptomatic" hyperparathyroidism is nothing but subtly symptomatic disease to which the patient has adapted), and two, that long-term complications are thus avoided. We do not really know what the consequences of chronic calcium overload in organ systems all over the body may be, but Freaney et al.[266] have suggested that the effect on the kidney may be a gradual but irreversible loss of function. They evaluated renal function before and approximately 2 years after parathyroidectomy in 40 patients with primary hyperparathyroidism classified according to their serum calcium at the time of presentation. There was a clear tendency for creatinine clearance to fall as serum calcium rose: mean clearance was 91 ml/min for the patients with calcium under 11.1 mg/dl, 68 ml/min for those with calcium of 11.1–12.0, 51 ml/min for those with calcium of 12.1–13.0, and 39 ml/min for those with calcium over 13. Even more striking is their finding that in almost none of these patients had creatinine clearance significantly improved 2 years after successful parathyroidectomy.

Despite anecdotal reports of the efficacy of propranolol and cimetidine, the proper treatment for almost all patients with primary hyperparathyroidism is still surgery performed by an experienced parathyroid surgeon. Traditional surgery calls for identification of all four glands, removal of a solitary adenoma or removal of three and one-half glands (subtotal parathyroidectomy) in the case of hyperplasia. More recently, some surgeons have advocated routine subtotal parathyroidectomy, on the grounds that late, recurrent hyperparathyroidism may thereby be prevented; Attie et al.[267] have reviewed the abundant arguments against the need for and safety of this course (it increases the incidence of postsurgical hypoparathyroidism) and concluded, as we do, that it is unwarranted. Only visibly enlarged glands should be removed.[267] There has been some debate over whether multiple parathyroid adenomas exist as a separate entity, or whether patients with more than one enlarged gland should be considered to have hyperplasia; Harness et al.[268] have presented convincing evidence that multiple adenomas can occur and that patients with them can be successfully treated by removal of the enlarged glands only.

Three groups have reported methods for making the pathologic distinction between adenomatous and hyperplastic or hyperplastic and normal glands intraoperatively, to help the surgeon decide how vigorous an exploration and how extensive an operation may be needed. Ljungberg and Tibblin[269] reported a modification of the fat-staining technique of Roth and Gallagher (see Ref. 28) that proved very helpful in their hands. Wang and Rieder[270] and Akerstrom et al.[271] evaluated density tests. Akerstrom et al. reported in 1977 that the fall of parathyroid glands in density gradient columns correlated with their percentage of parenchymal cells; since the ratio of parenchymal to fat cells increases early in the evolution of pathologic glands, Akerstrom et al. felt the density test had great potential for intraoperative detection. Wang and Rieder have taken this test further: they used a standardized mannitol solution with a density range between 1.049 and 1.069 and reported that "whereas the normal parathyroid tissue floated, the diseased tissue invariably sank." Using this test, which they feel is a more accurate indicator of pathology than is gland size, they were able to limit surgery to a unilateral neck exploration in 64% of their patients with parathyroid adenomas; all these patients proved to have one adenomatous and one normal gland (of which a small biopsy was tested for density) on the first side explored, so the other glands were not sought. There is certainly some benefit to the patient in limiting surgery as much as is reasonably possible; Wang and Rieder, however, discount the possibility of multiple adenomas, an entity they do not believe in. We are still inclined to think that for most patients, a bilateral neck exploration with an attempt to identify all four glands must be held to be the best policy.

Autotransplantation of parathyroid tissue from the neck to a peripheral muscle is still being studied and reported. We see no justification for its use as a routine procedure to guard against postoperative hypoparathyroidism or to make reoperation, if necessary, easier, as some have advocated. Ohman et al.[272] found that the procedure did not adequately protect patients undergoing total thyroidectomy from postoperative hypoparathyroidism and recommended, instead, that every effort be made to preserve the parathyroids *in situ*. Both Brennan et al.[273] and Penn and Haase[274] have reported recurrent hyperparathyroidism in patients who had portions of adenomas transplanted to the arm during parathyroid surgery. Since cryopreservation can preserve functional parathyroid tissue for at least 1–2 years,[275] it seems reasonable that some tissue be cryopreserved both from patients undergoing second-look surgery, who have already had normal glands removed, and from patients undergoing subtotal parathyroidectomies. If postsurgical hypoparathyroidism develops, autotransplantation can then be performed. Brennan *et al.*[276] have reported apparently successful treatment of postsurgical hypoparathyroidism in six patients by autotransplantation of their own preserved parathyroid tissue. It will be interesting to see if these patients remain "euparathyroid" on long-term follow-up.

What about medical treatment of hyperparathyroidism—not just to lower the serum calcium, as phosphate does, but to reduce PTH secretion? Published case reports do suggest that in an occasional patient, cimetidine[221] or propranolol[217] will reduce both PTH secretion and serum calcium to normal; the response probably depends on the idiosyncratic biologic properties of the individual tumor. Even in the responsive patients, however, the dose of drug required may be high and will carry its own risks and side effects; in addition, the risk of the patient's being lost to follow-up and of the drug ceasing to control the illness will still be present. It may be that for an occasional patient who is a poor surgical risk, a trial of propranolol or cimetidine or both will be indicated, and the option of drug treatment should, perhaps, be outlined to all patients. However, we still feel that for almost every patient, surgery remains the treatment of choice.

7.7.5. Renal Osteodystrophy

In chronic dialysis patients, classical, severe secondary hyperparathyroidism with osteitis fibrosa and widespread ectopic calcification is much less common than it once was. Its decline can probably be ascribed to two treatment practices: better control of serum phosphate, which has followed wider appreciation of the adverse effects of hyperphosphatemia, and more frequent and earlier prescription of cholecalciferol and its derivatives, especially 1α-hydroxy- and 1,25-dihydroxycholecalciferol.

Opinions differ as to the relative importance in early renal failure (GFR 50–75% of normal) of retained phosphate versus disturbed vitamin D metabolism (both 1,25- and 24,25-dihydroxycholecalciferol deficiency[277]) in the genesis of osteodystrophy. The different opinions are set out in two companion editorials published in 1978.[278,279] Although the theory of ever-increasing phosphate leading to ever-worsening secondary hyperparathyroidism has a certain neatness, there is really no evidence that phosphate retention is a problem in early human renal failure; if anything, these patients, along with slightly low serum calcium, have *low* serum phosphate, excrete a phosphate load as well or better than normal subjects, and have marked hypocalciuria and high PTH, the profile of vitamin D deficiency. The theory that early renal failure leads to 1,25-$(OH)_2D$ deficiency fits the facts, but is not fully proven. Proof turns upon the accurate measurement of 1,25-(OH)$_2$D levels in blood at various stages of renal failure. Slatopolsky et al.[278] have stated that 1,25-(OH)$_2$D levels are normal in early renal failure, but others have reported low levels[279] and have demonstrated both osteomalacia and decreased intestinal calcium absorption in patients with a GFR as high as 75% of normal.[280] Whichever factor one takes to be preeminent, it is clear that they overlap in inducing secondary hyperparathyroidism and that any tendency to retain phosphate will be detrimental to the patient, further suppressing 1,25-(OH)$_2$D production (by inhibiting the 1α-hydroxylation) and enhancing soft tissue deposition of calcium phosphate. There is evidence that diets that restrict phosphate can retard the development of bone disease.[281]

A wealth of studies testifies to the value of the newly available 1α-hydroxycholecalciferol and 1,25-dihydroxycholecalciferol in raising serum calcium, lowering PTH, and correcting both hyperparathyroid bone disease and osteomalacia in patients with chronic renal failure,[282–288] although good comparative studies with the older vitamin D preparations are, for the most part, lacking. There are definite risks to vitamin D therapy, however, and these must be watched for, most carefully with the most potent new derivatives. Vitamin D will increase intestinal absorption, not just of calcium but also of phosphate, increasing the body phosphate burden. The risk of hypercalcemia is high; it developed in 5 of 15,[284] 19 of 22,[285] 6 of 11,[288] and 7 of 8[289] subjects in recently reported clinical trials of the new vitamin D derivatives. Although the hypercalcemia produced by the new derivatives generally does not last as long as that produced by older products, it still may persist for several days even with treatment.[288] Christiansen et al.[289] reported a definite deterioration in renal function in nondialyzed patients (creatinine clearance less than 35 ml/min) treatment with 1,25-dihydroxycholecalciferol; a like decline was not seen in matched patients treated with vitamin D$_3$. Such reports must give us pause in embracing 1,25-dihydroxycholecalciferol as a miraculous adjunct to treatment of chronic renal failure, at least for patients who still have renal function to preserve. At any rate, it is clear that these new vitamin D products must be used with extreme care and watchfulness.

Recently, there has been described a new form of dialysis bone disease that looks like severe osteomalacia, with little or no osteitis fibrosa.[290,291] The incidence of this disease varies greatly between different countries and regions and appears to be highest in its most severe form in Newcastle, England (it has been called "Newcastle osteodystrophy"). Patients with this disease have normal alkaline phosphatase and may have normal or low PTH. Treatment with vitamin D or its derivatives commonly produces marked hypercalcemia but no beneficial effect on the bone disease. Coburn et al.[292] have shown that this bone disease may be a manifestation of chronic aluminum intoxication. It is associated with a high incidence of "dialysis dementia," which may also be a product of aluminum intoxication, and the aluminum may inhibit PTH secretion, blunting the PTH response to hypocalcemic stimuli. The aluminum in these cases comes from the water supply, not from aluminum-containing antacids, and the only known treatment is to change the water system used for drinking and dialysis, deionizing to remove aluminum.

CT levels are almost always high in chronic renal failure, there being an inverse correlation between creatinine clearance and CT level.[293] The high levels, thought to be due to decreased renal metabolism of CT, occur despite hypocalcemia, which should theoretically inhibit CT secretion. There is some slight evidence that osteodystrophy may be worse in patients who do not develop high CT levels.[294] Feletti and Bonomini[295] have attempted to treat osteodystrophy with a 6-month course of synthetic salmon CT. Bone pain disappeared in eight of their ten cases, alkaline phosphatase levels fell to normal, and bone biopsies showed a slight increase in osteoblastic and a significant decrease in osteoclastic activity. Serum phosphate levels fell significantly within 20 days, perhaps reflecting decreased bone resorption. Their promising results suggest that this treatment should be more widely tested. We also need better studies of why endogenous serum CT is elevated in renal failure and what, if anything, its elevation accomplishes.

Parathyroidectomy still has a place in the treatment of severe secondary hyperparathyroidism. Pruritus, bone pain, depression and confusion, and ectopic calcification may be positively affected. Quality of life can improve tremendously for some patients, and life may even be prolonged for some as the rate of ectopic vascular calcification decreases.

Ectopic calcification is a severe problem for the dialysis patient. Zucchelli et al.[296] followed with soft tissue microradiographs 94 uremic patients who started dialysis between 1968 and 1977; most began dialysis with arterial calcifications, and these progressed strikingly over the 10-year period of study. These authors attempted to treat nine uremic patients with widespread calcifications with the diphosphonate EHDP for 5 to 9 months. The treatment was well tolerated, and periarticular calcifications decreased in two patients, but arterial calcification decreased in only one of the nine (though progressing in none). Since no treatment other than parathyroidectomy has previously been found to reverse vascular calcification, diphosphonate therapy is worthy of further study. It should be noted, however, that diphosphonates can produce osteomalacia, and it is not clear that their long-term use will not prove to be of greater harm than benefit.

7.8. Hypoparathyroidism

7.8.1. Presentation and Diagnosis

"Hypoparathyroidism" is a composite entity comprising several disorders, some clinically and some only biochemically distinguishable. We are beginning to sort these out more accurately as our knowledge of PTH physiology and our ability to test it have increased. Table V, from a recent review of hypoparathyroidism,[297] outlines a proposed pathophysiologic classification of the hypoparathyroid disorders. The most important distinction is that between PTH deficiency and PTH resistance; only one patient has been described who produced normal amounts of an "ineffective" form of PTH.[298]

The clinical presentation will not distinguish primary (hormone deficiency) hypoparathyroidism from pseudo- (hormone resistant) hypoparathyroidism. Even the combination of hypocalcemia with Albright's osteodystrophy (short stature, round face, short neck, and short metacarpals and metatarsals) does not unequivocally indicate pseudohypoparathyroidism, since we now recognize that the PTH resistance and the somatic features once thought to be inseparable from it are inherited independently. The hypoparathyroid patient presents with some degree of hypocalcemia, sometimes with hyperphosphatemia, and often with some neurologic consequence of hypocalcemia, most commonly tetany (the symptoms of which may be very subtle), or seizures.[299] Ten of twenty-eight patients of Lewin et al.[299] presented with seizures; seven had been treated with anticonvulsants for 2 or more years before hypocalcemia was discovered. Graham et al.[300] reported two interesting cases of idiopathic hypoparathyroidism, which may occur at any age, presenting as new-onset seizures in elderly patients; one of their patients, at 85, is the oldest reported patient to present with hypoparathyroidism. Less common neuropsychiatric presentations have occurred in some patients with mild to severe hypocalcemia, sometimes in the absence of any of the more common neurologic signs. Slyter[301] recently reported the case of a 32-year-old man who presented with a gradually progressive dementia as his sole neurologic finding, despite a serum calcium of 4.5. Preskorn and Reveley[302] described a patient with pseudohypoparathyroidism and mild hypocalcemia who presented with Capgras' syndrome, a psychosis whose sufferers believe that close relatives have been replaced by physically indistinguishable impostors.

It is interesting that although hypocalcemia is a fairly common un-

Table V. Classification of Hypoparathyroid Disorders[a]

Category	Old terminology	Proposed terminology
PTH-deficient hypocalcemia		
Lack of hormone	Hypoparathyroidism	Hormone-deficient hypoparathyroidism
Ineffective hormone	Pseudoidiopathic hypoparathyroidism	Hormone-ineffective hypoparathyroidism
PTH-resistant		Hormone-resistant hypoparathyroidism
With hypocalcemia	Pseudohypoparathyroidism	Hypocalcemic phase
With normocalcemia	Pseudopseudohypoparathyroidism or normocalcemic pseudohypoparathyroidism	Normocalcemic phase
Normocalcemia (no PTH resistance)	Pseudopseudohypoparathyroidism	Albright's osteodystrophy

[a] Reproduced with permission from Breslau and Pak.[297]

expected finding on routine biochemical screens, hypoparathyroidism is rarely the cause. Parfitt,[303] in an excellent, clear, and inclusive review of the manifestations of hypoparathyroidism, notes that no previously unrecognized case was uncovered at the Henry Ford Hospital in the first 2 years of routine multichannel screening, "which suggests that completely asymptomatic hypoparathyroidism is exceedingly uncommon."

In any form of hypoparathyroidism that goes untreated for long enough, small cerebral calcifications, most commonly in the basal ganglia, may develop, sometimes with evidence of an extrapyramidal disorder such as Parkinsonism, dystonia, or athetosis. The calcification has been tentatively ascribed to a longstanding increase in the calcium–phosphorus product. Nyland and Skre[304] have reported an interesting family in which five out of nine members in one generation developed a midlife encephalopathy with massive calcifications in the basal ganglia, dentate nuclei, and cerebral sulci. Serum calcium and phosphate were normal; only a subnormal phosphorus diuresis in response to PTH indicated the presence of a hypoparathyroid state. Thus, the calcification could not be ascribed to chronic abnormal divalent ion metabolism. Perhaps it reflects a congenital vascular abnormality in these areas of the brain permitting calcification.

The diagnosis of hypoparathyroidism involves, first, determining that a patient presenting with symptomatic hypocalcemia has some form of hypoparathyroidism rather than another cause for hypocalcemia, such as vitamin D deficiency; and second, distinguishing between hormone-deficient and hormone-resistant hypoparathyroidism. Lewin et al.[299] and Werder et al.[305] correctly classified 68 patients as having either primary hypoparathyroidism, pseudohypoparathyroidism type 1 (with a deficient cAMP response to PTH), or pseudohypoparathyroidism type 2 (with deficient response to PTH beyond the step of cAMP activation) by measuring serum calcium and PTH levels and the urinary cAMP response to PTH infusion. In primary hypoparathyroidism, PTH is either undetectable or clearly below the level expected for the serum calcium,[303] while in pseudohypoparathyroidism PTH levels are high because of end-organ resistance. If high PTH levels are found, the urinary cAMP response will differentiate type 1 from type 2 pseudohypoparathyroidism.

EDTA infusion has been used to test PTH reserve and thereby to estimate the severity of primary hypoparathyroidism. However, this test carries some risk to the patient, should never be necessary in the clinical setting, and can virtually always be replaced in the research setting by the nephrogenous cAMP measurement.[306]

Magnesium deficiency produces a "secondary hypoparathyroidism" with hypocalcemia. The hypocalcemia results partly from a change in bone crystal structure that decreases responsiveness to PTH and partly from reduced PTH secretion. Rude et al.[307] found that magnesium infusion into magnesium-deficient patients produced an immediate PTH secretory response that peaked within 5 to 15 min. Since hormone synthesis takes at least 15 to 20 min, their results suggest that magnesium depletion impairs PTH secretion rather than its synthesis.

Mennes et al.[308] reported three patients hospitalized with chronic renal failure and severe hypocalcemia (serum calcium 3.6–4.7 mg/dl) who were found to have severe magnesium depletion. With magnesium replacement alone, serum calcium rose to virtually normal levels. Although severe hypomagnesemia is rare in chronic renal failure, this report reminds us that it should be looked for in any patient with renal failure who has unexpectedly severe hypocalcemia.

7.8.2. Pseudohypoparathyroidism

Like hypoparathyroidism, the term pseudohypoparathyroidism covers a spectrum of disease. All patients exhibit some resistance to PTH, and almost all have elevated PTH levels. The resistance is commonly incomplete, and it is clear that in at least some patients the high PTH levels do have some effect in overcoming target cell resistance.[309] It is equally clear that the degree of resistance of the various target cell types varies from patient to patient. Patients have been described in whom the skeleton (at least, the osteoclasts) appears to be responsive to PTH while the kidney, at least as regards phosphate excretion, is resistant,[310,311] and others in whom only the renal 1α-hydroxylase system for vitamin D appears to be resistant and other target cells responsive.[312]

Parfitt[313] found PTH-responsive renal tubular *calcium* reabsorption to be within normal limits in six of six unrelated patients with pseudohypoparathyroidism. Whether one believes that different patients really do have extremely selective disorders, or rather that the basic cellular defect is always present in all PTH target cells but is simply variably expressed,[314] the fact remains that the clinical presentations of these patients, in terms of their serum calcium and phosphate levels, their degree of bone disease, their measured serum 1,25-dihydroxycholecalciferol, and their renal cAMP and phosphaturic responses to PTH, do vary a great deal.

The pathophysiology of pseudohypoparathyroidism is complex, and at this point there is no acceptable unitary explanation available. For those interested in trying to make their own sense of it, the data to be accounted for are reviewed through 1979 by Breslau and Pak.[297] We can see three concepts of unifying value emerging from recent work: the importance of low calcium in mediating PTH refractoriness, the importance of $1,25-(OH)_2D$ deficiency, and the possibility that a defect in hormone-stimulated GTP mobilization underlies the subnormal cAMP response to PTH seen in pseudohypoparathyroidism type 1.

Calcium infusion has long been known to induce phosphaturia in patients with postsurgical hypoparathyroidism[315]; the fall in serum phosphate that occurs when hypoparathyroid patients are treated with vitamin D is probably due to the rise in serum calcium that vitamin D produces rather than to any direct effect of vitamin D on the kidney. Breslau and Moses[316] reported that in 15 patients with pseudohypoparathyroidism there was a significant correlation between the serum calcium and the increase in PTH-stimulated renal cAMP production. One can, of course, draw the obvious conclusion that the higher serum calcium and greater cAMP response were parallel manifestations of a less severe state of PTH refractoriness; however, a less obvious possibility is that the higher calcium increased cAMP responsiveness to PTH. This hypothesis is consistent with the known fact that PTH produces some of its effect by increasing calcium entry into its target cells, although it must be admitted that *in vitro* PTH-stimulated cAMP production is apparently independent of calcium. Duck *et al.*[311] have reported a patient with pseudohypoparathyroidism type 2 in whom correction of hypocalcemia with vitamin D lowered PTH levels to normal and resulted in normal cAMP and phosphaturic responses to PTH. Yamada *et al.*[309] studied two patients with pseudohypoparathyroidism type 1 and one with type 2 in whom renal cAMP and phosphaturic responses were improved by combined calcium and PTH infusion, as well as by PTH infusion after vitamin D treatment. Baron *et al.*[317] reported that acetazolamide treatment, which increased serum ionized calcium, produced a 100% increase in fractional phosphate excretion in four type 1 patients (although curiously, in contrast to other investigators, they found that calcium infusion had the opposite effect).

Low 1,25-(OH)$_2$D levels have been reported in pseudohypoparathyroidism, and at least one patient has been described whose only PTH-resistant system appeared to be the renal 1α-hydroxylase.[312] Lawayin et al.[318] have described another patient with a partially responsive 1α-hydroxylase in whom normal levels of 1,25-(OH)$_2$D and normocalcemia were induced by treatment with high-dose PTH infusions for 4 days. Although 1,25-(OH)$_2$D deficiency cannot be the sole defect in all pseudohypoparathyroid patients, as replacement with this hormone does not always effect a complete return to normal, it is probably an important contributor to hypocalcemia in virtually all cases. Subnormal 1,25-(OH)$_2$D levels may result from either inherent resistance of the renal 1α-hydroxylase to PTH or inhibition of the 1α-hydroxylase by hyperphosphatemia, or both; there may be patients whose only significant cellular defect is resistance of renal tubular phosphate transport to PTH, with resultant hyperphosphatemia, inhibition of 1,25-(OH)$_2$D production, and hypocalcemia due to both 1,25-(OH)$_2$D deficiency and the effect of high phosphate on the blood–bone equilibrium for calcium.

The suggestion of Drezner and Burch[205] and of Levine et al.[206] that a defect in the GTP coupling of PTH to adenylate cyclase is the basic cellular fault in pseudohypoparathyroidism is an exciting one. As we said above (Section 7.4), Levine et al. hypothesized that this defect should be a generalized one, and did indeed find evidence of it in red cells. A few case reports do describe endocrine abnormalities outside of the PTH system; Carlson et al.[319] found evidence of impaired prolactin secretion in six members of two families with hypoparathyroidism, and Wolfsdorf et al.[320] described a pseudohypoparathyroid patient with partial ovarian resistance to gonadotropins and a subnormal plasma cAMP response to glucagon. It is likely that pseudohypoparathyroidism is, in fact, a more generalized disorder than has been appreciated, and that subtle defects in many endocrine and even nonendocrine systems might be found in most patients if vigorously sought. An obvious question that arises about the postulated guanine nucleotide defect is why more widespread clinical manifestations would not be readily apparent, since the defect is such a basic one. We expect within the next few years to see much greater clarification of the pathophysiology of this intriguing disorder.

7.8.3. Treatment

The basic treatment for hypoparathyroidism of all kinds is still vitamin D. Despite the enormous interest generated by the newly available "active" forms, 1α-hydroxy- and 1,25-dihydroxycholecalciferol, there is no clear evidence that any form of vitamin D is "best." All can be used effectively.[321] 1α-hydroxy and 1,25-dihydroxycholecalciferol have the advantages of rapid action and of rapid metabolism, so that if they induce hypercalcemia it disappears relatively quickly when they are discontinued; however, they induce hypercalcemia very commonly.[284,285,288,289] Treatment with vitamin D should begin with a high dose for quick correction of hypocalcemia,[322] but most patients will need the dose decreased sharply when normocalcemia is reached; if this principle is not kept in mind, patients may become hypercalcemic very rapidly.

Several patients, reported by Lewin et al.,[299] had been treated with anticonvulsants, most commonly dilantin, for years before hypocalcemia was detected. As dilantin probably inhibits movement of calcium into bone as well as into brain, it may interfere with vitamin D treatment. In addition, since dilantin induces the liver enzymes involved in vitamin D metabolism, the dose requirement for vitamin D may change when dilantin is decreased or discontinued. Lewin et al. stress that particular care must be taken with patients receiving 1α-hydroxycholecalciferol and any of the anticonvulsants—dilantin, phenobarbital, and mysoline—which induce liver enzymes; since 1α-hydroxycholecalciferol is activated in the liver by 25-hydroxylation, these anticonvulsants may dramatically affect its metabolism, and reduction in anticonvulsant therapy may result in hypercalcemia.

Porter et al.[323] treated seven patients with mild hypoparathyroidism (mean serum calcium 8.2 mg/dl) with chlorthalidone and salt restriction; mean serum calcium rose to 9.3, though two patients were not rendered normocalcemic. Porter et al. suggest that chlorthalidone may be preferable to vitamin D therapy for selected patients because it does not produce the hypercalciuria "that often results in nephrocalcinosis, nephrolithiasis, and renal failure"[323]; their statement of the dire consequences of vitamin D-induced hypercalciuria is incorrect, however. The hypercalciuria of well-treated hypoparathyroid patients is not usually troublesome. It rarely produces stones and does not result in either nephrocalcinosis or renal failure. At this point we still consider vitamin D the treatment of choice for hypoparathyroid hypocalcemia.

Acetazolamide, as suggested by Baran et al.,[317] has promise as an adjunct to vitamin D therapy. By increasing ionized calcium, it may decrease the requirement for vitamin D and the risk of hypercalcemia. Its use deserves wider testing.

7.9. Calcitonin

Calcitonin is, to us, a hormone much more interesting in theory than in practice. Since thyroidectomized patients, as well as patients markedly hypercalcitonemic from medullary carcinoma of the thyroid (MCT), have normal calcium metabolism, it is obvious that CT can play no very important role in adult human calcium metabolism. We still hold to the opinion that CT is largely a vestigial hormone in man.

7.9.1. Origins, Embryology, Structure, and Metabolism

CT is a much older hormone than PTH, first appearing in saltwater fish.[324] The future CT-producing cells originate in the neural crest and migrate to the area of the fourth branchial pouch, there coming to be associated with either the ultimobranchial body or, in mammals, the thyroid gland.[325] The neural crest origin of CT may explain its relatively high content in brain, where it may have some effects on behavior.

Although the thyroid gland harbors most mammalian C-cells, CT has also been identified in parathyroid and thymus glands of several species, including man.[326,327] Silva et al.[328] have shown that almost all patients have detectable levels of serum CT after total thyroidectomy; levels in thyroidectomized men were significantly lower than in normal controls, while levels in women were near control levels. This finding has implications for interpretation of the CT assay (see below).

Mammalian and nonmammalian CTs have similar but not identical structures. Nonmammalian CTs are from 10 to 50 times more potent than human in the standard hypocalcemic rat bioassay,[324] and this greater potency can be demonstrated in clinical applications of the hormone in man as well. Knowledge of the amino acid sequence of the hormone, now determined for eel, three species of salmon, pig, cow, sheep, rat, and man,[324] permits prediction of the secondary structure. Ultimobranchial CTs can be predicted to have a much greater degree of helical structure than mammalian CTs, and the predicted degree of helical structure parallels the hypocalcemic potency.[329] In patients with MCT, and probably in other subjects, CT circulates in plasma in three to five immunoreactive forms. The 32-amino-acid peptide, "calcitonin monomer," whose sequence is known, may comprise as little as 20% of the hormone measured by RIA.[330] Heath and Sizemore[330] did a careful study of CT in tumor, tumor venous effluent, and peripheral blood of two patients with MCT. Under basal conditions, approximately one-third of the CT measured by RIA was CT monomer; the proportion increased to 53% during calcium infusion. The profiles of immunochemical heterogeneity were similar in tumor extract, tumor effluent, and peripheral blood, indicating that the various CT species were secreted from the gland and that the heterogeneity could not be ascribed to protein binding or peripheral metabolism.

The metabolic fate of CT in humans is not very clear. It is likely that it is cleared and degraded primarily by the kidney.[331] Baylin et al.[332]

have shown that some degradation occurs in plasma, probably by non-specific proteases, but this degradation does not appear to be quantitatively significant.

7.9.2. Assay

There have been many problems with the CT assay. Only in the past few years have immunoassays sensitive enough to detect immunoreactive CT in most normal human subjects been available.[333-335] In some studies, sera from thyroidectomized patients have been assumed to be appropriate CT-free controls—an invalid assumption, as Silva et al.[328] have shown. Because CT appears to circulate in many forms, and different antisera preferentially detect different forms, CT measurements vary enormously from laboratory to laboratory,[336] and serial studies on any given patient *must* be done in the same laboratory for any valid inferences to be drawn from the results. Immunoreactive heterogeneity also complicates the interpretation of studies of changes in CT secretion, since probably only CT monomer is biologically active.[333,337] A sensitive bioassay of CT is badly needed. Since CT, like PTH, acts by activating adenylate cyclase and appears to require the mediation of GTP to do so,[338] it may prove possible to exploit this dependence for a bioassay. At present, the only clinical uses of the CT radioassay are in the diagnosis of MCT and the detection of CT produced by some tumors (see below).

7.9.3. Secretion and Its Control

Pont[331] has reviewed this subject quite completely. As he points out, most of our knowledge of control of CT secretion has been derived from work in animals, which may not be very relevant to human physiology, and in patients with MCT. In the past few years, with the new, more sensitive radioassay, it has been possible to examine changes in CT secretion in normal men and women, and several such studies have been published. These studies appear to have established that CT does circulate in normal man, roughly within the concentration range of 5 to 100 pg/ml.[333] There is a large interindividual variation. Hillyard et al.[335] observed a marked circadian periodicity in CT levels in all subjects, with troughs in the early morning and peaks at midday. Heath and Sizemore[334] and Hillyard et al.[339] have observed that CT levels in women are significantly lower than those in men, although these authors disagree about the size of the difference. Mulder et al.[340] reported much higher CT levels in their West Indian black subjects than in their Dutch white subjects.

CT was first conceptualized as a hypocalcemic factor, and calcium was presumed to regulate its secretion. Supraphysiologic changes in serum calcium will induce appropriate changes in CT secretion in patients with MCT;[31] the question is whether physiologic changes in serum calcium will affect CT secretion in normal subjects. Heath and Sizemore[334] studied the effect of a standard 4-hr calcium infusion in 45 young adult men and women. Serum calcium increased by 1 to 6 mg/dl. Eighteen of twenty men, but only fourteen of twenty-five women, responded with an increase in serum CT concentration. Correlation between the increases in calcium and CT was poor. Vora et al.[341] reported a parallel increase in serum calcium and CT with calcium infusion in an unspecified number of normal men. Austin et al.[342] demonstrated dose-related increases in serum CT in response to oral calcium ingestion in ten normal young men; serum calcium and CT levels rose in parallel, peaking at 2–4 hr.

Hillyard et al.[335] measured serum CT in 21 hypercalcemic subjects. Although mean CT concentration in these subjects was higher than that in normal subjects, the values overlapped considerably, and in one patient, CT was undetectable.

Several gastrointestinal hormones may influence CT secretion; of these, gastrin seems to have the greatest and most consistent effect. The use of pentagastrin stimulation to detect MCT is by now familiar. Similarly, patients with hypergastrinemia secondary to Zollinger–Ellison syndrome often have high CT.[343] Again, as with calcium, the question is whether endogenous gastrin, under physiologic conditions, affects CT secretion. Owyang et al.[344] say no. They studied pentagastrin stimulation and serum gastrin and CT levels after low- and high-calcium meals in nine normal men. Pentagastrin produced an increase in CT in eight of the nine; however, the dose required to produce the minimum detectable increase was at least five times greater than the maximal gastrin level observed with feeding. With the various meals, gastrin levels increased in all subjects, but CT levels did not change at all. These findings are consistent with those of Austin et al.,[342] who found that gastrin levels in normal subjects peaked 30 min after a meal and fell to baseline by 120 min, while CT levels took 120 to 240 min to peak.

Conflicting data on the effects of secretin and glucagon as CT secretagogues have been reported. There is no evidence for a significant regulatory role of these hormones.

CT secretion, like that of many other hormones derived from neural crest tissue, seems to be inhibited by somatostatin. In rats,[345] rabbits,[346] and in human MCT, though not in normal human thyroids,[347] somatostatin can be detected in C-cells. In high doses, somatostatin decreased basal, calcium-, and pentagastrin-stimulated CT secretion in pigs,[348] suppressed basal CT secretion in rats and monkeys,[349] and inhibited pentagastrin-induced CT secretion in three of four patients with MCT.[350] The significance of the somatostatin effect is unknown.

A few other influences on CT secretion have been recognized. Peng et al.[351] found that iodine-deficient rats who developed goiters also developed C-cell hyperplasia and hypercalcitoninemia. Although the same effect is not seen in humans, a case of MCT in which thyroid hormone treatment induced remission has been reported.[352] Alcohol induces CT secretion in patients with MCT[353] or chronic renal failure[354] via an as yet mysterious, but possibly β-adrenergic, mechanism unrelated to calcium or gastrin. L-Dopa appears to suppress CT release,[355] as it does that of other hormones derived from APUD cells. Hillyard et al.[339] observed that CT levels in pregnant women and women taking oral contraceptives were elevated to the normal male range, suggesting an effect of sex steroids on CT production.

In several studies in various animals, CT has been secreted in response to cAMP and to catecholamines.[331,356] Vora et al.[357] found that both isoproterenol and phentolamine stimulated CT release in normal men, while propranolol inhibited release. These authors suggest that the adrenergic system "may play an important physiological role in control of CT secretion in man" and, by extension, "in the moment to moment adjustment of calcium homeostasis by its reciprocal modification of both PTH and CT secretion." The problem with this argument, as we stated in Section 7.3, is that there is no good evidence that the adrenergic nervous system plays any significant role in regulating the serum calcium.

7.9.4. Does Calcitonin Have a Physiologic Role in Man?

This is still an open question. Many roles have been suggested, but the evidence is not strong for any of them.

1. *To prevent hypercalcemia:* Since hypercalcemia can be life-threatening and the parathyroid glands are relatively helpless against it, it would be of survival value to have a hypocalcemic hormone. However, hypercalcemia does not occur in normal man, even in the virtual absence of CT, and is not prevented in pathologic states by its presence. There is good evidence that in fish[358] and in tadpoles[359] CT protects against hypercalcemia in high-calcium environments by limiting calcium absorption through the gills. In rats, CT prevents the acute rise in serum calcium seen in the early phase of fasting,[360] appears to prevent prostaglandin-induced hypercalcemia,[361] and may prevent postprandial hypercalcemia.[362] Infused CT has a rapid hypocalcemic effect in rats, which kinetic studies have suggested is due to decreased calcium efflux from bone ECF;[363] in support of this contention, Norimatsu et al.[364] have performed elegant electron microscopic studies that show that in the rat, CT has a marked effect on bone-lining cells within 5 min. Despite these experimentally demonstrable effects—greater than can be shown

in any other species—even the rat appears to adapt within a few weeks to the absence of CT.[362] Cutler et al.[365] found that changes in dietary calcium did not affect CT synthesis and release in chickens.

What of human hypercalcemia? When Heath and Sizemore[334] infused calcium into young adults, they found that those who failed to respond with CT secretion seemed to dispose of the excess calcium just as efficiently as those who did respond, i.e., the serum calcium levels reached by the two groups were not different. Further, there is no evidence that CT has any protective effect in chronic hypercalcemia. Although Lambert et al.[367] found evidence of decreased CT secretory reserve in hyperparathyroid patients, they also found no difference in serum CT levels between hyperparathyroid and normal subjects, nor between pre- and postoperative samples from the same patients.

2. *To prevent postprandial hypercalcemia:* Since CT is intimately involved in a complex interrelationship with the gastrointestinal hormones, particularly gastrin, and since it seems to be released in response to feeding,[368] it has been suggested that the main role of CT in mammals may be to prevent postprandial hypercalcemia by channeling absorbed calcium into bone. Talmage et al.[369] found that thyroidectomized rats receiving a normal calcium diet had much higher postprandial urinary calcium than normal rats did.[369] They suggest that the action of CT may be to conserve dietary calcium and make it available to the animal during periods of fasting. Cooper et al.[370] reported that suckling markedly increases CT secretion in the baby rat, and they also suggest that CT functions in this setting both to conserve ingested calcium and to guard against postprandial hypercalcemia. Austin et al.[342] believe that CT may serve the same function in man, since calcium ingestion in their normal male volunteers induced significant CT secretion. Calcium in the gastrointestinal tract seems to induce CT secretion by a mechanism that is independent of any rise in the serum calcium, so the findings of Austin et al. are not inconsistent with the less impressive CT response reported to i.v. calcium infusion.[334] It has yet to be shown, however, that euthyroid humans after thyroidectomy, or women with very weak CT secretory responses, have excessive postprandial hypercalcemia or urinary calcium wasting. The mere demonstration of a CT secretory response to physiologic oral calcium loads does not prove that this response accomplishes anything.

3. *To preserve skeletal integrity:* We have mentioned that women appear to have a relative CT deficiency[339] and generally minimal CT response to hypercalcemia.[334] The response to CT secretagogues also decreases with aging in both men and women.[334,371,372] Hillyard et al.[339] found that although plasma CT levels in normal women were less than 25% of those in men under most circumstances, women who were pregnant or taking

combination estrogen–progesterone birth control pills had levels equal to or greater than those in males. These authors suggest that CT deficiency may be involved in the pathogenesis of postmenopausal osteoporosis. Milhaud *et al.*[373] reported that women with significant osteoporosis have lower CT levels than do age-matched controls. If we hypothesize that the postprandial urinary calcium wasting that Talmage *et al.*[369] found in thyroidectomized rats is duplicated in normal women, a contribution of CT deficiency to osteoporosis certainly becomes plausible. Further studies should show more definitively whether one in fact exists.

Pregnancy and lactation, as we have previously discussed (Section 7.4), make potentially serious demands on the maternal skeleton. CT could conceivably help protect the maternal skeleton by maximally conserving ingested calcium. Pregnant and lactating women have been reported to have elevated CT levels.[136,339,374] Toverud *et al.*[137] have reported that in lactating rats, postprandial CT levels are two to three times higher than in nonlactating rats, and CT secretion is much more readily stimulated by calcium ingestion. It is likely that CT plays an important protective role in this animal. However, as Toverud *et al.* point out, "the rate of calcium loss to the milk relative to body weight is approximately 50 times higher in the rat than in the lactating woman."[137] It remains to be shown (and the difficulties of such a demonstration are evident) that CT is needed to protect the maternal skeleton in humans.

4. *In the gastrointestinal tract:* CT has a variety of effects on the feeding process, on hormones involved in digestion, and on the gastrointestinal tract. Freed *et al.*[375] showed that subcutaneous and intracerebral CT injections in rats inhibited feeding, probably by a direct effect on the CNS. Their findings are particularly interesting in light of all the recent work that has demonstrated several gastrointestinal peptides (many, like CT, of neural crest origin) in the CNS. CT has been shown to inhibit gastrin secretion in the pig,[376] gastrin and gastric acid secretion in the rat,[377] and basal and stimulated insulin secretion in man.[378] In the rat[379] and in man,[380] CT at supraphysiologic levels decreases small intestinal sodium absorption and induces chloride secretion, and in the rabbit CT increases intestinal sodium, water, and bicarbonate secretion.[381] Because of these findings, many have suggested that CT produces the watery diarrhea found in about one-third of patients with MCT.[381]

There is little we can say at this point about the role of CT in gastrointestinal physiology, other than that the wide range of findings suggest this hormone does have some part to play, at least in animals, and that this should emerge with continued work. At present, there is no conclusive evidence supporting a role for CT in normal human gastrointestinal physiology.

7.9.5. Calcitonin as a Tumor Marker

We can turn now from the vexing question of the physiologic role of CT to its somewhat more clear-cut diagnostic and therapeutic uses; we will first discuss its usefulness as a tumor marker.

The first type of cancer in which hypercalcitoninemia was demonstrated was, of course, MCT.[382] Goltzman *et al.*[383] reported that CT levels could be used postoperatively to determine whether or not complete tumor removal had been accomplished in MCT. The serum CT in patients with MCT is extraordinarily heterogeneous by immunoassay, and Becker *et al.*[384] believe it is possible to distinguish metastatic MCT from primary bronchogenic carcinoma with ectopic CT production by the degree of immunochemical heterogeneity demonstrated by the serum CT.

Over the past several years, it has become clear that serum CT is quite frequently elevated in patients with cancer. In individual cases, CT production by pancreatic somatostatinoma,[385] pheochromocytoma,[386] carcinoid,[387] myeloma,[388] and paraganglioma[389] has recently been reported. Silva *et al.*[390] reported ectopic CT secretion in two cases of oat-cell carcinoma in 1974. Since then it has been shown that this is a common phenomenon; serum CT is elevated in approximately two-thirds of all patients with oat-cell carcinoma.[391–393] In one series, 25% of such patients had a CT level in the MCT range, and 3 of 19 responded to pentagastrin stimulation with a significant increase,[391] indicating that a positive pentagastrin test is not diagnostic of MCT.

Although the incidence of hypercalcitoninemia in nonthyroid cancer appears to be highest in oat-cell carcinoma, Silva *et al.*[394] found high CT levels in 52% of all patients with bronchogenic cancer. They used selective thyroid venous sampling to determine whether CT in these patients was coming from the thyroid or the tumor; interestingly, only oat-cell carcinomas produced ectopic CT, while in other tumor types the CT was coming from the thyroid. CT levels did not correlate with the presence of bone metastases.

Silva *et al.*[393] have reviewed their experience with CT measurements in all types of cancer. They found elevated CT levels in 38% of lung cancers, 24% of colon cancers, 38% of breast cancers, 42% of pancreatic cancers, and 30% of gastric cancers. CT levels were also elevated in renal failure, acute gastrointestinal bleeding, and sometimes COPD. They also found no correlation between CT levels and either hypercalcemia or bone metastases.

Opinions differ as to the potential usefulness of CT as a tumor marker. It seems clear that, except perhaps in MCT, CT levels do not necessarily reflect body tumor burden.[392–395] There probably are some patients, however, whose CT levels will accurately mirror their clinical course and in whom serial measurements might be useful. We expect to see further evaluation of this in the future.

7.9.6. Therapeutic Uses of Calcitonin

7.9.6.1. Paget's Disease

Symptomatic Paget's disease is the strongest indication for the therapeutic use of CT; the response to treatment is impressive. Martin[396] has published a very useful review of this topic. His indications for CT treatment are bone pain, widespread, active disease in relatively young patients with or without symptoms, immobilization, high-output cardiac failure, neurologic compression signs, some types of fractures through Pagetic bone, and preparation for surgery on involved bone. Although controlled studies that would support these indications have not all been done as yet, reasoning and many impressive anecdotal reports provide, we think, an adequate basis for recommending a trial of CT therapy in all these situations. Good relief of pain in up to 90% of patients has clearly been demonstrated,[396] as has reduction in high skeletal blood flow and cardiac output in two recent studies.[397,398] In many cases, signs of neurologic compression have clearly been relieved.[396]

The usefulness of CT may be inhibited by the development of antibodies. Approximately 40% of patients treated with salmon CT will develop measurable antibodies. Hosking et al.,[399] however, found that these antibodies did not necessarily affect the hypocalcemic response to CT, i.e., the mere presence of measurable anti-CT antibodies does not mean further treatment will be unavailing. For those patients who do develop antibody-mediated resistance to salmon or porcine CT, human CT can still be used effectively.[400] It is likely that human CT will be more readily and inexpensively available in the future.

7.9.6.2. Hypercalcemia

Since the mid-1960s, when its use was first reported, CT has become an accepted treatment for hypercalcemia, although we think that the contention of Nilsson et al.[401] that CT should be considered first-line treatment for hypercalcemia is too strong. Wisneski et al.[75] reported good results in a series of 24 patients treated for hypercalcemia. Seventeen of these patients had hypercalcemia of malignancy, five hyperparathyroidism, and two multiple myeloma. Serum calcium decreased significantly in more than 75% of the patients and became normal within 2 hr of treatment in 50%. However, only 30% still had normal or near-normal calcium 96 hr after treatment. Patients with hypercalcemia of malignancy responded best; two out of five hyperparathyroid patients did not respond at all. The only significant side effect was nausea and vomiting, which occurred in three patients and was intolerable to one. No patient became hypocalcemic.

7.9.6.3. Osteoporosis

Osteoporosis is a major problem in our elderly population, and an effective treatment is badly needed. Since CT decreases bone resorption, some groups have tested it as a treatment for osteoporosis. Very preliminary results have not been overly encouraging. Wallach et al.[252] treated 25 patients with salmon CT and calcium supplements for 10 to 29 months. Total body calcium increased by a mean of 9% in 12, and back pain decreased in 75%, eventually disappearing in 50%. Standard X rays did not show any evidence of improvement, although no significant fractures occurred. Side effects were transient and insignificant. Jowsey et al.[306] treated 26 patients either with calcium, vitamin D, and CT, or with calcium and vitamin D alone for 15 months. CT did not seem to bring any additional therapeutic benefit to the vitamin D and calcium regimen; moreover, 10 of 26 patients suffered significant side effects.

References

1. Ordal, G. W., 1977, Calcium ion regulates chemotactic behavior in bacteria, *Nature (London)* **270**:66–67.
2. Golub, E. E., and Bronner, F., 1974, Bacterial calcium transport: Energy-dependent calcium uptake by membrane vesicles from *Bacillus megaterium*, *J. Bacteriol.* **119**:840–843.
3. Parfitt, A. M., and Kleerekoper, J., 1980, The divalent ion homeostatic system—Physiology and metabolism of calcium, phosphorus, magnesium, and bone, in: *Clinical Disorders fo Fluid and Electrolyte Metabolism* (M. H. Maxwell and C. R. Kleeman, eds.), 3rd ed., pp. 269–398, McGraw–Hill, New York.
4. Kretsinger, R. H., 1979, The informational role of calcium in the cytosol, *Adv. Cyclic Nucleotide Res.* **11**:1–26.
5. Loewenstein, W. R., and Rose, B., 1978, Calcium in functional intercellular communication and a thought on its behavior in intracellular communication, *Ann. N.Y. Acad. Sci.* **307**:285–307.
6. Blaustein, M. P., Ratzlaff, R. W., and Kendrick, N. K., 1978, The regulation of intracellular calcium in presynaptic nerve terminals, *Ann. N.Y. Acad. Sci.* **307**:195–212.
7. Martonosi, A. N., Chyn, T. L., and Schibeci, A., 1978, The calcium transport of sarcoplasmic reticulum, *Ann. N.Y. Acad. Sci.* **307**:148–159.
8. Carafoli, G., and Crompton, M., 1978, The regulation of intracellular calcium by mitochondria, *Ann. N.Y. Acad. Sci.* **307**:269–284.

9. Lehninger, A. L., Reynafarje, B., Vercesi, A., and Tew, W. P., 1978, Transport and accumulation of calcium in mitochondria, *Ann. N.Y. Acad. Sci.* **307:**160–176.

10. Akerman, K. E. O., 1978, Changes in membrane potential during calcium ion influx and efflux across the mitochondrial membrane, *Biochim. Biophys. Acta* **502:**359–366.

11. Bockaert, J., Roy, C., and Jard, S., 1972, Oxytocin-sensitive adenylate cyclase in frog bladder epithelial cells: Role of calcium, nucleotides, and other factors in hormonal stimulation, *J. Biol. Chem.* **247:**7073–7081.

12. Campbell, B. J., Woodward, G., and Borberg, V., 1972, Calcium-mediated interactions between the antidiuretic hormone and renal plasma membranes, *J. Biol. Chem.* **247:**6167–6175.

13. Keutmann, H. T., Sauer, M. M., Hendy, G. N., O'Riordan, J. L. H., and Potts, J. T., Jr., 1978, Complete amino acid sequence of human parathyroid hormone, *Biochemistry* **17:**5723–5729.

14. Brewer, H. B., Jr., 1972, Chemistry and conformation of bovine parathyroid hormone, in: *Endocrinology 1971: Proceedings of the Third International Symposium* (S. Taylor, ed.), pp. 324–332, Heinemann Press, London.

15. Fiskin, M. A., Cohn, D. V., and Peterson, G. S., 1977, A model for the structure of bovine parathormone derived by dark field electron microscopy, *J. Biol. Chem.* **252:**8261–8268.

16. Habener, J. F., and Potts, J. T., Jr., 1979, Cleavage-associated enhancement of an antigenic site in the biologically active NH_2-terminal region of parathyroid hormone, *Endocrinology* **105:**115–119.

17. Mahaffey, J. E., Rosenblatt, M., Shepard, G. L., and Potts, J. T., Jr., 1979, Parathyroid hormone inhibitors: Determination of minimum sequence requirements, *J. Biol. Chem.* **254:**6496–6498.

18. Tregear, G. W., van Rietschoten, J., Greene, E., Keutmann, H. T., Niall, H. D., Parsons, J. A., and Potts, J. T., Jr., 1974, Principles and recent applications in the solid-phase synthesis of peptide hormones, in: *Endocrinology 1973: Proceedings of the Fourth International Symposium* (S. Taylor, ed.), pp. 1–16, Heinemann Press, London.

19. Kronenberg, H. M., Roberts, B. E., Habener, J. F., Potts, J. T., Jr., and Rich, A., 1977, DNA complementary to parathyroid mRNA directs synthesis of pre-proparathyroid hormone in a linked transcription–translation system, *Nature (London)* **267:**804–807.

20. Habener, J. F., and Kronenberg, H. M., 1978, Parathyroid hormone biosynthesis: Structure and function of biosynthetic precursors, *Fed. Proc.* **37:**2561–2566.

21. Palade, G., 1975, Intracellular aspects of the process of protein synthesis, *Science* **189:**347–358.

22. Blobel, G., and Sabatini, D. P., 1971, Ribosome–membrane interaction in eukaryotic cells, *Biomembranes* **2:**193–195.

23. Habener, J. F., Rosenblatt, M., Kemper, B., Kronenberg, H. M., Rich, A., and Potts, J. T., Jr., 1978, Pre-proparathyroid hormone: Amino acid sequence, chemical synthesis, and some biological studies of the precursor region, *Proc. Natl. Acad. Sci. USA* **75:**2616–2620.

24. Habener, J. F., and Potts, J. T., Jr., 1979, Subcellular distributions of parathyroid hormone, hormonal precursors, and parathyroid secretory protein, *Endocrinology* **104**:265–275.

25. Dorner, A. J., and Kemper, B., 1978, Conversion of pre-proparathyroid hormone to proparathyroid hormone by dog pancreatic microsomes, *Biochemistry* **17**:5550–5555.

26. MacGregor, R. R., Hamilton, J. W., and Cohn, D. V., 1978, The mode of conversion of proparathormone to parathormone by a particulate converting enzymic activity of the parathyroid gland, *J. Biol. Chem.* **253**:2012–2017.

27. Mayer, G. P., and Hurst, J. G., 1978, Sigmoidal relationship between parathyroid hormone secretion rate and plasma calcium concentration in calves, *Endocrinology* **102**:1036–1042.

28. Kleeman, K., and Kleeman, C. R., 1978, Parathyroid hormone and calcitonin, in: *The Year in Endocrinology 1977* (S. H. Ingbar, ed.), pp. 109–160, Plenum Medical, New York.

29. Smith, D. L., and Boime, I., 1977, Reversible calcium inhibition of the membrane-dependent cleavage of pre-placental lactogen in ascites cell-free extracts, *FEBS Lett.* **84**:115–118.

30. Habener, J. F., Kemper, B. W., Potts, J. T., Jr., and Rich, A., 1974, Calcium-independent intracellular conversion of proparathyroid hormone to parathyroid hormone, *Endocr. Res. Commun.* **1**:239–246.

31. Habener, J. F., and Potts, J. T., Jr., 1978, Biosynthesis of parathyroid hormone, *N. Engl. J. Med.* **299**:580–585, 635–644.

32. Habener, J. F., Kemper, B., and Potts, J. T., Jr., 1975, Calcium-dependent intracellular degradation of parathyroid hormone: A possible mechanism for the regulation of hormone stores, *Endocrinology* **97**:431–441.

33. Silverman, R., and Yalow, R. S., 1973, Heterogeneity of parathyroid hormone: Clinical and physiologic implications, *J. Clin. Invest.* **52**:1958–1971.

34. Flueck, J. A., Di Bella, F. P., Edis, A. J., Kehrwald, J. M., and Arnaud, C. D., 1977, Immunoheterogeneity of parathyroid hormone in venous effluent serum from hyperfunctioning parathyroid glands, *J. Clin. Invest.* **60**:1367–1375.

35. Di Bella, F. P., Gilkinson, J. B., Flueck, J., and Arnaud, C. D., 1978, Carboxyl-terminal fragments of human parathyroid hormone in parathyroid tumors: Unique new source of immunogens for the production of antisera potentially useful in the radioimmunoassay of parathyroid hormone in human serum, *J. Clin. Endocrinol. Metab.* **46**:604–612.

36. Dambacher, M. A., Hunziker, W., Born, W., Moran, J., and Fischer, J. A., 1978, Circulating forms of immunoreactive parathyroid hormone (PTH) in control subjects and in patients with primary and secondary hyperparathyroidism, *Acta Endocrinol. [Suppl.] (Copenhagen)* **87**(Suppl. 215):110–111.

37. Mayer, G. P., Keaton, J. A., Hurst, J. G., and Habener, J. F., 1979, Effects of plasma calcium concentration on the relative proportion of hormone and carboxyl fragments in parathyroid venous blood, *Endocrinology* **104**:1778–1783.

38. Morrissey, J. J., and Cohn, D. V., 1979, Regulation of secretion of para-thormone and secretory protein-I from separate intracellular pools by cal-cium, dibutyryl cyclic AMP, and (1)-isoproterenol, *J. Cell Biol.* **83**:93–102.

39. Brown, G. M., Hurwitz, S., and Aurbach, G. D., 1976, Preparation of usable isolated bovine parathyroid cells, *Endocrinology* **99**:1582–1588.

40. Brown, G. M., Brennan, M. F., Hurwitz, S., Windeck, R., Marx, S. J., Spiegel, A. M., Koehler, J. O., Gardner, D. G., and Aurbach, G. D., 1978, Dispersed cells prepared from human parathyroid glands: Distinct calcium sensitivity of adenomas vs. primary hyperplasia, *J. Clin. Endocrinol. Metab.* **46**:267–275.

41. Blum, J. W., Mayer, G. P., and Potts, J. T., Jr., 1974, Parathyroid hormone response during spontaneous hypocalcemia and induced hypercalcemia in cows, *Endocrinology* **95**:84–92.

42. Mayer, G. P., Habener, J. F., and Potts, J. T., Jr., 1976, Parathyroid hor-mone secretion *in vivo:* Demonstration of a calcium-independent nonsup-pressible component of secretion, *J. Clin. Invest.* **57**:678–683.

43. Neer, R. M., 1979, Calcium and inorganic phosphate homeostasis, in: *En-docrinology,* Volume 2 (L. J. DeGroot, G. F. Cahill, Jr., W. D. Odell, L. Martini, J. T. Potts, Jr., D. H. Nelson, G. Steinberger, and A. I. Winegrad, eds.), pp. 699–692, Grune & Stratton, New York.

44. Brown, E. M., Brennan, M. F., Broadus, A. E., Marx, S. J., Gardner, D. G., Spiegel, A. M., Downs, R. W., Jr., Attie, M. F., and Aurbach, G. D., 1979, Human parathyroid autografts: Comparison of function *in vivo* and *in vitro, J. Clin. Endocrinol. Metab.* **48**:648–654.

45. Broadus, A. E., Deftos, L. J., and Bartter, F. C., 1978, Effects of the intravenous administration of calcium on nephrogenous cyclic AMP: Use as a parathyroid suppression test, *J. Clin. Endocrinol. Metab.* **46**:477–487.

46. Brown, E. M., Gardner, D. G., Windeck, R. A., and Aurbach, G. D., 1978, Relationship of intracellular 3′,5′-adenosine monophosphate accumulation to parathyroid hormone release from dispersed bovine parathyroid cells, *Endocrinology* **103**:2323–2332.

47. Matsuzaki, S., and Dumont, J. E., 1972, Effect of calcium ion on horse parathyroid gland adenyl cyclase, *Biochim. Biophys. Acta* **284**:227–234.

48. Rodriguez, H. J., Morrison, A., Slatopolsky, E., and Klahr, S., 1978, Aden-ylate cyclase of human parathyroid gland, *J. Clin. Endocrinol. Metab.* **47**:319–325.

49. Ramp, W. K., Cooper, C. W., Ross, A. J., III, and Wells, S. A., Jr., 1979, Effects of calcium and cyclic nucleotides on rat calcitonin and parathyroid hormone secretion, *Mol. Cell. Endocrinol.* **14**:205–215.

50. Tsuchiya, T., and Tamate, H., 1979, Ultrastructural localization of adenyl cyclase activity in sheep parathyroid gland, *Acta Histochem. Cytochem.* **12**:356–360.

51. Gardner, D. G., Brown, E. M., Windeck, R., and Aurbach, G. D., 1979, Prostaglandin $F_{2\alpha}$ inhibits 3′,5′-adenosine monophosphate accumulation and parathyroid hormone release from dispersed bovine parathyroid cells, *Endocrinology* **104**:1–7.

52. Gardner, D. G., Brown, E. M., Windeck, R., and Aurbach, G. D., 1978, PGE$_2$ stimulation of cAMP accumulation and PTH release in dispersed bovine parathyroid cells, *Endocrinology* **103**:577–582.

53. Licata, A. A., Au, W. Y., Vera, J., and Bartter, F. C., 1979, Effects of prostaglandin E$_1$ on the metabolism in rat parathyroid gland in vitro, *Biochim. Biophys. Acta* **582**:59–66.

54. Boquist, L., 1975, Occurrence of oxyphil cells in suppressed parathyroid glands, *Cell Tissue Res.* **163**:465–470.

55. Carafoli, E., and Lehninger, A. L., 1971, A survey of the interaction of calcium ions with mitochondria from different tissues and species, *Biochem. J.* **122**:681–690.

56. Carafoli, E., 1979, The calcium cycle of mitochondria, *FEBS Lett.* **104**:1–5.

57. Crompton, M., Moser, R., Ludi, H., and Carafoli, E., 1978, The interrelations between the transport of sodium and calcium in mitochondria of various mammalian tissues, *Eur. J. Biochem.* **82**:25–31.

58. Nicholls, D. G., 1978, Calcium transport and proton electrochemical potential gradient in mitochondria from guinea-pig cerebral cortex and rat heart, *Biochem. J.* **170**:511–522.

59. Lee, N. H., and Shapiro, I. M., 1978, Ca^{2+} transport by chondrocyte mitochondria of the epiphyseal growth plate, *J. Membr. Biol.* **41**:349–360.

60. Glick, D. M., and Mockel, J., 1980, The disposition of calcium within parathyroid tissue, *Horm. Metab. Res.* **12**:475–480.

61. Bruce, B. R., and Anderson, N. C., Jr., 1979, Hyperpolarization in mouse parathyroid cells by low calcium, *Am. J. Physiol.* **236**:C15–C21.

62. Petersen, O. H., 1976, Electrophysiology of mammalian gland cells, *Physiol. Rev.* **56**:535–577.

63. Heath, H., III, 1980, Biogenic amines and the secretion of parathyroid hormone and calcitonin, *Endocr. Rev.* **1**:319–338.

64. Sherwood, L. M., and Abe, M., 1972, Adrenergic receptors and the release of parathyroid hormone, *J. Clin. Invest.* **51**:88a.

65. Brown, E. M., Hurwitz, S., and Aurbach, G. D., 1977, Beta-adrenergic stimulation of cyclic AMP content and parathyroid hormone release from isolated bovine parathyroid cells, *Endocrinology* **100**:1696–1702.

66. Brown, E. M., Gardner, D. G., Windeck, R. A., Hurwitz, S., Brennan, M. F., and Aurbach, G. D., 1979, β-Adrenergically stimulated adenosine 3′,5′-monophosphate accumulation in and parathyroid hormone release from dispersed human parathyroid cells, *J. Clin. Endocrinol. Metab.* **48**:618–626.

67. Mayer, G. P., Hurst, J. G., Barto, J. A., Keaton, J. A., and Moore, M. P., 1979, Effect of epinephrine on parathyroid hormone secretion in calves, *Endocrinology* **104**:1181–1187.

68. Hanley, D. A., Takatsuki, K., Birnbaumer, M. E., Schneider, A. B., and Sherwood, L. M., 1980, In vitro perfusion for the study of parathyroid hormone secretion: The effects of extracellular calcium concentration and beta-adrenergic regulation on bovine parathyroid hormone secretion, *Calcif. Tissue Int.* **32**:19–27.

69. Kukreja, S. C., Williams, O. A., Hargis, G. K., Bowser, E. N., Banerjee, P.,

Vora, N. M., and Henderson, W. J., 1979, Dual control of suppressibility of parathyroid hormone by calcium and by beta-adrenergic blockade, *Miner. Electrolyte Metab.* **2:**316–322.

70. Brown, E. M., Hurwitz, S. H., and Aurbach, G. D., 1978, Beta-adrenergic inhibition of adenosine 3′,5′-monophosphate accumulation and parathyroid hormone release from dispersed bovine parathyroid cells, *Endocrinology* **103:**893–899.

71. Blum, J. W., Guillebeau, A., Binswanger, V., Kunz, P., Da Prada, M., and Fischer, J. A., 1978, Effects of alpha-adrenergic stimulation and blockade on plasma parathyroid hormone concentrations in cows, *Acta Endocrinol. (Copenhagen)* **88:**535–544.

72. Harney, A. N., Kukreja, S. C., Hargis, G. K., Jonson, P. A., Bowser, E. N., and Williams, G. A., 1978, Effect of long-term administration of epinephrine and propranolol on serum calcium, parathyroid hormone, and calcitonin in the rat, *Proc. Soc. Exp. Biol. Med.* **159:**266–269.

73. Heath, H., III, 1980, Provocative tests of parathyroid and C cell function in adrenalectomized and chemically sympathectomized rats, *Endocrinology* **107:**977–981.

74. Blum, J. W., Bianca, W., Naf, F., Kunz, P., Fischer, J. A., and Da Prada, M., 1979, Plasma catecholamine and parathyroid hormone responses in cattle during treadmill exercise at simulated high altitude, *Horm. Metab. Res.* **11:**246–251.

75. Wisneski, L. A., Croom, W. P., Silva, O. L., and Becker, K. L., 1978, Salmon calcitonin in hypercalcemia, *Clin. Pharmacol. Ther.* **24:**219–222.

76. Arnaud, C. D., Tsao, H. S., and Littledike, T., 1971, Radioimmunoassay of human parathyroid hormone in serum, *J. Clin. Invest.* **50:** 21–34.

77. Sinha, T. K., Miller, S., Fleming, J., Khairi, R., Edmondson, J., Johnston, C. C., Jr., and Bell, N. H., 1975, Demonstration of a diurnal variation in serum parathyroid hormone in primary and secondary hyperparathyroidism, *J. Clin. Endocrinol. Metab.* **41:**1009–1013.

78. Kripke, D. F., Lavie, P., Parker, D., Huey, L., and Deftos, L. J., 1978, Plasma parathyroid hormone and calcium are related to sleep stage cycles, *J. Clin. Endocrinol. Metab.* **47:**1021–1027.

79. Urist, M. R., 1976, Biogenesis of bone: Calcium and phosphorus in the skeleton and blood in vertebrate evolution, in: *Handbook of Physiology*, Section F, Volume VII (G. D. Aurbach, ed.), pp. 183–213, American Physiological Society, Washington, D. C.

80. Wendelaar Bonga, S. E., and Greve, J. A. A., 1978, The relationship between prolactin cell activity, environmental calcium, and plasma calcium in the teleost *Gasterosteus aculeatus:* Observations on stanniectomized fish, *Gen. Comp. Endocrinol.* **36:**90–101.

81. Pang, P. K. T., Schreibman, M. P., Balbontin, F., and Pang, R. K., 1978, Prolactin and pituitary control of calcium regulation in the killifish, *Fundulus heteroclitus, Gen. Comp. Endocrinol.* **36:**306–316.

82. MacIntyre, I., Colston, K. W., Szelke, M., and Spanos, E., 1978, A survey

of the hormonal factors that control calcium metabolism, *Ann. N.Y. Acad. Sci.* **307:**345–355.

83. Mahajan, K. K., Robinson, C. J., and Horrobin, D. F., 1975, The role of prolactin in hypercalcemia, *Br. J. Surg.* **62:**161.

84. Parsons, J. A., Gray, D., Rafferty, B., and Zanelli, J. M., 1978, Evidence for a hypercalcemic factor in the fish pituitary immunologically related to mammalian parathyroid hormone, in: *Endocrinology of Calcium Metabolism* (D. H. Copp and R. V. Talmage, eds.), pp. 111–114, Excerpta Medica, Amsterdam.

85. Lee, S. W., Halstead, L. R., and Avioli, L. V., 1978, Hypothalamic hypocalcemic factors, *Miner. Electrolyte Metab.* **1:**247–252.

86. Kleeman, K., and Kleeman, C. R., 1979, Parathyroid hormone, in: *Contemporary Endocrinology*, Volume 1 (S. H. Ingbar, ed.), pp. 305–339, Plenum Medical, New York.

87. Wecksler, W. R., Henry, H. L., and Norman, A. W., 1977, Studies on the mode of action of calciferol: Subcellular localization of 1,25-dihydroxyvitamin D_3 in chicken parathyroid glands, *Arch. Biochem. Biophys.* **183:**168–175.

88. Hughes, M. R., and Haussler, M. R., 1978, 1,25-Dihydroxyvitamin D_3 receptors in parathyroid glands, *J. Biol. Chem.* **253:**1065–1073.

89. Stumpf, W. E., Sar, M., Reid, F. A., Tanaka, Y., and DeLuca, H. F., 1979, Target cells for 1,25 dihydroxyvitamin D_3 in intestinal tract, stomach, kidney, skin, pituitary, and parathyroid, *Science* **206:**1188–1190.

90. Finco, D., Olgaard, K., Rothstein, M., Schwartz, J., Korkor, A., Teitelbaum, S., Klahr, S., and Slatopolsky, E., 1980, Lack of a direct effect of 24,25 $(OH)_2D_3$ on PTH secretion in studies *in vitro* or *in vivo*, *Proceedings of the 7th International Conference on Calcium-Regulating Hormones*.

91. Care, A. D., Pickard, D. W., Papapoulos, S. E., O'Riordan, J. L. H., and Redel, J., 1978, Inhibitory effect of 25,26-dihydroxycholecalciferol on the rate of secretion of parathyroid hormone in goats, *J. Endocrinol.* **78:**303–304.

92. Canterbury, J. M., Lerman, S., Claflin, A. J., Henry, H., Norman, A., and Reiss, E., 1978, Inhibition of parathyroid hormone secretion by 1,25-dihydroxycholecalciferol and 24,25-dihydroxycholecalciferol in the dog, *J. Clin. Invest.* **61:**1375–1383.

93. Dietel, M., Dorn, G., Montz, R., and Altenahr, E., 1979, Influence of vitamin D_3 on parathyroid hormone secretion, adenosine 3',5'-monophosphate release, and ultrastructure of parathyroid glands in organ cultures, *Endocrinology* **105:**237–245.

94. Golden, P., Mazey, R., Greenwalt, A., Martin, K., and Slatopolsky, E., 1979, Vitamin D: A direct effect on the parathyroid gland, *Miner. Electrolyte Metab.* **2:**1–6.

95. Oldham, S. B., Smith, R., Hartenbower, D. K., Henry, H. L., Norman, A. W., and Coburn, J. W., 1979, The acute effects of 1,25-dihydroxycholecalciferol on serum immunoreactive parathyroid hormone in the dog, *Endocrinology* **104:**248–254.

96. Oldham, S. B., Fischer, J. A., Shen, L. H., and Arnaud, C. D., 1974, Isolation and properties of a calcium-binding protein from porcine parathyroid gland, *Biochemistry* **13:**4790–4796.

97. Oldham, S. B., Arnaud, C. D., and Jowsey, J., 1973, Influence of vitamin D on canine parathyroid glands, *Clin. Res.* **21**:254A.
98. Oldham, S. B., Mitnick, S. A., and Coburn, J. W., 1980, Intestinal and parathyroid calcium-binding proteins in the dog: Comparison of biochemical properties and responses to vitamin D, *J. Biol. Chem.* **255**:5789–5794.
99. Brown, E. M., Carroll, R. J., and Aurbach, G. D., 1977, Dopaminergic stimulation of cyclic AMP accumulation and parathyroid hormone release from dispersed bovine parathyroid cells, *Proc. Natl. Acad. Sci. USA* **74**:4210–4213.
100. Williams, G. A., Longley, R. S., Hargis, G. K., Bowser, E. N., Kukreja, S. C., Johnson, P. A., Jackson, B. L., and Kawahara, W. J., 1979, Effect of histamine on parathyroid hormone, *Clin. Res.* **27**:704A.
101. Windeck, R., Brown, E. M., Gardner, D. G., and Aurbach, G. D., 1978, Effect of gastrointestinal hormones on isolated bovine parathyroid cells, *Endocrinology* **103**:2020–2026.
102. Deftos, L. J., Lorenzi, M., Bohanon, N., Tsalakian, E., Schneider, V., and Gerich, J. E, 1976, Somatostatin does not suppress plasma parathyroid hormone, *J. Clin. Endocrinol. Metab.* **43**:205–207.
103. Metz, S. A., Deftos, L. J., Baylink, D. J., and Robertson, R. P., 1978, Neuroendocrine modulation of calcitonin and parathyroid hormone in man, *J. Clin. Endocrinol. Metab.* **47**:151–159.
104. Hargis, G. K., Williams, G. A., Reynolds, W. A., Chertow, B. S., Kukreja, S. C., Bowser, E. N., and Henderson, W. J., 1978, Effect of somatostatin on parathyroid hormone and calcitonin secretion, *Endocrinology* **102**:745–750.
105. Williams, G. A., Hargis, G. K., Ensinck, J. W., Kukrega, S. C., Bowser, E. N., Chertow, B. S., and Henderson, W. J., 1979, Role of endogenous somatostatin in the secretion of parathyroid hormone and calcitonin, *Metabolism* **28**:950–954.
106. Brown, E. M., Gardner, D. G., and Aurbach, G. D., 1980, Effects of the calcium ionophore A23187 on dispersed bovine parathyroid cells, *Endocrinology* **106**:133–138.
107. Watterson, D. M., and Vicenzi, F. F. (eds.), 1980, *Calmodulin and Cell Functions, Ann. N.Y. Acad. Sci.* **356.**
108. Satir, B. H., Garofalo, R. S., Gilligan, D. M., and Maihle, N. J., 1980, Possible functions of calmodulin in protozoa, *Ann. N.Y. Acad. Sci.* **356**:83–91.
109. Oldham, S. B., Lipson, L. G., and Tiefjen, G. E., 1980, Evidence for calmodulin in parathyroid tissue, *Proceedings of the 7th International Conference on Calcium-Regulating Hormones.*
110. Martin, K. J., Hruska, K. A., Freitag, J. J., Klahr, S., and Slatopolsky, E., 1979, The peripheral metabolism of parathyroid hormone, *N. Engl. J. Med.* **301**:1092–1098.
111. Neuman, M. W., Neuman, W. F., and Lane, K., 1979, Formation and serum disappearance of fragments of parathyroid hormone in the infused dog, *Calcif. Tissue Int.* **28**:79–81.
112. Barret, P. Q., Teitelbaum, A., and Neuman, W. F., 1978, The heterogeneity of parathyroid hormone in rat plasma, *Metab. Bone Dis. Relat. Res.* **1**:263–267.
113. Papapoulos, S. E., Hendy, G. N., Tomlinson, S., Lewin, I. G., and O'-

Riordan, J. L. H., 1977, Clearance of exogenous parathyroid hormone in normal and uraemic man, *Clin. Endocrinol.* **7**:211–225.

114. D'Amour, P., Segre, G. V., Roth, S. I., and Potts, J. T., Jr., 1979, Analysis of parathyroid hormone and its fragments in rat tissues, *J. Clin. Invest.* **63**:89–98.

115. Hunziker, W. H., Blum, J. W., and Fischer, J. A., 1977, Plasma kinetics of exogenous bovine parathyroid hormone in calves, *Pfluegers Arch.* **371**:185–192.

116. Segre, G. F., D'Amour, P., and Rosenblatt, M., 1978, Heterogeneity and metabolism of parathyroid hormone, in: *Endocrinology of Calcium Metabolism* (D. H. Copp and R. V. Talmage, eds.), pp. 329–332, Excerpta Medica, Amsterdam.

117. Rosenblatt, M., Segre, G. V., and Potts, J. T., Jr., 1977, Synthesis of a fragment of parathyroid hormone, bPTH-(28–48): An inhibitor of hormone cleavage *in vivo, Biochemistry* **16**:2811–2816.

118. Freitag, J. J., Martin, K. J., Conrades, M. B., and Slatopolsky, E., 1979, Metabolism of parathyroid hormone by fetal rat calvaria, *Endocrinology* **104**:510–515.

119. Oldham, S. B., Finck, E. J., and Singer, F. R., 1978, Parathyroid hormone clearance in man, *Metabolism* **27**:993–1001.

120. Barrett, P. Q., Teitelbaum, A., Neuman, W. F., and Neuman, M. W., 1978, The role of the liver in the peripheral metabolism of parathyroid hormone, in: *Endocrinology of Calcium Metabolism* (D. H. Copp and R. V. Talmage, eds.), pp. 324–328, Excerpta Medica, Amsterdam.

121. Canterbury, J. M., Bricker, L. A., Levey, J. S., Kozlovskis, P. L., Ruiz, E., Zull, J. E., and Reiss, E., 1975, Metabolism of bovine parathyroid hormone: Immunological and biological characteristic of fragments generated by liver perfusion, *J. Clin. Invest.* **55**:1245–1253.

122. Martin, K. J., Hruska, K. A., Lewis, J., Anderson, C., and Slatopolsky, E., 1977, The renal handling of parathyroid hormone: Role of peritubular uptake and glomerular filtration, *J. Clin. Invest.* **60**:808–814.

123. Freitag, J., Martin, K. J., Hruska, K. A., Anderson, C., Conrades, M., Ladenson, J., Klahr, S., and Slatopolsky, E., 1978, Impaired parathyroid hormone metabolism in patients with chronic renal failure, *N. Engl. J. Med.* **298**:29–32.

124. Goltzman, D., Peytremann, A., Callahan, G. N., Segre, G. V., and Potts, J. T., Jr., 1976, Metabolism and biological activity of parathyroid hormone in renal cortical membranes, *J. Clin. Invest.* **57**:8–19.

125. Goltzman, D., 1978. Examination of the requirement for metabolism of parathyroid hormone in skeletal tissue before biological action, *Endocrinology* **102**:1555–1562.

126. Martin, K. J., Freitag, J. J., Conrades, M. B., Hruska, K. A., Klahr, S., and Slatopolsky, E., 1978, Selective uptake of the synthetic amino terminal fragment of bovine parathyroid hormone by isolated perfused bone, *J. Clin. Invest.* **62**:256–261.

127. Parsons, J. A., and Robinson, G. J., 1968, A rapid indirect hypercalcemic action of parathyroid hormone demonstrated in isolated perfused bone,

in: *Parathyroid Hormone and Thyrocalcitonin,* (R. V. Talmage and L. F. Belanger, eds.), pp. 329–331, Excerpta Medica, Amsterdam.

128. Mueller, W. J., Brubaker, R. L., Gay, C. V., and Boelkins, J. N., 1973, Mechanisms of bone resorption in laying hens, *Fed. Proc.* **32:**1951–1954.

129. Parsons, J. A., 1979, The physiology of parathyroid hormone, in: *Endocrinology,* Volume 2 (L. J. DeGroot, G. F. Cahill, Jr., W. D. Odell, L. Martini, J. T. Potts, Jr., D. H. Nelson, E. Steinberger, and A. I. Winegrad, eds.), pp. 621–630, Grune & Stratton, New York.

130. Wittle, L. W., and Dent, J. N., 1979, Effects of parathyroidectomy and of parathyroid extract on levels of calcium and phosphate in the blood and urine of the red-spotted newt, *Gen. Comp. Endocrinol.* **37:**428–439.

131. Rader, J. I., Baylink, D. J., Hughes, M. R., Safilian, E. F., and Haussler, M. R., 1979, Calcium and phosphorus deficiency in rats: Effects on PTH and 1,25 dihydroxyvitamin D_3, *Am. J. Physiol.* **236:**E118–E122.

132. Haldimann, B., Bonjour, J. P., and Fleisch, H., 1977, Role of parathyroid hormone in regulation of main calcium fluxes in rats, *Am. J. Physiol.* **232:**E535–E541.

133. Pitkin, R. M., 1979, Calcium metabolism during pregnancy and its effects on the fetus and newborn, *Pediatr. Adolesc. Endocrinol.* **5:**67–87.

134. Pitkin, R. M., Reynolds, W. A., Williams, G. A., and Hargis, G. K., 1979, Calcium metabolism in normal pregnancy: A longitudinal study, *Am. J. Obstet. Gynecol.* **133:**781–790.

135. Kumar, R., Cohen, W. R., Silva, P., and Epstein, F. H., 1979, Elevated 1,25-dihydroxyvitamin D plasma levels in normal human pregnancy and lactation, *J. Clin. Invest.* **63:**342–344.

136. Toverud, S. U., Becker, D. I., Boass, A., Cooper, C. W., Hirsch, P. F., Outjes, D. A., Peng, T.-C., and Ramp, W. K., 1978, Hormonal control of calcium metabolism in lactation, in: *Endocrinology of Calcium Metabolism* (D. H. Copp and R. V. Talmage, eds.), pp. 126–133, Excerpta Medica, Amsterdam.

137. Toverud, S. U., Cooper, C. W., and Munson, P. L., 1978, Calcium metabolism during lactation: Elevated blood levels of calcitonin, *Endocrinology* **103:**472–479.

138. Peck, W. A., 1978, The specialization of bone cells, in: *Endocrinology of Calcium Metabolism* (D. H. Copp and R. V. Talmage, eds.), pp. 237–240, Excerpta Medica, Amsterdam.

139. Wong, G. L., 1979, Basal activities and hormone responsiveness of osteoclast-like and osteoblast-like bone cells are regulated by glucocorticoids, *J. Biol. Chem.* **254:**6337–6340.

140. Baud, C. A., and Boivin, G., 1978, Effects of hormones on osteocyte function and perilacunar wall structure, *Clin. Orthop. Relat. Res.* **136:**270–281.

141. Norimatsu, H., Vander Wiel, C. J., and Talmage, R. V., 1979, Morphological support of a role for cells lining bone surfaces in maintenance of plasma calcium concentration, *Clin. Orthop. Relat. Res.* **138:**254–262.

142. Holtrop, M. E., King, G. J., Cox, K. A., and Reit, B., 1979, Time-related changes in the ultrastructure of osteoclasts after injection of parathyroid hormone in young rats, *Calcif. Tissue Int.* **27:**29–135.

143. Miller, S. C., 1978, Rapid activation of the medullary bone osteoclast cell surface by parathyroid hormone, *J. Cell Biol.* **76:**615–618.
144. Vander Wiel, C., Matthews, J. L., and Talmage, R. V., 1978, Intracellular calcium localization in cells lining bone surfaces following parathyroid hormone injection, in: *Endocrinology of Calcium Metabolism* (D. H. Copp and R. V. Talmage, eds.), p. 355, Excerpta Medica, Amsterdam.
145. Parfitt, A. M., 1976, The actions of parathyroid hormone on bone: Relation to bone remodeling and turnover, calcium homeostasis, and metabolic bone disease. II. PTH and bone cells: Bone turnover and plasma calcium regulation, *Metabolism* **25:**904–955.
146. Baud, C. A., and Boivin, G., 1978, Effects of hormones on osteocyte function and perilacunar wall structure, *Clin. Orthop. Relat. Res.* **136:**270–281.
147. Burger, E. H., Matthews, J. L., and Doty, S. B., 1978, Intracellular calcium distribution in parathyroid-hormone treated fetal bones, in: *Endocrinology of Calcium Metabolism* (D. H. Copp and R. V. Talmage, eds.), p. 356, Excerpta Medica, Amsterdam.
148. Schulz, A., Bressel, M., and Delling, G., 1977, Activity of osteoclastic bone resorption in primary human hyperparathyroidism: A comparative electron microscopic and histomorphometric study, *Calcif. Tissue Res.* **22**(Suppl):307–310.
149. Krempien, B., Friedrich, G., Geger, G., and Ritz, E., 1977, Factors influencing the effect of parathyroid hormone on endosteal cell morphology, *Calcif. Tissue Res.* **22**(Suppl.):164–168.
150. Bonucci, E., Lo Cascio, V., Adami, S., Cominacini, L., Galvanini, G., and Scuro, A., 1978, The ultrastructure of bone cells and bone matrix in human primary hyperparathyroidism, *Virchows Arch. A* **379:**11–23.
151. Meunier, P. J., Bressot, C., and Edouard, C., 1978, Dynamics of bone remodeling in primary hyperparathyroidism: Histomorphometric data, in: *Endocrinology of Calcium Metabolism* (D. H. Copp and R. V. Talmage, eds.), p. 415, Excerpta Medica, Amsterdam.
152. Will, M. R., 1970, Fundamental physiologic role of parathyroid hormone in acid base homeostasis, *Lancet* **2:**802–804.
153. Fraley, D. S., and Adler, S., 1979, An extrarenal role for parathyroid hormone in the disposal of acute acid loads in rats and dogs, *J. Clin. Invest.* **63:**985–997.
154. Lechene, C. P., and Warner, R. R., 1977, Ultramicroanalysis: X-ray spectrometry by electron probe excitation, *Annu. Rev. Biophys. Bioeng.* **6:**57–85.
155. Evers, C., Murer, H., and Kinne, R., 1978, Effect of parathyrin on the transport properties of isolated renal brush-border vesicles, *Biochem. J.* **172:**49–56.
156. Gmaj, P., Murer, H., and Kinne, R., 1979, Calcium ion transport across plasma membranes isolated from rat kidney cortex, *Biochem. J.* **178:**549–557.
157. Stoll, R., Kinne, R., and Murer, H., 1979, Effect of dietary phosphate intake on phosphate transport by isolated rat renal brush-border vesicles, *Biochem. J.* **180:**465–470.
158. Tenenhouse, H. S., and Scriver, C. R., 1979, Renal brushborder membrane adaptation to phosphorus deprivation in the Hyp/Y mouse, *Nature (London)* **281:**225–227.

159. Suki, W. N., 1979, Calcium transport in the nephron, *Am. J. Physiol.* **237:**F1–F6.

160. Rouse, D., and Suki, W. N., 1978, Calcium transport in the superficial straight proximal tubule (SPT), *Clin. Res.* **26:**544A.

161. Shareghi, G. R., and Stoner, L. C., 1978, Calcium transport across segments of the rat distal nephron *in vitro*, *Am. J. Physiol.* **235:**F367–F375.

162. Greger, R., Lang, F., and Oberleithneu, H., 1978, Distal site of calcium reabsorption in the rat nephron, *Pfluegers Arch.* **374:**153–157.

163. Agus, Z. S., Chiu, P. J. S., and Goldberg, M., 1977, Regulation of urinary calcium excretion in the rat, *Am. J. Physiol.* **232:**F545–F549.

164. Grabie, M., Lau, K., Agus, Z. S., Goldberg, M., and Goldfarb, S., 1978, Role of parathyroid hormone in the hypercalciuria of chronic phosphate depletion, *Miner. Electrolyte Metab.* **1:**279–287.

165. Costanzo, L. S., and Windhager, E. E., 1978, Calcium and sodium transport by the distal convoluted tubule of the rat, *Am. J. Physiol.* **235:**F492–F506.

166. Christensson, T., Hellstrom, K., and Wengle, B., 1977, Hypercalcemia and primary hyperparathyroidism, *Arch. Intern. Med.* **137:**1138–1141.

167. Mohamadi, M., Bivins, L., and Becker, K. L., 1979, Effect of thiazides on serum calcium, *Clin. Pharmacol. Ther.* **26:**390–394.

168. Lechene, C., Colindres, R., and Knox, F. G., 1978, Electron probe microanalysis of the renal effect of parathyroid hormone, in: *Endocrinology of Calcium Metabolism* (D. H. Copp and R. V. Talmage, eds.), pp. 230–233, Excerpta Medica, Amsterdam.

169. Pastoriza-Munoz, E., Colindres, R. E., Lassiter, W. E., and Lechene, C., 1978, Effect of parathyroid hormone on phosphate reabsorption in rat distal convolution, *Am. J. Physiol.* **235:**F321–F330.

170. Sraer, J., Sraer, J. D., Chansel, D., Jueppner, H. J., Hesch, R. D., and Ardaillou, R., 1978, Evidence for glomerular receptors for parathyroid hormone, *Am. J. Physiol.* **235:**F96–F103.

171. Sraer, J., Ardaillou, R., Loreau, N., and Sraer, J. D., 1974, Evidence for parathyroid hormone sensitive adenylate cyclase in rat glomeruli, *Mol. Cell. Endocrinol.* **1:**285–294.

172. Dousa, T. P., Barnes, L. D., Ong, S. H., and Steiner, A. L., 1977, Immunohistochemical localization of 3′,5′-cyclic AMP and 3′,5′-cyclic GMP in rat renal cortex: Effect of parathyroid hormone, *Proc. Natl. Acad. Sci. USA* **74:**3569–3573.

173. Humes, H. D., Ichikawa, I., Troy, J. L., and Brenner, B. M., 1978, Evidence for a parathyroid-hormone dependent influence of calcium on the glomerular ultrafiltration coefficient, *J. Clin. Invest.* **61:**32–40.

174. Ichikawa, I., Humes, H. D., Dousa, T. P., and Brenner, B. M., 1978, Influence of parathyroid hormone on glomerular ultrafiltration in the rat, *Am. J. Physiol.* **234:**F393–F401.

175. Lins, L.-E., 1979, Renal function in primary hyperparathyroidism and in non-hyperparathyroid hypercalcemia, *Acta Med. Scand.* **205:**607–613.

176. Levine, B. S., Brautbar, N., and Coburn, J. W., 1978, Does vitamin D affect the renal handling of calcium and phosphorus? *Miner. Electrolyte Metab.* **1:**295–302.

177. Bernstein, D., Kleeman, C. R., Dowling, J. T., and Maxwell, M. H., 1959,

The renal clearance of diffusible calcium associated with clinical and experimental alterations in parathyroid function, *Clin. Res.* **7:**246.

178. Hugi, K., Bonjour, J.-P., and Fleisch, H., 1979, Renal handling of calcium: Influence of parathyroid hormone and 1,25-dihydroxy vitamin D_3, *Am. J. Physiol.* **236:**F349–F356.

179. Forte, L. R., Nichols, R. A., and Anast, C. S., 1976, Renal adenylate cyclase and the interrelationship between parathyroid hormone and vitamin D in the regulation of urinary phosphate and adenosine cyclic 3′,5′-monophosphate excretion, *J. Clin. Invest.* **57:**559–568.

180. Kakuta, S., Sato, C., Suda, T., Kimura, N., Araki, N., Ono, Y., and Nagata, N., 1978, Relationship between parathyroid hormone and adenosine 3′,5′-monophosphate metabolism in the kidney of vitamin D-deficient rats, *Biochim. Biophys. Acta* **539:**173–180.

181. Adams, N. D., Gray, R. W., and Lemann, J., Jr., 1979, The effects of oral $CaCO_3$ loading and dietary calcium deprivation on plasma 1,25-dihydroxy vitamin D concentrations in healthy adults, *J. Clin. Endocrinol. Metab.* **48:**1008–1016.

182. Gray, R. W., Caldas, A. E., Wilz, D. R., Lemann, J., Jr., Smith, G. A., and DeLuca, H. F., 1978, Metabolism and excretion of ^3H-1,25-$(OH)_2$-vitamin D_3 in healthy adults, *J. Clin. Endocrinol. Metab.* **46:**756–765.

183. Hughes, M. R., Brumbaugh, P. F., Haussler, M. R., Wergedal, J. E., and Baylink, D. T., 1975, Regulation of serum 1α,25-dihydroxy vitamin D_3 by calcium and phosphate in the rat, *Science* **190:**578–580.

184. Ribovich, M. L., and DeLuca, H. F., 1978, Adaptation of intestinal calcium absorption: Parathyroid hormone and vitamin D metabolism, *Arch. Biochem. Biophys.* **188:**157–163.

185. Kaplan, R. A., Haussler, M. R., Deftos, L. J., Bone, H., and Pak, C. Y. C., 1977, The role of 1α,25-dihydroxyvitamin D in the mediation of intestinal hyperabsorption of calcium in primary hyperparathyroidism and absorptive hypercalciuria, *J. Clin. Invest.* **59:**756–760.

186. Bone, H. G., III, Zerwekh, J. E., Haussler, M. R., and Pak, C. Y. C., 1979, Effect of parathyroidectomy on serum 1α,25-dihydroxyvitamin D and intestinal calcium absorption in primary hyperparathyroidism, *J. Clin. Endocrinol. Metab.* **48:**877–879.

187. Peacock, M., Heyburn, P. J., Barnett, M. J., Brown, W. B., Davies, A., and Taylor, G. A., 1980, Relative importance of plasma parathyroid hormone, calcium and phosphate in regulating 1,25$(OH)_2$ vitamin D in primary hyperparathyroidism, *Proceedings of the 7th International Conference on Calcium-Regulating Hormones.*

188. Broadus, A. E., Horst, R. L., Lang, R., Littledike, E. T., and Rasmussen, H., 1980, The importance of circulating 1,25-dihydroxyvitamin D in the pathogenesis of hypercalciuria and renal-stone formation in primary hyperparathyroidism, *N. Engl. J. Med.* **302:**421–426.

189. Malluche, H. H., Goldstein, D. A., and Massry, S. G., 1979, Osteomalacia and hyperparathyroid bone disease in patients with nephrotic syndrome, *J. Clin. Invest.* **63:**494–500.

190. Weisbrode, S. E., Capen, C. C., and Norman, A. W., 1978, Ultrastructural evaluation of the effects of 1,25-dihydroxyvitamin D_3 on bone of thyroparathyroidectomized rats fed a low-calcium diet, *Am. J. Pathol.* **92:**459–472.

191. Nissenson, R. A., and Arnaud, C., 1979, Properties of the parathyroid hormone receptor–adenylate cyclase system in chicken renal plasma membranes, *J. Biol. Chem.* **254:**1469–1475.

192. Segre, G. V., Rosenblatt, M., Reiner, B. L., Mahaffey, J. E., and Potts, J. T., Jr., 1979, Characterization of parathyroid hormone receptors in canine renal cortical plasma membranes using a radioiodinated sulfur-free hormone analogue, *J. Biol. Chem.* **254:**6980–6986.

193. Mohr, H., and Hesch, R. D., 1978, Parathormone degrading activity in basal lateral membranes of the bovine renal cortex, *Acta Endocrinol. [Suppl.](Copenhagen)* **87**(Suppl. 25):107–108.

194. Mazzuoli, G. F., D'Erasmo, E., Scarda, A., Minisola, S., Mancini, D., and Aliberti, L. M., 1979, Significance of early increase in stable and radioactive plasma calcium after parathyroidectomy in primary hyperparathyroidism, *Calcif. Tissue Int.* **29:**185–191.

195. Borle, A. B., and Uchikawa, T., 1978, Effects of parathyroid hormone on the distribution and transport of calcium in cultured kidney cells, *Endocrinology* **102:**1725–1732.

196. Borle, A. B., and Uchikawa, T., 1979, Effects of adenosine 3′,5′-monophosphate, dibutyryl adenosine 3′,5′-monophosphate, aminophylline, and imidazole on renal cellular calcium metabolism, *Endocrinology* **104:**122–129.

197. Dziak, R., and Stern, P. H., 1975, Calcium transport in isolated bone cells, *Endocrinology* **97:**1281–1287.

198. Nagata, N., Ono, Y., and Kimura, N., 1977, Inhibition by cholera toxin of parathyroid hormone-induced calcium release from bone in culture, *Biochem. Biophys. Res. Commun.* **78:**819–826.

199. Kakuta, S., Suda, T., Sasak, S., Kimura, N., and Nagata, N., 1975, Effects of parathyroid hormone on the accumulation of cAMP in bone of vitamin D-deficient rats, *Endocrinology* **97:**1288–1293.

200. Carnes, D. L., Anast, C. S., and Forte, L. R., 1978, Impaired renal adenylate cyclase response to parathyroid hormone in the calcium-deficient rat, *Endocrinology* **102:**45–51.

201. Mears, D. C., 1971, Effects of parathyroid hormone and thyrocalcitonin on the membrane potential of osteoclasts, *Endocrinology* **88:**1021–1028.

202. Dietrich, J. W., Mundy, G. R., and Raisz, L. G., 1979, Inhibition of bone resorption in tissue culture by membrane-stabilizing drugs, *Endocrinology* **104:**1644–1648.

203. Baxter, J. D., and Funder, J. W., 1979, Hormone receptors, *N. Engl. J. Med.* **301:**1149–1161.

204. Goltzman, D., Callahan, E. N., Tregear, G. M., and Potts, J. T., Jr., 1978, Influence of guanyl nucleotides on parathyroid hormone-stimulated adenylyl cyclase activity in renal cortical membranes, *Endocrinology* **103:**1352–1360.

205. Drezner, M. K., and Burch, W. M., Jr., 1978, Altered activity of the nu-

cleotide regulatory site in the parathyroid hormone-sensitive adenylate cyclase from the renal cortex of a patient with pseudohypoparathyroidism, *J. Clin. Invest.* **62**:1222–1227.

206. Levine, M., Downs, R., Singer, M., Marx, S., Aurbach, G., and Spiegel, A., 1980, Deficiency of guanine nucleotide regulatory protein: Postreceptor site of defect in pseudohypoparathyroidism, *Proceedings of the 7th International Conference on Calcium-Regulating Hormones.*

207. Walling, M., Marvaso, V., and Bernard, G. W., 1978, Stimulation of guanylate cyclase activity in cultured osteogenic murine calvarial mesenchymal cells by PTH, calcitonin and insulin, *Biochem. Biophys. Res. Commun.* **83**:521–527.

208. Wrenn, R. W., Currie, M. G., and Biddulph, D. M., 1978, Influence of calcium, parathyroid hormone and ionophore A-23187 on cyclic nucleotide concentrations of isolated renal tubules, *Mol. Cell. Endocrinol.* **10**:263–276.

209. Araki, N., Nagata, N., and Kimura, N., 1977, Effects of parathyroid hormone and prostaglandin E_1 in vitro on release of cyclic AMP from kidney cortical tissue, *Endocrinol. Jpn.* **24**:581–587.

210. Currie, M. G., and Biddulph, D. M., 1979, Metabolism of cyclic AMP in isolated renal tubules: Effects of prostaglandins and parathyroid hormone, *Prostaglandins* **17**:211–222.

211. Biddulph, D. M., Currie, M. G., and Wrenn, R. W., 1979, Effects and interactions of parathyroid hormone and prostaglandins on adenosine 3′,5′-monophosphate concentrations in isolated renal tubules, *Endocrinology* **104**:1164–1171.

212. Marcus, R., and Orner, F. B., 1977, Cyclic AMP production in rat calvaria in vitro: Interaction of prostaglandins with parathyroid hormone, *Endocrinology* **101**:1570–1578.

213. Goldring, S. R., Dayer, J.-M, and Krane, S. M., 1979, Regulation of hormone-induced cyclic AMP response to parathyroid hormone and prostaglandin E_2 in cells cultured from human giant cell tumors of bone, *Calcif. Tissue Int.* **29**:193–200.

214. Brown, G. M., Broadus, A. E., Brennan, M. F., Gardner, D. G., Marx, S. J., Spiegel, A. M., Downs, R. W., Jr., Attie, M., and Aurbach, G. D., 1979, Direct comparison in vivo and in vitro of suppressibility of parathyroid function by calcium in primary hyperparathyroidism, *J. Clin. Endocrinol. Metab.* **48**:604–610.

215. Kukreja, S. C., Williams, G. A., Vora, N. M., Hargis, G. K., Bowser, E. N., and Henderson, W. J., 1980, Parathyroid hormone secretion in primary hyperparathyroidism: Retained control by calcium with impaired control by β-adrenergic system, *Miner. Electrolyte Metab.* **3**:98–103.

216. Habener, J. F., 1978, Responsiveness of neoplastic and hyperplastic parathyroid tissues to calcium in vitro, *J. Clin. Invest.* **62**:436–450.

217. Caro, J. F., and Besarab, A., 1978, Propranolol therapy for hyperparathyroidism, *Lancet* **1**:827.

218. Fournier, A., Coevoet, B., de Fremont, J. F., Gueris, J., Caillens, G., Desplan, C., Calmette, C., and Moukhtar, M. S., 1978, Propranolol therapy for seconday hyperparathyroidism in uremia, *Lancet* **2**:50–51.

219. Caro, J. F., Burke, J. F., Besarab, A., and Glennon, J. A., 1978, A possible role for propranolol in the treatment of renal osteodystrophy, *Lancet* **2:**451–454.
220. Caro, J. F., Castro, J. H., and Glennon, J. A., 1979, Effect of long-term propranolol administration on parathyroid hormone and calcium concentration in primary hyperparathyroidism, *Ann. Intern. Med.* **91:**740–741.
221. Sherwood, J., Reinhard, D., and Garcia, M., 1979, Does cimetidine inhibit parathyroid hormone secretion?, *N. Engl. J. Med.* **300:**200–201.
222. Palmer, F. J., Sawyers, T. M., and Wierzbinski, S. J., 1980, Cimetidine and hyperparathyroidism, *N. Engl. J. Med.* **302:**692.
223. Jacob, A. I., Lanier, D., Jr., Canterbury, J., and Bourgoignie, J. J., 1980, Reduction by cimetidine of serum parathyroid hormone levels in uremic patients, *N. Engl. J. Med.* **302:**671–674.
224. Christensson, T., 1978, Hyperparathyroidism and radiation therapy, *Ann. Intern. Med.* **89:**216–217.
225. Tisell, L.-E, Hansson, G., Lindberg, S., and Ragnhult, I., 1978, Occurrence of previous neck radiotherapy among patients with associated non-medullary thyroid carcinoma and parathyroid adenoma or hyperplasia, *Acta Chir. Scand.* **144:**7–11.
226. Russ, J. E., Scanlon, E. F., and Sener, S. F., 1979, Parathyroid adenomas following irradiation, *Cancer* **43:**1078–1083.
227. Erkocak, E. V., and Taylor, S., 1978, Hyperparathyroidism after radiotherapy, *Br. Med. J.* **2:**327–328.
228. Christensson, T., and Einarsson, K., 1977, Cholelithiasis in subjects with hypercalcemia and primary hyperparathyroidism detected in a health screening, *Gut* **18:**543–546.
229. Linos, D. A., Van Heerden, J. A., Abboud, C. F., and Edis, A. J., 1978, Primary hyperparathyroidism and peptic ulcer disease, *Arch. Surg.* **113:**384–386.
230. McCarthy, D. M., Peikin, S. R., Lopatin, R. N., Long, B. W., Spiegel, A., Marx, S., and Brennan, M., 1979, Hyperparathyroidism—A reversible cause of cimetidine-resistant gastric hypersecretion, *Br. Med. J.* **1:**1765–1766.
231. Christensson, T., 1977, Serum urate in subjects with hypercalcemic hyperparathyroidism, *Clin. Chim. Acta* **80:**529–533.
232. Akgun, S., and Ertel, N. H., 1978, Hyperparathyroidism and coexisting diabetes mellitus, *Arch. Intern. Med.* **138:**1500–1502.
233. Marx, S. J., Spiegel, A. M., Brown, E. M., and Aurbach, G. D., 1977, Family studies in patients with primary parathyroid hyperplasia, *Am. J. Med.* **62:**698–706.
234. Marx, S. J., Spiegel, A. M., Brown, E. M., Koehler, J. O., Gardner, D. G., Brennan, M. F., and Aurbach, G. D., 1978, Divalent cation metabolism: Familial hypocalciuric hypercalcemia versus typical primary hyperparathyroidism, *Am. J. Med.* **635:**235–242.
235. Marx, S. J., Spiegel, A. M., Brown, E. M., Windeck, R., Gardner, D. G., Downs, R. W., Jr., Attie, M., and Aurbach, G. D., 1978, Circulating parathyroid hormone activity: Familial hypocalciuric hypercalcemia versus typical primary hyperparathyroidism, *J. Clin. Endocrinol. Metab.* **47:**1190–1197.

236. Massry, S. G., and Goldstein, D. A., 1978, Role of parathyroid hormone in uremic toxicity, *Kidney Int.* **13**(Suppl. 8):S39–S42.
237. Cogan, M. G., Covey, C. M., Arieff, A. I., Wisniewski, A., and Clark, O. H., 1978, Central nervous system manifestations of hyperparathyroidism, *Am. J. Med.* **65**:963–970.
238. Guisado, R., Arieff, A. I., and Massry, S. G., 1975, Changes in the electroencephalogram in acute uremia: Effects of parathyroid hormone and brain electrolytes, *J. Clin. Invest.* **55**:738–745.
239. Goldstein, D. A., and Massry, S. G., 1978, Effect of parathyroid hormone administration and its withdrawal on brain calcium and electroencephalogram, *Miner. Electrolyte Metab.* **1**:84–91.
240. Cooper, J. D., Lazarowitz, V. C., and Arieff, A. I., 1978, Neurodiagnostic abnormalities in patients with acute renal failure, *J. Clin. Invest.* **61**:1448–1455.
241. Goldstein, D. A., Chui, L. A., and Massry, S. G., 1978, Effect of parathyroid hormone and uremia on peripheral nerve calcium and motor nerve conduction velocity, *J. Clin. Invest.* **62**:88–93.
242. Avram, M. M., Feinfeld, D. A., and Huatuco, A. H., 1978, Search for the uremic toxin: Decreased motor nerve conduction velocity and elevated parathyroid hormone in uremia, *N. Engl. J. Med.* **298**:1000–1003.
243. Arieff, A. I., and Schmidt, R. W., 1978, Parathyroid hormone as a uremic neurotoxin, *N. Engl. J. Med.* **299**:362–363.
244. Avram, M. M, Iancu, M., Morrow, P., Feinfeld, D., and Huatuco, A., 1979, Uremic syndrome in man: New evidence for parathormone as a multisystem neurotoxin, *Clin. Nephrol.* **11**:59–62.
245. Sauerwein, H. P., and Krediet, R. T., 1978, Parathyroid hormone as a uremic neurotoxin, *N. Engl. J. Med.* **29**:362.
246. diGiulio, S., Chkoff, N., Lhoste, F., Zingraff, J., and Drueke, T., 1978, Parathormone as a nerve poison in uremia, *N. Engl. J. Med.* **299**:1134–1135.
247. Massry, S. G., Goldstein, D. A., Procci, W. R., and Kletzky, O. A., 1977, Impotence in patients with uremia: A possible role for parathyroid hormone, *Nephron* **19**:305–310.
248. Ladenson, J. H., Lewis, J. W., McDonald, J. M., Slatopolsky, E., and Boyd, J. C., 1978, Relationship of free and total calcium in hypercalcemic conditions, *J. Clin. Endocrinol. Metab.* **48**:393–397.
249. Conceicao, S. C., Weightman, D., Smith, P. A., Luno, J., Wared, M. K., and Kerr, D. N. S., 1978, Serum ionised calcium concentration: Measurement versus calculation, *Br. Med. J.* **1**:1103–1105.
250. Larsson, L., and Ohman, S., 1979, Serum calcium ion activity: Some aspects of methodological differences and intraindividual variation, *Clin. Biochem.* **12**:138–141.
251. Parthemore, J. G., Roos, B. A., Parker, D. C., Kripke, D. F., Avioli, L. V., and Deftos, L. J., 1978, Assessment of acute and chronic changes in parathyroid hormone secretion by a radioimmunoassay with predominant specificity for the carboxy-terminal region of the molecule, *J. Clin. Endocrinol. Metab.* **47**:284–289.
252. Wallach, S., Cohn, S. H., Atkins, H. L., Ellis, K. J., Kohberger, R., Aloia, J. F., and Zanzi, I., 1977, Effect of salmon calcitonin on skeletal mass in osteoporosis, *Curr. Ther. Res.* **22**:556–572.

253. Christensen, M. S., 1979, Radioimmunoassay of human parathyroid hormone, *Dan. Med. Bull.* **26:**157–174.
254. Broadus, A. E., Deftos, L. J., and Bartter, F. C., 1978, Effects of the intravenous administration of calcium on nephrogenous cyclic AMP: Use as a parathyroid suppression test, *J. Clin. Endocrinol. Metab.* **46:**477–487.
255. Chambers, D. J., Schafer, H., Laughorn, J. A., Jr., Johnstone, J., Zanelli, J. M., Parsons, J. A., Bitensky, L., and Chayen, J., 1978, Dose-related activation by PTH of specific enzymes in various regions of the kidney, in: *Endocrinology of Calcium Metabolism* (D. H. Copp and R. V. Talmage, eds.), pp. 216–220, Excerpta Medica, Amsterdam.
256. Chambers, D. J., Dunham, J., Zanelli, J. M., Parsons, J. A., Bitensky, L., and Chayen, J., 1978, A sensitive bioassay of parathyroid hormone in plasma, *Clin. Endocrinol.* **9:**375–379.
257. Fenton, S., Somers, S., and Heath, D. A., 1978, Preliminary studies with the sensitive cytochemical assay for parathyroid hormone, *Clin. Endocrinol.* **9:**381–384.
258. Karo, J. J., Maas, L. C., Kaine, H., and Gelzayed, E. A., 1978, Ultrasonography and parathyroid adenoma, *J. Am. Med. Assoc.* **239:**2163–2164.
259. Crocker, E. F., Jellins, J., and Freund, J., 1979, Parathyroid lesions localized by radionuclide subtraction and ultrasound, *Radiology* **130:**215–217.
260. Shimshak, R. R., Schoenrock, G. J., Taekman, H. P., Cianci, P., and Chambers, R. F., 1979, Preoperative localization of a parathyroid adenoma using computed tomography and thyroid scanning, *J. Comput. Assist. Tomogr.* **3:**117–119.
261. Fagerberg, G., 1978, Angiographic localization of parathyroid adenomas, *Acta Radiol. Diagn.* **19:**7–16.
262. Brote, L., Fagerberg, G., Gillquist, J., and Larson, L., 1978, Parathyroid localization in patients with previous neck surgery, *Acta Chir. Scand.* **144:**445–449.
263. Wang, C.-A., 1977, Parathyroid re-exploration: A clinical and pathological study of 112 cases, *Ann. Surg.* **186:**140–145.
264. Sofianides, T., Chang, Y.-S., Leary, J. S., and Nichols, F. X., 1978, Localization of parathyroid adenomas by cervical esophagram. *J. Clin. Endocrinol. Metab.* **46:**587–592.
265. Van Vroonhoven, T. J., and Muller, H. J., 1978, Causes of failure in the surgical treatment of primary hyperparathyroidism: Lessons from 51 successful reoperations, *Br. J. Surg.* **65:**297–300.
266. Freaney, R., Casey, O. M., and Muldowney, F. P., 1978, The long-term effect of parathyroidectomy on renal function, *Ir. J. Med. Sci.* **147:**205–209.
267. Attie, J. N., Wise, L., Mir, R., and Ackerman, L. V., 1978, The rationale against routine subtotal parathyroidectomy for primary hyperparathyroidism, *Am. J. Surg.* **136:**437–444.
268. Harness, J. K., Ramsburg, S. R., Nishiyama, R. H., and Thompson, N. W., 1979, Multiple adenomas of the parathyroid: Do they exist?, *Arch. Surg.* **114:**468–474.
269. Ljungberg, O., and Tibblin, S., 1979, Perioperative fat staining of frozen sections in primary hyperparathyroidism, *Am. J. Pathol.* **95:**633–645.
270. Wang, C.-A, and Rieder, S. V., 1978, A density test for the intraoperative

differentiation of parathyroid hyperplasia from neoplasia, *Ann. Surg.* **187**:63–67.

271. Akerstrom, G., Grimelius, L., Johansson, H., and Lundqvist, H., 1977, Estimation of the parenchymal cell content of the parathyroid gland using density-gradient columns, *Acta Pathol. Microbiol. Scand. Sect. A* **85**:555–557.

272. Ohman, V., Granberg, P.-O., and Lindell, B., 1978, Function of the parathyroid glands after total thyroidectomy, *Surg. Gynecol. Obstet.* **146**:773–778.

273. Brennan, M. F., Brown, E. M., Marx, S. J., Spiegel, A. M., Broadus A. E., Doppman, J. L., Webber, B., and Aurbach, G. D., 1978, Recurrent hyperparathyroidism from an autotransplanted parathyroid adenoma, *N. Engl. J. Med.* **299**:1057–1059.

274. Penn, I., and Haase, G. M., 1979, Autotransplantation of parathyroid adenoma, *N. Engl. J. Med.* **300**:1489.

275. Brennan, M. F., Brown, E. M., Sears, H. F., and Aurbach G. D., 1978, Human parathyroid cryopreservation: In vitro testing of function by parathyroid hormone release, *Ann. Surg.* **187**:87–90.

276. Brennan, M. F., Brown, E. M., Spiegel, A. M., Marx, S. J., Doppman, J. L., Jones, D. C., and Aurbach, G. D., 1979, Autotransplantation of cryopreserved parathyroid tissue in man, *Ann. Surg.* **189**:139–142.

277. Taylor, C. M., Mawer, E. B., Wallace, J. E., St. John, J., Cochran, M., Russell, R. G. G., and Kanis, J. A., 1978, The absence of 24,25-dihydroxycholecalciferol in anephric patients, *Clin. Sci. Mol. Med.* **55**:541–547.

278. Slatopolsky, E., Rutherford, W. E., Hruska, K., Martin, K., and Klahr, S., 1978, How important is phosphate in the pathogenesis of renal osteodystrophy?, *Arch. Intern. Med.* **138**:848–852.

279. Massry, S. G., and Ritz, E., 1978, The pathogenesis of secondary hyperparathyroidism of renal failure: Is there a controversy?, *Arch. Intern. Med.* **138**:853–856.

280. Malluche, H. H., Werner, E., and Ritz, E., 1978, Intestinal absorption of calcium and whole body calcium retention in incipient and advanced renal failure, *Miner. Electrolyte Metab.* **1**:263–270.

281. Fiaschi, E., Maschio, G., D'Angelo, A., Bonucci, E., Tessitore, N., and Messa, P., 1978, Low protein diets and bone disease in chronic renal failure, *Kidney Int.* **13**(Suppl. 8):S79–S82.

282. Bordier, P., Zingraff, J., Gueris, J., Jungers, P., Marie, P., Pechet, M., and Rasmussen, H., 1978, The effect of $1\alpha(OH)D_3$ and $1\alpha,25(OH)_2D_3$ on the bone in patients with renal osteodystrophy, *Am. J. Med.* **64**:101–107.

283. Chesney, R. W., Moorthy, A. V., Eisman, J. A., Jax, D. K., Mazess, R. B., and DeLuca, H. F., 1978, Increased growth after long-term oral $1\alpha,25$-vitamin D_3 in childhood renal osteodystrophy, *N. Engl. J. Med.* **298**:238–242.

284. Berl, T., Berns, A. S., Huffer, W. E., Hammill, K., Alfrey, A. C., Arnaud, C. D., and Schrier, R. W., 1978, 1,25 dihydroxycholecalciferol effects in chronic dialysis, *Ann. Intern. Med.* **88**:774–780.

285. Madsen, S., and Olgaard, K., 1978, Long-term trial of 1-alpha-hydroxycholecalciferol in adults with chronic renal failure, *Eur. J. Clin. Pharmacol.* **13**:401–408.

286. Goldstein, D. A., Malluche, H. H., and Massry, S. G., 1979, Management

of renal osteodystrophy with 1,25(OH)$_2$D$_3$. I. Effects on clinical, radiographic and biochemical parameters, *Miner. Electrolyte Metab.* **2:**35–47.

287. Malluche, H. H., Goldstein, D. A., and Massry, S. G., 1979, Management of renal osteodystrophy with 1,25(OH)$_2$D$_3$. II. Effects on histopathology of bone: Evidence for healing of osteomalacia, *Miner. Electrolyte Metab.* **2:**48–55.

288. Binswanger, U., Fischer, J. A., Iselin, H., Oswald, N., Keusch, G., Frei, D., and Willimann, P., 1979, 1,25-dihydroxycholecalciferol treatment of clinically asymptomatic renal osteodystrophy, *Miner. Electrolyte Metab.* **2:**103–115.

289. Christiansen, L., Rodbro, P., Christensen, M. S., Hartnack, B., and Transbol, I., 1978, Deterioration of renal function during treatment of chronic renal failure with 1,25-dihydroxycholecalciferol, *Lancet* **2:**700–703.

290. Feest, T. G., Ward, M. K., Ellis, H. A., Conceicao, S., Pierides, A. M., Aird, E., Simpson, W., Cook, D. B., and Kerr, D. N. S., 1977, Renal bone disease—What is it and why does it happen?, *Clin. Endocrinol.* **7**(Suppl.):19s–23s.

291. Alvarez-Ude, F., Feest, T. G., Ward, M. K., Pierides, A. M., Ellis, H. A., Peart, K. M., Simpson, W., Weightman, D., and Kerr, D. N. S., 1978, Hemodialysis bone disease: Correlation between clinical, histologic, and other findings, *Kidney Int.* **14:**68–73.

292. Coburn, J. W., personal communication.

293. Nielsen, H. E., Christensen, C. K., and Olsen, K. J., 1979, Serum calcitonin in patients with chronic renal disease, *Acta Med. Scand.* **205:**615–618.

294. Heynen, G., Kanis, J. A., Oliver, D., Ledingham, J. G. G., and Russel, R. G. G., 1976, Evidence that endogenous calcitonin protects against renal bone disease, *Lancet* **2:**1322–1325.

295. Feletti, C., and Bonomini, V., 1979, Effect of calcitonin on bone lesions in chronic dialysis patients, *Nephron* **24:**85–88.

296. Zucchelli, P., Fusaroli, M., Fabbri, L., Pavlica, P., Casanoa, S., Viglietta, G., and Sasdelli, M., 1978, Treatment of ectopic calcification in ureia, *Kidney Int.* **13:**(Suppl. 8):S-86–S90.

297. Breslau, N. A., and Pak, C. Y. C., 1979, Hypoparathyroidism, *Metabolism* **28:**1261–1276.

298. Nusynowitz, M. L., and Klein, M. H., 1973, Pseudoidiopathic hypoparathyroidism: Hypoparathyroidism with ineffective parathyroid hormone, *Am. J. Med.* **55:**677–686.

299. Lewin, I. G., Papapoulos, S. E., Tomlinson, S., Hendy, G. N., and D'Riordan, J. L. H., 1978, Studies of hypoparathyroidism and pseudohypoparathyroidism, *Q. J. Med.* **47:**533–548.

300. Graham, K., Williams, B. O., and Rowe, M. J., 1979, Idiopathic hypoparathyroidism: A cause of fits in the elderly, *Br. Med. J.* **1:**1460–1461.

301. Slyter, H., 1979, Idiopathic hypoparathyroidism presenting as dementia, *Neurology* **29:**393–394.

302. Preskorn, S. H., and Reveley, A., 1978, Pseudohypoparathyroidism and Capgnas' syndrome, *Br. J. Psychiatry* **133:**34–37.

303. Parfitt, A. M., 1979, Surgical, idiopathic, and other varieties of parathyroid hormone-deficient hypoparathyroidism, in: *Endocrinology*, Volume 2 (L. J. DeGroot, G. F. Cahill, Jr., W. D. Odell, L. Martin, J. T. Potts, Jr., D. H.

Nelson, E. Steinberger, and A. I. Winegrad, eds.), pp. 755–768, Grune & Stratton, New York.

304. Nyland, H., and Skre, H., 1977, Cerebral calcinosis with late onset encephalopathy: unusual type of pseudo-pseudohypoparathyroidism, *Acta Neurol. Scand.* **56:**309–325.

305. Werder, E. A., Fischer, J. A., Illig, R., Kind, H. P., Bernasconi, S., Fanconi, A., and Brader, A., 1978, Pseudohypoparathyroidism and idiopathic hypoparathyroidism: Relationship between serum calcium and parathyroid hormone levels and urinary cyclic adenosine-3′,5′-monophosphate response to parathyroid extract, *J. Clin. Endocrinol. Metab.* **46:**872–879.

306. Parfitt, A. M., 1979, Testing for hypoparathyroidism, *N. Engl. J. Med.* **300:**1163.

307. Rude, R. K., Oldham, S. B., Sharp, C. F., Jr., and Singer, F. R., 1978, Parathyroid hormone secretion in magnesium deficiency, *J. Clin. Endocrinol. Metab.* **47:**800–806.

308. Mennes, P., Rosenbaum, R., Martin, K., and Slatopolsky, E., 1978, Hypomagnesemia and impaired parathyroid hormone secretion in chronic renal disease. *Ann. Intern. Med.* **88:**206–209.

309. Yamada, K., Tamura, Y., Yamamoto, M., and Kumagai, A., 1978, Effect of calcium administration on renal responsiveness to parathyroid hormone in pseudohypoparathyroidism type I and II in comparison with normals, idiopathic and surgical hypoparathyroidism, *Endocrinol. Jpn.* **26:**147–157.

310. Frame, B., Hanson, C. A., Frost, H. M., Block, M., and Arnstein, A. R., 1972, Renal resistance to parathyroid hormone with osteitis fibrosa: "Pseudohypohyperparathyroidism," *Am. J. Med.* **52:**311–321.

311. Duck, S. C., Rosenberg, E. M., Ratzan, S. K., and Haymond, M. W., 1978, Renal-resistant hormonoplethoric hypoparathyroidism with evidence for a defective response to cAMP, *J. Clin. Endocrinol. Metab.* **47:**640–646.

312. Metz, S. A., Baylink, D. J., Hughes, M. R., Haussler, M. R., and Robertson, R. P., 1977, Selective deficiency of 1,25-dihydroxycholecalciferol: A case of isolated skeletal resistance to parathyroid hormone, *N. Engl. J. Med.* **297:**1084–1090.

313. Parfitt, A. M., 1978, Tubular reabsorption of calcium in pseudohypoparathyroidism, in: *Endocrinology of Calcium Metabolism* (D. H. Copp and R. V. Talmage, eds.), p. 409, Excerpta Medica, Amsterdam.

314. Potts, J. T., Jr., 1979, Pseudohypoparathyroidism, in: *Endocrinology* (L. T. DeGroot, G. F. Cahill, Jr., W. D. Odell, L. Martin, J. T. Potts, Jr., D. H. Nelson, E. Steinberger, and A. I. Winegrad, eds.), pp. 769–776, Grune & Stratton, New York.

315. Eisenberg, E., 1965, Effect of serum calcium level and parathyroid extract on phosphate and calcium excretion in hypoparathyroid patients, *J. Clin. Invest.* **44:**942–946.

316. Breslau, N., and Moses, A., 1977, Studies on renal calcium reabsorption in patients with pseudo- and pseudopseudohypoparathyroidism, Endocrine Society Meeting, Chicago.

317. Baran, D. T., Klahr, S., Slatopolsky, E., and Avioli, L. V., 1979, Effect of acetazolamide on calcium and phosphate metabolism in type I pseudo-

hypoparathyroidism: Interaction with parathyroid hormone, *J. Clin. Endocrinol. Metab.* **48:**766–770.

318. Lawayin, S., Norman, D. A., Zerwekh, J. E., Breslau, N. A., and Pak, C. Y. C., 1979. A patient with pseudohypoparathyroidism with increased serum calcium and 1α,25-dihydroxyvitamin D after exogenous parathyroid hormone administration, *J. Clin. Endocrinol. Metab.* **49:**783–786.

319. Carlson, H. E., Brickman, A. S., and Bottazzo, G. F., 1977, Prolactin deficiency in pseudohypoparathyroidism, *N. Engl. J. Med.* **296:**140–144.

320. Wolfsdorf, J. T., Rosenfield, R. L., Fang, V. S., Kobayashi, R., Razdan, A. K., and Kim, M. H., 1978, Partial gonadotrophin resistance in pseudohypoparathyroidism, *Acta Endocrinol. (Copenhagen)* **88:**321–328.

321. Parfitt, A. M., 1978, Adult hypoparathyroidism treatment with calcifediol, *Arch. Intern. Med.* **138:**874–881.

322. Kind, H. P., Handysides, A., Kooh, S. W., and Fraser, D., 1977, Vitamin D therapy in hypoparathyroidism and pseudohypoparathyroidism: Weight-related dosages for initiation of therapy and maintenance therapy, *J. Pediatr.* **91:**1006–1010.

323. Porter, R. H., Cox, B. G., Heaney, D., Hostetter, T. H., Stinebaugh, B. J., and Suki, W. N., 1978, Treatment of hypoparathyroid patients with chlorthalidone, *N. Engl. J. Med.* **298:**577–581.

324. Copp, D. H., 1979, Calcitonin: Comparative endocrinology, in: *Endocrinology*, Volume 2 (L. J. DeGroot, G. F. Cahill, Jr., W. D. Odell, L. Martin, J. T. Potts, Jr., D. H. Nelson, E. Steinberger, and A. I. Winegrad, eds.), pp. 637–640, Grune & Stratton, New York.

325. Fontaine, J., 1979, Multistep migration of calcitonin cell precursors during ontogeny of the mouse pharynx, *Gen. Comp. Endocrinol.* **37:**81–92.

326. Kameda, Y., 1971, The occurrence and distribution of the parafollicular cells in the thyroid, parathyroid -IV and thymus -IV in some mammals, *Arch. Histol. Jpn.* **33:**283–299.

327. Galante, L., Gudmundsson, T. V., Matthews, E. W., Tse, A., Williams, E. D., Woodhouse, N. J. Y., and MacIntyre, I., 1968, Thymic and parathyroid origin of calcitonin in man, *Lancet* **2:**537–538.

328. Silva, O. L., Wisneski, L. A., Cyrus, J., Snider, R. H., Moore, C. F., and Becker, K. L., 1978, Calcitonin in thyroidectomized patients, *Am. J. Med. Sci.* **275:**159–164.

329. Merle, M., Lefevre, G., and Milhaud, G., 1979, Predicted secondary structure of calcitonin in relation to the biological activity, *Biochem. Biophys. Res. Commun.* **87:**455–460.

330. Heath, H., III, and Sizemore, G. W., 1979, Immunochemical heterogeneity of calcitonin in tumor, tumor venous effluent, and peripheral blood of patients with medullary thyroid carcinoma, *J. Lab. Clin. Med.* **93:**390–401.

331. Pont, A., 1979, Secretion and metabolism of calcitonin in man, in: *Endocrinology*, Volume 2 (L. J. DeGroot, G. F. Cahill, Jr., W. D. Odell, L. Martin, J. T. Potts, Jr., D. H. Nelson, E. Steinberger, and A. I. Winegrad, eds.), pp. 641–645, Grune & Stratton, New York.

332. Baylin, S. E., Bailey, A. J., Hsu, T.-H., and Foster, G. V., 1977, Degradation of human calcitonin in human plasma, *Metabolism* **26:**1345–1354.

333. Parthemore, J. G., and Deftos, L. G., 1975, The regulation of calcitonin in normal human plasma as assessed by immunoprecipitation and immunoextraction, *J. Clin. Invest.* **56**:835–841.

334. Heath, H., III, and Sizemore, G. W., 1977, Plasma calcitonin in normal man, *J. Clin. Invest.* **60**:1135–1140.

335. Hillyard, C. J., Cooke, T. J. C., Coombes, R. C., Evans, I. M. A., and MacIntyre, I., 1977, Normal plasma calcitonin: Circadian variation and response to stimuli, *Clin. Endocrinol.* **6**:291–298.

336. Deftos, L. J., and O'Riordan, J. L. H., 1978, Problems in radioassays of the calcitropic hormones, in: *Endocrinology of Calcium Metabolism* (D. H. Copp and R. V. Talmage, eds.), pp. 345–348, Excerpta Medica, Amsterdam.

337. Becker, K. L., Bivins, L. E., Radfor, R. H., Snider, R. H., Moore, C. F., and Silva, O. L., 1978, Study of calcitonin heterogeneity using a radioreceptor assay, *Horm. Metab. Res.* **10**:457–458.

338. Loreau, N., Lajotte, C., Wahbe, F., and Ardaillou, R., 1978, Effects of guanyl nucleotides on calcitonin-sensitive adenylate cyclase and calcitonin binding in rat renal cortex, *J. Endocrinol.* **76**:533–545.

339. Hillyard, C. J., Stevenson, J. C., and MacIntyre, I., 1978, Relative deficiency of plasma calcitonin in normal women, *Lancet* **1**:961–962.

340. Mulder, H., Hackeng, W. H. L., and Silberbusch, J., 1979, Racial difference in serum calcitonin, *Lancet* **2**:154.

341. Vora, N. M., Williams, G. A., Hargis, G. K., Bowser, E. N., Kawahara, W., Jackson, B. L., Henderson, W. J., and Kukreja, S. C., 1978, Comparative effect of calcium and of the adrenergic system on calcitonin secretion in man, *J. Clin. Endocrinol. Metab.* **46**:567–571.

342. Austin, L. A., Heath, H., III, and Go, V. L. W., 1979, Regulation of calcitonin secretion in normal man by changes of serum calcium within the physiologic range, *J. Clin. Invest.* **64**:1721–1724.

343. Sizemore, G. W., Go, V. L. W., Kaplan, E. L., Sanzenbacher, L. J., Holtermuller, K. H., and Arnaud, C. D., 1973, Relations of calcitonin and gastrin in the Zollinger–Ellison syndrome and medullary carcinoma of the thyroid, *N. Engl. J. Med.* **288**:641–644.

344. Owyang, C., Heath, H., III, Sizemore, G. W., and Go, V. L. W., 1978, Comparison of the effects of pentagastrin and meal-stimulated gastrin on plasma calcitonin in normal man, *Dig. Dis.* **23**:1084–1088.

345. Van Noorden, S., Polak, J. M., and Pearse, A. G., 1977, Single cellular origin of somatostatin and calcitonin in the rat thyroid gland, *Histochemistry* **53**:243–247.

346. Buffa, R., Chayvialle, J. A., Fontana, P., Uselli, L., Capella, C., and Solcia, E., 1979, Parafollicular cells of rabbit thyroid store both calcitonin and somatostatin and resemble gut D cells ultrastructurally, *Histochemistry* **62**:281–288.

347. Capella, C., Bordi, C., Monga, G., Buffa, R., Fontana, P., Bonfanti, S., Bussolati, G., and Solcia, E., 1978, Multiple endocrine cell types in thyroid medullary carcinoma, *Virchows Arch. A* **377**:111–128.

348. Linehan, W. M., Cooper, C. W., Bolman, R. M., III, and Wells, S. A., Jr., 1979, Inhibition of in vivo secretion of calcitonin in the pig by somatostatin and calcitonin in the rat thyroid gland, *Histochemistry* **53**:243–247.

349. Hargis, G. K., Williams, G. A., Reynolds, W. A., Chertow, B. S., Kukreja, S. C., Bowser, E. N., and Henderson, W. J., 1978, Effect of somatostatin on parathyroid hormone and calcitonin secretion, *Endocrinology* **102**:745–750.

350. Gordin, A., Lamberg, B.-A., Pelkonen, R., and Almquist, S., 1978, Somatostatin inhibits the pentagastrin-induced release of serum calcitonin in medullary carcinoma of the thyroid, *Clin. Endocrinol.* **8**:289–293.

351. Peng, T-C., Cooper, C. W., Garner, S. C., and Bolpert, E. M., 1978, Hypercalcitoninism and C-cell hyperplasia in rats with goiters produced by a low iodine diet or propylthiouracil, *J. Pharmacol. Exp. Ther.* **206**:710–717.

352. Didoklar, M. S., and Moore, G. E., 1974, Hormone-dependent medullary carcinoma of the thyroid, *Am. J. Surg.* **128**:100–102.

353. Wells, S. A., Cooper, C. W., and Ontjos, D. A., 1975, Stimulation of thyrocalcitonin secretion by ethanol in patients with medullary thyroid carcinoma—an effect apparently not mediated by gastrin, *Metabolism* **24**:1215–1219.

354. Kanis, J. A., Adams, N. D., Cecchettin, M., Luizetto, G., Gaspar, S., and Heymen, G., 1979, Ethanol induced secretion of calcitonin in chronic renal disease, *Clin. Endocrinol.* **10**:155–161.

355. Baylin, S. B., Hsu, T.-H., Stevens, S. A., Kallman, C. H., Trump, D. L., and Beaven, M. A., 1979, The effects of L-dopa on in vitro and in vivo calcitonin release from medullary carcinoma of the thyroid, *J. Clin. Endocrinol. Metab.* **48**:408–414.

356. Cooper, C. W., Ramp, W. K., Becker, D. I., and Ontjes, D. A., 1977, In vitro secretion of immunoreactive rat thyrocalcitonin, *Endocrinology* **101**:304–311.

357. Vora, N. M., Williams, G. A., Hargis, G. K., Bowser, E. N., Kawahara, W., Jackson, B. L., Henderson, W. J., and Kukrega, S. C., 1978, Comparative effect of calcium and of the adrenergic system on calcitonin secretion in man, *J. Clin. Endocrinol. Metab.* **46**:567–571.

358. Milhaud, G., Rankin, J. C., Bolis, L., and Benson, A. A., 1977, Calcitonin: Its hormonal action on the gill, *Proc. Natl. Acad. Sci. USA* **74**:4693–4696.

359. Sasayama, Y., 1978, Effects of implantation of the ultimobranchial glands and the administration of synthetic salmon calcitonin on serum Ca concentrations in ultimobranchialectomized bullfrog tadpoles, *Gen. Comp. Endocrinol.* **34**:229–233.

360. Kalu, D. N., 1978, Acute effect of calcitonin deficiency on plasma calcium in fasted young rats, *Horm. Metab. Res.* **10**:72–75.

361. Robertson, R. P., and Baylink, D. J., 1977, Hypercalcemia induced by prostaglandin E_2 in thyroparathyroidectomized but not intact rats, *Prostaglandins* **13**:1141–1145.

362. Kalu, D. N., 1977, Acute and longterm effects of thyroidectomy on plasma calcium in rats, *Endocrinology* **101**:1665–1669.

363. Grubb, S. A., Markham, T. C., and Talmage, R. V., 1977, Effect of salmon

calcitonin infusion on plasma concentrations of recently administered ^{45}Ca, *Calcif. Tissue Res.* **24:**201–208.

364. Norimatsu, H., Vander Wiel, C. J., and Talmage, R. V., 1979, Electron microscopic study of the effects of calcitonin on bone cells and their extracellular milieu, *Clin. Orthop. Relat. Res.* **139:**250–258.

365. Cutler, G. B., Jr., Habener, J. F., and Potts, J. T., Jr., 1977, Biosynthesis and secretion of calcitonin by avian ultimobranchial glands, *Endocrinology* **100:**537–548.

366. Jowsey, J., Riggs, B. L., Kelly, P. J., and Hoffman, D. L., 1978, Calcium and salmon calcitonin in treatment of osteoporosis, *J. Clin. Endocrinol. Metab.* **47:**633–639.

367. Lambert, P. W., Heath, H., III, and Sizemore, G. W., 1979, Pre- and postoperative studies of plasma calcitonin in primary hyperparathyroidism, *J. Clin. Invest.* **63:**602–608.

368. Talmage, R. V., Doppelt, S. H., and Cooper, C. W., 1975, Relationship of blood concentrations of calcium, phosphate, gastrin and calcitonin to the onset of feeding in the rat, *Proc. Soc. Exp. Biol. Med.* **149:**855–859.

369. Talmage, R. V., Vander Wiel, C. J., Decker, S. A., and Grubb, S. A., 1979, Changes produced in postprandial urinary calcium excretion by thyroidectomy and calcitonin administration in rats on different calcium regimens, *Endocrinology* **105:**459–464.

370. Cooper, C. W., Obie, J. F., Toverud, S. U., and Munson, P. L., 1977, Elevated serum calcitonin and serum calcium during suckling in the baby rat, *Endocrinology* **101:**1657–1664.

371. Parthemore, J. G., and Deftos, L. J., 1979, Calcitonin secretion in primary hyperparathyroidism, *J. Clin. Endocrinol. Metab.* **49:**223–226.

372. Shamonki, I. M., Frumar, A. M., Tataryn, J. V., Meldrum, D. R., Davidson, B. H., Parthemore, J. G., Judd, H. L., and Deftos, L. J., 1980, Age-related changes of calcitonin secretion in females, *J. Clin. Endocrinol. Metab.* **50:**437–439.

373. Milhaud, G., Benezich-Lefevre, M., and Mouktar, M. S., 1978, Deficiency of calcitonin in age-related osteoporosis, *Biomed. Exp.* **29:**272–276.

374. Samaan, N. A., Anderson, G. D., and Adam-Mayne, M. E., 1975, Immunoreactive calcitonin in the mother, neonate, child and adult, *Am. J. Obstet. Gynecol.* **121:**622–625.

375. Freed, W. J., Perlow, M. J., and Wyatt, R. J., 1979, Calcitonin: Inhibitory effect on eating in rats, *Science* **206:**850–852.

376. Bolman, R. M., III, Cooper, C. W., Garner, S. C., Munson, P. L., and Wells, S. A., Jr., 1977, Stimulation of gastrin secretion in the pig by parathyroid hormone and its inhibition by thyrocalcitonin, *Endocrinology* **100:**1014–1021.

377. Ito, H., Sakurada, T., and Orimo, H., 1977, Role of endogenous calcitonin in the secretion of gastrin and gastric acid in rats, *Horm. Metab. Res.* **9:**89–92.

378. Cantalamessa, L., Catania, A., Reschini, E., and Peracchi, M., 1978, Inhibitory effect of calcitonin on growth hormone and insulin secretion in man, *Metabolism* **27:**987–992.

379. Walling, M. W., Brasitus, T. A., and Kimberg, D. V., 1977, Effects of

calcitonin and substance P on the transport of Ca, Na, and Cl across rat ileum in vitro, *Gastroenterology* **73**:89–94.

380. Gray, T. K., Brannan, P., Juan, D., Morawski, S. G., and Fordtran, J. S., 1976, Ion transport changes during calcitonin-induced intestinal secretion in man, *Gastroenterology* **71**:392–398.

381. Kisloff, B., and Moore, E. W., 1977, Effects of intravenous calcitonin on water, electrolyte, and calcium movement across in vivo rabbit jejunum and ileum, *Gastroenterology* **72**:462–468.

382. Clark, M. B., Boyd, G. W., Byfield, P. G. H., and Foster, G. V., 1969, A radioimmunoassay for human calcitonin, *Lancet* **2**:74–77.

383. Goltzman, D., Potts, J. T., Jr., Ridgway, E. C., and Maloof, F., 1974, Calcitonin as a tumor marker, *N. Engl. J. Med.* **290**:1035–1039.

384. Becker, K. L., Snider, R. H., Silva, O. L., and Moore, C. F., 1978, Calcitonin heterogeneity in lung cancer and medullary thyroid cancer, *Acta Endocrinol. (Copenhagen)* **89**:89–99.

385. Galmiche, J. P., Colin, R., DuBois, P. M., Chayvialle, J. A., Descos, F., Paulin, C., and Geffroy, Y., 1978, Calcitonin secretion by a pancreatic somatostatinoma, *N. Engl. J. Med.* **299**:1252.

386. Kalager, T., Gluck, E., Heimann, P., and Myking, O., 1977, Pheochromocytoma with ectopic calcitonin production and parathyroid cyst, *Br. Med. J.* **2**:21.

387. Dayal, Y., Tashjian, A. H., and Wolfe, H. J., 1979, Immunocytochemical localization of calcitonin-producing cells in a stromal carcinoid with amyloid stroma, *Cancer* **43**:1331–1338.

388. Rousseau, J. J., Franck, G., Grisar, T., Reznik, M., Heynen, G., and Salmon, J., 1978, Osteosclerotic myeloma with polyneuropathy and ectopic secretion of calcitonin, *Eur. J. Cancer* **14**:133–140.

389. White, M. C., and Hickson, B. R., 1979, Multiple paragangliomata secreting catecholamines and calcitonin with intermittent hypercalcemia, *J. R. Soc. Med.* **72**:532–538.

390. Silva, O. L., Becker, K. L., Primack, A., Doppman, J., and Snider, R. H., 1974, Ectopic secretion of calcitonin by oat-cell carcinoma, *N. Engl. J. Med.* **290**:1122–1124.

391. Hansen, M., Hansen, H. H., and Tryding, N., 1978, Small cell carcinoma of the lung: Serum calcitonin and serum histaminase (diamine oxidase) at basal levels and stimulated by pentagastrin, *Acta Med. Scand.* **204**:257–261.

392. Hansen, M., Rehfeld, J. F., and Stadil, F., 1979, Small cell carcinoma of the lung: Relation of calcitonin to bone marrow metastases, parathormone and gastrin, *Acta Med. Scand.* **206**:215–218.

393. Silva, O. L., Broder, L. E., Doppman, J. L., Snider, R. H., Moore, C. F., Cohen, M. H., and Becker, K. L., 1979, Calcitonin in non thyroidal cancer, *J. Clin. Endocrinol. Metab.* **49**:438–444.

394. Silva, O. L., Broder, L. E., Doppman, J. L., Snider, R. H., Moore, C. F., Cohen, M. H., and Becker, K. L., 1979, Calcitonin as a marker for bronchogenic carcinoma, *Cancer* **44**:680–684.

395. Baylin, S. B., Weisburger, W. R., Eggleston, J. C., Mendelsohn, G., Beaven,

M. A., Abeloff, M. D., and Ettinger, D. S., 1978, Variable content of histaminase, L-dopa decarboxylase and calcitonin in small-cell carcinoma of
the lung, *N. Engl. J. Med.* **299:**105–110.

396. Martin, T. J., 1979, Treatment of Paget's disease with the calcitonins, *Aust.
N.Z. J. Med.* **9:**36–43.

397. Wooton, R., Reeve, J., Spellacy, E., and Tellez-Yudilevich, M., 1978, Skeletal blood flow in Paget's disease and its response to calcitonin therapy,
Clin. Sci. Mol. Med. **54:**69–74.

398. Henley, J. W., Croxson, R. S., and Ibbertson, H. K., 1979, The cardiovascular system in Paget's disease of bone and the response to therapy with
calcitonin and diphosphonate, *Aust. N.Z. J. Med.* **9:**390–397.

399. Hosking, D. J., Denton, L. B., Cadge, B., and Martin, T. J., 1979, Functional
significance of antibody formation after long-term salmon calcitonin therapy, *Clin. Endocrinol.* **10:**243–252.

400. Rojanasathit, S., Rosenberg, E., and Haddad, J. G., Jr., 1974, Paget's bone
disease: Response to human calcitonin in patients resistant to salmon calcitonin, *Lancet* **2:**1412–1415.

401. Nilsson, O., Almqvist, S., and Karlberg, B. E., 1978, Salmon calcitonin in
the acute treatment of moderate and severe hypercalcemia in man, *Acta
Med. Scand.* **204:**249–252.

Ectopic Hormone Syndromes

Louis M. Sherwood

8.1. Etiology and Mechanisms of Ectopic Hormone Production

While enormous progress has been made in recognizing the production of hormones by tumors, the pathogenesis of this phenomenon still remains obscure.[1] Inherent in a complete understanding of the mechanisms is a fuller appreciation of the processes of normal cell proliferation, maturation, and differentiation. Any hypothesis satisfactory to explain the process must account for the following observations:

1. Polypeptide hormone production is extremely widespread in both normal tissues and tumors. [1-4]
2. There are distinct histologic associations between tumor type and the nature of the hormone produced (see Table I).
3. Biosynthesis of hormones by tumors appears not to be the expression or activation of abnormal genes but of known genes for recognized polypeptide hormones or their precursors.

In considering pathogenesis, the following concepts must be considered:

1. The suggestion that nonendocrine tumors that synthesize hormones do so because their cells have amine precursor uptake and de-

LOUIS M. SHERWOOD • Department of Medicine, Albert Einstein College of Medicine, Bronx, New York 10461.

Table I.   Relationship of Tumor Type to Hormone Production

Hormone	Tumor type
ACTH and lipotropin (β-MSH, endorphin, and enkephalin)	Oat-cell carcinoma of the lung
	Thymoma
	Islet-cell tumor
	Bronchial carcinoid
	Also ovarian tumors, pheochromocytoma, gastrointestinal, prostate, neurogenic, and parotid tumors, and medullary thyroid carcinoma
	Inactive "big" ACTH in a wide variety of tumors
Growth hormone-releasing hormone	Bronchial carcinoid, pancreatic carcinoid
Human placental lactogen	Undifferentiated carcinoma of the lung
	Hepatoma
	Lymphoma
	Pheochromocytoma
Prolactin (rare)	Renal-cell carcinoma
	Undifferentiated carcinoma of the lung
	Breast carcinoma
Thyrotropin	Choriocarcinoma, hydatidiform mole
	Epidermoid carcinoma of the lung
	Mesothelioma
Gonadotropin	Choriocarcinoma of male and female, other testicular tumors; hydatidiform mole
	Hepatoblastoma, pancreatic, other gastrointestinal tumors
	Adenocarcinoma and other carcinomas of the lung
	Islet-cell tumors (malignant)
	Breast carcinoma
	Melanoma
	Normal tissues (liver and colon)
hCG β subunit	Adenocarcinoma of the pancreas
	Islet-cell tumors (malignant)
hCG α subunit	Carcinoid
	Islet-cell tumors (malignant)
Vasopressin	Oat-cell carcinoma of the lung
	Pancreatic adenocarcinoma
Calcium-mobilizing peptide hormones	Epidermoid carcinoma of the lung
	Renal-cell carcinoma
	Hepatoma, pancreatic, and gastrointestinal carcinoma
	Other epidermoid tumors
	Lymphoma
Prostaglandin E_2	Renal-cell carcinoma
	Lung tumors

Table I. (Continued)

Hormone	Tumor type
Osteoclast-activating factor	Multiple myeloma
	Burkitt's and other lymphomas
Calcitonin	Oat-cell carcinoma of the lung
	Breast, pancreatic, and other carcinomas
Somatomedin (NSILA, IbF)	Mesodermal and mesenchymal tumors
	Adrenal carcinoma
Glucagon	Nonbeta islet-cell tumors
	Undifferentiated lung cancer
Gastrin	Nonbeta islet-cell tumor
	Duodenal wall carcinoma
	Ovarian carcinoma
Vasoactive intestinal peptide	Nonbeta islet-cell tumor
	Carcinoma of the lung
	Pheochromocytoma and
	ganglioneuroblastoma
Erythropoietin	Renal-cell carcinoma
	Cerebellar hemangioblastoma
	Pheochromocytoma
	Hepatoma
	Uterine fibroids
Renin	Juxtaglomerular tumor
	Wilms's tumor
	Renal-cell carcinoma
Serotonin and 5-hydroxytryptophan	Nonbeta islet-cell tumor
	Oat-cell carcinoma of the lung
	Carcinoid (also growth hormone-
	releasing activity)
	Pancreatic adenocarcinoma

carboxylation characteristics (APUD) explains only some cases. Similar histologic and ultrastructural characteristics in tumors such as small cell carcinoma of the lung and carcinoma of the pancreatic islet, adrenal medulla, argentaffin cells (carcinoid), and thyroid (medullary) fit this category. Although it was believed earlier that such cells could be derived only from the neural crest, it now appears that cells of endodermal tissues, by mechanisms poorly understood, may develop the distinct structural and biochemical characteristics of APUD cells and produce hormones of this type. (See Refs. 1, 5, and 6 for detailed analysis of the APUD hypothesis.)

2. Recent progress in molecular biology and in understanding the biosynthesis and processing of polypeptide hormones has been helpful in evaluating the pathogenesis of ectopic hormone syndromes. From a

consideration of the biosynthesis of proteins destined for secretion (both polypeptide hormones and other secreted peptides, such as albumin), it is apparent that the initial product of biosynthesis is a preprotein or prehormone that has a "leader" or "signal" sequence of hydrophobic amino acids at the N terminus, varying in length from 15 to 30 residues.[7] This prepeptide is necessary to allow transport of the newly synthesized hormone through the endoplasmic reticular membrane into the subcellular transport systems of the cell. During transport, the signal "sequence" is cleaved, perhaps even while the new peptide is still on the ribosome. In the biosynthesis of some hormones, such as parathyroid hormone, ACTH, insulin, glucagon, gastrin, and somatostatin, prehormone is converted to one or more prohormone precursors that are then modified to mature hormones in other parts of the cell (see Fig. 1). Specify cytoplasmic enzymes are necessary in the appropriate cellular location to carry out such posttranslational processing.[7] Furthermore, for the glycoprotein hormones, posttranslational glycosylation is an essential feature in the development of the mature hormone.

In analyzing the production of hormones by ectopic tumors, it is apparent that it consists of the biosynthesis of known polypeptides. There is no evidence as yet for abnormal gene activation or for the production by tumors of peptides not known to exist in normal endocrine glands.[6] These studies suggest, therefore, that the differences between peptide expression in endocrine glands and in some tumors may be differences

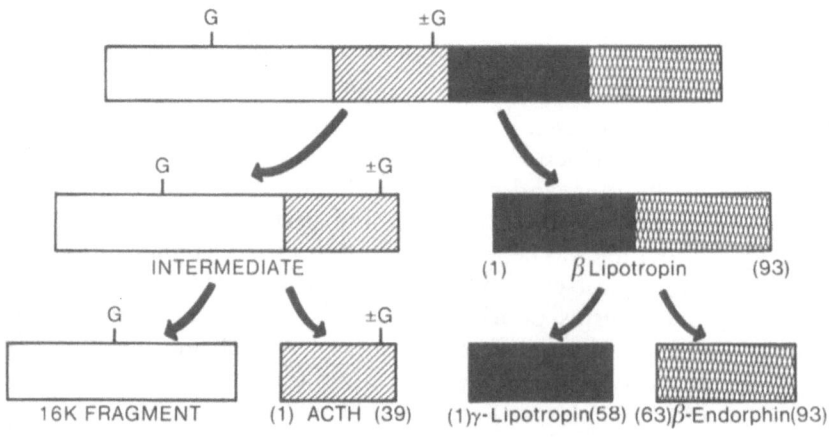

Fig. 1. Conversion of proACTH/endorphin 30K precursor to ACTH, lipotropins, and endorphin. G refers to glycosylation. Numbers refer to residues in peptide sequence. Function of 16K fragment is presently unknown. From Eipper and Mains (1980).

in posttranslational processing,[8] rather than differences in synthesis of the peptide hormone itself. The presence or absence of critical cytoplasmic enzymes or granules (as in APUD-type cells) may be the critical factor in determining whether normal processing takes place or not.

It has been traditional to suggest that derepression of DNA or dedifferentiation of cells in the course of malignancy may explain the production of hormones by tumors.[5] Although this hypothesis is very attractive, there is little or no experimental evidence to support it. Baylin and Mendelsohn[6] have proposed a new model for ectopic production of hormones by tumors; this is based on observations in medullary carcinoma of the thyroid, neuroblastoma, and small cell carcinoma. They suggest that hormone-producing cells result from altered differentiation or "dysdifferentiation" of cells, rather than the more commonly suggested mechanism of dedifferentiation or of derepression of DNA. The development of multipotential tumor cells would therefore be similar to that in the hemopoietic system, in which a primitive "stem cell" differentiates along multiple lines (e.g., producing erythrocytes, granulocytes, thrombocytes, or histiocytes) and sometimes leading to malignancy.[9] Primitive tumor cells are capable of both expressing fetal antigens or hormones and maturing to phenotypic cells that look like epithelial cells or hormone-producing cells, depending on their state of proliferation and maturation. Fetal cells have either the capacity to produce trophoblastic-type proteins, such as chorionic gonadotropin (hCG) or placental lactogen, or alternatively, the capacity to produce α-fetoprotein or carcinoembryonic antigen (the latter proteins being derived primarily from yolk sac epithelium). Cells with APUD characteristics need not be derived solely from the neural crest but could also arise from epithelial cells that differentiate along these lines. Since the production of various fetal proteins or placental hormones by tumors is not random, but rather a highly specific event in certain types of tumors, there is plausibility to this hypothesis. However, as the authors explain, it is a highly speculative model whose confirmation requires more data. Most embryologic models suggest that differentiation involves progressive specialization or irreversible suppression of DNA as developmental stages proceed. Baylin and Mendelsohn[6] support a forward-moving model in which there are different lines of development for primitive tumor cells, with factors in the local environment affecting development. Malignancy at each stage of differentiation would thus come from a clone of transformed tumor cells. Rather than being a "universal concomitant of neoplasia,"[10] production of peptide hormones and fetal antigens would be the result of progressive cell differentiation.

That the tumors represent a heterogeneous population of cells is supported by immunochemical and immunoperoxidase studies of tumor tissues, which show the presence of various tumor markers and hormones in different cells within the same tumor.[11,12] The development of APUD characteristics may be one of only several directions open to immature and as yet uncommitted epithelial cells. The production of onco-placental proteins and hormones by tumors is not random. Gonadal tumors are most likely to produce such hormones, particularly when there are trophoblastic elements.[13,14] Perturbations of endodermal epithelial cell surfaces by either benign or neoplastic processes may increase the level of differentiation and result in production of specific hormones. The appearance of distinct proteins and antigens implies a certain stage of differentiation, not necessarily dedifferentiation. Antigens expressed by the yolk sac, primitive liver, and gastrointestinal tract include α-fetoprotein and carcinoembryonic antigen. Germ cell tumors are often heterogeneous, and the antigens or hormones they express are determined by their histologic type.

It was believed previously that the K or Kultschitzky cell led to small cell carcinoma of the lung, but this is now less clear.[6,15] Small cell carcinoma of the lung may not differ from epidermoid carcinoma in origin. It is also the lung tumor that is most likely to produce ectopic hormones, and there may be heterogeneity of cells, even in the small cell tumor.[16] It is usually an advanced tumor when first diagnosed, but is characterized by variability and heterogeneity. The content of histaminase and calcitonin (CT) in small cell carcinoma is greater than in normal lung. Dopa-decarboxylase is also generally high, but there is much variability. These differences are quantitative, not qualitative. In medullary carcinoma, CT, dopa-decarboxylase, and histaminase are usually found, whereas in C-cell hyperplasia, histaminase is not usually present.[11] These findings are similar to those of Kahn *et al.*[17] who found that expression of hCG or its subunits by a pancreatic neoplasm indicated that it was malignant rather than benign.

Brown[18] has recently reviewed mechanisms currently thought to be operative in gene expression of eukaryotic organisms. These mechanisms involve both those in which the genes themselves are altered by diminution, amplification, rearrangement, or modification and those in which there is a change or modulation in gene expression through control mechanisms during transcription, posttranscription, or translation. The exact relationship of genetic control mechanisms to expression of hormones by tumor cells is probably extraordinarily important. Future studies should clarify the precise ways in which tumor cells are altered at various control sites so that variations in gene expression can be documented in these disorders.

8.2. Recent Developments in Specific Hormone Syndromes

8.2.1. Ectopic Production of Corticotropin

There has been considerable growth in our understanding of the pathogenesis of this disorder, in part through the progress that has been made in the molecular biology and biochemistry of ACTH and related peptides. There is new and convincing evidence that ACTH is synthesized through a higher-molecular-weight precursor known as proopiomelanocortin (POMC), which is glycosylated and contains the sequences of ACTH and the β- and γ-lipotropins[8] (see Fig. 1). The sequence of β-lipotropin (91 residues) includes the structure of γ-lipotropin (1–58), β-endorphin (61–91), and the enkephalins.

The data supporting the structure of the ACTH and lipotropin gene and precursor come from two major sources. One approach used radioactive amino acid incorporation to show that animal or human pituitary cells in tissue culture synthesized higher-molecular-weight forms of ACTH.[8,19] Several forms of ACTH-related peptides were detected within cells and medium, and other studies showed that higher-molecular-weight forms could be converted to ACTH by trypsin-like enzymes. A precursor–product relationship could not be demonstrated on the base of size and structural data alone, and it was therefore necessary to show in radioactive pulse–chase experiments that the higher-molecular-weight precursor was converted to the smaller forms. The incorporation studies in cells were supported by work with ACTH mRNA in cell-free systems, which demonstrated the existence of a 29K precursor.[20] A second major approach by Nakanishi et al.[21] involved determination of the structure of cloned cDNA for bovine ACTH–lipotropin that includes the codons for the above peptides (see Fig. 1). In addition, there is a 16K peptide N-terminal to the ACTH sequence whose function has not yet been determined. This 16K region is preceded by the "signal" sequence for the prePOMC molecule.[8] These studies have pointed definitively to the existence of a common precursor for the pituitary peptides of the ACTH family. These findings are of considerable importance in understanding both normal physiologic function of the pituitary as well as the pathogenesis of the ectopic ACTH syndrome.

In addition to data supporting a common precursor, there is also evidence that the metabolism of the precursor may vary in different tissues.[3,22,23] For example, it appears that the normal pituitary can process POMC to make ACTH, β-lipotropin, and β-endorphin.[8] This is supported by the fact that levels of ACTH, lipotropin, and endorphin are elevated in patients with Addison's disease and Nelson's syndrome.

In the pars intermedia of animal pituitary glands, a different type of cleavage takes place in which α-MSH and corticotropin-like intermediate peptide (CLIP) are produced. Various permutations of posttranslational processing are possible, depending on the tissue in which the precursor is present and presumably the presence of different enzymes, sites of processing, or secretory granules in which processing can take place. Although the precursor protein in various tissues could theoretically vary, there is no evidence for this. There has been no evidence for activation of abnormal genes or the production of peptides not known to be synthesized in normal tissues. More likely is variable metabolism in different tissues and tumors.

Earlier studies by Gewirtz and Yalow,[24] and subsequently by Odell *et al.*,[25] indicated that ACTH was present by radioimmunoassay in many tumors of patients who did not have clinical Cushing's syndrome. Furthermore, these studies suggested that the form of ACTH that might be synthesized and released was higher in molecular weight than 39-amino-acid ACTH and could be converted to ACTH by trypsin. Furthermore, this material had little or no biologic activity and was presumably an ACTH precursor. Wolfsen and Odell[26] have examined both plasma and extracts of lung cancer for the presence of proACTH by column chromatography and radioimmunoassay. In 100 patients who were admitted with abnormal chest X rays, 53 of 74 with lung cancer had increased plasma ACTH. The remaining 26 patients had benign disease and normal plasma ACTH. In evaluating 101 patients with chronic obstructive lung disease, 5 of 20 with increased ACTH and only 2 of 81 with normal ACTH developed lung cancer within 2 years. The mean level of ACTH in the patients with cancer was 131.8, compared with 52.5 pg/ml in normal subjects. Of the 74% of patients with cancer who exceeded the normal level, all had values about 107 pg/ml (mean plus 2 S.D.). The patients with benign lung disease had a mean level of 55. Immunoreactive ACTH was increased in the serum of patients with lung cancer and tumors of other organs, including the colon, breast, kidney, and pancreas, although concentrations by radioreceptor assay were within the normal range. This immunoreactive ACTH was believed to be a precursor form of ACTH since it eluted in the void volume of Sephadex G-50 and did not react in the receptor assay. In normal subjects, plasma values for ACTH by radioimmunoassay and radioreceptor assay were equivalent. Radiation therapy and chemotherapy lowered plasma ACTH in patients with lung cancer (values falling from a mean of 131.8 initially to 87.0 pg/ml in treated patients).

When tumor extracts were assayed, 38 lung cancer specimens each contained more than 1 ng/g of ACTH-like immunoreactivity, most containing more than 5 ng. Normal lung at postmortem from patients who died without cancer contained less than 2 ng/g. Chromatography of tissue extracts showed that more than 50% of the ACTH immunoreactivity was in the void volume, with little or no immunoreactivity in the area of elution of ACTH[1-39]. The molecular weight of the proACTH in these studies was 20K or greater.[26]

There have been recent reports of interesting and unusual cases of the ectopic ACTH syndrome. Hashimoto et al.[27] described a 5-year-old girl in whom a nephroblastoma produced ACTH, β-LPH, β-endorphin, and corticotropin-releasing hormone activity. The tumor contained 505 ng/g wet wt immunoreactive ACTH and 85 ng/g biologically active ACTH. Corticotropin-releasing activity was demonstrated in tumor extracts using pituitary cell cultures and was equivalent to 0.83 ng equivalent/mg wet wt. In this patient, slight responses of plasma ACTH and urinary 17-hydroxysteroids to metyrapone were observed; the responsiveness could have been due to preservation of the hypothalamic–pituitary–adrenal axis or to the response of the tumors to metyrapone. Pituitary–adrenal function returned to normal within 1 month after removal of the tumor.

Gomi et al.[28] described two patients who had a combination of ectopic ACTH and amylase production. The latter was reflected in zymogen granules present in the tumor. These cases raised interesting questions about possible relationships between neurosecretory-type granules and zymogen granules, not previously known to be associated. Chin[29] described an interesting patient with a lateral neck mass and Cushing's syndrome who had ectopic ACTH production. The mRNA extracted directly from the tumor directed the translation of a precursor of CT in a cell-free system, leading to the ultimate diagnosis of medullary carcinoma of the thyroid. Thus, the techniques of molecular biology were used to identify the tumor type. Although the authors were looking for the translation of an ACTH precursor from the tumor tissue, they found a dominant protein of 15K that was immunoprecipitated by antibodies to human CT. They also identified a small amount of higher-molecular-weight precursor to ACTH. Extraction of the tissue showed high levels of ACTH and CT by radioimmunoassay, and thus several criteria for ectopic hormone production, including in vitro biosynthesis, were fulfilled. The tumor was also positive for carcinoembryonic antigen.

Matsuyama et al.[30] reported an argyrophil cell carcinoma of the uterine cervix that produced ACTH, LPH, serotonin, histamine, and amylase. Several patients with ACTH secretion from pheochromocytoma have also been described.[31-34] In one case, episodes of secretion of ACTH and catecholamines followed each other. Review of the literature of ACTH production by pheochromocytoma by Forman et al.[32] revealed a mortality of over 50% in these patients, and it was suggested that all patients with ectopic ACTH or with Cushing's syndrome be screened for cathecholamine production. ACTH secretion was also described from carcinoma of the breast[35] and prostate,[36] from carcinoid in a child with multiple endocrine neoplasia,[37] and from pulmonary tumorlets (small peripheral nodules in the lung field that bear an uncertain relationship to the bronchial carcinoid[38]). In a patient with medullary carcinoma of the thyroid and ectopic ACTH production described by Rosenberg et al.,[39] senile osteoporosis was the presenting manifestation, and the course was more chronic and indolent than in most other reports of the syndrome. Drasin et al.[40] described a patient with mediastinal lipomatosis masquerading as a mediastinal tumor in a patient with ectopic ACTH production due to bronchial carcinoid. Although the latter has been well described in Cushing's syndrome, it has not previously been reported in the ectopic ACTH syndrome.

Findling et al.[41] emphasized the use of selective venous sampling for ACTH in differentiating Cushing's disease from the ectopic ACTH syndrome. They performed selective venous catheterization and sampling for ACTH in six patients with Cushing's disease and four patients with ectopic tumors. In five patients with the former, in whom the inferior petrosal sinus could be catheterized, ACTH was higher than in peripheral blood, the ratio varying from 2.2 to 16.7. In three patients with the ectopic ACTH syndrome, the ratio was less than 1.5. Ratios obtained at the level of the jugular bulbar vein were not diagnostic, and blood from the inferior petrosal sinus was felt to be much more reliable. In a fourth patient, an arteriovenous gradient of 6.8 across the pulmonary circulation was found in a patient with a bronchial carcinoid tumor. In a review by Singer et al.[42] of 164 autopsies of patients with bronchogenic carcinoma, ten were found who had had pathologic evidence of the ectopic ACTH syndrome, all occurring in oat-cell carcinoma and constituting 19% of the group. The features identified at postmortem included hyperplasia of the adrenals (zona fasciculata) and Crooke's hyaline changes in the pituitary. The syndrome had been diagnosed antemortem in only four of the ten patients.

Gold[43] reviewed Cushing's syndrome and current views of differential diagnosis and treatment. Spontaneous remission[44] and intermittent disease[45] are important causes of confusion in differential diagnosis. Crapo[46] also reviewed the diagnostic tests in Cushing's syndrome and suggested that the overnight dexamethasone suppression test was the best screening test. He emphasized the importance of urinary free cortisol determinations and late evening plasma cortisol with the 2-mg daily test dose of dexamethasone. Luton et al.[47] and Cooper and Shucart[48] emphasized the value of ortho,para-DDD in the treatment of Cushing's disease, a method that is useful in patients with the ectopic ACTH syndrome, particularly in combination with aminoglutethimide and metyr-apone.[49]

8.2.2. Ectopic Production of Lipotropin

Odell et al.[25] found evidence of increased lipotropin in tumor extracts and in the serum of the same patients whose tumors produced ACTH. The frequency of its occurrence was not as great as that of ACTH,[26] but was significant nonetheless. Comparative statistics were as follows: In lung cancer, 72% of patients had increased plasma proACTH and 36% had increased LPH. In colon cancer, comparable values were 27 and 10% respectively, in pancreatic cancer 92 and 25%, in gastric or esophageal cancer 54 and 14%, and in breast cancer 41 and 0%. In 79 acetic acid extracts of carcinoma of the lung, colon, stomach, esophagus, and breast, LPH concentrations greater than those in blood were found in 61. LPH was also present in larger amounts than in control tissues from patients without cancer. Thus, LPH was frequently increased in the blood and tumor tissue of patients with various types of carcinoma and seemed a useful marker of ectopic production.

Jeffcoate et al.[50] developed a specific radioimmunoassay for human β-LPH. Animals were immunized with β-hLPH isolated from human pituitary glands, and the plasma for assay was extracted with ground glass. Normal levels of β-hLPH in the morning were 25 and in the evening 20 to 80 pg/nl. In normal subjects, there was a rise in secretion following the administration of metyrapone and a fall after dexamethasone; insulin-induced hypoglycemia increased values to 200 pg/ml. In patients with Cushing's disease, Nelson's syndrome, and the ectopic ACTH syndrome, there was excellent correlation between ACTH and β-hLPH, supporting the concept that they were cosecreted. The function of lipotropin has not yet been determined, although it has been suggested that β-hLPH is the precursor of β-endorphin. The potential role of β-hLPH in the control and awareness of pain, appetite, release of other hormones, and etiology of mental disorders has not yet been defined. There is great interest in the potential importance of the endorphin–enkephalin peptides in these areas.

Immunoperoxidase studies of β-endorphin in the human pituitary gland show a somewhat parallel distribution of β-LPH and ACTH immunoreactivity, although the peptides are not necessarily present in cells at the same time.[51] Previous studies using immunocytochemical techniques showed that ACTH and β-MSH were present within the same cells, but β-MSH is now known to be an artifact and part of β-LPH[1]. Guillemin et al.[52] showed that ACTH and β-endorphin in the rat were cosecreted by the pituitary. Tanaka et al.[53] also suggested that the enkephalin–endorphin peptides and ACTH were secreted in parallel during both physiologic and pathologic conditions. Studies by Deftos et al.[54] suggested that immunoreactive CT might be present within the anterior lobe of the rat pituitary gland and could be part of the 31K precursor molecule for ACTH and β-LPH, but this has not been confirmed. Mendelsohn et al.[51] were unable to demonstrate CT in normal human pituitary glands using conditions that demonstrated it in medullary carcinoma; they were also unable to find any evidence of immunoreactive β-LPH in medullary carcinoma of the thyroid. Xavier et al.[55] recently reported a small cell carcinoma of the lung that made both CT and ACTH, and there was evidence for separate biosynthetic precursors.

Ueda et al.[56] used antibodies against β-MSH and α-endorphin to evaluate extracts of human pituitaries and ectopic tumors producing ACTH. On gel filtration, β-LPH was identified by antibodies developed against both β-MSH and α-endorphin, while γ-LPH was identified only by antibodies to β-MSH. Gel filtration studies of extracts of five normal human pituitary glands showed both β- and γ-LPH peaks, but no peak of β-MSH. Gel filtration studies of seven ectopic ACTH-producing tumors showed both β-MSH and γ-LPH peaks, but a clear β-LPH peak was observed in only three tumor extracts. β-MSH comprised 3 to 55% of total immunoreactive β-LPH. Whether these studies show that β-MSH was actually present in some of the tumors has not yet been determined. Differing enzyme characteristics of tumors compared with normal tissues may have accounted for these findings. Whether these are physiologic effects or nonspecific effects due to protease activity remains to be determined.

It appears that β-LPH is a major opioid-like peptide in human pituitary glands and in the plasma of normal human subjects.[57,58] High concentrations of β-endorphin are present in the plasma of patients with endocrine disorders associated with increased ACTH and β-LPH, but the latter is not completely converted to β-endorphin in vivo in normal subjects. Studies of pituitary adenomas in patients with Cushing's syndrome showed that the conversion of β-LPH to β-endorphin was enhanced in ACTH/β-LPH-producing adenomas.[59] β-Endorphin in the normal pituitary gland is more likely to exist in the β-LPH form. Wiedemann et al.[60] developed a specific radioimmunoassay for human β-endorphin in unextracted plasma in which there was minimal cross-reaction with β-LPH. In normal fasting subjects, morning levels ranged from 5 to 45 pg/ml, and β-endorphin was elevated in patients with untreated Cushing's disease, Nelson's syndrome, and a patient with bronchogenic carcinoma. In normal subjects with an intact pituitary–adrenal axis, endorphin was undetectable following dexamethasone administration and increased after metyrapone and insulin-induced hypoglycemia.

It thus appears to respond to the same stimuli as ACTH and β-LPH. Patients in remission from pituitary–adrenal disease had normal levels. Pullan et al.[61] looked for Met-enkephalin and β-endorphin in tissue extracts of nonendocrine tumors. High concentrations of the two peptides that were undetectable in control lung tissue were identified in three carcinoid tumors from patients with the ectopic ACTH syndrome. In one patient, the Met-enkephalin concentration in veins draining the tumor was twice that in a peripheral vein. The presence of increased quantities of neural peptides in the tumors and blood of patients with malignancy suggests that some of the confusing and diverse paraneoplastic syndromes associated with malignancy could be related to such peptides. In patients with renal failure, levels of both γ- and β-LPH may be significantly elevated and they must be considered possible factors in causing some of the clinical phenomena.[62]

Pullan et al.[63] studied extracts from seven tumors. Four tumors contained the complete family of peptides, including ACTH, LPH, α-MSH, CLIP, β-endorphin, and Met-enkephalin, although the proportions varied in different tumors. In addition, high-molecular-weight forms of ACTH and Met-enkephalin were observed. None of these peptides was detectable in normal lung tissue. These data suggested that the common precursor was synthesized by all tumors, but that the subsequent pattern of metabolism depended on the particular enzyme activity present in the particular tumor. There was a high-molecular-weight enkephalin-like peptide that reacted in the Met-enkephalin assay but not in the β-endorphin assay, supporting the concept that the precursor for Met-enkephalin might be distinct from that for ACTH and LPH.[64] The presence of enkephalin, as well as precursors for the ACTH–LPH genes for these polypeptides, might have resulted either from gene duplication or from genes closely related to each other in structure. Whether these non-ACTH peptides have physiologic effects in cancer patients remains to be determined, but they may have a number of important actions, including stimulation of insulin secretion (by CLIP), production of analgesia (by β-endorphin and Met-enkephalin), as well as behavioral effects. Recently, it has been shown by Grossman et al.[65] that an analog of Met-enkephalin may inhibit vasopressin release during hyperosmolar stimulation of vasopressin secretion. Thus, these peptides might suppress release of osmotically mediated vasopressin. In the past, it has been suggested that baroreceptor-mediated release of ADH may be stimulated by morphine and related peptides, since they cause antidiuresis. More detailed studies suggested that the antidiuretic effect of opiates is only seen when there are associated hemodynamic changes, and that the primary effect of morphine or β-endorphin or Met-enkephalin may be to suppress rather than stimulate vasopressin release. The multiple effects of β-LPH and the endorphins in a wide variety of physiologic systems, such as hormone release,[65,66] stress-induced eating,[67,68] blood pressure control,[69] exercise,[70] and behavior,[71] suggest that in the future these peptides will likely be shown to be responsible for important clinical phenomena. Their effects could potentially explain a number of clinical phenomena in cancer patients.

8.2.3. Ectopic Production of GH and GHRH

There has been new information documenting the association of acromegaly with nonpituitary tumors that produce GH-releasing factor and stimulate the normal pituitary gland to release GH, causing acromegaly. Saeed et al.[72] described a patient with a bronchial carcinoid and acromegaly, pituitary enlargement, and elevated GH. Symptoms of active acromegaly and elevated GH persisted for 11 years after hypophysectomy, and resection of the pulmonary tumor reduced GH to normal levels. No GH was present in the carcinoid tumor, but when extracts of it were added to isolated pituitary cells in culture, GH-releasing activity was noted. Frohman et al.[73] recently reported work on a number of additional tumors containing GH-releasing activity. They studied extracts of a pancreatic islet tumor that contained a large amount of activity, as did extracts of a small cell carcinoma of the lung and carcinoid. Each of the tumors also contained somatostatin-like immunoreactivity, but the levels did not correlate with the biologic activity of the tumor. The material with GH-releasing activity had a molecular weight greater than 6000, was adsorbed on DEAE-cellulose at low ionic strength and removed at higher ionic strength. When purified further by HPLC, the preparation increased GH release by pituitary monolayer cultures up to 5 times baseline. The activity was resistant to exopeptidase digestion but could be destroyed by trypsin and chymotrypsin. It was suggested that this finding could explain the possible presence of pituitary tumors in some patients with multiple endocrine neoplasia type 1. The stimulatory effects of the GH-releasing factor were inhibited by somatostatin. It had not been clear whether the releasing hormone was the same peptide produced by the median eminence of the hypothalamus; there were differences between them in size and chromatographic behavior, although the tumor material might be a precursor. Recent purification and chemical characterization of the peptides now suggests that they are the same.

It has been suggested that the possibility of an extrapituitary tumor be considered in every patient with acromegaly. The presence of pituitary tumors suggests that prolonged stimulation of GH release can cause tumor formation, supporting the possibility that pituitary acromegaly might be primarily a hypothalamic disease. Clemens et al.[74] and others[75–78] focused on the radioimmunoassay of somatomedin C as a highly reliable means for confirming the diagnosis of acromegaly and assessing clinical disease activity, since it correlated extremely well with GH concentrations. The mean fasting levels were 6.8 U/ml in acromegalic patients and 0.67 U/ml in normal subjects. Following therapy, somatomedin C measurements were extremely useful as an index of improvement.[74]

To follow up earlier observations that GH itself might be produced ectopically, Kaganowicz et al.[79] examined surgically removed human ovaries and found that 8 of 118 contained GH in concentrations up to 50 ng/g. The highest concentration was in an ovarian metastasis from an adenocarcinoma of the breast. The specimens were all positive, by both radioreceptor and radioimmunoassay. The examination of two extracts on Sephadex showed a major peak of immunologic activity that was coincident with monomeric hGH. GH was not being secreted into the blood in a clinically significant quantity, as indicated by the absence of signs of acromegaly in any of the patients. GH levels in ovarian vein blood, when available, were normal.

8.2.4. Ectopic Production of Gonadotropin

In recent years, there has been great interest in the production of gonadotropins, particularly hCG, by both nontrophoblastic tumors and normal cells.[80] hCG is a primary secretory product of the trophoblast, and is known to be elevated early in pregnancy. In the past, its measurement was used principally for documentation of pregnancy and for the diagnosis, evaluation, and follow-up of patients with gestational neoplasms, particularly hydatidiform mole and choriocarcinoma. It is also elevated in males with histologically related tumors of the testis. Recent progress in this field has depended on the development of radioimmunoassays that are specific for the β subunit of hCG and that differentiate the placental marker protein from its closely related structural homolog, pituitary LH. This permits measurement of concentrations of hCG as low as 1 ng in the presence of physiologic quantities of LH. Braunstein et al.[81] first called attention to an hCG-like substance in extracts of normal human testicular tissue. This protein was parallel with hCG standard in the radioimmunoassay, cochromatographed with hCG on gel filtration and was adsorbed to Con A. In subsequent studies by several workers, hCG-like substances were identified in a number of other tissues. Yoshimoto et al.[82] identified β-hCG by radioimmunoassay and radioreceptor assay in extracts of normal colon and liver, although they found that the material did not bind Con A well and suggested that it might have less carbohydrate. Using an antibody against the unique C-terminal portion of hCG, Chen et al.[83] found evidence in normal subjects of a protein that had physical, immunologic, and biologic similarities to hCG. Borkowski and Muquardt[84] extracted hCG from human plasma in normal nonpregnant subjects and found a level of 18 pg/ml in the plasma of 13 normal men. More recently, Braunstein et al.[80,85] have identified hCG-like protein in numerous normal human tissues, including the ovary, pituitary, lung, liver, kidney, spleen, stomach, placenta, and small intestine. The techniques used involve both highly specific radioimmunoassays and radioreceptor assays. The concentrations varied between 1 and 11 ng/g in normal tissues, over 5000 ng/g in the placenta, and over 20,000 ng/g in the pituitary. The pituitary material was felt to be distinct from LH. The antiserum used in the assay had previously been passed through an immunosorbant column containing human LH. During Con A-binding studies, the extracts of various tissues varied widely in the degree of adsorption of the immunoreactive substance to the lectin. More of the material present in testes, ovaries, placenta, or small intestine adsorbed to Con A than was the case with the material in lung, liver, or kidney. These findings were similar to those of Yoshimoto et al.,[82] who identified hCG-like material in all extracts of normal human tissues studied (colon, liver, and lung) at concentrations varying from 1.2 to 7 ng/g.

Given that hCG production may be common to a variety of normal tissues, there has been extensive interest in examining the production of even larger amounts of this protein by a variety of tumors. Prior to the development of specific assays for hCG, there were relatively few reports of ectopic hCG production by tumors. Braunstein et al.[86] studied sera from 906 patients with nontrophoblastic neoplasms and found that 11.4% had detectable hCG. A number of other investigators examined multiple human sera, and the highest frequency of positives was found in patients with gynecologic, breast, lung, and gastrointestinal tract tumors, as well as melanoma, with an average of approximately 19%. The actual production of hCG by these tumors may be more frequent than that. Yoshimoto et al.[82] found that 7 of 30 tumors studied contained hCG-like material in amounts greater than those in normal tissue; the rest containing it in amounts similar to these in normal tissue. The values in cancer patients varied from 1 to greater than 100 ng/g. In their studies, Con A bound 92.5% of hCG from the placenta, 31% of cancer tissue hCG, and only 6% of hCG from normal tissues. The discrepancy between the frequency of positive assays for hCG in serum and in tumor tissues may be related to defective glycosylation or the short half-life of desialylated hCG in the circulation.

The levels of hCG in the circulation of cancer patients are low, usually in the range of 1 to 5 ng/ml (at the lower limit of detection of the β-hCG assay). The presence of hCG in serum is not absolutely specific for cancer, since 2.6% of control subjects were found to have detectable hCG.[87] Further close follow-up of these positive controls may show some to harbor an occult neoplasm, but this needs to be determined. Recently, Braunstein et al.[86] examined serum samples from 1150 patients for the presence of the β subunit, and found it to be present in 11.6% of 876 patients with nontrophoblastic tumors and 1.5% of 1074 patients with benign disorders. There were no significant differences in age, race, or histologic type of tumor between patients with neoplasms who had hCG present and those who did not. More of the patients with metastatic disease who were positive were women. Patients over 50 years of age with benign disorders were more likely to have false-positive tests. The majority of patients had values between 1 and 4 ng/ml, while no patient with a benign disorder had levels greater than 10, and 13% of patients with tumor production of hormone had levels above this. Thus, serum hCG measurements were of limited usefulness in screening for nontrophoblastic malignancies.

Hattori et al.[88] found hCG in 10 of 100 plasma samples from patients with malignancy and in none of 56 control subjects. In tumor tissues, hCG was identified in 42%, and it was suggested that APUD tumors might contain smaller amounts of hCG than non-APUD tumors. Papapetrou et al.[89] studied hCG in both serum and urine in patients with malignant disease. They found 17.1% of patients positive in serum and 44.3% in urine; 20 patients were positive only for urine. The hCG immunoreactive material in the urine was mostly a species smaller than hCG and β-hCG, although its nature was not further known. Weymann and Nisula[90] studied the renal clearance rates of subunits of hCG in man and found that excretion of unaltered subunit accounts for a very small fraction of the total metabolic removal of hCG. Twelve hours after injection of the β-hCG subunit, 90% of the immunoreactivity in the urine was in a fragment that contained carbohydrate and had a molecular weight about 25% that of the injected peptide. Within the first 4 hr after injection, most of the material was intact.

Goldenberg et al.[91] used antibodies to hCG coupled to ^{125}I in an attempt to localize tumor tissue. In several patients this showed promise, and excision of one of the metastatic tumors located by this method indicated a tumor/nontumor radioactive ratio of 39. There are many technical issues, including sensitivity, that have to be resolved, but the use of this advanced technology shows promise in locating tumor tissue. On the other hand, the status of hormone production by the tumors may or may not be related to the amount of tumor tissue present. A similar approach has been used for tumors producing carcinoembryonic antigen.[92]

Production of hormones may also vary at different times in the life cycle of the tumor. In a patient who had large cell carcinoma of the lung and gynecomastica reported by Metz et al.,[93] preoperative levels of hCG were 109 ng/ml, with the α and β subunit concentrations being 3.2 and 21 ng/ml, respectively; after complete tumor resection and resolution of gynecomastia, hCG titers remained elevated at 3.3 ng/ml, indicating tumor recurrence. During this time, administration of LHRH produced a markedly delayed increase in pituitary gonadotropins. Subsequent chemotherapy, helped by the use of hCG measurements, reduced it to undetectable levels, and the response to LHRH was then normal.

In attempting to define the specificity of the antibodies to hCG, it is useful to look at antigenic sites in the molecule. Swaminathan and Braunstein[94] concluded tentatively that a major antigenic site for the β subunit is present between residues 21 and 23 with the disulfide bond connecting cysteine-23 or 26 with residues further down the peptide chain. Ghai et al.[95] made a number of chemical and enzymatic modifications of the β subunit and suggested, as others have previously, that the carbohydrate is not a significant factor in immunologic activity. They concluded from their studies that the antigenic determinants were primarily in the polypeptide chain as a result of conformation and that there were two types of antigenic determinants, those unique to hCG and those common to hCG and LH. Reduction and alkylation of the β subunit produced derivatives that had significant cross-reactivity in the β-hCG system but little activity in the LH system and were therefore more specific antigens. Matsumura et al.[96] used synthetic peptide analogs of the C-terminal peptide of the β subunit to generate specific antisera.

Considerable work in recent years has defined mechanisms for the biosynthesis of the subunits of hCG and other glycoprotein hormones.[97–99] These studies have established the separate synthesis of the two subunits and identified posttranslational processing that involves carbohydrate addition. A variety of different-sized products may be produced, and, in some cases, the released α subunit may be larger than the one in the cells due to carbohydrate addition.[100–103] These findings may have ultimate implications for the kinds of subunits and intact molecules produced by tumors.

A major problem at present is the fact that normal tissues can produce hCG, and in a small percentage of normal subjects, there will be detectable hCG in blood. Although hCG measurements may be useful as a screening agent, they certainly do not prove cancer, but the patient with a positive assay needs to be followed up carefully. Further information on these points is necessary in order to improve the care of patients with hCG-producing tumors.

Braunstein et al.[80] maintained in culture an ovarian carcinoma cell line that produced hCG and released neither free α nor β subunits.

Studies suggested that the material produced *in vitro* was very similar to that made *in vivo*, and studies by Kanabus *et al.*[104] showed that sodium butyrate could enhance release of this material markedly *in vitro*. Tralka *et al.*[105] studied the effects of sodium butyrate on the production of hCG and its α subunit in a cell line from a human bronchogenic carcinoma. They found that butyrate caused elongation or flattening of cells on light microscopy, while electron microscopy showed enhanced adhesion of cells to glass and changes in ultrastructure that included increases in perinuclear tonofilaments, smooth endoplasmic reticulum vesicles, dense mitochondrial inclusions, and lipid granules. There was a marked decrease in condensed chromatin clumps, which may reflect modification in chromatin and increased transcription.

8.2.5. Ectopic Production of Thyrotropin

Since hCG has been postulated to be the thyrotropic factor in trophoblastic and nontrophoblastic neoplasms associated with hyperthyroidism, further studies have been performed on the thyroid-stimulating capabilities of hCG. Amir *et al.*[106] studied the interaction of both crude and purified hCG with receptors in human thyroid membranes by examining the binding of iodinated TSH and adenylate cyclase activation. These studies showed that crude preparations of hCG contained a factor that inhibited the binding of iodinated bovine TSH to human thyroid. There was also a factor in the crude preparations that inhibited the stimulation of adenylate cyclase by bovine TSH. Purified hCG did not stimulate adenylate cyclase directly or inhibit its response to bovine TSH. Pekonen and Weintraub[107,108] conducted similar studies and found that the cross-reactivity in a TSH radioreceptor assay using bovine TSH and thyroid membranes was very great with crude hCG but very limited with the purified preparation. However, when "physiologic" conditions were used, the crude and purified preparations behaved similarly, and the effect of the other protein inhibitors was abolished. Based on these studies, the authors concluded that the thryotropic activity of 1 IU of hCG was equivalent to 0.5–0.8 μIU of bovine TSH. With the very high levels of hCG present in choriocarcinoma or hydatidiform mole, there would be sufficient thyrotropic activity to account for the hyperthyroid response.

The association of mild hyperthyroidism with trophoblastic neoplasms has been known for 25 years. Recently, Higgins and Hirschman[109] studied 20 patients with hydatidiform mole and found that 12 were euthyroid, while 6 were severely and 2 mildly hyperthyroid. The six patients with more severe disease had clinical signs and symptoms, and all had palpable goiter. Two patients developed supraventricular tachycardia and pulmonary edema, while a number of the other patients had significant symptoms. In the past, most studies showed that the patients were clinically euthyroid even though their circulating levels of free thyroid hormone were increased. Molar pregnancy is much more common in the Far East, being ten times as frequent as in the West. The current data still point to hCG as the pathogenic factor in the disease although human chorionic thyrotropin has been theoretically identified. hCG increases adenylate cyclase activity in human thyroid membranes, although its effects are very slight. Harada and Hirschman[110] extracted human term placentas and failed to obtain significant evidence for human chorionic thyrotropin.

An interesting variant of TSH has been found in plasma by Kourides et al.[111] and Spitz et al.[112]; this is of higher molecular weight than the normal protein. In the three patients in whom a large form of TSH was described, the higher molecular weight of TSH could be related to posttranslational processing and probably does not represent a precursor. The patients studied by Spitz et al.[112] were euthyroid with an elevated TSH level. The material showed normal binding to TSH receptor but decreased stimulation of adenylate cyclase. No studies in patients with tumors have yet been performed.

8.2.6. Ectopic Production of Vasopressin

Recent studies by radioimmunoassay have shown an increased frequency of vasopressin secretion by tumors in patients with malignant disease, particularly those with bronchogenic tumors of the small cell variety. Robertson[113] described a number of patients with elevated plasma levels of tumor vasopressin in the absence of a clinical syndrome. Because of the close physiologic tie between serum osmolality and vasopressin, the magnitude of vasopressin secretion must be assessed in relation to serum osmolality. Normal physiologic regulation involves a flat response of vasopression secretion until the critical threshold of osmolality is reached, following which a large increase in secretion is observed. In carcinoma patients, relatively inappropriate levels of vasopressin are seen at lower than normal levels of serum osmolality. The syndrome (SIADH) represents inappropriate secretion of vasopressin from the tumor. Its production by tumors has been well documented both by direct synthesis in vitro and by the more recent studies of Kondo et al.[114] showing cell-free translation of mRNA for vasopressin and neurophysin.

Recent studies of Padfield et al.[115,116] showed that the patterns of vasopressin secretion in patients with ectopic ADH production may be quite variable. In some cases, the physiologic response to changes in osmolality is normal, but the osmostat appears to be set at an abnormal level. In the patient with malignant disease, a number of factors may cause SIADH, and it is important to differentiate potential tumor production of ADH from the multiple other causes, which include disease of the chest and lungs, pulmonary infection, meningitis, metastatic disease, pain, stress, morphine, and various drugs such as chlorpropamide and vincristine. Perks et al.[117,118] described a patient with malignant mesothelioma and the SIADH syndrome who had increased serum and urine concentrations of arginine vasopressin, but no vasopressin in the tumor. It appears more likely that nonosmotic stimuli related to the patient's extensive chest disease may have been factors in stimulating ADH, working through pulmonary baroreceptors or the vagus nerve. Skrabanek and Powell[119] reviewed the evidence for ectopic ADH production and suggested that it was still incomplete. They suggested that there was no clear evidence for arteriovenous gradients of ADH across a tumor bed and that the low levels in tumors might possibly be accounted for by binding of neurophysin, which is produced in the same tissue. Pettingill et al.,[120] however, reported a cell line from an oat-cell carcinoma that produced small amounts of immunoreactive arginine vasopressin in vitro.

Kondo et al.[114] obtained tumor tissue at autopsy from a 58-year-old man with bronchogenic oat-cell carcinoma and SIADH. The tumor tissue was transplanted serially in nude mice, with 20 passages over more than 4 years, and the plasma levels of vasopressin in the mice were 24–50 pg/ml and in the tumor tissue, 1.3 ng/g. Furthermore, neurophysin was detected in both plasma and tumor tissues (7.5 ng/ml and 2.8 μg/g, respectively). The nude mice had water retention, with high sodium concentrations in the urine, and when they were hydrated, they had decreased water clearance. They did not become hyponatremic because they drank less. When loaded with water, they developed a marked decrease in plasma sodium concentration. This tumor obviously produced ADH and induced SIADH in the nude mice. It is a useful experimental model and provides further convincing evidence for ectopic ADH production by human tumors.

Padfield et al.[116] studied 17 patients with the SIADH syndrome associated with bronchogenic carcinoma and found that plasma AVP levels were elevated in most. In 14 patients with tumors but without overt SIADH, levels were also significantly higher than normal. This finding, together with the lower than normal osmolality, suggested that ADH excess might be more common than believed. The usual positive correlation between osmolality and plasma AVP is reversed in SIADH associated with ectopic tumors. Kelly and Morton[121] examined tumor tissues from 32 patients with carcinoma of the bronchus and found immunologic activity in only three, all of whom had small cell tumors and two of whom had hyponatremia. AVP levels varied between 28 and 164 pg/mg wet wt. These findings argue against the conclusion that ectopic secretion is the cause of raised ADH in patients with carcinoma of the bronchus and a normal serum sodium. However, the study was not conclusive, since plasma levels were not known, and there could have been tissue destruction. In another study, Morton et al.[115,121] found immunologic activity only in tumors of the small cell type. Perks et al.[118] studied 29 patients with histologically proven mesotheliomas and found 62% with hyponatremia. It was felt by the authors that the hyponatremia was not only caused by ectopic production of ADH but could also be due to reflex effects through the vagus nerve. Compression of pulmonary baroreceptors or infiltration of the vagus nerve by the mesothelioma could lead to reflex secretion of ADH.

Hansen et al.[122,123] studied ACTH, ADH, and CT as markers of small cell carcinoma of the lung. No significant or consistent changes in these three hormones were found following lysis of tumor cells by cytotoxic agents. After the tumor had responded, plasma ACTH, ADH, and CT became normal in most patients, but recurrent or progressive disease was not always followed by increases in plasma ACTH or ADH. In 12 patients with disease progression, however, CT increased in 10 and plasma ADH in 11, although the changes were only moderate. Furthermore, in some patients, CT concentrations were found to be increased after tumor regression. Therefore, decisions concerning patient treatment cannot be based exclusively on the concentrations of these hormones, as the amounts may vary greatly at different times in the life cycle of the tumor. Hansen et al.[123] also examined the pattern of metabolites in small cell tumors in relation to stage and subtype. Approximately one-third had the ectopic ADH syndrome. Twenty-nine percent had elevated plasma ACTH, and 64% elevated serum calcitonin. Gastrin concentrations were increased in 20% but only marginally. There was no elevation of glucagon, insulin, secretin, VIP, GH, hCG, hPL, or VMA. The concentrations of ACTH, CT, and urine ADH were found not to be correlated with the stage of the disease, and no correlation with histologic subtypes of small cell carcinoma was identified.

Comis et al.[124] evaluated 41 patients with small cell carcinoma of the lung for water abnormalities using a standard water loading test; 68% had abnormalities. They found these abnormalities in 47% of patients with carcinoma in one hemithorax and in 86% with more extensive disease. Forty-six percent had SIADH. Zerbe et al.[125] reviewed the various types of vasopressin release in patients with SIADH, and discussed the multiple possible mechanisms for SIADH in patients with cancer other than ectopic hormone production. These included hypovolemia, obstruction of the vena cava, invasion of the vagus nerve, metastases to the hypothalamus, drug administration, carcinomatous neuropathy, as well as ectopic production of a vasopressin-releasing factor.

North et al.[126] used the radioimmunoassay for two human neurophysins to study 61 patients with small cell carcinoma of the lung. They found that plasma levels of one or both of these proteins were elevated to levels more than three times normal in 62% of patients before the beginning of therapy. Presumably, these elevations were the result of production and release by the tumor. Eighteen patients who had elevated values prior to therapy were followed, and there was an excellent correlation between decreases in neurophysin concentrations and the clinical response of the patient. Partial or complete response in 12 patients was associated with a marked reduction in circulating concentrations and with a rise during progression. Relapse was associated with an increase over earlier values. Thus, the radioimmunoassay of neurophysins may be an extremely useful guide to the management of patients with small cell carcinoma of the lung.

Recent treatment of SIADH involves the use of demeclocycline or lithium. Decaux et al.[127] have described treatment with exogenous urea, the latter lowering urinary sodium excretion and increasing plasma sodium as long as the value was less than 130 mEq/liter. Urea also induced a persistent osmotic diuresis, allowing a normal daily intake of water. Up to 30 g of urea per day was administered over a number of weeks, and this was suggested as an alternative to other therapy. The potential risk of this therapy is dehydration if the patient does not drink enough. Demeclocycline is not well tolerated by some patients because of potential nephrotoxicity, although it is felt to be superior to lithium. Short-term treatment with urea[127] and chronic administration of oral furosemide together with adequate salt intake[128] have also been used in the syndrome.

8.2.7. Ectopic Production of Nonsuppressible Insulin-like Activity

Recent studies have suggested that bioassayable insulin activity in plasma consists of a mixture of true pancreatic insulin and a larger portion known as nonsuppressible insulin-like activity (NSILA). This concept is based on the failure of anti-insulin antibodies to neutralize most of the biologic activity in plasma. Using the criterion of acid alcohol solubility, two components of NSILA have been identified. These are NSILA-s, a lower-molecular-weight component soluble in acid alcohol, and NSILA-p, a higher-molecular-weight protein precipitable by acid alcohol. NSILA-s consists of two polypeptides of approximately 7500 daltons, termed insulin-like growth factors I and II (IGF 1 and 2).[129] These peptides have growth-promoting effects on chick embryo fibroblasts and have extensive homology with the amino acid sequence of human proinsulin, suggesting a common molecular precursor. The structural homology extends to the tertiary structure and accounts for its cross-reactivity with the insulin receptor. In adipose tissue, IGF 1 and 2 have 1/60th the biologic activity of insulin and demonstrate weak affinity for the insulin receptor. In muscle and fibroblast, biologic activity is much greater and is mediated by high-affinity interaction with the insulin receptor. Synthesis of these peptides occurs in the liver and is under the influence of GH. These peptides are closely related to or identical with the somatomedins, peptides that are mediators of GH action on various target tissues. IGF 1 appears to be very similar to or identical with somatomedin C.[130] Like the somatomedins, IGF 1 and 2 stimulate the sulfation of cartilage and their synthesis is GH dependent.

NSILA-s has been suggested as the pathogenic factor causing hypoglycemia in some patients with non-islet cell tumors, but more specific assays have not always confirmed this. The variety of assays used for NSILA-s may account for the findings of different investigators. Megyesi et al.[131] used a radioreceptor assay that detects predominantly IGF 2 and identified increased NSILA-s in some patients. Gorden et al.[132] recently reviewed the variety of tumor types associated with nonislet tumor hypoglycemia, using an assay for multiplication-stimulating activity of a gel filtration eluate in acid. Nineteen of fifty-two samples had IGF-like levels greater than 150% of controls. Elevations were found in patients with hemiangiopericytoma (6 of 7), hepatoma (2 of 4), adrenocortical carcinoma (1 of 3), and pheochromocytoma (2 of 2). Patients with lymphoma and hypoglycemia had distinctly low values. This material was thought to be similar to IGF 2. Daughaday et al.,[133] using a new radioreceptor assay for IGF 2 with rat placental membranes, showed increased circulating levels in 10 of 14 sera from patients with tumor-related hypoglycemia. IGF 1, on the other hand, was low or unmeasurable. A variety of insulin-like growth factors, including IGF 1 (somatomedin C), somatomedin A, multiplication-stimulating activity, and IGF 2 are able to lower blood glucose.[134,135] Additional studies are necessary to clarify the frequency with which various insulin-related peptides may be associated with hypoglycemia.

NSILA-p has also been reported to cause hypoglycemia.[136] This is a 90,000-dalton serum glycoprotein that exhibits insulin-like activity and has been characterized only partially. It apparently accounts for the major portion of serum insulin-like activity in bioassays. NSILA-p is not considered a member of the somatomedin family since it has limited or no sulfation factor activity. NSILA-p levels increase moderately in pregnancy, and elevations have been found in patients with various types of cancer.[136]

8.2.8. Ectopic Production of Calcium-Mobilizing Substances

Hypercalcemia is perhaps the most common metabolic problem associated with cancer. It is generally due either to the physical presence of tumor cells in bone, causing osteolytic destruction and mobilizing calcium into the extracellular fluid, or alternatively, to the production of humoral factors by tumors that mobilize calcium from bone. Even where tumor cells are actually present in bone, it is possible that such lysis is mediated by one or more known factors responsible for local bone destruction such as prostaglandin E_2 (PGE_2),[137] osteoclast-activating factor,[138,139] epidermal growth factor,[140] or direct lysis of bone by tumor cells,[141] monocytes,[142] or macrophages.[143]

In those patients without metastases to bone (and even in some of those with), it has been suggested that a humoral factor produced by the tumor itself and released into the circulation might mediate the hypercalcemia, causing increased bone resorption, calcium mobilization into the circulation, and the resultant clinical disorder.[144] There has been considerable controversy concerning the factor(s) responsible for such calcium mobilization. The first candidate to be studied intensively was parathyroid hormone (PTH), as the well-recognized disorder of primary hyperparathyroidism is associated with similar biochemical abnormalities. There has been intensive study of the production of PTH or PTH-like substances of tumors. In early studies by complement fixation inhibition and radioimmunoassay,[145] it was shown that PTH or PTH-like peptides could be extracted from tumors. There is also evidence for the net synthesis of PTH by tumors, as judged from positive arteriovenous gradients across a tumor bed[146] and the direct biosynthesis of hormone *in vitro* by tumor tissues.[147] On the other hand, confusing evidence has been provided in recent years by the extensive application of radioimmunoassays for PTH (both N and C terminal) to the serum of many patients with cancer and hypercalcemia. While most of these studies have shown detectable levels of PTH in the circulation, they have, in general, been relatively low or normal.[144] When elevated hormone levels occur as they do occasionally, they suggest PTH production by the tumor or, more commonly, coexisting primary hyperparathyroidism. These observations have been complicated somewhat by the complex metabolism of PTH and the persistence of biologically inert but immunoreactive C-terminal fragments with a relatively long half-life in the circulation.[148] Nevertheless, if PTH itself were the usual mediator of tumor hypercalcemia, consistent elevation of PTH peptides in the circulation should be found. One cannot account for the lack of elevation of PTH in these patients by renal dysfunction or by abnormal metabolism of PTH by the tumors. From the well-understood biosynthesis of PTH, it is highly unlikely that precursors or other factors could explain the phenomenon, since proPTH is not known to enter the circulation and is also relatively inert biologically. Because of the paucity of evidence supporting more than the occasional ectopic production of PTH in these clinical syndromes, there has been an intensive search for other possible factors.

Prostaglandins were first shown to cause local bone resorption in an *in vitro* system by Klein and Raisz in 1970.[149] Their studies showed that the PGE compounds were the most potent in mobilizing calcium, and that they caused osteoclastic bone resorption. In the mediation of bone resorption by PG, it was also shown that there was increased collagenase activity and cAMP production. Subsequent exciting studies by Tashjian and colleagues[150] suggested in two animal models, fibrosarcoma in the mouse and VX_2 carcinoma in the rabbit, that PG production accounted for the hypercalcemic state. These studies showed that tumor production of PG resulted in systemic hypercalcemia, that there was an arteriovenous difference in PG concentration across the tumor bed, and that the PG could be synthesized by the tumor *in vitro* as well. Similarly, inhibitors of PG synthesis ameliorated the hypercalcemia and decreased the circulating levels. Increased osteoclastic bone resorption was noted at sites distant from the tumor. They also provided evidence that PGE_2 infusion into rats produced a hypercalcemic state.[151]

A number of clinical studies since 1974 have suggested that PG may account for hypercalcemia in some patients with malignancy. [152–154] Robertson *et al.* [153] reported a patient with renal cell carcinoma and hypercalcemia who had low PTH, elevations of both plasma PGE and tissue PGE. Indomethacin-responsive hypercalcemia in patients with tumors was also described by others.[144] Seyberth[154] described 14 patients with hypercalcemia and malignancy who had increased PG metabolites in the urine (PGE-M), while patients with primary hyperparathyroidism and hypercalcemia had normal levels of urinary metabolites. In later studies, Robertson *et al.*[155] found increased levels of plasma PGE in a number of patients with hypercalcemia, and Cummings and Robertson[156] showed that renal cell carcinoma in monolayer tissue culture synthesized PGE. Furthermore, Atkins *et al.*[157] reported that hypernephroma in coculture with mouse calvarium caused indomethacin-reversible bone resorption. In a recent review by Metz *et al.*,[137] 10 of 33 hypercalcemic patients with cancer had elevated levels of PGE and PGE metabolites in venous blood, although levels were not as high as those reported in the animal studies. In a review of the three largest series of human subjects studied, a total of 63 patients with this syndrome have been described.[137] There is considerable variability in the methods used to detect the PG in these studies, and the prevalence of elevated levels varies considerably. Problems to be resolved in this kind of work include the possible role of PG and metabolites other than PGE, the source of the PG, the importance of location of the tumor (because of the metabolism of PGE on first pass through the liver and lung), and the potential site of PG production that causes bone resorption. It is not known whether the problem is due to release of PG itself from the tumor or, as Minkin et al.[158] have suggested, to local production of PG in bone in response to a circulating humoral factor such as epidermal growth factor.[159] In addition to PTH and PG, Mundy and Raisz[139] have suggested that osteoclast-activating factor might be involved in the development of hypercalcemia in patients with certain types of malignancy, such as multiple myeloma and some lymphomas.

Considering the prevalence of tumor-related hypercalcemia,[144] the etiologic factors described above do not seem adequate to account for the frequency of the phenomenon. In recent studies,[144,160–162] it has become apparent that immunoreactive PTH in the circulation is often normal or low in patients with cancer and hypercalcemia, although urinary cAMP or nephrogenous cAMP may be increased. cAMP in the urine had been considered to be the hallmark of PTH activity,[163] and thus the studies seem paradoxical. Stewart et al.[162] recently investigated such patients in detail. On evaluating 50 consecutive individuals with cancer and hypercalcemia, they found that nephrogenous cAMP excretion was elevated in 41 and suppressed in 9 (5.85 vs. 0.51 nmole/100 ml glomerular filtrate). They compared the group of patients with elevated nephrogenous cAMP with a group of 15 patients with primary hyperparathyroidism and found the following: the group with hypercalcemia, cancer, and increased nephrogenous cAMP had reduced tubular reabsorption of phosphorus like the patients with primary hyperparathyroidism, but unlike the latter, they had increased fasting calcium excretion (0.66 vs. 0.25 mg/100 ml glomerular filtrate), substantial reduction in circulating levels of 1,25-dihydroxyvitamin D_3 (20 vs. 83 pg/ml), and low levels of immunoreactive PTH in four different radioimmunoassays (which measured both N- and C-terminal portions of the molecule). Thus, the patients appeared on the surface to behave as if they had increased PTH, but the low levels of 1,25-dihydroxyvitamin D_3 and the increased fractional calcium excretion, as well as diminished or absent PTH, suggested that some factor other than PTH itself was responsible for increased urinary cAMP. On further evaluation, they showed increased cytochemical bioactivity in the peripheral plasma of 10 of 16 of these patients.[164] This is a highly sensitive bioassay that depends on the activation of glucose-6-phosphate dehydrogenase in renal tubular cells (which is known to be stimulated by PTH and cAMP). The patients with hypercalcemia and cancer, like patients with primary hyperparathyroidism, had increased activity in their serum of a material that mimics PTH. When this activity was fractionated by gel filtration, however, it appeared in a number of sera to elute from the column at a molecular weight higher than that of PTH. Furthermore, antiserum to PTH only partially neutralized the biologic activity in the serum, whereas it neutralized completely the activity in patients with primary hyperparathyroidism. In similar studies by Rude et al.,[161] plasma and urinary cAMP were determined in 91 patients with hypercalcemia and malignancy. Plasma cAMP was elevated in cancer patients with both hypercalcemia and normocalcemia, but not in patients with primary hyperparathyroidism. The mean urinary cAMP was increased at least twofold in all patient groups. They found increased nephrogenous cAMP in 46% of the patients with hypercalcemia and malignancy who had bone metastases and 60% of the patients with normocalcemia and malignancy. Increased urinary cAMP was most likely to be found in patients with squamous cell carcinoma of the lung, upper gastrointestinal tumors, and renal cell carcinomas, although it was not completely specific for these tumors. Only 4 of 91 patients had detectable IPTH, 3 of these having coexisting primary hyperparathyroidism. In further studies, Minkin et al.[158] utilized extracts of tumors from patients with this syndrome to examine bone resorption in vitro from labeled mouse calvaria. Extracts of three of five tumors caused a significant increase in ^{45}Ca release, and bone resorption was blocked by indomethacin. Further studies by Stewart et al.[165] evaluated bone histomorphometry in these subjects. Compared with patients with primary hyperparathyroidism, those with humoral hypercalcemia or malignancy showed a threefold increase in bone resorption coupled with reduction in bone formation, decreased bone volume, and the appearance of uncoupling of osteoclast and osteoblast activity. In these patients, 10.6% of the bone surface was covered with osteoclasts, compared with 2.7% in primary hyperparathyroidism and 0.5% in controls.

The above studies thus point to the possibility that a new factor, not previously identified, may account for the clinical disorder. It is possible that these effects may be mediated by a humoral factor that stimulates the local production in bone of PG or related metabolites of arachidonic acid. Tumor-stimulated resorption was blocked by inhibitors of PG synthesis and related metabolites of arachidonic acid, whereas resorption stimulated by PTH, PGE_2, and 1,25-dihydroxyvitamin D_3 was not.[158] There was insufficient PTH or PGE_2 in tumor extracts to account for the degree of resorption. One of the problems in the current studies is that the tumors themselves have not been examined extensively. With some of the newer techniques available, it is highly likely that a factor will be isolated from such tumors that accounts for the clinical disorder. Of considerable interest is the likelihood that a potent hypercalcemic factor (not known previously to exist) is present in these tumors. From what is known about the synthesis of hormones and gene activation (vide *supra),* it is highly likely that this is a physiologic regulator (not a new hormone) whose site of origin and presence were not previously known. Of interest is a recent report by Saito *et al.*[166] in which a squamous cell carcinoma of the thyroid associated with hypercalcemia and leukocytosis was transplanted into athymic nude mice. The mice also developed marked leukocytosis and hypercalcemia.

Animal models of ectopic hypercalcemia currently being pursued include a Leydig cell tumor of the rat[167] and adenocarcinoma of the dog.[168] Whether these tumors produce substances similar to those produced in man is unknown. As Sherwood[144] and Skrabanek *et al.*[169] have emphasized, multiple factors are likely responsible for the hypercalcemic syndrome.

8.2.9. Ectopic Production of Calcitonin

There have been numerous reports of the ectopic production of CT by tumors other than medullary carcinoma of the thyroid.[170–173] As in patients with medullary carcinoma,[174] those with ectopic CT usually have no clinical effects from the production of the hormone. It is the association of the disorder with the production of other proteins or substances by medullary carcinoma or by the ectopic tumor that leads to clinical consequences or symptoms, if they are present at all. Schwartz *et al.*[173] performed a prospective study to determine the value of CT as a tumor marker. In these studies, elevated concentrations of plasma CT were found in a number of common cancers such as those of the lung (38%), colon (24%), breast (38%), pancreas (42%), and stomach (30%). In patients with small cell carcinoma of the lung, 58% had elevated CT, and immunologic activity was detected in 14% of tumor extracts, but not in normal tissue outside of the thyroid. There was no clinical correlation of hypercalcemia with increased CT secretion, and control studies with [^{125}I]hCT suggested that the measurements were not an artifact of label degradation. That CT is not an absolute marker for neoplastic disease, however, was shown by elevations in some patients with renal failure, gastrointestinal bleeding, and chronic obstructive lung disease. It is known that CT secretion responds physiologically to calcium, gastrin, glucagon, and catecholamines. Silva *et al.*[175] did a similar prospective study in 61 patients with bronchogenic cancer. Fifty-two percent of these patients exhibited increased plasma CT without any correlation with particular histologic type, and 78% of those with increased CT remained normacalcemic, there being no correlation between CT concentrations and the presence of bony metastases. Release of CT from tumors was either ectopic or due to thyroidal release, the ectopic type being more closely correlated with small cell tumors.[175] With appropriate therapy, circulating concentrations decreased. A similar study of immunoreactive CT in lung cancer by Roos *et al.*[176] examined these issues in a more detailed way since they not only measured plasma CT by radioimmunoassay but also validated it by immunoextraction and gel filtration. In their studies, plasma CT appeared to be elevated in 18% of basal samples from patients with epidermoid or anaplastic cancer, although unequivocal increases in CT were not found in any of these patients. However, in patients with small cell or adenocarcinoma, unequivocal increases were found in 27%, and the form of CT recovered in these latter patients was larger than the CT monomer.

In *in vitro* studies, Bertagna *et al.*[22] studied a line of human small cell carcinoma in culture producing ACTH, lipotropin, endorphin, and CT. After gel exclusion chromatography, two forms of CT were found at 7000 and 14,000 daltons. These appeared to be high-molecular-weight forms of CT that did not cross-react with ACTH antibodies; they supported the release of high-molecular-weight forms of CT from small cell carcinoma, but *not* the existence of a common precursor of ACTH and CT. Immunoperoxidase staining has also been useful in documenting the presence of CT in lung cancer. In the study of Roof *et al.*,[171] the staining was positive only in patients with adenocarcinoma and oat-cell carcinoma. Baylin and Mendelsohn[6] found increased quantities of L-dopa-decarboxylase in small cell and adenocarcinoma of the lung, but not in other types of lung cancer.

In a study by Hansen *et al.*,[170] both basal and pentagastrin-stimulated levels of CT and serum histaminase were examined in a group of 79 patients with small cell carcinoma of the lung. Serum CT was increased in 68% (54 of 79 patients), 20 patients having a level as high as that usually found in medullary carcinoma of the thyroid gland. Levels of histaminase were no different from control. In 3 of 19 patients who had pentagastrin stimulation, CT was significantly increased.

Roos *et al.*[172] also examined small cell carcinoma for the presence of somatostatin-like immunoreactivity. In 15 control subjects, the upper limit of normal of plasma somatostatin was 37 pg/mg. Of 26 patients with small cell lung cancer, 4 had significant elevations in the range of 136–6150 pg/mg, while none of 19 patients with epidermoid lung cancer had an increase. Immunoadsorbant chromatography confirmed that the plasma measurements were due to true measurement of somatostatin-like activity, although there was evidence on gel filtration for at least three species in the range of 13,000, 4000 and 1600 daltons. It was also detectable in extracts of five of nine small cell lung cancers in the range of 14–441 pg/mg compared with concentrations of 60–9200 pg/mg in medullary carcinoma of the thyroid, and was not detectable in normal lungs or in epidermoid lung cancer. The presence of higher-molecular-weight forms may represent biosynthetic precursors. Baylin and Mendelsohn[6] also examined the contents of histaminase, L-dopa-decarboxylase, and CT in small cell carcinoma of the lung. These three markers have regularly been used for medullary carcinoma of the thyroid. There was evidence that histaminase was increased in six lung tumors (to 3–14,000 times control), L-dopa-decarboxylase in four of six (to 6 to 30 times), and CT in one of one. In some metastatic lesions, low or absent levels of these markers were found despite high values in the primary tumor lesions. Since the concentration of tumor markers varied between primary tumors and metastases, circulating levels may not correlate very well with the tumor burden. Samaan *et al.*[177] studied patients with bronchogenic and breast cancer both before and after pentagastrin stimulation and compared the patients with those with medullary carcinoma of the thyroid. They found a number of patients with either bronchogenic tumors or breast cancer with increased CT. In some patients with normal basal CT, the level was abnormally high after pentagastrin stimulation. The degree of response was significantly less than that seen in patients with medullary carcinoma of the thyroid, however. CT has also been shown to be elevated in several patients with VIPomas.[1,178]

The evidence for CT and related peptides in ectopic tumors, particularly small cell carcinoma, is interesting when viewed in relation to new developments in the area of CT physiology and medullary carcinoma of the thyroid.[179,180] For over 20 years, research on CT has focused on the issue of its physiologic role. Despite a great deal of investigation, this is not clear, even though CT is a useful agent in the management of Paget's disease, and measurement of CT is useful in the diagnosis of medullary carcinoma of the thyroid. Emphasis has shifted to the potential role of CT as a hormone related to gastrointestinal function in conserving calcium taken in through the diet. Calcitonin, like other polypeptide hormones of similar molecular weight, is derived through synthesis of a higher-molecular-weight precursor.[181,182] Some variability of the assay of CT in normal plasma is related to the difference between serum samples and plasma, hemolysis, and other variations also account for differing values seen in various laboratories. Some of these factors affect the values obtained in plasma of patients with various tumors (*vide supra*). Furthermore, there is heterogeneity of plasma CT on gel filtration, and immunoassay reveals several peaks of CT-like immunoreactivity. Heterogeneity of the hormone may also be found in the plasma of patients with nonthyroid cancers that produce CT.[182] Whether these multiple forms are the result of peripheral metabolism or of the synthesis of different peptides including precursors has not yet been resolved. Although monomeric CT equivalents are being measured, the value may actually represent the aggregate of multiple forms of CT. Thus, the values for CT from any one laboratory must be interpreted in relation to the normal values from the same laboratory. Goltzman and Tischler[183] showed that the only form of CT having biologic activity in a radioreceptor assay was equivalent to the CT monomer. Of interest in relation to the issue of ectopic production is the controversial evidence concerning the normal presence of extrathyroidal CT activity.[179] It has been well documented in man that C cells of the thyroid actually contain CT although some results have suggested that it might also be present in many other tissues.

Plasma CT appears to be higher in neonates and pregnant women than in others, and estrogen administration may also increase its release. Males have higher basal and stimulated secretion than women, and CT responses to calcium may diminish with age. Parthemore and Deftos[184] studied CT secretion in normal subjects and found greater stimulation by pentagastrin and calcium in males than in females; they suggested that women might have decreased CT reserve. The decreased secretion of CT with age in females noted by Shamonki *et al.*[185] could possibly be related to decrease bone mass and osteoporosis with age in women.

There is no evidence that the total absence of CT (as after thyroidectomy) leads to any problems with plasma calcium homeostasis. Likewise, marked excess of CT, as in medullary carcinoma or ectopic tumors, does not appear to cause any significant problems. Values up to 20,000 times the physiologic can generally be tolerated without hypocalcemia. A variety of studies have suggested that the inhibitory effect of calcitonin on bone is transient and is characterized by an "escape" phenomenon that may be related to down-regulation of receptors. The absence of significant physiologic effects from deficient or excessive CT does not rule out its usefulness as a therapeutic agent in bone that is turning over very rapidly, however. CT has a reasonably secure place in the treatment of Paget's disease, and recent studies suggest that it may be very useful in life-threatening or symptomatic hypercalcemia.[186] Between 75 and 90% of patients with hypercalcemia secondary to cancer appear to have some response to therapeutic levels of salmon CT. Usually there is a plateau within several hours after CT injection, the serum calcium seldom returning to normal. There is one report[187] that the administration of glucocorticoid together with CT may prevent the escape phenomenon.

The role of CT in plasma calcium homeostasis appears to be minor, and it could conceivably have a more important role in preventing bone resorption (particularly since women appear to have lower levels than men). This effect may well be subtle and connected to long-term maintenance of skeletal mass and balance.

8.2.10. Metabolic Bone Diseases Associated with Tumors

The association of osteomalacia with tumors has been well documented. The initial report by McCance[188] described a 15-year-old girl with osteomalacia that was improved following the removal of a degenerating osteoid tumor of the femur. The subsequent 20 or more patients have essentially all had mesodermal tumors that included sclerosing hemangiomas, giant-cell tumors of bone, fibromas, ossifying mesenchymomas, hemangiopericytomas, and a mesenchymal tumor of the pharynx. In these patients there is a common syndrome consisting of hyperphosphaturia and hypophosphatemia, normocalcemia, elevated serum alkaline phosphatase, and osteomalacia associated with bone pain and pseudofractures on X ray.[1,189–191] Most of these cases appeared in childhood, and some were familial. In 1977, Drezner and Feinglos[192] described a 42-year-old woman with a giant-cell tumor of the iliac bone who had osteomalacia and aminoaciduria. This patient had low levels of $1\alpha,25$-dihydroxyvitamin D_3, and it was suggested by these authors that a defect in the conversion of 25-hydroxy D_3 to the dihydroxy derivative might be an important part of the picture. Deficiency of the metabolite is known to contribute to renal phosphate loss, but the degree of hypophosphatemia and phosphaturia in these patients is inappropriately high. Daniels and Weisenfeld[189] recently reported a middle-aged man with sclerosing hemangiomas of bone who showed marked improvement following the administration of oral phosphate (1.5 g phosphorus) and 100,000 U/day of vitamin D. Fukumoto et al.[191] described a patient with a benign osteoblastoma associated not only with osteomalacia but also with marked proximal renal tubular dysfunction that included generalized aminoaciduria and glucosuria. The level of 1,25-dihydroxy D_3 was less than 4 pg/ml in this patient, and the 25-hydroxy D_3 level was normal. The patient was treated with 1α-hydroxy D_3, and despite levels of 1,25 that were in the high-normal range, hypophosphatemia and phosphaturia persisted (suggesting that 1,25 deficiency was not the sole pathogenic defect). Correction of the abnormal tubular reabsorption of phosphorus and hypophosphatemia followed very quickly removal of the tumor. It is possible that a proximal renal tubular defect may explain both the phosphaturia and the vitamin D metabolite deficiency, since conversion to 1,25-dihydroxy D_3 occurs in the proximal tubule. In a patient described by Sweet et al.,[193] correction of vitamin D concentrations and serum phosphorus following removal of a hemangiopericytoma occurred within 1 day and was essentially complete by 4 to 5 days.

Lyles et al.[194] emphasized that hypophosphatemic osteomalacia may be associated not only with mesenchymal tumors but also with prostatic carcinoma and endodermal malignancy. They described two patients with hypophosphatemia associated with metastatic prostatic carcinoma who had significant osteomalacia; this abnormality has not been described in prostatic cancer. They were unable to remove the metastatic tumor and effect cure of the clinical problem. On bone biopsy, there was unequivocal osteomalacia demonstrated by excessive osteoid covering trabecular bone surfaces and inadequate mineralization. The level of 1,25-dihydroxy D_3 was 15 pg/ml, and there was significant renal phosphate wasting. This association is worth pursuing further because of the frequency of prostatic carcinoma and the possibility that osteomalacia might be contributing to the bone pain in this disease. Frame and Parfitt[190] reviewed osteomalacia and described the increasing number of factors responsible, emphasizing the importance of more frequent bone biopsies with tetracycline labeling in evaluating these conditions. The pathogenesis of osteomalacia in relation to vitamin D deficiency is an area undergoing active investigation, and there is some evidence that 1,25-dihydroxy D_3 may not be the only important vitamin D metabolite for proper mineralization and bone healing. Some evidence has accumulated that 24,25-dihydroxy D_3 may also be important.

Atkinson et al.[195] presented an interesting patient with stage 4B Hodgkin's disease (nodular sclerosis) who had hypertrophic pulmonary osteoarthropathy that was completely reversed by chemotherapy, including evidence of periosteal new bone formation in the tibia. They reviewed 13 additional cases of Hodgkin's disease associated with similar findings. The majority were patients with advanced disease (stage 3B or 4), and mediastinal involvement was present in all. The mechanism remains obscure.

Goodman et al.[196] studied abnormal endocrine function in 18 patients with primary osteosarcoma. In 14, there were abnormal glucose, insulin, and GH responses during oral glucose tolerance tests; elevated somatomedin values were noted in 13. These abnormalities were not consistent over time in any one patient and are not necessarily correlated with the activity of the tumor. This may be a new paraneoplastic syndrome associated with mesodermal tumors.

Golde et al.[197] reviewed recent data concerning a variety of growth factors related to various cellular phenomena. In the sections of this review concerning hypoglycemia, the potential importance of somatomedins or insulin-like growth factors was emphasized. Two very important growth factors that were originally identified in male mouse submaxillary glands may be important in man. One is nerve growth factor, which appears to consist of three distinct subunits, the β subunit of which is biologically active and consists of a dimer of two identical polypeptides of 118 amino acids.[198] Human nerve growth factor has now been purified from human placental tissue,[199] and it has a distinct structural homology with insulin. Although it cannot substitute for insulin action, it appears to have important effects on the growth of nerve cells *in vitro* and *in vivo* and may also have important effects on tyrosine hydroxylase. Both nerve growth factor and its receptors have been found on human melanoma cells, but no definite relationship has been identified as yet between overproduction or deficiency of nerve growth factor and a human disease. Subsequent studies by radioimmunoassay may change this perspective. A second important growth factor also originally identified in mouse submaxillary tissue is a protein that causes early eyelid opening and incisor tooth eruption in animals that were used for the bioassay of nerve growth factor. This peptide (epidermal growth factor) was subsequently purified and shown to consist of 53 amino acids and its amino acid sequence has been determined.[125] Epidermal growth factor has been identified in human urine, and receptors have been identified in a number of target tissues including human cornea, fibroblasts, glial cells, and granulosa cells.[200] It has been an important agent in the study of down-regulation of peptides using radiolabeled peptide. Its possible relationship to human disease, including cancer, remains to be explored.

8.2.11. Ectopic Production of Tumors Associated with Diarrhea

8.2.11.1. Gastrointestinal Hormones

The syndromes associated with production of tumors by pancreatic islets have been well defined.[1,201] Pancreatic cholera, one of the most well-recognized syndromes, may be associated with a number of factors in addition to VIP, particularly pancreatic polypeptide (PP).[202] While secretin and cholecystokinin are important regulators of pancreatic exocrine function, there is little evidence that they account for much clinical disease. Glucagon-producing tumors have a well-defined syndrome and may be cured by tumor resection.[203] Gastrinoma and insulinoma syndromes will not be discussed here, having been reviewed earlier.[1]

Pancreatic cholera is also known as Verner–Morrison syndrome, WDHA (watery diarrhea, hypokalemia, and achlorhydria), WDHH (watery diarrhea, hypokalemia, and hypochlorhydria), diarrheagenic tumor, and VIPoma. VIP, discovered by Said and Mutt in 1970,[204] is a member of the secretin family and has secretin-like effects on the gastrointestinal tract, as well as inotropic and vasodilator type actions. Tumors causing pancreatic cholera often contain VIP, but not exclusively so. Extrapancreatic tumors of neural crest origin may also produce the syndrome, and thus the term "pancreatic cholera" may not always be appropriate.

The most prominent symptoms consist of very watery, massive diarrhea, often including explosive outbursts but relatively few cramps or increased peristaltic activity. There is frequently a high potassium and bicarbonate concentration in the stool. Two-thirds of the patients have basal achlorhydria and the rest normal acid production. Pentagastrin causes a minimal or no rise in gastric acid, although histamine causes more acid to be produced. Over 50% of these tumors are malignant, and if the tumor is untreated, there is a high mortality because of acidosis, dehydration, or renal failure. A significant number of patients have hypercalcemia for unknown reasons. Occasionally, hyperglycemia is also present, and both metabolic abnormalities will be relieved by removal of the tumors.[203,205]

The etiology appears to be multifactorial. VIP has probably been associated with more of these tumors than any other single agent, although many of the tumors contain more than one peptide or agent. Prostaglandins have also been noted to be elevated.[206,207] Some of the agents produced by these tumors may act locally (paracrine) rather than systemically as endocrine factors. VIP is related structurally to glucagon, secretin, and gastric inhibitory peptide. It contains 28 amino acids, the others containing 29 (glucagon), 27 (secretin) and 43 (GIP). Common pharmacologic features of these peptides include inhibition of gastric acid production and increased water and electrolyte release by the mucosa of the small bowel. Other substances may also have similar effects on gut secretion, and prostaglandins and CT specifically may be involved with production of diarrhea in certain patients with pancreatic as well as nonpancreatic tumors.

The diagnosis in patients with diarrhea requires ruling out laxative or diuretic abuse and confirmation that stool volumes in excess of 0.5 to 1 liter/day are maintained during fasting. Net secretion of water, sodium, and chloride can be documented in the jejunum, a finding that is very rare in diseases other than cholera or related syndromes. Measurement of VIP, if available, and other substances may be helpful. Current noninvasive diagnostic techniques facilitate the diagnosis of pancreatic tumors. There are some patients who have a pseudo-Verner–Morrison syndrome with normal levels of VIP and no pancreatic tumor, but there are also reports of improvement in the syndrome after partial or total pancreatic resection when no tumor could be identified. PP is not known to have any significant effect on intestinal secretion, but it is not infrequently present in the tumors of patients with pancreatic cholera and may be a useful marker.[207–209] Watery diarrhea may be mediated by different hormones in families having multiple endocrine neoplasia, the etiology varying in different members of the family.[202]

The exact physiologic role of PP has not been determined. The cell of origin of PP appears to be distinct from the α, β, and δ cells of the pancreas, and it is found not only in the islets of Langerhans but also in acinar tissue and duct epithelium. It has been shown that PP stimulates basal acid secretion from the stomach, but inhibits acid secretion stimulated by gastrin; that it inhibits pancreatic secretion stimulated by secretin and cholecystokinin; and that it relaxes the gallbladder while stimulating the biliary duct.[210] Postprandial increases in PP can be measured, but the factors responsible for this release are controversial. Vagotomy apparently abolishes the response of PP to a meal. Since vagal stimulation increases PP release, and it is diminished by atropine and stimulated by cholinomimetics, the hypothesis that the release of PP is vagal–cholinergic dependent seems likely. In addition, there is evidence that other hormones such as secretin might stimulate PP release.

The principal clinical interest in PP is that of a tumor marker for APUDomas of the pancreas and other tissues. Taylor et al.[209] studied PP concentrations in 41 patients with Zollinger–Ellison (ZE) syndrome and 100 control subjects. Four of the patients had PP concentrations greater than 240 pm/liter, but three control subjects did as well. In patients with ZE who had increased PP, evaluation of the tumor extracts showed high concentrations of gastrin as well as PP. Bloom et al.[211] recently studied PP concentrations in patients with gastrinomas and insulinomas and reported increased values in 26 and 22%, respectively, but they found elevated levels in 77% of patients with VIPomas. Larsson et al.[212] found elevated PP in three of four patients with the watery diarrhea syndrome, and three of the four tumors contained both PP and VIP cells. Of 18 APUDomas, 10 contained more than one cell type. It appears that PP is principally a tumor marker in patients with the watery diarrhea syndrome and otherwise is no more frequent a tumor marker than elevated concentrations of insulin, gastrin, or glucagon. There also appears to be a direct correlation of normal basal serum concentrations of PP with age, and this needs to be taken into consideration in relation to the tumor marker issue.

8.2.11.2. Glucagon-Producing Tumors

A distinctive syndrome in which there are increased levels of glucagon associated with α-cell tumors of the pancreas has been identified. Mallinson et al.[213] reported nine patients with pancreatic tumors who had a clinical complex consisting of diabetes mellitus, stomatitis, anemia, and a necrolytic migratory skin rash. In addition to the effects of glucagon on carbohydrate tolerance, it also has effects on the gastrointestinal tract; these include inhibition of gastric and pancreatic secretion, increased fluid production from the gut, and suppression of gastrin. More than 50 patients with the glucagonoma syndrome have now been reported. Higgins et al.[205] and Stacpoole[203] have reviewed the syndrome and all the cases reported up until that time. Reports of probable glucagonoma syndrome go back as far as 1942, but documentation of glucagon production has awaited the availability of the radioimmunoassay. The first documented report of excess glucagon production was actually by McGavran et al. in 1966.[214] In the review by Higgins et al.,[205] the age span of patients ranged from 20 to 73 years, with a mean age of 56, although many of the patients had had a long history of symptoms before diagnosis. A slight preponderance of females to males is recorded in the literature. Weight loss was recorded in more than half of the patients, and in many of the patients metastases were present at the time of diagnosis. The majority of tumors arose in the body and tail of the pancreas, were at least 3 cm in diameter, and had malignant characteristics. The distinctive skin lesion, necrolytic migratory erythema, led to the diagnosis in many of the cases. The characteristic lesion in the skin evolves over 7–14 days, the center of each erythematous macule or papule becoming paler, purpuric, blistering, and then becoming necrotic. If lesions are extensive, they may be mistaken for the "scalded skin syndrome." Crusting after oozing from the central erosion may occur, while the edge that is erythematous spreads peripherally. Crops of lesions or joining of lesions may occur in areas of friction. Skin lesions show focal parakeratoses, which are vesicles in the superficial epidermis with subcorneal separation. There may also be swollen, pale, vacuolated cells with pyknotic nuclei. In one-third of patients there was glossitis or stomatitis, and diabetes was present in the majority.

When plasma glucagon is studied, the major component is a molecule of 9000 to 20,000 daltons, in striking contrast to the 3500 daltons of normal glucagon.[1] Whether this is a precursor of glucagon is unknown. Decreased plasma amino acids that may be related to the rash[215] have been reported in a number of patients as well as a normocytic normochromic anemia in the majority. Ingemansson et al.[216] located these tumors by obtaining samples from various pancreatic veins through percutaneous catheterization. Samples obtained from the inferior vena cava or abdominal aorta were useful for preoperative diagnosis.

Stacpoole[203] has reviewed the glucagonoma syndrome and described a family with multiple endocrine neoplasia type I in which three members had pancreatic cell tumors. In his report, secretin directly stimulated secretion of glucagon by the tumor, and somatostatin caused hyperglycemia, presumably from inhibition of insulin secretion. The response to secretin was documented in vitro. These tumors, even when malignant, tend to be slow growing and may be treated effectively with streptozotocin. Diaminotriazenoimidazole carboximide (DITC) has been used successfully in a patient who showed no response to streptozotocin.

8.2.11.3. Somatostatin-Producing Tumors

Somatostatin, originally identified in the brain as a peptide responsible for inhibiting GH secretion, has been shown to be widely present throughout the gastrointestinal tract, particularly in the pancreatic islet.[211,217,218] Somatostatin production by tumors, particularly the pancreas, has been well documented. The so-called "somatostatinoma" syndrome has recently been reviewed by Krejs et al.[219] They described a 50-year-old patient with diabetes mellitus, steatorrhea, and cholelithiasis who had a tumor pressing on the duodenum. Plasma somatostatin in this patient varied from 9 to 13 ng/ml (normal = 0.088) and existed in several molecular forms. Somatostatin-like immunoreactivity (SLI) was present in the primary tumor, and there was also evidence that the plasma as well as the tumor contained increased quantities of CT as well. Five previous cases had been described, some being discovered accidentally at the time of cholecystectomy.[1]

In the patient described by Krejs et al.,[219] a preoperative diagnosis was made, and careful physiologic studies were performed. These studies indicated the following: The predominant elution profile of plasma SLI showed no bound SLI, but smaller forms in three peaks, the largest being that of free somatostatin itself. (It is known that plasma SLI is bound to components of very high molecular weight, although smaller amounts of free somatostatin can be found.) The former can be dissociated with acetic acid. The primary tumor contained concentrations of SLI between 1.2 and 5 μg/mg, these concentrations being markedly in excess of the normal pancreas. On immunofluorescent staining, there were some cells that contained both somatostatin and CT in the same secretory granules, although the majority of cells contained SLI activity and not CT. Preoperatively, a glucose tolerance test caused a fourfold stimulation in SLI (not normally increased by glucose), and there was no suppression of the rise of immunoreactive glucagon or C-peptide. Similarly, arginine infusion caused a rise in SLI. The response of GH secretion to hypoglycemia or arginine infusion was abolished. The release of TSH in response to TRH was not suppressed in this patient. β-Cell function in this patient was only moderately impaired, and the patient's basal glucagon secretion was not impaired.

Somatostatin is known to suppress the release of gastrin, cholecystokinin, secretin, gastric inhibitory peptide, and glucagon-like immunoreactivity; theoretically, this should cause hypochlorhydria, indigestion and fullness, eructation, abdominal pain and vomiting, poor digestion with diarrhea and steatorrhea, and susceptibility to cholelithiasis. In the six reported cases five had malignant disease with metastases to the liver at the time of diagnosis, and three of the patients died shortly after surgery. Only the patient with benign disease[220] appears to have been cured. It was emphasized by Krejs et al.[219] that early diagnosis was difficult. Administration of a potent stimulator of pancreatic release of SLI such as tolbutamide may be necessary, and the classical triad of features, dyspepsia, mild diabetes, and cholelithiasis, are rather common and nonspecific findings. Clearly, measurement of SLI in plasma is important and essential for early diagnosis. With the development of highly sensitive noninvasive diagnostic methods, such as computerized axial tomography and ultrasound, these tumors should be easier to identify in the future.

Somatostatin content in pancreatic endocrine tumors was evaluated by Bloom et al.,[207] who examined 28 pancreatic tumors, incuding 5 of neural origin and 23 pancreatic endocrine tumors. All tumors contained extractable SLI activity that diluted in parallel with the standard curve. Gastrinomas contained considerable quantities of somatostatin while VIPomas contained relatively small amounts. None of these tumors contained predominantly somatostatin. These studies emphasize the point that most pancreatic endocrine tumors contain a mixed population of cells.

The production of SLI by pancreatic islet cell tumors is eutopic; Szabo et al.[221] have described the ectopic production of this hormone by small cell carcinoma of the lung. They examined 11 cultures of human pulmonary small cell carcinoma, and 8 were demonstrated to secrete quantities of SLI varying from 0.07 to 27 ng/ml of culture medium over 4 days. SLI was also identified in an extract of one of three small cell carcinomas obtained at autopsy. The characteristics of one of the cell line-produced proteins was evaluated in detail. The peptide released was entirely parallel to synthetic somatostatin in the radioimmunoassay and revealed multiple molecular forms, the largest being about 12,000 daltons. The low-molecular-weight form coeluted with synthetic hormone, while the high-molecular-weight form in cultures had a much longer half-life and was biologically active. The material released from lysed cells or after 1-hr incubation consisted predominantly of monomeric peptide. Thus, somatostatin was well documented in cells presumably derived from APUD-type tumor cells. These same authors have identified SLI in a number of carcinoid tumors, which are histologically related. It is believed that the high-molecular-weight forms of SLI seen in these studies are probably precursors, since there is evidence to support the presence of higher-molecular-weight biosynthetic precursors. Their virtual absence within cell lysates, however, suggests that they may be converted very rapidly to somatostatin monomer in the cells. Furthermore, they do not change in size in the presence of dissociating or reducing conditions, indicating that they do not result from noncovalent aggregation or disulfide interchange. There is no evidence as yet that the production of somatostatin by small cell carcinoma leads to the clinical manifestations described above for the pancreatic somatostatinoma; nonetheless, SLI in serum could potentially be most useful as a tumor marker.

Another patient with somatostatinoma was reported by Pipeleers *et al.*[220] Somatostatin was increased 40-fold in an insulin-treated diabetic with disseminated pancreatic carcinoma. Of interest was the fact that 75% of the plasma SLI was 67,000 daltons and 25% was monomer, while the increased urinary fraction was almost exclusively of higher molecular weight. The increase in somatostatin was associated with reduced basal and stimulated pancreatic hormone levels. Plasma SLI increased 50% following insulin withdrawal and tenfold after tolbutamide, as well as falling 30% after diazoxide. In this patient, insulin-induced hypoglycemia was not associated with increased glucagon and PP, and a protein meal did not elevate PP. During arginine infusion, plasma glucagon increased only slowly. After injection of tolbutamide, peripheral C-peptide increased twofold, but there was no decrease in plasma glucose. Plasma SLI increased progressively, reaching almost ten times the control values. No such increase was observed with tolbutamide in normal subjects or insulin-treated diabetics. Diazoxide caused a fall of 30% in SLI in 15 min; this lasted for 24 hr. This patient was treated successfully with streptozotocin.

Somatostatin has also recently been identified in the cytotrophoblast of the early human placenta, not the syncytiotrophoblast, which contains placental lactogen and hCG.[222] There is no evidence that it affects secretion of these hormones *in vitro*, but its presence inside the trophoblast may imply some physiologic role.[223]

Analogs of somatostatin have been used clinically in attempts to inhibit some of the clinical manifestations of various secreting pancreatic tumors because of the known effect of somatostatin to inhibit secretion of these peptides normally.[224] Specifically, this approach was used to suppress the secretion of insulin, glucagon, and gastrin by tumors known to produce these peptides. These tumors are often metastatic when first identified, and the use of the analogs of somatostatin may prove of clinical benefit. It has also been used to inhibit diarrhea in the carcinoid syndrome.[225,226]

8.2.12. Disorders Due to Ectopic Erythropoietin Production

The development of a highly sensitive radioimmunoassay for the hormone in human blood should allow its application to patients with a variety of neoplastic and other disorders.[227] Production of erythropoietin by renal tumors is not thought to be ectopic in nature, but whether hormone production in other organs such as the liver (which may be a source of normal hormone production) or cerebellum is ectopic is not certain. Anagnostou et al.[228] reported an interesting young woman who had several recurrences of a cerebellar hemangioblastoma. Elevated plasma erythropoietin levels were found, and these became normal after resection of the tumor. Hormone concentrations were also found to be high in a saline extract of the tumor. These studies were done by bioassay not radioimmunoassay. Erslev et al.[229] used a bioassay technique that involved concentrating plasma from patients who required phlebotomy for primary or secondary polycythemia. Levels were 5 mU/ml in all patients with primary polycythemia. In a variety of other patients with secondary polycythemia, including patients with tumors, the levels were up to 3000 mU/ml. Normal subjects were between 5 and 18. By radioimmunoassay,[230] values in normal subjects were 0.25 ng/ml, in anemic subjects up to 16 ng/ml. Further work on serum and tumors needs to be performed.

8.2.13. Ectopic Production of Renin

Further studies of renin produced by tumors have been hampered by incomplete information on the biosynthesis of renin in the kidney and other tissues and by the presence of inactive renin in the plasma, the latter being highly labile.[231,232] The active enzyme has been quantitated principally by the generation from substrate of its product angiotensin I. From studies of renal renin, the molecular weight appears to be approximately 40,000, while less-active higher-molecular-weight forms can be extracted from the kidney of several species.[233] By cell-free synthesis, Poulsen et al.[234] identified preprorenin as a 50,000-dalton protein in the mouse submaxillary gland. This suggests that there is a precursor form of renin, at least in extrarenal sites. Higher-molecular-weight forms of renin have also been purified from hog kidney, consisting of forms with molecular weights of 140,000 and 60,000 with only minimal enzymatic activity.[231,235] Whether these represent precursor forms or binding to a larger protein is not clear. Further studies of the biosynthesis and isolation of specific mRNA are necessary in order to clarify these issues. Because renin is still present in the plasma of anephric patients, it will be necessary to do substantial further work before one is able to determine its status in tumors.

8.2.14. Ectopic Production of Other Proteins by Tumors

As described above, and in the studies of Rosen *et al.*[236] in many human tumor cell lines, widespread production of polypeptide hormones by tumor has been extraordinarily well documented. Likewise, a variety of immune disorders have been associated with the production of tumor antigens and appropriate immune responses.[1] It is highly likely that future studies will produce even more data suggesting that specific clinical or biochemical syndromes associated with cancer are due to proteins that are produced by the tumors themselves. More problematic is the cause(s) of this phenomenon, but the tremendous advances in molecular biology coupled with an intense interest in tumor cells *in vitro* should assist in resolving the remaining mysteries.

Acknowledgment

The author wishes to express his gratitude and appreciation to Ms. Luciana Lesch for her excellent assistance in the preparation of the manuscript.

References

1. Sherwood, L. M., 1979, Ectopic hormone syndromes, in: *Contemporary Endocrinology*, Volume 1 (S. H. Ingbar, ed.), pp. 341–386, Plenum Medical, New York.
2. Odell, W. D., and Wolfsen, A. R., 1980, Hormones from tumors: Are they ubiquitous?, *Am. J. Med.* **68:**317–318.
3. Krieger, D. T., and Martin, J. B., 1981, Brain peptides, *N. Engl. J. Med.* **304:**876–885, 944–951.
4. Roth, J., LeRoith, D., Shiwach, J., Rosenweig, J. L., Lesniak, M. A., and Havrankova, J., 1982, The evolutionary origins of hormones, neurotransmitters, and other extracellular–chemical messengers: Implications for mammalian biology, *N. Engl. J. Med.* **306:**523–527.
5. Sherwood, L. M., 1976, Ectopic hormone syndromes, in: *The Year in Endocrinology 1975–1976* (S. H. Ingbar, ed.), pp. 249–276, Plenum Medical, New York.
6. Baylin, S. B., and Mendelsohn, G., 1980, Ectopic (inappropriate) hormone production by tumors, mechanisms involved and the biological and clinical implications, *Endocr. Rev.* **1:**45–235.

7. Zimmerman, M., Mumford, R. A., and Steiner, D. P. (eds.), 1980, *Precursor Processing in the Biosynthesis of Proteins, Ann. N.Y. Acad. Sci.* **343**:1–449.

8. Eipper, B. A., and Mains, R. E., 1980, Structure and biosynthesis of proadrenocorticotropinendorphin and related peptides, *Endocr. Rev.* **1**:1–27.

9. Quensenberry, P. and Levitt, L., 1979, Hematopoietic stem cells, *N. Engl. J. Med.* **301**:755–760, 819–823, 868–872.

10. Odell, W., Wolfsen, A., Yoshimoto, Y., Weitzman, R., Fisher, D., and Hirose, F., 1977, Ectopic peptide synthesis: A universal concomitant of neoplasia, *Trans. Assoc. Am. Physicians* **90**:204–227.

11. Baylin, S. B., Mendelsohn, G., Weisburger, W. R., Gann, D. S., and Eggleston, J. C., 1979, Levels of histaminase and L-dopa decarboxylase activity in the transition from C-cell hyperplasia to familial medullary thyroid carcinoma, *Cancer* **44**:1315–1321.

12. Abeloff, M. D., Eggleston, J. C., Mendelsohn, G., Ettinger, D. S., and Baylin, S. B., 1979, Changes in morphologic and biochemical characteristics of small cell carcinoma of the lung—A clinicopathologic study, *Am. J. Med.* **66**:757–764.

13. Abelev, G. I., 1974, α-Fetoprotein as a marker of embryo-specific differentiation in normal and tumor tissues, *Transplant. Rev.* **20**:3–37.

14. Kurman, R. J., Scardino, P. T., McIntire, K. R., Waldmann, T. A., and Javadpour, N., 1977, Cellular localization of alpha-fetoprotein and human chorionic gonadotropin in germ cell tumors of the testis using an indirect immunoperoxidase technique, *Cancer* **40**:2136–2151.

15. Bonikos, D. S., and Bensch, K. G., 1977, Endocrine cells of bronchial and bronchiolar epithelium, *Am. J. Med.* **63**:765–771.

16. Berger, C. L., Goodwin, G., Mendelsohn, G., Eggleston, J. C., Abeloff, M. D., Aisner, S., and Baylin, S. B., 1981, Endocrine-related biochemistry in the spectrum of human lung carcinoma, *J. Clin. Endocrinol. Metab.* **53**:422–429.

17. Kahn, C. R., Rosen, S. W., Weintraub, B. D., Fajans, S. S., and Gurdon, P., 1977, Ectopic production of chorionic gonadotropin and its subunits by islet-cell tumors, *N. Engl. J. Med.* **297**:565–569.

18. Brown, D. D., 1981, Gene expression in eukaryotes, *Science* **211**:667–674.

19. Mains, R. E., and Eipper, B. A., 1976, Biosynthesis of the adrenocorticotropic hormone in mouse pituitary tumor cells, *J. Biol. Chem.* **251**:4115–4120.

20. Roberts, J. L., and Herbert, E., 1977, Characterization of a common precursor to corticotropin and β-lipotropin peptides and their arrangement relative to corticotropin in the precursor synthesized in a cell-free system, *Proc. Natl. Acad. Sci. USA* **74**:5300–5304.

21. Nakanishi, S., Inoue, A., Kita, T., Nakamura, M., Chang, A. C. Y., Cohen, S. N., and Numa, S., 1979, Nucleotide sequence for bovine corticotropin-beta-lipotropin precursor, *Nature* **278**:423–427.

22. Bertagna, X. Y., Nicholson, W. E., Sorenson, G. D., Pettengill, O. S., Mount, C. D., and Orth, D. N., 1978, Corticotropin, lipotropin and β-endorphin production by a human nonpituitary tumor in culture: Evidence for a common precursor, *Proc. Natl. Acad. Sci. USA* **75**:5160–5164.

23. Orth, D. N., Guillemin, R., Ling, N., and Nicholson, W. E., 1978, Immunoreactive endorphins, lipotropins, and corticotropins in a human non-

pituitary tumor: Evidence for a common precursor, *J. Clin. Endocrinol. Metab.* **46:**849–852.

24. Gewirtz, G., and Yalow, R. S., 1974, Ectopic ACTH production in carcinoma of the lung, *J. Clin. Invest.* **53:**1022–1032.

25. Odell, W. D., Wolfsen, A. R., Bachelot, I., and Hirose, F., 1979, Ectopic production of lipotropin by cancer, *Am. J. Med.* **66:**631–638.

26. Wolfsen, A. R., and Odell, W. D., 1979, ProACTH: Use for early detection of lung cancer, *Am. J. Med.* **66:**765–772.

27. Hashimoto, K., Takahara, J., Ogawa, N., Yunoki, S., Ofuji, T., Arata, A., Kanda, S., and Terada, K., 1980, Adrenocorticotropin, beta-lipotropin, beta-endorphin and corticotropin-releasing factor-like activity in an adrenocorticotropin-producing nephroblastoma, *J. Clin. Endocrinol. Metab.* **50:**461–465.

28. Gomi, K., Kameya, T., Tsumuraya, M., Shimosato, Y., Zexe, F., Abe, K., and Yoneyama, T., 1976, Ultrastructural, histochemical and biochemical studies of two cases with amylase, ACTH, and beta-MSH producing tumor, *Cancer* **38:**1645–1654.

29. Chin, W. W., 1981, Medullary thyroid carcinoma identified by cell-free translation of tumor messenger ribonucleic acid in a patient with a neck mass and the syndrome of ectopic adrenocorticotropin, *J. Clin. Endocrinol. Metab.* **52:**572–575.

30. Matsuyama, M., Inoue, T., Ariyoshi, Y., Doi, M., Suchi, T., Sato, T., Tashiro, K., and Chiara, T., 1979, Argyrophil cell carcinoma of the uterine cervix with ectopic production of ACTH, beta-MSH, serotonin, histamine and amylase, *Cancer* **44:**1813–1823.

31. Forman, B. H., 1979, ACTH-secreting pheochromocytoma, *N. Engl. J. Med.* **301:**1399.

32. Forman, B. H., Marban, E., Kayne, R. D., Passarelli, N. M., Bobrow, S. N., Livolsi, V. A., Merino, M., Minor, M., and Farber, L. R., 1979, Ectopic ACTH syndrome due to pheochromocytoma: Case report and review of the literature, *Yale J. Biol. Med.* **52:**181–189.

33. Ganguly, A., Henry, D. P., Yune, K. Y., Pratt, J. H., Grim, C. E., Donohue, J. P., and Weinberger, M. H., 1979, Diagnosis and localization of pheochromocytoma: Detection by measurement of urinary norepinephrine excretion during sleep, plasma norepinephrine concentration and computerized axial tomography (CT-scan), *Am. J. Med.* **67:**21–26.

34. Spark, R. F., Connolly, P. B., Gluckin, D. S., White, R., Sacks, B., and Landsberg, L., 1979, ACTH secretion from a functioning pheochromocytoma, *N. Engl. J. Med.* **301:**416–418.

35. Cohle, S. D., Tschen, J. A., Smith, F. E., Lane, M., and McGavran, M. H., 1979, ACTH-secreting carcinoma of the breast, *Cancer* **43:**2370–2376.

36. Molland, E. A., 1978, Prostatic adenocarcinoma with ectopic ACTH production, *Br. J. Urol.* **50:**358.

37. Amano, S., Hazama, F., Haebara, H., Tsurusawa, M., and Kaito, H., 1978, Ectopic ACTH-MSH producing carcinoid tumor with multiple endocrine hyperplasia in a child, *Acta Pathol. Jpn.* **28:**721–730.

38. Rodgers-Sullivan, R. F., Weiland, L. H., Palumbo, P. J., and Hepper, N. G. G., 1978, Pulmonary tumorlets associated with Cushing's syndrome, *Am. Rev. Respir. Dis.* **117:**799–806.
39. Rosenberg, E. M., Hahn, T. J., Orth, D. N., Deftos, L. J., and Tanaka, K., 1978, ACTH secreting medullary carcinoma of the thyroid presenting as severe idiopathic osteoporosis and senile purpura, *J. Clin. Endocrinol. Metab.* **47:**255–262.
40. Drasin, G. F., Lynch, T., and Temes, G. P., 1978, Ectopic ACTH production and mediastinal lipomatosis, *Radiology* **127:**610.
41. Findling, J. W., Aron, D. C., Tyrrell, J. B., Shinsako, J. H., Fitzgerald, P. A., Norman, D., Wilson, C. B., and Forsham, P. H., 1981, Selective venous sampling for ACTH in Cushing's syndrome, *Ann. Intern. Med.* **94:**647–652.
42. Singer, W., Kovacs, K., Ryan, N., and Horvath, E., 1978, Ectopic ACTH syndrome: Clinicopathological correlations, *J. Clin. Pathol.* **31:**591–598.
43. Gold, E. M., 1979, The Cushing syndrome: Changing views of diagnosis and treatment, *Ann. Intern. Med.* **90:**829–844.
44. Kammer, H., and Barter, M., 1979, Spontaneous remission of Cushing's disease: A case report and review of the literature, *Am. J. Med.* **67:**519–523.
45. Bochner, F., Burke, C. J., Lloyd, H. M., and Nurnberg, B. E., 1979, Intermittent Cushing's disease, *Am. J. Med.* **67:**507–510.
46. Crapo, L., 1979, Cushing's syndrome: A review of diagnostic tests, *Metabolism* **28:**955–977.
47. Luton, J. P., Mahoudeau, J. A., Bouchard, P. H., Thieblot, P. H., Hautecouverture, M., Simon, D., Laudat, M. H., Touitou, Y., and Bricaire, H., 1979, Treatment of Cushing's disease with o,p′DDD: Survey of 62 cases, *N. Engl. J. Med.* **300:**459–464.
48. Cooper, P. R., and Shucart, W. A., 1979, Treatment of Cushing's disease with o,p′DDD, *N. Engl. J. Med.* **301:**48–49.
49. Orth, D. N., 1978, Metyrapone is useful only as adjunctive therapy in Cushing's disease, *Ann. Intern. Med.* **89:**128–130.
50. Jeffcoate, W. J., Rees, L. H., Lowry, P. J., and Besser, G. M., 1978, A specific radioimmunoassay for human β-lipotropin, *J. Clin. Endocrinol. Metab.* **47:**160–167.
51. Mendelsohn, G., D'Agostino, R., Eggleston, J. C., and Baylin, S. B., 1979, Distribution of β-endorphin immunoreactivity in normal human pituitary, *J. Clin. Invest.* **63:**1297–1301.
52. Guillemin, R. T., Vargo, M., Rossi, R. J., Minick, F., Ling, N., Riviera, C., Vale, W., and Bloom, F., 1977, Beta endorphin and adrenocorticotropin are secreted concomitantly by the pituitary gland, *Science* **197:**1367–1369.
53. Tanaka, K., Nicholson, W. E., and Orth, D. N., 1978, The nature of the immunoreactive lipotropin in human plasma and tissue extracts, *J. Clin. Invest.* **62:**94–104.
54. Deftos, L. J., Burton, D., Catherwood, B. D., Bone, H. G., Parthemore, J. G., Guillemin, R., Watkins, W. B., and Moore, R. Y., 1978, Demonstration by immunoperoxidase histochemistry of calcitonin in the anterior lobe of the rat pituitary, *J. Clin. Endocrinol. Metab.* **47:**457–458.

55. Xavier, Y. B., Nicholson, W. E., Pettengill, O. S., Sorenson, G. D., Mount, C. D., and Orth, D. N., 1978, Ectopic production of high molecular weight calcitonin and corticotropin by human small cell carcinoma cells in tissue culture: Evidence for separate precursors, *J. Clin. Endocrinol. Metab.* **47:**1390–1393.
56. Ueda, M., Takeuchi, T., Abe, K., Miyakawa, S., Ohnami, S., and Yanaihara, N., 1980, Beta-melanocyte-stimulating hormone immunoreactivity in human pituitaries and ectopic adrenocorticotropin-producing tumors, *J. Clin. Endocrinol. Metab.* **50:**550–556.
57. Liotta, A. S., Suda, T., and Krieger, D. T., 1978, Beta-lipotropin is the major opioid-like peptide of human pituitary and rat pars distalis: Lack of significant beta endorphin, *Proc. Natl. Acad. Sci. USA* **75:**2590–2954.
58. Suda, T., Liotta, A. S., and Krieger, D. T., 1978, Beta endorphin is not detectable in plasma from normal human subjects, *Science* **202:**221–223.
59. Suda, T., Abe, Y., Demura, H., Demura, R., Shizume, K., Tamahashi, N., and Sasano, N., 1979, ACTH beta-LPH and beta-endorphin in pituitary adenomas of the patients with Cushing's disease: Activation of beta-LPH conversion to beta-endorphin, *J. Clin. Endocrinol. Metab.* **49:**475–477.
60. Wiedemann, E., Saito, T., Linfoot, J. A., and Li, C. H., 1979, Specific radioimmunoassay of human beta-endorphin in unextracted plasma, *J. Clin. Endocrinol. Metab.* **49:**478–480.
61. Pullan, P. T., Clement-Jones, V., Corder, R., Lowry, P. J., Rees, G. M., Rees, L. H., Besser, G. M., Macedo, M. M., and Galvao-Telles, A., 1980, Ectopic production of methionine enkephalin and beta-endorphin, *Br. Med. J.* **1:**758–759.
62. Bertagna, X. Y., Stone, W. J., Nicholson, W. E., Mount, C. D., and Orth, D. N., 1981, Simultaneous assay of immunoreactive β-lipotropin, α-lipotropin and β-endorphin in plasma of normal human subjects, patients with ACTH/lipotropin hypersecretory syndromes and patients undergoing chronic hemodialysis, *J. Clin. Invest.* **67:**124–133.
63. Pullan, P. T., Clement-Jones, V., Corder, R., Lowry, P. J., Besser, G. M., and Rees, L. H., 1980, ACTH, LPH and related peptides in the ectopic ACTH syndrome, *Clin. Endocrinol.* **13:**437–445.
64. Clement-Jones, V., Corder, R., and Lowry, P. J., 1980, Isolation of human Met-enkephalin and two groups of putative precursors (2K-pro-met-enkephalin) from an adrenal medullary tumor, *Biochem. Biophys. Res. Commun.* **95:**665–672.
65. Grossman, A., Besser, G. M., Milles, J. J., and Baylis, P. H., 1980, Inhibition of vasopressin release in man by an opiate peptide, *Lancet* **2:**1108–1110.
66. Matsuoka, H., Mulrow, P. J., and Li, C. H., 1980, β-Lipotropin: A new aldosterone-stimulating factor, *Science* **209:**307–309.
67. McCloy, J., and McCloy, R. F., 1979, Enkephalins, hunger and obesity, *Lancet* **2:**156.
68. Margules, D. L., Moisset, B., Lewis, M. J., Shibuya, H., and Pert, C. B., 1978, Beta-endorphin is associated with overeating in genetically obese mice (*ob/ob*) and rats (*fa/fa*), *Science* **202:**988–991.

69. Holaday, J. W., O'Hara, M., and Faden, A. I., 1981, Hypophysectomy alters cardiovascular variables: Central effects of pituitary endorphins in shock, *Am. J. Physiol.* **241:**479–485.

70. Carr, D. B., Bullen, B. A., Skrinar, G. S., Arnold, M. A., Rosenblatt, M., Beitins, I. Z., Martin, J. B., and McArthur, J., 1981, Physical conditioning facilitates the exercise induced secretion of beta-endorphin and beta lipotropin in women, *N. Engl. J. Med.* **305:**560–563.

71. Davis, G. G., Buchsbaum, S., and Bunney, W. E., Jr., 1981, Opiates, opioid peptides and psychiatry, *Ann. N.Y. Acad. Sci.* **362:**67–75.

72. Saeed, U. Z., Zafar, M., Mellinger, R. C., Fine, G., Szabo, M., and Frohman, L., 1979, Acromegaly associated with a bronchial carcinoid tumor: Evidence for ectopic production of growth hormone releasing activity, *J. Clin. Endocrinol. Metab.* **48:**66–71.

73. Frohman, L. A., Szabo, M., Berelowitz, M., and Stachura, M., 1980, Partial purification and characterization of a peptide with growth hormone-releasing activity from extrapituitary tumors in patients with acromegaly, *J. Clin. Invest.* **65:**43–54.

74. Clemens, D. R., Van Wyk, J. J., Ridgway, E. C., Kliman, B., Kjellberg, R. N., and Underwood, L. E., 1979, Evaluation of acromegaly by radioimmunoassay of somatomedin-C, *N. Engl. J. Med.* **301:**1138–1142.

75. Daughaday, W. H., 1979, New criteria for evaluation of acromegaly, *N. Engl. J. Med.* **301:**1175–1176.

76. Bala, R. M., and Bhaumick, B., 1979, Radioimmunoassay of a basic somatomedin: Comparison of various assay techniques and somatomedin levels in various sera, *J. Clin. Endocrinol. Metab.* **49:**770–777.

77. Horner, J. M., and Hintz, R. L., 1979, Further comparisons of the [125I]somatomedin A and the [125I]somatomedin C radioreceptor assays of somatomedin peptide, *J. Clin. Endocrinol. Metab.* **48:**959–963.

78. Phillips, L. S., and Vassilopouloul-Sellin, R., 1980, Somatomedins, *N. Engl. J. Med.* **302:**371–380.

79. Kaganowicz, A., Farkouh, N. H., Frantz, A. G., and Blaustein, A. U., 1979, Ectopic human growth hormone in ovaries and breast cancer, *J. Clin. Endocrinol. Metab.* **48:**5–8.

80. Braunstein, G. D., Kamdar, V., Rasor, J., Swaminathan, N., and Wade, M. E., 1979, Widespread distribution of a chorionic gonadotropin-like substance in normal human tissues, *J. Clin. Endocrinol. Metab.* **49:**917–925.

81. Braunstein, G. D., Rasor, J., and Wade, M. E., 1975, Presence in normal human testes of a chorionic-gonadotrophin-like substance distinct from human luteinizing hormone, *N. Engl. J. Med.* **293:**1339–1343.

82. Yoshimoto, Y., Wolfsen, A. R., and Odell, W. D., 1979, Glycosylation, a variable in the production of hCG by cancers, *Am. J. Med.* **67:**414–420.

83. Chen, H. C., Hodgen, G. D., Matsuura, S., Lin, J. L., Gross, E., Reichert, L. E., Birken, S., Canfield, R. E., and Ross, G. T., 1976, Evidence for gonadotropin from nonpregnant subjects that has physical, immunological and biological similarities to human chorionic gonadotropin, *Proc. Natl. Acad. Sci. USA* **73:**2885–2889.

84. Borkowski, A., and Muquardt, C., 1979, Human chorionic gonadotropin in the plasma of normal, nonpregnant subjects, *N. Engl. J. Med.* **301**:298–302.

85. Braunstein, G. D., 1979, Human chorionic gonadotropin in nontrophoblastic tumors and tissues, in: *Recent Advances in Reproduction and Regulation of Fertility* (G. P. Talwar, ed.), pp. 389–397, Elsevier, Amsterdam.

86. Braunstein, G., Rasor, J., Thompson, R., Van Scoy-Mosher, M., and Wade, M. D., 1981, Prospective evaluation of serum chorionic gonadotrophin measurements for the immunodiagnosis of cancer, *Clin. Res.* **29**:90–98.

87. Braunstein, G. D., Rasor, J., and Wade, M. E., 1980, Presence of an HCG-like substance in non-pregnant humans, in: *Chorionic Gonadotropin* (S. J. Segal, ed.), pp. 303–409, Plenum Press, New York.

88. Hattori, M., Fukase, M., Yoshimi, H., Matsukura, S., and Imura, H., 1978, Ectopic production of human chorionic gonadotropin in malignant tumors, *Cancer* **42**:2328–2333.

89. Papapetrou, P. D., Sakarelov, N. P., Braouzi, H., and Fessas, P. H., 1980, Ectopic production of human chorionic gonadotropin by neoplasm, *Cancer* **45**:2583–2592.

90. Weymann, R. E., and Nisula, B. C., 1979, Renal clearance rates of the subunits of human chorionic gonadotropin in man, *J. Clin. Endocrinol. Metab.* **49**:674–679.

91. Goldenberg, D. M., Kim, E. E., DeLand, F. H., Van Nagell, J. R., and Javadpour, N., 1980, Clinical radioimmunodetection of cancer with radioactive antibodies to human chorionic gonadotropin, *Science* **208**:1284–1286.

92. Goldenberg, D. M., DeLand, F., Kim, E., Bennett, S., Pririus, F. J., Van Nagell, J. R., Estes, N., De Simone, P., and Rayburn, P., 1978, Use of radiolabelled antibodies to carcinoembryonic antigen for the detection and localization of diverse cancers by external photoscanning, *N. Engl. J. Med.* **298**:1384–1388.

93. Metz, S. A., Weintraub, B., Rosen, S. W., Singer, J., and Robertson, R. P., 1978, Ectopic secretion of chorionic gonadotropin by a lung carcinoma, *Am. J. Med.* **65**:325–333.

94. Swaminathan, N., and Braunstein, G. D., 1978, Location of major antigen sites of the β-subunit of human chorionic gonadotropin, *Biochemistry* **17**:5832–5838.

95. Ghai, R. D., Mise, T., Pandian, M. R., and Bahl, J. P., 1980, Immunological properties of the β-subunit of human chorionic gonadotropin. I. Effect of chemical and enzymatic modifications, *Endocrinology* **107**:1556–1558.

96. Matsumura, S., Ohashi, M., Chen, H-C., and Hodgen, G. D., 1979, A human chorionic gonadotropin-specific antiserum against synthetic peptide analogs to the carboxyl-terminal peptide for its beta-subunit, *Endocrinology* **104**:396–401.

97. Bielinska, M., and Boime, I., 1978, mRNA-dependent synthesis of a glycosylated subunit of hCG in cell-free extracts derived from the ascites tumor cells, *Proc. Natl. Acad. Sci. USA* **75**:1768–1772.

98. Birken, S., and Canfield, R. E., 1978, Structural and immunochemical properties of human choriogonadotropin, in: *Structure and Function of the Gonadotropins* (K. W. McKerns, ed.), pp. 47–60, Plenum Press, New York.

99. Boime, I., Landefeld, T., McQueen, S., and McWilliams, D., 1978, The biosynthesis of chorionic gonadotropin and placental lactogen in first- and third-trimester human placenta, in: *Structure and Function of the Gonadotropins* (K. W. McKerns, ed.), pp. 235–257, Plenum Press, New York.

100. Benveniste, R., Conway, M. C., Puett, D., and Rabinowitz, D., 1979, Heterogeneity of the human chorionic gonadotropin alpha subunit secreted by cultured choriocarcinoma (JEG) cells, *J. Clin. Endocrinol. Metab.* **48:**85–91.

101. Benveniste, R., Lindner, J., Puett, D., and Rabin, D., 1979, Human chorionic gonadotropin alpha subunit from cultured choriocarcinoma (JEG) cells: Comparison of the subunit secreted free with that prepared from secreted human chorionic gonadotropin, *Endocrinology* **105:**581–587.

102. Dean, D. J., Weintraub, B. D., and Rosen, S. W., 1980, *De novo* synthesis and secretion of heterogeneous forms of human chorionic gonadotropin and its free alpha-subunit in the human choriocarcinoma clonal cell line JEG-3, *Endocrinology* **106:**849–858.

103. Quigley, M. M., Tyrey, L., and Hammond, C. B., 1980, Alpha-subunit in sera of choriocarcinoma patients in remission, *J. Clin, Endocrinol. Metab.* **50:**98–102.

104. Kanabus, J., Braunstein, G. D., Emry, P. K., DiSaia, P. H., and Wade, M. E., 1978, Kinetics of growth and ectopic production of human chorionic gonadotropin by an ovarian cystadenocarcinoma cell line maintained *in vitro, Cancer Res.* **38:**765–770.

105. Tralka, T. S., Rosen, S. W., Weintraub, B. D., Lieblich, J. M., Engel, L. W., Wetzel, B. K., Kingsbury, E. W., and Rabson, A. S., 1979, Ultrastructural concomitants of sodium butyrate-enhanced ectopic production of chorionic gonadotropin and its alpha subunit in human bronchogenic carcionoma (ChaGo) cells, *J. Natl. Cancer Inst.* **62:**45–61.

106. Amir, S. M., Sullivan, R. C., and Ingbar, S. H., 1980, In vitro response to crude and purified HCG in human thyroid membranes, *J. Clin. Endocrinol. Metab.* **51:**51–58.

107. Pekonen, F., and Weintraub, B. D., 1978, Thyrotropin binding to cultured lymphocytes and thyroid cells, *Endocrinology* **103:**1668–1677.

108. Pekonen, F., and Weintraub, B. D., 1980, Interaction of crude and pure chorionic gonadotropin with the thyrotropin receptor, *J. Clin. Endocrinol. Metab.* **50:**280–285.

109. Higgins, H. P., and Hirschman, J. M., 1978, The hyperthyroidism due to trophoblastic hormone, *Clin. Endocrinol. Metab.* **7:**167–175.

110. Harada, A., and Hirschman, J. M., 1978, Extraction of human chorionic thyrotropin from term placentas: Failure to recover thyrotropic activity, *J. Clin. Endocrinol. Metab.* **47:**681–685.

111. Kourides, I., Weintraub, B. D., and Maloof, F., 1978, Large molecular weight TSH-β in certain human sera, *J. Clin,. Endocrinol. Metab.* **47:**24–33.

112. Spitz, M., LeRoth, D., Hirsch, H., Carayon, P., Pekonen, F., Liel, Y., Sobel, R., Chorer, Z., and Weintraub, B., 1981, Increased high-molecular-weight thyrotropin with impaired biologic activity in a euthyroid man, *N. Engl. J. Med.* **304:**278–282.

113. Robertson, G. L., 1977, The regulation of vasopressin in function in health and disease, *Recent Prog. Horm. Res.* **33:**333–385.

114. Kondo, Y., Mizumoto, Y., Katayaman, S., Murase, T., Yamaji, T., Ohsawa, N., and Kosaka, K., 1981, Inappropriate secretion of antidiuretic hormone in nude mice bearing a human bronchogenic oat-cell carcinoma, *Cancer Res.* **41**:1545–1548.

115. Morton, J. J., Kelly, P., and Padfield, P. L., 1978, Antidiuretic hormone and bronchogenic carcinoma, *Clin. Endocrinol.* **9**:357–370.

116. Padfield, P. L., Morton, J. J., Brown, J. J., Lever, A. F., Robertson, J. I. S., Wood, H., and Fox, R., 1976, Plasma arginine vasopressin in the syndrome of antidiuretic hormone excess associated with bronchogenic carcinoma, *Am. J. Med.* **61**:825–831.

117. Perks, W. H., Crow, J. C., and Green, M., 1978, Mesothelioma associated with the syndrome of inappropriate secretion of antidiuretic hormone, *Am. Rev. Respir. Dis.* **117**:789–794.

118. Perks, W. H., Stanhope, R., and Green, M., 1979, Hyponatremia and mesothelioma, *Br. J. Dis. Chest* **73**:89–90.

119. Skrabanek, P., and Powell, O., 1980, Is the evidence for ectopic antidiuretic hormone watertight?. *Med. Hypotheses* **2**:193–197.

120. Pettingill, O. F., Faulkner, C. S., Wurster-Hill, D. H., Maurer, L. H., Sorenson, G. D., Robinson, A. G., and Zimmerman, E. A., 1977, Isolation and characterization of a hormone-producing cell line of human small-cell anaplastic carcinoma of the lung, *J. Natl. Cancer Inst.* **58**:511–516.

121. Kelly, P., and Morton, J. J., 1980, Antidiuretic hormone immunoactivity in tumour tissue from patients with bronchogenic carcinoma: With and without hypernatremia, *Clin. Endocrinol.* **12**:99–101.

122. Hansen, M., Hammer, M., and Hummer, L., 1980, ACTH, ADH and calcitonin concentrations as markers for response and relapse in small cell carcinoma of the lung, *Cancer* **46**:2062–2067.

123. Hansen, M., Hansen, M. H., Hirsch, F. R., Arends, J., Christensen, J. D., Christensen, J. M., Hummer, L., and Kuhl, C., 1980, Hormonal polypeptides and amine metabolites in small cell carcinoma of the lung, with special reference to stage and subtypes, *Cancer* **45**:1432–1437.

124. Comis, R. L., Miller, M., and Ginsberg, S., 1980, Abnormalities in water homeostasis in small cell anaplastic lung cancer, *Cancer* **45**:2414–2421.

125. Zerbe, R., Stropes, L., and Robertson, G., 1980, Vasopressin function and the syndrome of inappropriate antidiuresis, *Annu. Rev. Med.* **31**:315–327.

126. North, W. G., Maurer, L. H., Baltin, H., and O'Donnell, J. F., 1980, Human neurophysins as potential tumor markers for small cell carcinoma of the lung: Application of specific radioimmunoassays, *J. Clin. Endocrinol. Metab.* **51**:892–896.

127. Decaux, G., Brimioulle, S., Genette, F., and Mockel, J., 1980, Treatment of the syndrome of inappropriate secretion of antidiuretic hormone by urea, *Am. J. Med.* **69**:99–106.

128. Decaux, G., Watercot, Y., Genette, F., and Mockel, J., 1981, Treatment of the syndrome of inappropriate secretion of antidiuretic hormone with furosemide, *N. Engl. J. Med.* **304**:329–330.

129. Zapf, J., Rinderknecht, E., Humbel, R. E., and Froesch, E. R., 1978, Nonsuppressible insulin-like activity (NSILA) from human serum: Recent accomplishments and their physiologic implications, *Metabolism* **27**:1803–1828.

130. Suoboda, M. E., Van Wyk, J. J., Klapper, D. G., Fellows, R. E., Grissom, F. E., and Schlueter, R. J., 1980, Purification of somatomedin C from human plasma, *Biochemistry* **19**:790–797.

131. Megyesi, K., Kahn, C. R., Roth, J., and Gorden, P., 1974, Hypoglycemia in association with extrapancreatic tumors: Demonstration of elevated plasma NSILA-α by a non radioreceptor assay, *J. Clin. Endocrinol. Metab.* **38**:931–934.

132. Gorden, P., Hendricks, C. M., Kahn, C. R., Megyesi, K., and Roth, J., 1981, Hypoglycemia associated with non-islet cell tumors and insulin-like growth factors: A study of the tumor types, *N. Engl. J. Med.* **305**:1452–1455.

133. Daughaday, W. H., Trivedi, B., and Kapadia, M., 1981, Measurement of insulin-like growth factor II by a specific radioreceptor assay in serum of normal individuals, patients with abnormal growth hormone secretion and patients with tumor-related hypoglycemia, *J. Clin. Endocrinol. Metab.* **53**:289–294.

134. Skrabanek, P., and Powell, D., 1978, Ectopic insulin and Occam's razor: Reappraisal of the riddle of tumour hypoglycaemia, *Clin. Endocrinol.* **9**:141–154.

135. Kahn, C. R., 1980, The riddle of tumour hypoglycaemia revisited, *J. Clin. Endocrinol. Metab.* **9**:335–360.

136. Plovnick, H., Ruderman, N. B., Aoki, T., Chideckel, E. W., and Poffenbarger, P. L., 1979, Non-β-cell tumor hypoglycemia associated with increased nonsuppressible insulin-like protein (NSILP), *Am. J. Med.* **66**: 154–159.

137. Metz, S. A., McRae, J. R., and Robertson, R. P., 1981, Prostaglandins as mediators of paraneoplastic syndromes: Review and update, *Metabolism* **30**:299–316.

138. Luben, R. A., Mohler, M. A., and Nedwin, G. E., 1979, Production of hybridomas secreting monoclonal antibodies against the lymphokine osteoclast-activating factor, *J. Clin. Invest.* **64**:337–341.

139. Mundy, G. R., and Raisz, L. G., 1977, Big and little forms of osteoclast-activating factor, *J. Clin, Invest.* **60**:122–128.

140. Raisz, L. G., Simmons, H. A., Sandbery, A. L., and Canaus, E., 1980, Direct stimulation of bone resorption by epidermal growth factor, *Endocrinology* **107**:270–273.

141. Eilon, G., and Mundy, G. R., 1978, Direct resorption of bone by human breast cancer cells in vitro, *Nature (London)* **276**:726–728.

142. Mundy, G. R., Altman, A. J., Gondek, M. D., and Bandelin, J. G., 1977, Direct resorption of bone by human monocytes, *Science* **196**:1109–1110.

143. Minkin, C., Posek, R., and Newbrey, J., 1981, Mononuclear phagocytes and bone resorption: Identification and preliminnary characterization of a bone-derived macrophage chemotactic factor, *Metab. Bone Dis. Relat. Res.* **2**:363–369.

144. Sherwood, L. M., 1980, The multiple causes of hypercalcemia in malignant disease, *N. Engl. J. Med.* **303**:1412–1413.

145. Wiske, P. S., Epstein, S., Bell, N. H., Queener, S. F., Edmondson, J., and Johnston, D. D., Jr., 1979, Increases in immunoreactive parathyroid hormone with age, *N. Engl. J. Med.* **30**:1419–1421.

146. Knill-Jones, R. T., Buckle, R. M., Parsars, V., Calne, R., and Williams, R., 1970, Hypercalcemia and increased parathyroid hormone activity in primary hepatoma, *N. Engl. J. Med.* **282**:704–708.

147. Hamilton, J. W., Hartman, C. R., McGregor, D. H., and Cohn, D. V., 1977, Synthesis of parathyroid hormone-like peptides by a human squamous cell carcinoma, *J. Clin. Endocrinol. Metab.* **45**:1023–1030.

148. Martin, K. J., Hruska, K. A., Freitag, J. J., Klahr, S., and Slatopolsky, E., 1979, The peripheral metabolism of parathyroid hormone, *N. Engl. J. Med.* **301**:1092–1098.

149. Klein, D. C., and Raisz, L. G., 1970, Prostaglandin: Stimulation of bone resorption in tissue culture, *Endocrinology* **86**:1436–1440.

150. Tashjian, A. H., Jr., 1978, Role of prostaglandins in the production of hypercalcemia by tumors, *Cancer Res.* **38**:4138–4141.

151. Franklin, R. D., and Tashjian, A. H., Jr. 1975, Intravenous infusion of prostaglandin E_2 raises plasma calcium concentration in the rat, *Endocrinology* **97**:240–243.

152. Demers, L. M., Allegra, J. C., Harvey, H. A., Lipton, A., Luderer, J. R., Mortel, R., and Brenner, D. E., 1977, Plasma prostaglandins in hypercalcemic patients with neoplastic disease, *Cancer* **39**:1559–1562.

153. Robertson, R. P., Baylink, D. J., Mariki, J. J., and Adkison, H. W., 1975, Elevated prostaglandins and suppressed parathyroid hormone associated with hypercalcemia and renal cell carcinoma, *J. Clin, Endocrinol. Metab.* **41**:164–167.

154. Seyberth, H. W., 1978, Prostaglandin-mediated hypercalcemia: A paraneoplastic syndrome, *Klin. Wochenschr.* **56**:373–387.

155. Robertson, R. P., Baylink, D. J., Metz, S. A., and Cummings, K. B., 1977, Plasma prostaglandin E in patients with cancer with and without hypercalcemia, *J. Clin. Endocrinol. Metab.* **43**:1330–1335.

156. Cummings, K. B., and Robertson, R. P., 1977, Prostaglandin: Increased production by renal cell carcinoma, *J. Urol.* **118**:720–723.

157. Atkins, D., Ibbotson, K. J., Hillier, K., Hunt, N. H., Hammonds, J. C., and Martin, T. J., 1977, Secretion of prostaglandin in bone-resorption by renal cortical carcinoma in culture, *Br. J. Cancer* **36**:601–607.

158. Minkin, C., Fredericks, R. S., Pokress, S., Rude, R. K., Sharp, C. F., Jr., Tung, M., and Singer, F., 1981, Bone resorption and humoral hypercalcemia of malignancy: Stimulation inhibited by prostaglandin synthesis inhibitors, *J. Clin. Endocrinol. Metab.* **53**:941–947.

159. Shupnik, M. A., and Tashjian, A. M., 1981, Functional receptors for epidermal growth factor on human osteosarcoma cells, *J. Cell. Physiol.* **109**:403–410.

160. Kukreja, S. C., Shemerdiak, W. P., Lad, T. E., and Johnson, P. A., 1980, Elevated nephrogenous cyclic AMP with normal serum parathyroid hormone levels in patients with lung cancer, *J. Clin. Endocrinol. Metab.* **51**:167–169.

161. Rude, R. K., Sharp, C. F., Jr., Fredericks, R. S., Oldham, S. B., Elbaum, N., Link, J., Irwin, L., and Singer, F., 1981, Urinary and nephrogenous cyclic AMP in the hypercalcemia of malignancy, *J. Clin. Endocrinol. Metab.* **52**:765–771.

162. Stewart, A. F., Horst, R., Deftos, L. J., Cadman, E. C., Lang, R., and Broadus, A. E., 1980, Biochemical evaluation of patients with cancer associated hypercalcemia, *N. Engl. J. Med.* **303:**1377–1383.

163. Broadus, A. E., Mahattey, J. E., Bartter, F. C., and Neer, R. M., 1977, Nephrogenous cyclic adenosine monophosphate as a parathyroid function test, *J. Clin. Invest.* **60:**771–783.

164. Goltzman, D., Stewart, A. F., and Broadus, A. E., 1981, Malignancy-associated hypercalcemia: Evaluation with a cytochemical bioassay for parathyroid hormone, *J. Clin. Endocrinol. Metab.* **53:**899–904.

165. Stewart, A. F., Vignery, A., Ravin, N. D., Gertner, J., Broadus, A. E., and Baron, R., 1981, Bone histomorphometry in humoral hypocalcemia of malignancy and uncoupling of bone cell activity, *Clin. Res.* **29:**423A.

166. Saito, K., Kuratomi, Y., Yamamoto, R., Saito, T., Kuzuya, T., Yoshida, S., Moriyama, S. I., and Takahashi, A., 1981, Thyroid cancer associated with marked leukocytosis and hypercalcemia, *Cancer* **48:**2080–2083.

167. Sica, D., Martodam, R., Aronon, J., and Mundy, G., 1981, The relationship between hypercalcemia and urinary cyclic AMP in the humoral hypercalcemia of malignancy, *Am. Soc. Bone Miner. Res.* **30A.**

168. Meuten, D. J., Cooper, B. J., Capen, C. E., Chew, D. J., and Kociba, G. J., 1981, Hypercalcemia associated with adenocarcinoma derived from the apacrine glands of the anal sac, *Vet. Pathol.* **18:**454–471.

169. Skrabanek, P., McPartun, J., and Powell, D., 1980, Tumor hypercalcemia and ectopic hyperparathyroidism, *Medicine (Baltimore)* **59:**262–282.

170. Hansen, M., Hansen, H. H., and Tryding, N., 1978, Small cell carcinoma of the lung: Serum calcitonin and serum histaminase (diamine oxidase) at basal levels and stimulated by pentagastrin, *Acta Med. Scand.* **204:**257–261.

171. Roof, B. S., O'Dell, R., Wrenn, J. D., and Spicer, S. S., 1980, Sequential levels of immunoreactive calcitonin (iCT) by radioimmunoassay in serum and by immunoperoxidase staining in cancerous tissues of patients with lung cancer, *Clin. Res.* **28:**420A.

172. Roos, B. A., Lindall, A. W., Baylin, S. B., O'Neil, J. A., Frelinger, A. L., Birnbaum, R. S., and Lambert, P. W., 1979, Plasma immunoreactive calcitonin in lung cancer, *J. Clin. Endocrinol. Metab.* **49:**659–666.

173. Schwartz, K. E., Wolfsen, A. R., Forster, B., and Odell, W. D., 1979, Calcitonin in nonthyroidal cancer, *J. Clin. Endocrinol. Metab.* **49:**438–444.

174. Graze, K., Spiler, I. J., Tashjian, A. H., Jr., Melvin, K. E. W., Cervi-Skinner, S., Gagel, R. F., Miller, H. H., Wolfe, H. J., DeLellis, R. A., Leape, L., Feldman, Z. T., and Reichlin, S., 1978, Natural history of familial medullary thyroid carcinoma, *N. Engl. J. Med.* **299:**980–985.

175. Silva, O. L., Broder, L. E., Duppman, J. L., Snider, R. H., Moore, C. F., Cohen, M. H., and Becker, K. L., 1979, Calcitonin as a marker for bronchogenic cancer, *Cancer* **44:**680–684.

176. Roos, B. A., Yoon, M. J., Frelinger, A. L., Pensky, A. E., Birnbaum, R. S., and Lambert, P. W., 1979, Tumor growth and calcitonin during serial transplantation of rat medullary thyroid carcinoma, *Endocrinology* **105:** 27–32.

177. Samaan, N. A., Castillo, S., Schultz, P. N., Khalil, K. G., and Johnston, D. A., 1980, Serum calcitonin after pentagastrin stimulation in patients with

bronchogenic and breast cancer compared to that in patients with medullary thyroid carcinoma, *J. Clin. Endocrinol. Metab.* **51**:237–241.

178. Galmiche, J. P., Colin, R., DuBois, P. M., Chayvialle, J. A., Descos, F., Paulin, C., and Geffroy, Y., 1978, Calcitonin secretion by a pancreatic somatostatinoma, *N. Engl. J. Med.* **299**:1252.

179. Austin, L. A., and Heath, H., 1981, Calcitonin: Physiology and pathophysiology, *N. Engl. J. Med.* **304**:269–278.

180. Austin, L. A., Heath, H., III, and Go, V. L. W., 1979, Regulation of calcitonin secretion in normal man by changes of serum calcium within the physiologic range, *J. Clin. Invest.* **64**:1721–1724.

181. Goodman, R. H., Jacobs, J. W., and Habener, J. R., 1979, Cell-free translation of messenger RNA coding for a precursor of human calcitonin, *Biochem. Biophys. Res. Commun.* **91**:932–938.

182. Heath, H., III, Sizemore, G. W., Larson, J. M., and Jerpak, C. M., 1979, Immunochemical heterogeneity of calcitonin in tumor tumor venous effluent, and peripheral blood of patients with medullary thyroid carcinoma, *J. Lab. Clin. Med.*. **93**:390–401.

183. Goltzman, D., and Tischler, N., 1978, Characterization of the immunochemical forms of calcitonin released by a medullary thyroid carcinoma in tissue culture, *J. Clin. Invest.* **61**:449–458.

184. Parthemore, J. G., and Deftos, L. J., 1979, Calcitonin secretion in primary hyperparathyroidism, *J. Clin. Endocrinol. Metab.* **49**:223–226.

185. Shamonki, I. M., Frumar, A. M., Tataryn, I. V., Meldrum, D. R., Davidson, B. H., Parthemore, J. G., Judd, H. L., and Deftos, L. J., 1980, Age-related changes of calcitonin secretion in females, *J. Clin. Endocrinol. Metab.* **50**:437–439.

186. Nilsson, O., Almquist, S., and Karlberg, B. E., 1978, Salmon calcitonin in the acute treatment of moderate and severe hypercalcemia in man, *Acta Med. Scand.* **204**:249–252.

187. Binstock, M. L., and Mundy, G. R., 1980, Calcitonin and glucocorticoids in combination on the hypercalcemia of malignancy, *Ann. Intern. Med.* **93**:269–271.

188. McCance, R. A., 1947, Osteomalacia with Looser's nodes (Milkman's syndrome) due to resistance to vitamin D acquired about the age of 15 years, *Q. J. Med.* **16**:33–46.

189. Daniels, R. A., and Weisenfeld, I., 1979, Tumorous phosphaturic osteomalacia: Report of a case associated with multiple hemangiomas of bone, *Am. J. Med.* **67**:155–159.

190. Frame, B., and Parfitt, A. M., 1978, Osteomalacia: Current concepts, *Ann. Intern. Med.* **89**:966–982.

191. Fukumoto, Y., Tarui, S., Tsukiyama, K., Ichihara, K., Moriwaki, K., Nonaka, K., Mizushima, T., Kobayashi, Y., Dokoh, S., Fukunaga, M., and Morita, R., 1979, Tumor-induced vitamin D-resistant hypophosphatemic osteomalacia associated with proximal renal tubular dysfunction and 1,25-dihydroxyvitamin D deficiency, *J. Clin. Endocrinol. Metab.* **49**:873–878.

192. Drezner, M. K., and Feinglos, M. M., 1977, Osteomalacia due to 1 alpha 25-dihydroxycholecalciferol deficiency: Association with a giant cell tumor of bone, *J. Clin. Invest.* **60**:1046–1053.

193. Sweet, R. A., Malles, J. L., Hamstra, A. J., and DeLuca, H. F., 1980, Vitamin D metabolite levels in oncogenic osteomalacia, *Ann. Intern. Med.* **93:**279–280.

194. Lyles, K. W., Berry, W. R., Haussler, M., Harrelson, J. M., and Drezner, M. K., 1980, Hypophosphatemic osteomalacia: Association with prostatic carcinoma, *Ann. Intern. Med.* **93:**275–278.

195. Atkinson, M. D., McElwain, T. J., Peckham, M. J., and Thomas, P. R. M.., 1976, Hypertrophic pulmonary osteoarthropathy in Hodgkin's disease, *Cancer* **38:**1729–1734.

196. Goodman, M. A., McMaster, J. H., Drash, A. L., Diamond, P. E., Kappakas, G. S., and Scranton, P. E., 1978, Metabolic and endocrine alterations in osteosarcoma patients, *Cancer* **42:**603–610.

197. Golde, D. W., Herschman, H. R., Lusis, A. J., and Groopman, J. E., 1980, Growth factors (UCLA Conference), *Ann. Intern. Med.* **92:**650–662.

198. Frazier, W. A., Angeletti, R. H., and Bradshaw, R. A., 1972, Nerve growth factor and insulin: Structural similarity is indicated in evolutionary relationship reflected by physiologic action, *Science* **176:**482–488.

199. Goldstein, L. B., Reynolds, C. T., and Perez-Polo, J. R., 1978, Isolation of human nerve growth factor from placental tissue, *Neurochem. Res.* **3:**175–183.

200. Ahronav, A., Truss, R. M., and Herschman, H. R., 1978, Epidermal growth factor: Relationship between the receptor regulation and mitogenesis in 3T3 cells, *J. Biol. Chem.* **253:**3970–3977.

201. Larsson, L.-I., 1978, Endocrine pancreatic tumors, *Hum. Pathol.* **9:**401–416.

202. Walsh, J. H., Tompkins, R. K., Taylor, I. L., Lechago, J., and Hansky, J., 1979, Gastrointestinal hormones in clinical disease: Recent developments, *Ann. Intern. Med.* **90:**817–828.

203. Stacpoole, P. W., 1981, The glucagonoma syndrome: Clinical features, diagnosis and treatment, *Endocr. Rev.* **2:**347–361.

204. Said, S. I., and Mutt, V., 1970, Polypeptide with broad biological activity: Isolation from small intestine, *Science* **169:**1217–1218.

205. Higgins, G. A., Recant, L., and Fischman, A. B., 1979, The glucagonoma syndrome: Surgically curable diabetes, *Am. J. Surg.* **137:**142–148.

206. Metz, S. A., McRae, T. R., and Robertson, R. P., 1981, Prostaglandins as mediators of paraneoplastic syndromes: Review and update, *Metabolism* **30:**299–316.

207. Bloom, S. R., Adrian, T. E., Bryant, M. G., and Polak, J. M., 1978, Pancreatic polypeptide: A marker for Zollinger–Ellison syndrome, *Lancet* **1:**1155.

208. Polak, J. M., Bloom, S. R., Adrian, T. E., Heitz, P., Bryant, M. G., and Pearse, A. G. E., 1976, Pancreatic polypeptide in insulinomas, gastrinomas, VIPomas and glucagonomas, *Lancet* **1:**328–330.

209. Taylor, I. L., Walsh, J. H., Rodder, J. M., and Passaro, E., Jr., 1978, Is pancreatic polypeptide a marker for Zollinger–Ellison syndrome?, *Lancet* **1:**845–848.

210. Walsh, J. H., Tompkins, R. K., Taylor, I. L., Lechago, J., and Hansky, J., 1979, Gastrointestinal hormones in clinical disease: Recent developments, *Ann. Intern. Med.* **90:**817–828.

211. Bloom, S. R., Polak, J. M., and West, A. M., 1978, Somatostatin content of pancreatic endocrine tumors, *Metabolism* **27:**1235–1238.

212. Larsson, L. I., Schwartz, T., Lundqvist, G., Chance, R. E., Sundler, F., Rehfeld, J. F., Grimelius, L., Fahrenkrug, J., Schaffalitzky De Muckadell, O., and Moon, N., 1976, Occurrence of human pancreatic polypeptide in pancreatic endocrine tumors, *Am. J. Pathol.* **86:**675–684.

213. Mallinson, C. N., Bloom, S. R., Warin, A. P., Salmon, P. R., and Cox, V., 1974, A glucagonoma syndrome, *Lancet* **2:**1–5.

214. McGavran, M. H., Unger, R. H., Recant, L., Polk, H. C., Kilo, C., and Levin, M. E., 1966, A glucagon-secreting alpha-cell carcinoma of the pancreas, *N. Engl. J. Med.* **274:**1408–1413.

215. Norton, J. A., Kahn, C. R., Schiebinger, R., Gorschboth, C., and Brenna, M. F., 1979, Amino acid deficiency and the skin rash associated with glucagonoma, *Ann. Intern. Med.* **91:**213–215.

216. Ingemansson, S., Holst, J., Larsson, L. I., and Lunderquist, A., 1977, Localization of the glucagonomas by catheterization of the pancreatic veins and with glucagon assay, *Surg. Gynecol. Obstet.* **145:**509–516.

217. Guillemin, R., 1978, Some thoughts on current research with somatostatin, *Metabolism* **27:**1453–1461.

218. Lundbaek, K., 1978, Somatostatin: Clinical importance and outlook, *Metabolism* **27:**1463–1469.

219. Krejs, G. J., Orci, L. Conlon, J. M., Ravazzola, M., Davis, G. R., Raskin, P., Collins, S. M., McCarthy, D. M., Baetens, D., Rubenstein, A., Aldor, T. A. M., and Unger, R. H., 1979, Somatostatinoma syndrome, *N. Engl. J. Med.* **301:**285–292.

220. Pipeleers, D., Somers, G., Gepts, W., De Nutte, N., and De Vroede, M., 1979, Plasma pancreatic hormone levels in a case of somatostatinoma: Diagnostic and therapeutic implications, *J. Clin. Endocrinol. Metab.* **49:**572–579.

221. Szabo, M., Berelowitz, M., Pettengill, O. S., Sorenson, G. D., and Frohman, L A., 1980, Ectopic production of somatostatin-like immuno- and bioactivity by cultured human pulmonary small cell carcinoma, *J. Clin. Endocrinol. Metab.* **51:**978–987.

222. Watkins, W. B., and Yen, S. S. C., 1980, Somatostatin in cytotrophoblast of the immature human placenta: Localization by immunoperoxidase cytochemistry, *J. Clin. Endocrinol. Metab.* **50:**969–970.

223. Fitz-Patrick, D. and Ptel, Y. C., 1979, Measurement, characterization and source of somatostatin-like immunoreactivity in human amniotic fluid, *J. Clin, Invest.* **64:**737–742.

224. Long, R. G., Adrian, T. E., Brown, M. R., Rivier, J. E., Barnes, A. J., Mallinson, C. N., Vale, W., Christofides, N. D., and Bloom, S. R., 1979, Suppression of pancreatic endocrine tumour secretion by long-acting somatostatin analogue, *Lancet* **2:**764–767.

225. Charmasthaphorn, K., Sherwin, R. S., Cataland, S., Jaffe, B., and Dobbins, J., 1980, Somatostatin inhibits diarrhea in the carcinoid syndrome, *Ann. Intern. Med.* **92:**68–69.

226. Thulin, L., Samnegard, H., Tyden, G., Long, D. H., and Efendic, S., 1978, Efficacy of somatostatin in a patient with carcinoid syndrome, *Lancet* **2:**43.

227. Sherwood, J. B., and Goldwasser, E. B., 1979, Radioimmunoassay for erythropoietin, *Blood* **54:**885–893.

228. Anagnostou, A., Chawla, M. S., Pololi, L., and Fried, W., 1979, Determination of plasma erythropoietin levels: An early marker of tumor activity, *Cancer* **44:**1014–1016.

229. Erslev, A. J., Caro, J., Kansu, E., Miller, O., and Cobbs, E. 1979, Plasma erythropoietin in polycythemia, *Am. J. Med.* **66:**243–247.

230. Goldwasser, E., and Sherwood, J. B., 1981, Radioimmunoassay of erythropoietin, *Br. J. Haematol.* **48:**359–363.

231. Slater, E. E., and Haber, E., 1979, Inactive renin—"Through a glass darkly," *N. Engl. J. Med.* **301:**429–430.

232. Sealey, J. E., Atlas, S. H., and Laragh, J. H., 1980, Prorenin and other large molecular weight forms of renin, *Endocr. Rev.* **1:**365–391.

233. Slater, E. E., and Haber, E., 1978, A large form of renin from normal human kidney, *J. Clin. Endocrinol. Metab.* **47:**105–109.

234. Poulsen, K., Vuust, J., Lykegaard, S., Nielsen, A. H/J., and Lund, T., 1979, Renin is synthesized as a 50,000 dalton single chain polypeptide in cell-free translation systems, *FEBS Lett.* **98:**135–138.

235. Murakami, K., and Ingami, T., 1979, Reversible conversion of big renin to renin in kidney extracts, *Int. Cong. Biochem.*, Toronto, p. 301.

236. Rosen, S. W., Weintraub, B. D., and Aaronson, S. A., 1980, Nonrandom ectopic protein production by malignant cells: Direct evidence in vitro, *J. Clin. Endocrinol. Metab.* **50:**834–841.

Vasopressin

Gary R. Robertson

9.1. Introduction

The past few years has been a time of rapid growth in our knowledge of vasopressin and neurohypophyseal function. In 1977, the major advances of the prior decade were represented by less than 150 papers.[1] In the last 5 years, more than 250 papers exploring new or controversial aspects of vasopressin function have appeared. While this new growth occurred in many areas, it was particularly pronounced in those pertaining to basic anatomy, biochemistry, physiology, and pharmacology of the system. Some advances also were made in pathophysiology, diagnosis, and treatment, but much of the new information in these areas served to confirm and consolidate existing concepts. In the following sections, these new developments will be reviewed, giving particular attention to those that seem the most important, well developed, or controversial. Wherever it seems particularly important or helpful to understanding, pertinent historical material will also be reviewed. For more complete background material, the reader is referred to the initial chapter in the series.[1]

GARY R. ROBERTSON ● University of Chicago School of Medicine, Chicago, Illinois 60637.

9.2. Anatomy

Histologic studies with new and improved immunocytochemical techniques have revealed that the CNS domain of vasopressinergic and oxytocinergic neurons is much more extensive than previously recognized.[2,3] In addition to dense accumulations in and around the supraoptic and paraventricular nuclei, multipolar cell bodies containing vasopressin and/or its neurophysin have been identified in the suprachiasmatic nuclei of humans[4] and other primates,[3] as well as most commonly used laboratory animals.[2,5] From these three origins, vasopressinergic fibers have been traced to diverse and widespread areas of the CNS. From the supraoptic nuclei, most if not all axons project to the posterior pituitary, from whence the hormone is secreted into the systemic circulation.[2,3] The paraventricular nucleus also sends some vasopressinergic axons to the neural lobe, but most of them project to other areas. One large division terminates in the median eminence, where hormone is secreted into portal blood and taken to the adenohypophysis.[2,3] Another division, somewhat smaller and anatomically separate, projects caudally to the medulla and spinal cord where, in primates[3] as well as other mammals,[5–7] the axons appear to terminate on other neurons in the nucleus tractus solitarius, substantia gelatinosa, and neighboring structures thought to be involved in the afferent control of cardiovascular and related autonomic functions. Still another division of the paraventricular nucleus projects through the stria terminalis to the lateral amygdala.[3] Finally, a few vasopressinergic neurons appear to terminate on the walls of the lateral and/or third ventricle, where the hormone is probably secreted directly into cerebrospinal fluid.[8] The vasopressinergic neurons that arise in the suprachiasmatic nuclei are of relatively fine caliber and lack any apparent vascular connections.[3] They seem to project exclusively to a variety of other neurons in the medial amygdala, lateral septum, and mediodorsal thalamus.[2,3,5]

The widespread distribution of vasopressin in the CNS has also been demonstrated by direct radioimmunoassay of tissue extracts.[9,10] The amounts recovered are quite small relative to those from the neural lobe, but are in a range that permits easy detection and characterization with the more sensitive immunoassays. These studies leave little doubt that neurons containing authentic vasopressin exist in many brain areas outside the hypothalamic–neurohypophyseal system.

Oxytocinergic cell bodies appear to be less numerous than those containing vasopressin and are found primarily in discrete areas in or around the paraventricular nuclei.[2] Some are also scattered throughout the supraoptic nuclei, but none have been found in the suprachiasmatic nuclei. Most of the oxytocinergic neurons in the supraoptic areas and a few of paraventricular origin project to the neural lobe of the pituitary. However, like vasopressinergic fibers, many also run to the organum vasculosum or the hypophyseal portal system of the zona externa of the median eminence. In addition, a relatively large paraventricular division runs in parallel with vasopressinergic fibers to the medulla and spinal cord, where it splits into multiple ramifications that terminate on or near the same neural elements.

The functions of the various extrahypophyseal projections of neurosecretory neurons are poorly understood compared with the much larger and more extensively studied neurohypophyseal divisions. Some information about the regulation of vasopressinergic pathways to the median eminence and cerebrospinal fluid is available but their purpose, if any, is still unclear. Even less is known about the functions of those pathways that project to other neurons, although a variety of nervous effects have been ascribed to vasopressin and related peptides (Section 9.5.3).

9.3. Biosynthesis

As noted in an earlier chapter in this series,[1] vasopressin and oxytocin are known to be synthesized, transported, stored, and secreted in close association with specific binding proteins known collectively as neurophysins. Recently, Brownstein and colleagues have obtained direct experimental evidence in rats confirming earlier suggestions[11] that vasopressin and its neurophysin are synthesized together as part of a larger peptide.[12,13] This common precursor, which they have isolated and named propressophysin, appears to have a molecular weight of approximately 20,000. In addition to neurophysin and vasopressin, it contains a relatively large glycosylated protein that originally was thought to occupy the N terminus of the molecule. However, it now seems clear from subsequent studies, including DNA cloning,[14] that AVP is preceded at the N terminus by a signal peptide, the glycoprotein occupies the C terminus, and neurophysin is situated in between them. As in many other propeptides, the various components are separated by lysine and/or arginine residues, which mark the point of cleavage by proteolytic enzymes. Oxytocin and its neurophysins also appear to be formed from a common precursor named prooxytocin, which, except for the absence of glycosylation, closely resembles propressophysin.[12,13] Both propressophysin and prooxytocin appear to be formed from still larger peptides synthesized in the cell bodies of their respective neurosecretory neurons. Presumably, these precursors undergo proteolysis within neurosecretory granules to yield the biologically active hormones and their neurophysins, as well as the glycoproteins. The synthesis of vasopressin and oxytocin in humans probably occurs by similar mechanisms, although the precursors have not been identified and may have different chemical structures.

These studies of vasopressin and oxytocin biosynthesis also produced some unexpected evidence suggesting the existence of a third or abnormal neurohypophyseal hormone in homozygous Brattleboro rats.[12,13] Consistent with other evidence that this strain can make oxytocin but not vasopressin,[15] Goldstein and colleagues found prooxyphysin, but not propressophysin. However, the supraoptic nuclei of these animals also yielded another cysteine-containing protein that could be hydrolyzed with trypsin to yield neurophysin and vasopressin-like peptides. These observations are consistent with a more recent preliminary report of low but readily detectable levels of vasopressin-like immunoactivity in the plasma and pituitary of homozygous Brattleboro rats.[16] It remains to be determined whether the vasopressin-like materials found in the biosynthesis and immunoassay studies are related to each other or to any other form of hormone production by the neurohypophysis. However, the discovery of a vasopressin-like material is particularly interesting in view of the still unexplained capacity of homozygous Brattleboro rats to concentrate their urine during water deprivation.[17]

9.4. Secretion

9.4.1. Osmoregulation

As reviewed in an earlier volume of this series,[1] the secretion of vasopressin from the neurohypophysis is regulated primarily by osmoreceptors that are exquisitely sensitive to changes in the plasma concentration of sodium and certain other solutes. The functional properties of this osmoregulatory system are known in some detail, even though there is still much uncertainty about its exact location and mode of operation. This state of affairs has changed only slightly in the last few years. Most of the new information obtained serves to confirm and solidify our current understanding of the system. However, certain ideas about its functional properties have been challenged, while other factors that influence it have been discovered.

The long-established concept of an osmotic "threshold" or "set point" for vasopressin release[1] has recently been questioned. By analyzing the relationship between plasma vasopressin and osmolality in sheep, Weitzman and colleagues conclude that it is best described by an exponential rather than a linear-threshold model.[18] This result would suggest that osmotically mediated vasopressin secretion is an infinitely continuous, rather than a discontinuous, process. However, as pointed out in a subsequent letter[19] and editorial,[20] the data are subject to alternative interpretations that, for various reasons, cannot be resolved at present. For one thing, the methods currently available are not sufficiently precise to distinguish between the relatively small differences in the plasma osmolality–vasopressin relationship that would be predicted from the "threshold" and "exponential" models of osmoreceptor function. To further complicate matters, the overall relationship may be distorted by concurrent nonosmotic influences, such as hemodynamic stimuli, changes in vascular clearance, or individual differences in the "set" or "sensitivity" of the osmostat.[21] Finally, even a precise and undistorted description of the plasma vasopressin–osmolality relationship may not provide a true picture of the stimulus–response pattern in individual neurons, since secretory activity may reflect the balance of multiple inhibitory as well as stimulatory influences from a bimodal osmoreceptor system (Section 9.6.1.2). For these reasons, it is currently a moot question whether the concept of an osmotic threshold for vasopressin release accurately represents the operation of the control mechanism at its most fundamental level. As a practical matter, however, the concept remains a valid and useful way of describing certain aspects of normal and abnormal osmoregulatory function as they present in the intact animal.

It also has been suggested that osmotic stimulation causes vasopressin to be released in spurts.[22] In sheep and dogs subjected to dehydration or bolus infusion of hypertonic saline, Weitzman and colleagues found that plasma vasopressin fluctuated widely and did not correlate with concurrent plasma osmolality or sodium concentration unless multiple values were integrated over a period of time. These findings differ from those obtained by others, who consistently find a close correlation between individual plasma vasopressin and osmolality in healthy people[21,23–25] and dogs (A. Melman and G. Robertson, unpublished observations). The reason for this discrepancy is unclear, but could be due to differences in the frequency and/or site of sampling. In the studies showing wide fluctuations in plasma vasopressin, blood was collected more often and nearer the source of secretion,[22] an approach that might be expected to provide a better picture of the temporal dynamics of neurohypophyseal secretion. However, collecting from the right atrium could also be misleading. If confluent streams of blood from the superior and inferior vena cavae do not mix uniformly, intermittent sampling from undiluted eddies of vasopressin-rich blood from the head could result in large sample-to-sample fluctuations in hormone concentration that mimic episodic secretion. Since the data currently available do not exclude this kind of artifact or that due to intermittent nonosmotic secretion, the issue of continuous *versus* episodic secretion of vasopressin remains unsettled.

The temporal pattern of vasopressin secretion by single neurons should not be confused with that displayed by the entire neurohypophysis. Recordings from individual, antidromically identified neurosecretory neurons show episodic bursts of electrical activity that increase in frequency in direct proportion to increases in plasma osmolality.[25] However, this kind of phasic firing by individual neurons would not be expected to manifest as episodic fluctuations in plasma vasopressin because it occurs with a periodicity of only about 20 sec and seems to be unsynchronized from unit to unit. Hence, only if a stimulus superimposes a slower synchronized rhythm upon a myriad of independent, phasically firing neurons could it induce discernible fluctuations in neurohypophyseal secretion. Whether or not such synchronized rhythms are induced by regulatory afferents remains an important question for understanding neurosecretion at its most basic level. However, uncertainty about this issue does not preclude meaningful studies of vasopressin regulation in the whole animal, since intermittent samples of peripheral venous plasma appear to provide a reliable picture of temporal changes in hormone secretion, as well as hormone concentration in the kidney and other effector organs.

Considerably more progress has been made toward resolving longstanding controversies concerning the location of the osmoreceptor vis-à-vis the blood–brain barrier. As reviewed previously,[1] vasopressin secretion is known to be quite sensitive to changes in the concentration of certain blood solutes like sodium, mannitol, and sucrose, but relatively insensitive to the concentration of others, such as urea and glucose. This specificity has been attributed to differences in the rate at which particular blood solutes enter the osmoreceptor neurons. Those that penetrate slowly or not at all are stimulatory because the resultant inequality of intra- and extracellular solute concentrations produces an osmotic gradient that dehydrates the osmoreceptor. Conversely, those solutes that penetrate rapidly do not have these effects. It has never been clear, however, whether the permeability of a solute is determined by the blood–brain barrier, the osmoreceptor cell membrane, or both.[23] Recently, three different laboratories have confirmed the differential effects of these solutes on vasopressin secretion in humans,[26] sheep,[27] and dogs[28] and also found a very similar specificity for the osmoregulation of thirst. More importantly, they also obtained the first convincing evidence that most, if not all, of the osmoreceptors are located in a part of the head that is outside of the blood–brain barrier. By exclusion, therefore, the specificity of the osmoreceptor must be determined by the permeability characteristics of the osmoreceptor itself.

The above findings would appear to invalidate previous suggestions that the osmoreceptor is actually a sodium receptor located near the cerebral ventricles or elsewhere within the blood–brain barrier,[29] However, because intraventricular injections of equiosmolar solutions of hypertonic saline and sucrose elicit different degrees of antidiuresis, McKinley and associates have suggested that juxtaventricular sodium receptors may coexist with primary osmoreceptors located outside the blood–brain barrier.[27] However, intravenous infusion of hypertonic urea or glucose raises the sodium concentration of cerebrospinal fluid but causes little or no stimulation of thirst or vasopressin.[27,28] Hence, unless these two solutes inhibit the system by some nonosmotic or toxic mechanism,[30] these putative juxtaventricular sodium receptors, if they exist at all, must be relatively unimportant for osmoregulation.

Progress has also been made in elucidating some of the factors that determine or modify specific aspects of osmoregulatory function. As noted previously, the sensitivity of the vasopressin response to osmotic stimuli varies markedly from person to person.[1] Studies in twins have now shown that this property is relatively constant in the same person and is determined largely by genetic influences.[31] However, the sensitivity of the system is not totally immutable since it seems to increase slightly with age[32] and may also be altered by certain drugs (Section 9.4.7). The threshold or "set" of the osmoreceptor is much more susceptible to outside influences. Along with hypotension and hypovolemia,[1] pregnancy must now be included as one of the factors that lowers the osmotic threshold for vasopressin release.[33] This shift occurs early in pregnancy and apparently is not attributable to a reduction in total blood volume or increased production of estrogen or progesterone. The effect is quite specific for the set of the osmoreceptor, since the sensitivity of the vasopressin response is not altered. Although not yet studied, human pregnancy is probably accompanied by a similar reduction in osmoreceptor threshold, since basal plasma osmolality falls 5 to 10 mOsm/kg in the first trimester and remains low until delivery.[34–36]

The anatomy of the osmoregulatory system remains ill-defined despite continued probing with refined, ablative techniques. As noted previously,[1] there is a great deal of circumstantial evidence that the osmoreceptor neurons are located somewhere in the anterior hypothalamus, near to but separate from, the perikarya of the neurosecretory neurons. In rats, electrolytic lesions anteroventral to the third ventricle (AV3V) selectively impair the dipsogenic and antidiuretic response to osmotic as well as angiotensin stimulation.[37,38] These animals exhibit pathophysiologic findings very similar to those in patients with adipsic hypernatremia (Section 9.6.1.2). However, it is not yet clear whether lesions of the AV3V area involve the osmoreceptor neurons *per se* or their afferent fibers in passage. Hence, the exact location of the sensing portion of the system remains uncertain.

Similar uncertainty surrounds the neurochemistry of the osmoregulatory neurons. In rats, injection of 6-OH dopamine destroys dopaminergic and noradrenergic neurons in the brain and markedly impairs the vasopressin response to osmotic and hemodynamic stimuli.[39] These findings suggest that inputs from osmoregulatory and baroregulatory systems are mediated in part by noradrenergic pathways. However, this interpretation must be viewed with caution since 6-OH dopamine causes widespread destruction of noradrenergic neurons in the brain and may also damage other pathways as a result of its relatively strong oxidizing effects.[40] Studies in explants of rat hypothalamic–neurohypophyseal tissue indicate that osmotically induced vasopressin release can be inhibited by addition of hexamethonium or other antagonists of nicotinic-cholinergic receptors, but is not affected by atropine, a muscarinic antagonist.[41] Since acetylcholine also causes vasopressin release from these explants,[42] at least some of the osmoreceptor afferents may be cholinergic. However, it is not yet clear whether the functional properties of these explants are similar to those of the intact system. Experiments performed *in vivo* have given inconsistent results concerning the effects of atropine and other cholinergic antagonists on vasopressin secretion,[43–46] but in these systems it is not always possible to distinguish primary and secondary effects. Further studies in conscious animals, with appropriate monitoring of blood pressure and other nonosmotic influences, are needed to further explore the role of adrenergic and cholinergic pathways in the osmoregulation of vasopressin secretion.

9.4.2. Baroregulation

Our understanding of the hemodynamic control of vasopressin secretion has advanced considerably in recent years. As reviewed previously,[1] an acute rise or fall in blood pressure and/or volume of more than 5 to 10% produces a decrease or increase in vasopressin secretion that is proportional to the magnitude of the hemodynamic disturbance. These effects appear to be mediated via neurogenic afferents that arise in pressure-sensitive receptors in the left atrium, aorta, and carotid sinus, and project via the vagus and glossopharyngeal nerves to the bed nuclei of the tractus solitarius in the medulla. From there, postsynaptic pathways that are partly noradrenergic project to magnacellular elements in the supraoptic and/or paraventricular nuclei.[47,48] These pathways appear to be closely associated with other ascending noradrenergic neurons that project to parvocellular portions of the paraventricular nuclei involved in the control of ACTH and autonomic function. Input from the baroreceptor appears to be predominantly negative or inhibitory under basal conditions, since vagotomy results in an acute rise in vasopressin and catecholamine secretion.[49] Thus, "stimulation" by hypovolemia or hypotension probably reflects a fall in tonic inhibitory input from the baroreceptors whereas the "suppression" produced by hypervolemia or hypertension reflects a rise in activity of these inhibitory pathways.

The exponential relationship between plasma vasopressin and blood volume or pressure that was originally demonstrated in rats and man[1] has also been found in monkeys.[50] Interestingly, the relationship between hypovolemia and vasopressin secretion may be altered quantitatively by changes in body temperature,[51] although it is not yet clear whether this thermal effect is due to an intrinsic change in sensitivity to hemodynamic influences or is due merely to secondary changes in peripheral resistance and blood pressure. In man, aging appears to result in diminished vasopressin responsiveness to hypotensive stimuli.[52] This loss may be due to interruption of inhibitory baroreceptor afferents since it is also associated with hypertension, increased plasma catecholamines, and increased vasopressin responsiveness to osmotic stimuli.

Hemodynamic influences appear to alter vasopressin secretion by raising or lowering the set of the osmostat, indicating that the two control systems converge and act on the same population of neurosecretory neurons.[1] This concept has recently received further support from electrophysiologic studies showing that most individual neurohypophyseal neurons of the rat alter firing rates in response to both osmotic and hemodynamic stimuli.[53] These same studies also showed that raising the pressure in the carotid sinus inhibited the electrical response to hypertonic stimuli, another result that agrees remarkably well with the *in vivo* secretory studies.[1] Like other electrophysiologists, Kannan and Yagi also found that a few neurosecretory neurons decreased their discharge rate in response to osmotic stimuli, a paradoxical response that is consistent with other findings suggesting a bimodal osmoregulatory system (Section 9.6.1.2).

The list of stimuli of vasopressin secretion shown to be mediated by baroreceptor pathways continues to lengthen. In addition to many drugs and hormones,[1] positive and expiratory ventilation[54] and vasovagal reactions[55] appear to increase vasopressin at least in part via their hemodynamic effects. The transiency of the hypotension associated with the vasovagal stimulus further emphasizes the importance of closely monitoring blood pressure in all studies of the mechanism of vasopressin stimuli.[1]

9.4.3. Nociceptive Influences

The debate concerning the effect of pain and other noxious "stresses" on vasopressin secretion[1] continues unabated. The persistence of this issue is due to many factors, including the very vagueness of the term "stress" and the paucity of well-controlled studies. A case in point is a recent report of patients seen in an emergency room.[56] Because those who complained of pain were found to have significantly higher levels of plasma vasopressin in the absence of any increase in plasma osmolality, the observed hormonal difference was attributed to nociceptive stimuli. Efforts were made to control for the effects of drugs, hypovolemia, and hypotension, but they were based solely on history, clinical impression, and exclusion of patients with blood pressures below an arbitrary limit. Such an approach is too crude to reliably exclude the effect of other nonosmotic stimuli such as a modest or transient reduction in blood volume or pressure.[1,55] Moreover, it failed to consider the possible role of nausea or other disorders known to influence vasopressin secretion (*vide infra*). Other studies tend to support previous findings that, in rats at least, vasopressin secretion is unaffected by a variety of noxious stresses.[57] The only exceptions were electric shock and abdominal compression, either of which could have acted by reducing blood pressure or effective blood volume. These two reports illustrate the need for more carefully controlled experiments designed specifically to answer fundamentally important questions about the effects of pain and other noxious sensations on vasopressin secretion.

9.4.4. Emetic Influences

It has recently been shown that nausea is an extremely potent stimulus to vasopressin secretion in man.[58] This study, which confirms a much older observation,[59] establishes for the first time that nausea acts by a mechanism independent of osmotic, hemodynamic, or other recognized stimuli. Vasopressin release appears to be triggered via the emetic center since it occurs when nausea is induced by vestibular mechanisms[60] as well as via the chemoreceptor trigger zone.[58] It can be blocked by pretreatment with antiemetics and, like most other nonosmotic stimuli, is attenuated by water loading. The purpose of this reflex is unknown, but the increase in plasma vasopressin customarily produced by nausea is probably great enough to cause contraction of smooth muscle in the uterus,[59] as well as the intestines and blood vessels (Section 9.5.2).

9.4.5. Glucopenic Stimuli

Recent studies revealed that acute insulin-induced hypoglycemia also causes vasopressin secretion.[61] This response does not seem to be mediated by any of the recognized osmotic or nonosmotic stimuli and is directly proportional to the degree of hypoglycemia achieved.[62] The mechanism of the effect is unknown. However, hypoglycemia appears to act only in concert with osmotic stimuli because its effect on vasopressin secretion is abolished totally by water loading.[63] The effect of insulin may be a direct result of deficient glucose metabolism in one or more parts of the brain because infusion of 2-deoxyglucose also increases vasopressin secretion.[64,65] The raison d'être for the glucopenic influence on vasopressin is uncertain. It may serve to reinforce the antidiuretic response to water deprivation since the latter is often associated with decreased intake of food and a fall in plasma glucose. It could also contribute in a minor way to glucose homeostasis because vasopressin appears to cause hepatic glycogenolysis and gluconeogenesis (Section 9.5.3).

9.4.6. Hypoxic Stimuli

Exposure to high altitude produces a variable array of changes in salt and/or water excretion.[66] In some cases, particularly that of healthy people subjected to moderate hypobaria and/or hypoxia, pronounced increases in salt and water excretion have been observed. In others, most notably anesthetized animals but also occasionally in conscious humans, acute hypoxia induces an intense and lenghty antidiuresis. The reason for the disparate responses, the role of vasopressin, and the relative importance of hypoxia and other factors in mediating them have long been unclear. Recent studies in anesthetized cats[67] and dogs[68] indicate that acute hypoxia without hypobaria consistently produces marked increases in plasma vasopressin that cannot be accounted for by recognized osmotic or hemodynamic stimuli. In contrast, conscious humans subjected to similar levels of acute normobaric hypoxia rarely exhibit a rise in plasma vasopressin[69] and may actually have a slight decrease.[70] Whether these disparate results are due to the anesthesia or to species difference has not been determined. However, recent studies indicate that conscious adults are more likely to exhibit a rise in vasopressin secretion if the hypoxia is accompanied by a reduction in blood pressure.[71] They also show that the resultant rise in vasopressin is related not to the hypoxia or hypobaria per se, but to the acute hypotension and/or nausea that these conditions induce in some but not all subjects. Hence, it seems clear that activation of chemoreceptors by a fall in arterial oxygen tension is not a primary stimulus to vasopressin secretion in conscious humans. Such an effect cannot be excluded in certain animals and/or in the presence of anesthesia, but, even there, a secondary effect via the emetic center remains a reasonable probability.

9.4.7. Pharmacological Influences

9.4.7.1. Opiates

Perhaps no aspect of neurohypophyseal function has undergone a greater revolution in recent years than our concepts of the way in which opiates influence vasopressin secretion. The pioneering studies of de Bodo performed more than 40 years ago[72] established quite clearly that large doses of morphine inhibited a water diuresis in dogs by stimulating release of an antidiuretic hormone from the neurohypophysis. These observations were confirmed by Duke, Pickford, and Watt who also found that the same antidiuretic effect could be elicited when morphine sulfate was given intravenously in smaller doses that did not cause "excitement or defecation" or when it was injected directly into the supraoptic nucleus at doses that caused "little or no alteration in systemic blood pressure."[73] These observations led to the conclusion that morphine stimulates the release of antidiuretic hormone by a direct effect on the hyothalamic neurohypophyseal tract, a view that has since become deeply entrenched by decades of reiteration in textbooks of pharmacology, physiology, and medicine.

Along the way, other investigators reported studies that seemed to tie up most of the remaining loose ends in this story. Application of the then relatively new bioassay techniques confirmed that administration of morphine to rats resulted in a rise in the urinary content of an antidiuretic substance with physiochemical properties indistinguishable from those of pituitary extracts.[74,75] It was also found that the antidiuretic effect of morphine could be prevented by pretreatment with the antagonist nalorphine[75,76] and, on repeat testing, exhibited the same kind of rapidly developing tolerance or resistance as other effects of the drug.[77] However, these papers also contained some incidental observations that at the time did not attract much attention but that, with the aid of the retrospectroscope, may be recognized as early warnings of possible flaws in the conventional view of the way in which morphine affects the neurohypophysis. For example, it was observed that antidiuresis also occurred following the administration of apomorphine,[75] a dopamine agonist whose only similarity to morphine is its name and ability to produce sedation, emesis, and orthostatic hypotension. Moreover, the antidiuresis produced by morphine in humans[76] and rats[77] was noted to be associated in many cases with emesis and/or hypotension, two stimuli that are now recognized to have potent effects on vasopressin release (Sections 9.4.2 and 9.4.4). Finally, there were a few scattered reports that, instead of antidiuresis, low doses of morphine produced a modest increase in urine flow[78–80] or inhibited the antidiuretic response to hypovolemic stimuli.[80] The latter reports also seemed to have little impact, however, probably because the data were rather sketchy or failed to permit a clear distinction between effects on vasopressin secretion or action, or both.

The modern era in the study of opiate actions on vasopressin secretion was ushered in by the studies of Miller.[81] Using a radioimmunoassay to measure urinary excretion of the hormone, he found that the administration of butorphanol, an opiate with mixed agonist/antagonist properties, suppressed vasopressin secretion and produced a diuresis in normal and dehydrated rats with partial deficiency of the hormone. Because of the then dominant view that opiates directly stimulated vasopressin release, the inhibitory–diuretic effect of butorphanol was attributed to its antagonist properties. This interpretation would suggest that endogenous opiates mediate the effects of osmotic or hypovolemic stimuli on vasopressin release. Consistent with this view were subsequent observations that intravenous[82–84] or intracerebroventricular injection[83,84] of β-endorphin or Leuenkephalin produces increases in plasma vasopressin and/or urine osmolality that could be blocked with naloxone. However, with the exception of one study in which arterial pressure was measured,[84] these reports did not provide any information on changes in osmotic or nonosmotic variables known to influence vasopressin secretion. In particular, no mention is made of the occurrence of emesis, although other studies have shown that vomiting regularly occurs in cats following intravenous administration of β-endorphin in doses comparable to those employed in the vasopressin studies.[85] Therefore, the idea quickly surfaced that the enkephalinergic neurons and receptors recently shown to be present in relatively high concentrations in the intermediate and posterior lobes of the pituitary[86–88] somehow mediated the effect of various stimuli on vasopressin release.[89]

Almost as soon as this concept was proposed, however, contradictory data appeared simultaneously from two laboratories. Working in conscious rats, Kamoi et al.[90] and Greidanus et al.[91] found that parenteral administration of morphine suppressed plasma vasopressin under basal conditions and inhibited the rise produced by osmotic stimulation. These inhibitory effects were equally marked after intraventricular injection of smaller doses of morphine,[91] were blocked completely by pretreatment with naloxone,[90,91] and appeared to be due to an elevation in the osmotic threshold for vasopressin release.[90] The effects of butorphanol were identical to those of morphine and also were blocked with naloxone,[90] indicating that its inhibitory action on vasopressin secretion was a property of its agonist rather than its antagonist properties. Interestingly, Greidanus *et al.* found that β-endorphin also inhibits vasopressin secretion in rats, but they could not prevent this effect by pretreatment with naloxone.[91] The significance of this finding is not yet clear, but it suggests that at least some endogenous opiates act via a class of receptors that are not naloxone-sensitive.[92-95]

These challenging observations were followed very quickly by a number of others that also indicated that opiates and their natural and synthetic analogs had an inhibitory effect on basal and stimulated vasopressin secretion.[96-99] Like the previous observations with β-endorphin,[91] the inhibitory effects of one enkephalin analog in humans were not prevented by naloxone.[97] However, those of a different analog were blocked.[98] These observations suggest that, though the neurohypophysis may contain different classes of opiate receptors that bind preferentially or specifically with particular agonists and antagonists, the ultimate effect of all of them is to inhibit vasopressin release. This hypothesis is consistent with recent studies of vasopressin secretion from neurohypophyses *in vitro*[100] and of firing rates of individual vasopressinergic neurons,[101] both of which show that local application of opiate agonists inhibits secretory or electrical activity.

Despite rapidly mounting evidence of the effects of exogenous opiates on vasopressin secretion, information about the role played by endogenous opiates remains scanty and conflicting. Administration of the μ receptor antagonist, naloxone, has been reported to enhance the vasopressin response to a hemodynamic stimulus.[102] However, another study observed an inhibitory effect,[103] while a third found only small and inconsistent potentiation of the vasopressin response to osmotic and hemodynamic stimuli.[90] These findings do not necessarily mean that endogenous opiates are unimportant in the regulation of vasopressin secretion. As noted above, the enkephalins and other endogenous opiates may bind preferentially to δ receptors, which are known to be unaffected by naloxone. Clarification of this question awaits the development and application of more effective δ receptor antagonists. Moreover, given recent findings concerning the inhibitory action of exogenous opiates, it may be more productive to examine the effect of antagonists on the suppression rather than the stimulation of vasopressin. Consistent with this idea is a recent preliminary report that naloxone partially prevents the inhibition of vasopressin release normally induced by ethanol.[104]

One of the more interesting questions in this saga is why virtually all of the studies published before 1979 report that opiates stimulate antidiuresis and/or vasopressin release while those published afterwards almost uniformly observe the reverse. Review of the literature suggests that a number of factors are probably involved. First, many of the early studies relied solely on urine flow as an index of antidiuretic hormone secretion, and it is now clear that morphine and other opiates can reduce urine output by mechanisms totally independent of vasopressin secretion.[105] Hence, the advent of radioimmunoassays and other methodologic improvements permitted contemporary workers to avoid this source of confusion. However, the nonspecificity of the methodology cannot be the only reason, since some of the early studies went to great lengths to verify the essential role of the posterior pituitary and to exclude the influence of reductions in glomerular filtration or solute excretion that might be confused with the antidiuretic effects of vasopressin.[72] Moreover, one recent study reported that opiates increase vasopressin secretion as determined by radioimmunoassay.[82] In these instances, the results may be explained at least in part by a failure to distinguish between primary and secondary effects of opiates. Hypotension and/or nausea are frequent side effects of medium to high doses of morphine and only recently have become widely recognized as potent stimuli of vasopressin release. Close rereading of the literature indicates that one or both of these factors probably were responsible for the results obtained in many of the older studies. Modern workers seem to have avoided this problem either because they were more aware of it, used lower doses of opiates and/or performed the studies in rats, which are relatively refractory to emetic influences.[58] However, even after all these factors are taken into account, one is left with a number of studies in which it is difficult, if not impossible, to reconcile experimental differences. Hence, there may be other as yet undiscovered factors that alter the influence of exogenous or endogenous opiates on vasopressin release.

9.4.7.2. Nicotine

Nicotine is another drug that, like the opiates, has long been associated with stimulation of vasopressin secretion. Theories concerning its mechanism of action have varied, but the dominant view until recently was that the drug acted directly on the hypothalamus via cholinergic receptors believed to be involved in the control of vasopressin release. Several years ago, Schrier and colleagues presented evidence that nicotine acted via peripheral receptors linked to the neurohypophysis via cervical parasympathetic nerves.[106] Shortly thereafter, Bisset *et al.* also reported that nicotine did not act directly on the hypothalamic–neurohypophyseal tract but via an area on the ventral brain stem that received vagal and other cervical parasympathetic afferents.[107] This effect could be dissociated from the hypotensive actions of nicotine which, nonetheless, may contribute to vasopressin release. Since the studies were performed in anesthetized animals, it is impossible to exclude a direct or indirect effect on the emetic center, a nicotine-sensitive medullary area with potent effects on vasopressin release.

It is still unclear how these observations relate to the effect of smoking or intravenous nicotine on vasopressin release in man. Previous studies indicate that, though intravenous nicotine consistently elicits an antidiuretic response, the dose and rate of administration required to do so almost always result in nausea, vomiting, or hypotension.[108–110] More recent studies indicate that the vasopressin response elicited by smoking is not due to emetic or hypotensive stimuli[111–113] and, in fact, is not even mediated by absorbed, bloodborne nicotine.[113] Taken as a whole, these results suggest that actions of nicotine on vasopressin secretion are complex and involve multiple sites and mechanisms, depending on the dose, rate and route of administration.

9.4.7.3. Other Drugs with Antidiuretic Effects

The controversy surrounding the mechanism by which chlorpropamide, clofibrate, and carbamazepine promote antidiuresis in patients with diabetes insipidus was reviewed in an earlier volume of this series.[1] The tentative conclusions advanced at that time have since received additional experimental support. In studies performed in healthy humans as well as rats, Pokracki et al.[114] found that administration of chlorpropamide consistently impaired the ability to maximally dilute the urine after a water load without altering the ability to suppress plasma vasopressin. They also found that chlorpropamide did not augment and may even have inhibited the vasopressin response to osmotic or nonosmotic stimuli. These results provide additional evidence that the antidiuretic effects of chlorpropamide are mediated not by an increase in vasopressin secretion but by some effect on the kidney. Similar conclusions probably apply to the antidiuretic actions of carbamazepine. In controlled studies performed in healthy volunteers, two different laboratories found that administration of the drug suppressed plasma[115] or urinary[116] vasopressin without decreasing plasma sodium. These findings agree with those reported previously[117] and suggest that the drug inhibits hormone secretion by raising the threshold or lowering the sensitivity of the osmostat. It should be noted, however, that in some patients, carbamazepine may have a paradoxical stimulatory effect since, in one patient, it caused inappropriate antidiuresis with elevations in plasma vasopressin.[118]

9.4.7.4. Drugs with Diuretic Effects

Treatment with lithium is known to block the antidiuretic actions of vasopressin (Section 9.5). Until recently, however, nothing was known about the effect of this drug on vasopressin secretion. Studies performed in patients receiving lithium carbonate for psychiatric disorders have now shown that the drug increases plasma vasopressin.[119,120] This potentiation occurs independently of any increase in plasma sodium, indicating that it is due to increased sensitivity and/or reduced threshold of the vasopressin osmostat. The mechanism by which this alteration occurs is unknown. However, it is interesting that the changes appear to be the opposite of those produced by other drugs, such as carbamazepine, that potentiate instead of inhibit the antidiuretic effects of vasopressin. These symmetrical, offsetting changes may be an unrelated coincidence or they may indicate the operation of some unrecognized, nonosmotic feedback system that alters the osmoregulation of vasopressin to compensate for abnormalities in its antidiuretic effects.

9.4.7.5. Miscellaneous

A variety of other drugs or hormones have recently been reported to influence vasopressin release. In anesthetized dogs and rats, intravenous administration of clonidine, an antihypertensive agent with central, α-adrenoreceptor actions, causes an acute increase in urine output. Studies performed by Humphreys and colleagues originally indicated that this diuresis was due to a decrease in vasopressin secretion that they suggested might be secondary to the hemodynamic effects of the drug.[121] Follow-up studies by Reid and colleagues confirmed by direct immunoassay that clonidine did in fact suppress vasopressin secretion, but also showed that this effect occurred independently of its pressor activity.[122] Subsequent work by Kimura *et al.* supported earlier suggestions[122] that the drug suppressed vasopressin secretion as well as blood pressure by stimulating α adrenoreceptors in the brain.[123] These observations are particularly interesting in light of recent findings that the central afferents that mediate baroregulatory influences on magnocellular neurons of the supraoptic nucleus are noradrenergic (Section 9.4.2). Whether or not conventional therapeutic doses of oral clonidine have similar effects on vasopressin secretion in conscious humans is unknown. Diuretic effects have not been reported, but they might be counteracted rapidly by a slight rise in plasma osmolality caused by the water loss.

Administration of TRH has been reported to suppress plasma vasopressin in euthyroid and hypothyroid people.[124] The findings indicate that the effect is not mediated by changes in plasma osmolality but they do not exclude other secondary influences such as increases in blood pressure. Further exploration of this effect seems indicated in view of reports that the neurohypophysis contains large quantities of TRH.[125,126]

In rats, Skowsky *et al.* observed that androgens inhibit and estrogens stimulate vasopressin secretion.[127] These effects occurred at physiologic levels of the steroids and could not be accounted for by changes in plasma osmolality. However, hemodynamic and other, nonosmotic influences were not monitored. In intact, virgin female rats, the administration of large doses of estrogen and/or progesterone does not seem to affect vasopressin secretion.[33] The results of these two studies would not be incompatible if vasopressin secretion were stimulated maximally by physiologic levels of estrogen. The relevance of these observations to humans is unclear. In normal man, estradiol administration has been reported to increase urinary excretion of vasopressin.[128] However, as reviewed previously,[1] it does not seem to stimulate secretion of the neurophysin associated with vasopressin, and there are no obvious differences in the regulation of plasma vasopressin in young men and women. It may be that the effects of estrogen and testosterone in young adults are subtle or are offset by other sex-related differences. Further study of this problem in postmenopausal women and older men may clarify this interesting problem.

Substance P is a widely distributed peptide that is suspected of playing a role in neurotransmission or neuromodulation in the brain and many other organs. Recently, the native hormone and several synthetic analogs were reported to produce a transient antidiuresis in ethanol-anesthetized rats.[129] Although this result could indicate a direct effect of substance P on the kidney, it could also be due to release of endogenous vasopressin, since substance P is a depressor, and ethanol is not a very effective inhibitor of vasopressin release. Consistent with this interpretation was the finding of a correlation between antidiuretic and hypotensive properties of various analogs.[129] Hence, rather than a direct effect on the kidney or neurohypophysis, substance P probably increases vasopressin secretion as a consequence of hemodynamic or other non-osmotic stimuli.

9.5. Biological Actions

9.5.1. Renal

The principal if not the only physiologic action of vasopressin in man is to promote concentration of the urine. The mechanism by which this antidiuresis is induced is an extensively studied topic whose complexity is beyond the scope of the present review. For a detailed overview of current concepts, the reader is referred to recent reviews.[130–132] However, there are also a number of new developments in this area that may be of particular interest to endocrinologists and others interested in a better understanding of antidiuretic function. In the following section, a few of the more interesting of these findings will be noted and, where possible, related to existing knowledge about the renal actions of vasopressin.

9.5.1.1. cAMP

There is general agreement that vasopressin promotes urinary concentration by increasing the hydroosmotic permeability of the mucosal epithelium. The exact mechanism by which the increased permeability occurs is unknown but by all accounts seems to involve interaction with receptors on the serosal surface followed by activation of adenylate cyclase and formation of cAMP. Recent studies in rats indicate that little if any of the cAMP formed in collecting tubules gains access to the urine.[133] Hence, measurements of cAMP in urine probably are not a reliable indicator of the renal actions of vasopressin. Infusion of the hormone has been reported to increase urinary cAMP as well as osmolality in water-loaded, healthy adults.[134] However, the doses of vasopressin used in this study were relatively large and could well have been acting on blood vessels or other extrarenal tissues. Hence, the observed increases in urinary cAMP may have come from plasma via glomerular filtration, rather than renal production. If so, the concept that some forms of nephrogenic diabetes insipidus are due to impaired renal formation of cAMP will require reevaluation.

9.5.1.2. Prostaglandins

There is also general agreement that vasopressin stimulates the production of prostaglandins by the kidney and that this increase in synthesis is reflected by a rise in their urinary excretion.[135] However, it is less clear how and where the increase in prostaglandin production occurs and what role, if any, it plays in the antidiuretic effects of vasopressin. Recent studies in cultured interstitial cells from renal medulla indicate that the increase in prostaglandins is due to the pressor rather than the antidiuretic properties of vasopressin.[136] On the other hand, prostaglandin excretion in rats with hereditary neurogenic diabetes insipidus appears to be stimulated equally by vasopressin and DDAVP, an analog with antidiuretic, but no pressor, actions.[137] Hence, it is still unknown whether the effect of vasopressin on prostaglandins is an integral or an incidental aspect of its effect on urine concentration. Similar uncertainty surrounds the consequences of renal prostaglandin production. Although there is general agreement that the antidiuretic action of vasopressin can be inhibited by the addition of prostaglandin E and potentiated by treatment with prostaglandin synthetase inhibitors,[131,135] it is by no means clear that either effect reflects the action of endogenous prostaglandins. Indomethacin has been observed to increase urine osmolality in the absence of vasopressin or significant changes in prostaglandin excretion.[137] In addition, there is reason to believe that some prostaglandin metabolites potentiate, while others inhibit, the hydroosmotic effects of vasopressin.[138] Because of these uncertainties, it is difficult at present to properly assess the putative role of renal prostaglandins in the physiology, pathology, or pharmacology of antidiuretic function (Section 9.6.1).

9.5.1.3. Kinins and Kallikreins

The distal nephron and urine contain large amounts of kallikrein, an enzyme that acts on kininogen to liberate kinins, hormones with a wide array of biological effects.[139,140] Recent studies suggest that this kallikrein–kinin system may be involved in the regulation of antidiuretic function. The urine of man and many other mammals contains large amounts of kinins, which appear to be formed primarily in the collecting tubules.[141] Their rate of excretion is suppressed by water loading and stimulated by vasopressin,[142] suggesting that the kinins are somehow involved in the regulation of antidiuretic function. Consistent with this view are *in vitro* observations that the hydroosmotic effects of vasopressin are antagonized by kininase inhibitors[143] or by bradykinin itself[144] and are potentiated by inhibitors of kallikrein.[143] Hence, it may be that locally generated kinins act as a negative feedback system to modulate the effects of vasopressin on the kidney. This effect could be mediated in part by stimulation of prostaglandin production.[145] However, definitive evidence linking the kallikrein–kinin system to the physiology or pathology of antidiuretic function is still lacking.

9.5.1.4. Calcium and Calmodulin

There is now considerable evidence that the antidiuretic effect of vasopressin is a calcium-dependent process. Verapamil, which inhibits the entry of calcium into cells, antagonizes the hydroosmotic effects of vasopressin.[146] A similar effect is seen in the presence of phenothiazines, which block the actions of calmodulin, a binding protein that mediates most of the actions of calcium.[147,148] Conversely, the antidiuretic effect of vasopressin in rats is enhanced by parathyroid hormone, and this effect can be blocked with verapamil.[149] It is not clear at which step in the antidiuretic response the calcium acts or whether these effects are related in any way to the clinical abnormalities in antidiuretic function often seen in patients with hypo- or hypercalcemia.

9.5.1.5. Somatostatin

Somatostatin, a peptide hormone with potent inhibitory effects on the secretion of many other hormones, is also capable of counteracting the antidiuretic actions of vasopressin.[150,151] Antagonism seems to be due to interference with the formation of cAMP, an effect common to many of its other inhibitory actions. It is doubtful whether this antidiuretic action is of any physiologic or pathophysiologic importance since somatostatin is not known to be present in mammalian kidney, and its concentration in blood is probably too low to appreciably influence the kidney. Nevertheless, it may prove to be of some relevance to the pharmacologic use of the hormone or in the rare case of somatostatin-producing tumors.

9.5.1.6. Vasopressin Antagonists

One recent development that is bound to have a major investigative if not therapeutic impact in the near future is the synthesis of the first truly effective antagonists of the antidiuretic actions of vasopressin.[152] These compounds are analogs of vasopressin in which β-mercapto-ββ-cyclopentamethylene-proprionic acid substitutes for cysteine in position 1 of the ring, valine replaces glutamine in position 4, and a methyl or ethyl group is attached to the ring of tyrosine in position 2. When given in the absence of vasopressin, they appear to be weak agonists. However, in the presence of exogenous or endogenous vasopressin, they competitively inhibit its antidiuretic effects. These antagonists may be particularly useful for investigating the cause of the hypovasopressinemic antidiuresis that has been observed in a variety of experimental and clinical settings (Sections 9.5.1.7, 9.6.3.1, and 9.6.3.2).

9.5.1.7. Other Factors

Recently, it has been shown that dehydration in homozygous rats with diabetes insipidus causes a urinary concentration in the absence of both vasopressin and a significant fall in glomerular filtration.[153] The mechanism of this effect is totally unknown. However, increases in papillary osmolality, a reduction in solute excretion, or the elaboration of oxytocin or some other as yet unrecognized antidiuretic hormone are reasonable possibilities. These observations are of more than usual interest in view of the clinical disorder distinguished by inappropriate antidiuresis in the presence of maximal suppression of plasma vasopressin (Section 9.6.3.1).

9.5.2. Vascular

Perhaps no aspect of posterior pituitary function has attracted more attention in recent years than its role in blood pressure regulation. As the name implies, vasopressin was found very early to cause the contraction of vascular smooth muscle.[154] In fact, this property was exploited for many years as a means of assaying the hormone. However, it was also generally recognized that the pressor assay was relatively insensitive unless the animal was pithed.[154] Similarly, the infusion of vasopressin at doses many times greater than those required to produce maximum antidiuresis was shown years ago to have no appreciable effect on arterial pressure in healthy or hypertensive humans.[155] This knowledge led to the idea that vasopressin does not play an important role in baroregulation unless plasma levels are extremely high or autonomic reflexes are impaired.[156]

In recent years, interest in this question revived, largely because of suggestions that vasopressin plays an important role in the pathogenesis of certain forms of hypertension (Section 9.6.3.4). Although the final word may not yet have been heard, these studies confirm to a remarkable degree the original views about the role of the neurohypophysis in baroregulation. Thus, in anesthetized animals, an inability to secrete vasopressin impairs the capacity to maintain arterial pressure during hemorrhage.[157–159] These results are consistent with the idea that large increases in vasopressin secretion contribute significantly to the maintenance of arterial pressure, at least in the presence of anesthesia or other conditions that impair autonomic reflexes. In conscious dogs or humans with intact baroregulatory reflexes, infusion of vasopressin fails to significantly alter the mean arterial pressure until plasma levels of the hormone are increased to more than 20 times normal.[160–163] Much lower vasopressin concentrations, ranging from two to five times basal levels, may produce other hemodynamic effects such as increased peripheral resistance,[160] but they do not raise arterial pressure, presumably because of reflex reductions in heart rate and cardiac output. Consistent with this interpretation are experiments showing that sensitivity to the pressor effect of vasopressin is greatly enhanced by denervation of the baroreceptors in dogs[160,161] or by defects in central vasomotor pathways in humans.[163]

Taken as a whole, these studies indicate that plasma vasopressin plays no more than a trivial role in baroregulation of healthy animals.

Such a result might have been anticipated from the older literature as well as from many years of clinical experience that fails to reveal a particular predisposition to hypotension in patients with neurogenic diabetes insipidus. However, they also confirm that the hormone may contribute to the maintenance of blood pressure under conditions in which the primary autonomic defense mechanisms are maximally stressed or largely inoperative. Whether these effects are of any clinical importance remains to be determined.

It should be noted that peripheral secretion may not be the only, or even the most important, route by which vasopressin can influence baroregulation. As noted in Section 9.1, some vasopressinergic and many oxytocinergic fibers project from the paraventricular nucleus to areas near the vasomotor center in the medulla. Moreover, electrical stimulation of the paraventricular and supraoptic nuclei appears to depress blood pressure and heart rate in anesthetized animals.[164] Hence, it may be that stimulating vasopressin and/or oxytocin secretion has complex baroregulatory consequences that reflect the balance of peripheral pressor and central depressor mechanisms.

9.5.3. Extrarenal, Extravascular

Vasopressin appears to have a number of actions besides its antidiuretic and pressor effects. For example, it acts on the liver to stimulate both glycogenolysis[165] and gluconeogenesis[166] and to inhibit ketogenesis.[167] The vasopressin concentrations required have not been established, but probably are well within the range elicited by nausea or severe hypotension. It also has a variety of effects on motor and secretory activity in the gastrointestinal tract,[168,169] which may play some role in the emetic reflex.

The vasopressin secreted into hypophyseal portal blood may also have significant effects on anterior pituitary function. Electrical stimulation of the paraventricular nucleus, a major source of the vasopressinergic fibers that terminate in the zona externa of the median eminence, causes release of both ACTH and vasopressin.[170] Hence, while vasopressin is almost certainly not the only or even the major corticotropin-releasing factor,[171–174] that portion secreted into portal blood may contribute to the release of ACTH. It may also influence secretion of β-endorphin.[175]

Vasopressin also appears to have multiple effects on the CNS. Besides altering the water content of brain,[176] it has been implicated in a variety of direct effects on neurons[177] including the enhancement of memory and other cognitive functions.[178,179] These observations are particularly interesting in light of the many extrahypophyseal projections of vasopressinergic neurons (Section 9.2), the presence of a separate pathway for secretion of vasopressin into cerebrospinal fluid,[8] and the finding of abnormalities in plasma or cerebrospinal fluid vasopressin in patients with certain affective disorders.[180] At present, however, it is totally unknown whether any of these neurologic effects and pathways play a role in normal or disordered states of central nervous function.

9.6. Pathology

9.6.1. Deficient Secretion

9.6.1.1. Neurohypophyseal Damage

Diagnostic differentiation of neurogenic diabetes insipidus from other causes of nonglucosuric polyuria has long been based on a variety of indirect measures of vasopressin secretion.[181,182] The advent of radioimmunoassay techniques has made it much easier to assess neurohypophyseal function by direct assay of the hormone in plasma.[1,24,183–185] Recently, comparative studies have shown that direct assay of vasopressin is also more accurate than the standard indirect test.[186] This advantage is most pronounced in differentiating between partial neurogenic diabetes insipidus and primary polydipsia, a situation in which the indirect test gives a wrong diagnosis at least 30% of the time. Analysis of the relationship between plasma vasopressin and urine osmolality in these patients revealed that the errors in the indirect test were due in part to a previously unrecognized increase in sensitivity to the antidiuretic effect of low concentrations of vasopressin in patients with partial neurogenic diabetes insipidus. This supersensitivity and the decrease in maximum concentrating capacity that results from polyuria *per se* combine to obscure the difference in the antidiuretic response to water deprivation and vasopressin administration that would be expected in the two kinds of patients. The cause of the renal hypersensitivity to vasopressin is not known, but it may be a manifestation of the increase in vasopressin receptors that has been observed in patients with chronic deficiency of the hormone.[187]

Whatever the mechanism, this alteration in renal sensitivity to vasopressin suggests that direct assay of the hormone should become a standard part of the diagnostic evaluation of all polyuric patients whose urine concentrates to any degree during water deprivation. The most physiologic way of doing this is to measure plasma vasopressin during water deprivation and to relate these values to the concurrent level of plasma and urine osmolality.[186] However, it is also possible to assess the hormone response to hypertonic saline or to a nonosmotic stimulus such as nausea.[185] The latter approach has the advantage of requiring a good deal less assay sensitivity and specificity but also is less discriminating, since the vasopressin values cannot be quantitatively related to stimulus strength.

The basic therapeutic approach to neurogenic diabetes insipidus has not changed in recent years.[1] Tests have been conducted on a new, sublingual form of DDAVP and an even more potent relative, DVDAVP,[188] but it is not yet clear whether either of these preparations is sufficiently more effective or convenient to warrant replacement of the intranasal DDAVP now used in America. Chlorpropamide remains an effective alternative mode of therapy in many patients with neurogenic diabetes insipidus. Efforts to understand its mechanism of action have received some help from studies indicating that the drug does not increase vasopressin secretion in healthy adults or rats[114] and may act by inhibiting the vasopressin-induced increase in renal prostaglandins.[189] However, as noted in Section 9.5.1.2, the inhibitory effect of renal prostaglandins on antidiuresis is still a complicated issue, and it is quite possible that they are not the ony way in which chlorpropamide promotes antidiuresis.

9.6.1.2. Osmoreceptor Damage

Deficiency of vasopressin secretion also occurs in patients with the entity variously referred to as adipsic or "essential" hypernatremia.[190] In this condition, the deficiency is due largely if not totally to destruction of the osmostat rather than the neurohypophysis because the hormone usually responds normally to nonosmotic stimuli. These patients can be distinguished clinically from those with diabetes insipidus by the absence of thirst and polyuria under hypertonic conditions. However, when efforts are made to correct their dehydration, many of them dilute their urine at inappropriately high levels of plasma osmolality. In all cases where this phenomenon has been adequately characterized, it has been shown to be due not to resetting of the osmostat but to a marked reduction in the sensitivity or gain of the system. Other patients fail to dilute their urine even under hypotonic conditions, suggesting that they may have lost the capacity to respond appropriately to osmotic suppression or stimulation. This combination of abnormalities suggests that osmoregulatory function is normally bimodal, i.e., maximum suppression of vasopressin requires inhibitory input as well as the absence of stimulation. If so, then the threshold or "set" of the osmostat would not correspond to the point of maximum vasopressin secretion, but to a somewhat higher value where activity of both inhibitory and stimulatory components is minimal. On close inspection, virtually all patients with adipsic hypernatremia have pathology in or around the hypothalamus, a finding consistent with the presumed location of the osmoreceptors (Section 9.4.1).

A number of new cases of this relatively rare syndrome have been reported in recent years.[191–195] Each of those appropriately tested was shown to be due to selective destruction of the osmoreceptor.[193,194] Treatment with chlorpropamide,[191,195] clofibrate, or carbamazepine[193] was reported to improve control of the hypernatremia in four patients, but had no effect on the other.[194] In two cases,[193,195] this improvement may have been due to reduction of the polyuria that often frustrates efforts at forced rehydration. In the other two,[191] it was attributed to stimulation of thirst. Whatever the mechanism, a therapeutic trial with one or more of these drugs would appear to be worthwhile in patients with this potentially devastating disorder.

9.6.2. Deficient Renal Response

Diabetes insipidus due to an absent renal response to plasma vasopressin can occur as a sex-linked inherited disorder.[196] Recently a variant of this nephrogenic disorder was discovered.[197] Unlike the classical form, in which affected males are totally refractory to the antidiuretic effects of vasopressin, the new variant is characterized by partial resistance or a shift in the dose–response curve to plasma vasopressin. Hence, although polyuria occurs in the presencce of normal levels of plasma vasopressin, these patients are able to concentrate their urine if plasma levels are raised 10- to 20-fold by such procedures as prolonged fluid deprivation or high doses of exogenous vasopressin. The existence of this variant of nephrogenic diabetes insipidus is important to recognize because it can be misdiagnosed as partial neurogenic diabetes insipidus by standard indirect tests.[181,182] Moreover, though unresponsive to standard therapeutic doses of antidiuretic hormone, the polyuria in this condition can be corrected totally by administration of pharmacologic doses of DDAVP. Whether acquired forms of nephrogenic diabetes insipidus also exist is uncertain, but recent studies in sarcoid[186] and lithium-induced forms (see below) suggest that they do.

Nephrogenic diabetes insipidus can also be caused by a variety of drugs.[198,199] Some of the most interesting and potentially important new information in this area relates to the effects of lithium.[200] Initial studies suggested that the drug caused nephrogenic diabetes insipidus by interfering with a step distal to the formation of cAMP in the collecting tubule.[201] However, it now appears that other defects in other parts of the nephron may also play a role. In rats treated with lithium at doses too small to produce basal polyuria, the administration of relatively large doses of vasopressin produces a paradoxical increase in urine flow that seems to be due at least in part to interference with the reabsorption of salt and water at a site proximal to the collecting tubule.[202] Equally fascinating is the report that polyuria induced by chronic lithium treatment in rats can be overcome by relatively high doses of DDAVP.[203] This analog was reported to be much more effective than native vasopressin, but the comparison is dubious because the latter was given in smaller amounts and no allowancce was made for the slower rate of degradation of DDAVP. Nevertheless, the finding that high doses of vasopressin in any form can overcome the polyuria of lithium-induced nephrogenic diabetes insipidus would suggest that the defect is partial or relative and occurs proximal to the formation of cAMP. Finally, a variety of structural lesions have also been found in renal biopsies from patients receiving chronic lithium therapy.[204] Hence, the nephrotoxic effects of lithium would appear to be protean, depending perhaps on factors such as dose of the drug, duration of therapy, and the amount and type of vasopressin present. Further studies of this phenomenon in man are needed to better define the characteristics of the defect.

A recent brief report indicates that neoplasms can also produce nephrogenic diabetes insipidus.[205] This association has not been observed previously and cannot be accounted for by any of the known causes of nephrogenic diabetes insipidus. Its discovery suggests the existence of unrecognized hormones or other humoral factors that can block the antidiuretic effects of vasopressin (Section 9.5.1).

9.6.3. Excessive Secretion

9.6.3.1. Inappropriate Antidiuresis

Much information about the pathophysiology of this syndrome has accumulated over the last 20 years. It is summarized in an earlier volume of this series[1] and in two subsequent reviews.[206,207] The following section will focus on more recent developments not covered in those sources.

The list of diseases associated with the syndrome of inappropriate antidiuresis continues to grow. To the more than two score conditions noted previously,[207] we may now add hypoplasia of the corpus callosum,[208] central pontine myelinosis,[209] and an idiopathic form associated with hypertension and inappropriate thirst.[210,211] In some of the latter patients, the hyponatremia and hypertension are associated with resetting of the osmostat and impaired hemodynamic control of vasopressin.[211] This constellation of abnormalities may be related since loss of baroregulatory input might be expected to remove a tonic inhibitory influence on the set of the osmostat, as well as on the vasomotor center (Section 9.4.2). It is not known if baroreceptor deafferentation occurs in any of the other forms of reset osmostat, a relatively common variant of the syndrome of inappropriate antidiuresis.[207] In these patients, as in those with most other types of abnormal vasopressin secretion,[207] the cause remains a complete mystery. Ectopic production by a neoplasm is a notable exception, but that mechanism is relatively uncommon even among cancer patients with inappropriate antidiuresis.[212,213] Like the nonmalignant forms of the syndrome, the mechanism by which tumors cause abnormal secretion from the neurohypophysis is unknown.

Abnormalities in water balance are also frequent in psychosis. The most common problem is uncomplicated compulsive water drinking.[214] For reasons that are not clear, however, many of these patients also have inappropriate antidiuresis, a particularly devastating combination that can result in severe water intoxication.[215-221] The finding of maximally dilute urine in some of these patients led to the suggestion that psychogenic water drinking alone might cause hyponatremia.[219] Although such a mechanism may suffice in the rare patients with truly astronomical rates of water intake (in excess of 20 liters a day), most cases of hyponatremia with maximally dilute urine under basal conditions prove on closer inspection to have primary polydipsia in conjunction with resetting of the vasopressin osmostat.[220] As in virtually all other forms of the syndrome, the cause of the vasopressin abnormality is a mystery, although orthostatic hypotension induced by psychotropic drugs may be responsible in some cases. Occasionally, therapy with lithium may further complicate matters by producing nephrogenic diabetes insipidus that can be confused with psychogenic polydipsia.

Hypothyroidism is another clinical condition traditionally associated with inappropriate antidiuresis. Until recently, however, the problem had not even been examined systematically using assays of vasopressin. Water loading tests have now confirmed that a very large proportion of patients with myxedema exhibit impaired urinary dilution and inadequate suppression of plasma vasopressin.[222] However, it also seems that impaired water excretion can occur in the absence of detectable abnormalities in vasopressin,[222-224] that inappropriate vasopressin secretion can occur in the absence of impaired urinary dilution,[222] and that myxedema can occur without detectable abnormalities in either water excretion or vasopressin secretion.[222] Hence, it is probably not hypothyroidism *per se* but several as yet unknown complications that cause variable abnormalities in the secretion and/or action of vasopressin.

Other studies also suggest that inappropriate antidiuresis is not always due to inappropriate secretion of vasopressin.[206] In about 10% of all patients who fulfill the clinical criteria for this syndrome, the osmoregulation of plasma vasopressin is found to be completely normal.[207] This "hypovasopressinemic" form of inappropriate antidiuresis has been observed in association with a variety of conditions other than hypothyroidism.[225,226] It may reflect production of some abnormal antidiuretic hormone or greatly increased renal sensitivity to normally suppressed levels of endogenous vasopressin. As noted above (Section 9.5.1.2), a decrease in renal prostaglandins has been shown to increase urinary concentration in both the absence and the presence of vasopressin. Moreover, many clinical features of the syndrome can be reproduced by administering indomethacin and ACTH to normal volunteers,[227] maneuvers that would not be expected to increase plasma vasopressin. Although indomethacin was not a factor in any of the patients with hypovasopressinemic inappropriate antidiuresis, it is possible that intrinsic defects in prostaglandin production with or without other abnormalities cause water retention in some cases.

Recent studies have also revived the concept of cerebral salt wasting as an alternative defect to the syndrome of inappropriate antidiuresis.[228] The basic issue is whether the hyponatremia and excessive sodium excretion that often occur in patients with neurologic disease is simply a manifestation of inappropriate vasopressin secretion and water intake, as generally believed, or is actually due to a primary defect in sodium excretion that leads secondarily to hypovolemia and a hemodynamically appropriate increase in vasopressin secretion. Data concerning blood volume recently obtained in these patients suggest that the latter is the case.[228] However, these measurements are fraught with difficulty and revealed certain abnormalities, such as a parallel reduction in red cell mass, which cannot be explained in terms of cerebral salt wasting. Hence, judgement on this intriguing question must be reserved pending the results of the kind of prospective balance studies needed to establish the volume changes present.

9.6.3.2. Adrenal Insufficiency

Urinary dilution is also impaired in most if not all patients with glucocorticoid or mineralocorticoid deficiency. Traditionally, this defect has been excluded from the category of inappropriate antidiuretic hormone either because an increase in vasopressin secretion could not be demonstrated[229–231] or was thought to be an appropriate response to the hypovolemia and/or hypotension that often results from the steroid deficiency.[232–234] Recent immunoassay studies confirm that adrenal insufficiency is, in fact, associated with osmotically inappropriate increases in plasma vasopressin.[235–240] In the case of isolated mineralocorticoid deficiency, the increase in vasopressin appears to be due largely if not totally to volume depletion[237] with resulting resetting of the osmostat.[240] In the case of isolated glucocorticoid deficiency, the increase in vasopressin secretion cannot be attributed to hypovolemia or hypotension,[235,238] although other baroreceptor-mediated stimuli arising from defects in cardiac output cannot be excluded.[235] In addition, there is also a vasopressin-independent mechanism that develops late and contributes to the impaired water excretion in isolated glucocorticoid deficiency.[239] Hence, these studies essentially confirm earlier observations that indicate that the antidiuresis of adrenal insufficiency is a complex phenomenon that, depending on the type, severity, and duration of the steriod deficiency, results from vasopressin-independent as well as vasopressin-dependent mechanisms.

9.6.3.3. Edema-Forming States

Cardiac, hepatic, and renal failure also result in hyponatremia and impaired water excretion. Like adrenal insufficiency, however, these conditions are routinely excluded from the category of inappropriate antidiuresis because at least part of the excretory defect is known to be due to excessive sodium retention.[241] In addition, the abnormal urinary concentration has been attributed to increases in vasopressin secretion stimulated by the "effective" hypovolemia that accompanies cardiac or hepatic failure. However, only recently have investigators begun to examine these concepts using radioimmunoassay and other sophisticated techniques. In rats with cirrhosis induced experimentally by bile duct ligation[242] or carbon tetrachloride,[243] urinary diluting capacity is impaired. This abnormality is probably due to abnormal vasopressin secretion since it does not occur in animals that lack the hormone[242] or is associated with plasma vasopressin levels that are inappropriately high for the hypoosmolality present.[243] The nonosmolar stimulus to vasopressin has not been precisely identified but it may be secondary to abnormal systemic hemodynamics. Plasma vasopressin is also inappropriately high in patients with congestive heart failure and hyponatremia.[244] As in the cases of the cirrhotic rats, the nonosmolar stimulus has not been identified with certainty but probably is hemodynamic in nature.

9.6.3.4. Diabetes Mellitus

Recent studies reveal that vasopressin secretion is increased in patients with insulin-dependent diabetes mellitus.[245,246] This abnormality is most marked in patients with ketoacidosis, but preliminary studies indicate that it also occurs to a lesser degree in patients who are well controlled and have no complications of the disease.[247,248] The finding was unexpected since hyperglycemia suppresses vasopressin in diabetics[247] as well as in healthy adults (Section 9.4.1). Its cause is unknown. In patients who are poorly controlled, it may be due in part to the associated hypovolemia, hypotension, and/or nausea. However, it could also be due in part to intracellular hypoglycemia (Section 9.4.5) or to a more direct effect of insulin on parts of the brain known to be intimately involved in the regulation of vasopressin secretion.[249] The significance of these abnormalities, particularly their relationship to the polydipsia and hyponatremia that often occur in uncontrolled diabetics, is still unknown.

9.6.3.5. Hypertension

The role of vasopressin in the pathogenesis of hypertension suddenly emerged as a very "hot" topic in recent years. The surge of investigative interest is difficult to explain, particularly in view of older data indicating that the hormone is only weakly pressor unless baroreceptor reflexes are inoperative (Section 9.5.2). Pursuit of this subject seems to have started with a paper by Möhring and colleagues in 1976.[250] They reported that, in rats with malignant hypertension induced by unilateral nephrectomy, administration of saline and desoxycorticosterone, plasma vasopressin was increased eightfold and the injection of vasopressin antisera transiently corrected their hypertension. In subsequent papers,[251-254] Möhring and colleagues elaborated on these observations. In essence, they observed that: (1) rats with spontaneous or malignant Goldblatt hypertension also exhibited increases in plasma vasopressin that correlated positively with increases in blood pressure; (2) injection of vasopressin antisera lowered blood pressure in most but not all rats with these three forms of hypertension; (3) raising plasma vasopressin to the same level in rats with diabetes insipidus did not produce an increase in arterial pressure. To explain these observations, they concluded that all three forms of hypertension were caused at least in part by hypersensitivity to the pressor effect of vasopressin. This hypersensitivity was attributed tentatively to loss of the buffering effect of some unknown baroregulatory reflex.[254]

Almost simultaneously, other laboratories took up the chase. Crofton *et al.* also reported higher levels of vasopressin in the plasma and urine of spontaneously hypertensive rats, but at the same time cautioned that the magnitude and timing of the increase seemed inadequate to account for the hypertension.[255] Pullan *et al.* observed a modest increase in plasma vasopressin in dogs with Goldblatt hypertension, but also concluded from infusion data that it was inadequate to account for the rise in blood pressure.[256] Finally, Rabito *et al.* all but finished the idea by showing that administration of dPVDAVP or cyclo-dVDAVP, highly effective antagonists of the pressor actions of AVP,[257] had no effect on blood pressure in rats with adrenal regeneration hypertension, malignant DOCA salt hypertension, or malignant Goldblatt hypertension.[258] As a whole, these data indicate that even though vasopressin may be elevated in several animal models of hypertension, it plays little or no role in the blood pressure abnormalities. Why vasopressin antisera lower blood pressure in some animals with similar forms of hypertension is unknown.

Vasopressin also appears to be unimportant in the genesis of human hypertension. Plasma vasopressin levels are low[259,260] or normal[261] and respond normally to osmotic stimuli in uncomplicated essential hypertension.[262] In malignant hypertension, plasma vasopressin may be elevated modestly,[259] but the increases are nowhere near the level required to affect blood pressure in healthy adults (Section 9.5.2). In primary hyperaldosteronism, plasma vasopressin tends to be low even though plasma osmolality and sodium are increased.[261] This combination is due to upward resetting of the osmostat, apparently as a consequence of the chronic hypervolemia associated with this condition. Hence, it seems likely that any vasopressin abnormalities in hypertension are the consequence rather than the cause of the underlying disturbance in blood volume or pressure.

References

1. Robertson, G. L., 1978, Vasopressin and water metabolism, in: *The Year in Endocrinology 1977* (S. H. Ingbar, ed.), pp. 205–231, Plenum Medical, New York.
2. Zimmerman, E. A., 1981, The organization of oxytocin and vasopressin pathways, in *Neurosecretion and Brain Peptides* (J. B. Martin, S. Reichlin, and K. L. Bick, eds.), pp. 63–75, Raven Press, New York.
3. Sofroniew, M. V., Weindl, A., Schrell, U., and Wetzstein, R., 1981, Immunohistochemistry of vasopressin, oxytocin and neurophysin in the hypothalamus and extrahypothalamic regions of the human and primate brain, *Acta Histochem. Suppl.* **24:**79–95.
4. Dierickx, K., and Vandesande, F., 1977, Immunocytochemical localization of the vasopressinergic and the oxytocinergic neurons in the human hypothalamus, *Cell Tissue Res.* **184:**15–27.
5. Sofroniew, M. V., and Weindl, A., 1978, Projections from the parvocellular vasopressin- and neurophysin-containing neurons of the suprachiasmatic nucleus, *Am. J. Anat.* **153:**391–430.
6. Swanson, L. W., 1977, Immunohistochemical evidence for a neurophysin-containing automatic pathway arising in the paraventricular nucleus of the hypothalamus, *Brain Res.* **128:**346–353.
7. Nilaver, G., Zimmerman, E. A., Wilkins, J., Michaels, J., Hoffman, D., and Silverman, A.-J., 1980, Magnocellular hypothalamic projections to the lower

brain stem and spinal cord of the rat: Immunocytochemical evidence for predominance of the oxytocin–neurophysin system compared to the vasopressin–neurophysin system, *Neuroendocrinology* **30:**150–158.

8. Luerssen, T. G., and Robertson, G. L., 1980, Cerebrospinal fluid vasopressin and vasotocin in health and disease, in: *Neurobiology of Cerebrospinal Fluid*, Vol. 1 (J. H. Wood, ed.), pp.613–623, Plenum Press, New York.

9. Glick, S. M., and Brownstein, M. J., 1980, Vasopressin content of rat brain, *Life Sci.* **27:**1103–1110.

10. Summy-Long, J. V., Keil, L. C., and Severs, W. B., 1978, Identification of vasopressin in the subfornical organ region: Effects of dehydration, *Brain Res.* **140:**241–250.

11. Sachs, H., Fawcett, P., Takabatake, Y., and Portanova, R., 1969, Biosynthesis and release of vasopressin and neurophysin, *Recent Prog. Horm. Res.* **25:**447–491.

12. Russell, J. T., Brownstein, M. J., and Gainer, H., 1980, Biosynthesis of vasopressin, oxytocin, and neurophysins: Isolation and characterization of two common precursors (propressophysin and prooxyphysin), *Endocrinology* **107:**1880–1891.

13. Brownstein, M. J., Russell, J. T., and Gainer, H., 1980, Synthesis, transport, and release of posterior pituitary hormones, *Science* **207:**373–378.

14. Land, H., Schütz, G., Schmale, H., and Richter, D., 1982, Nucleotide sequence of cloned cDNA encoding bovine arginine vasopressin-neurophysin II precursor, *Nature (London)* **295:**299–303.

15. Valtin, H., Sokol, H. W., and Sunde, D., 1975, Genetic approaches to the study of the regulation and actions of vasopressin, *Recent Prog. Horm. Res.* **31:**447–486.

16. Oiso, Y., Gaskill, M. B., Stamoutsos, B., Lindheimer, M., and Robertson, G. L., 1981, Vasopressin immunoactivity in Brattleboro rats with hereditary hypothalamic diabetes insipidus, *Clin. Res.* **29:**708A.

17. Edwards, B. R., Gellai, M., and Valtin, H., 1980, Concentration of urine in the absence of ADH with minimal or no decrease in GFR, *Am. J. Physiol.* **239:**F84–F91.

18. Weitzman, R. E., and Fisher, D. A., 1977, Log linear relationship between plasma arginine vasopressin and plasma osmolality, *Am. J. Physiol.* **233:**E37–E40.

19. Moses, A. M., 1978, Is there an osmotic threshold for vasopressin release?, *Am. J. Physiol.* **234:**E339–E340.

20. Rodbard, D., and Munson, P. J., 1978, Editorial comment, *Am. J. Physiol.* **234:**E340–E342.

21. Hammer, M., Ladegoged, J., and Olgaard, K., 1979, Relationship between plasma osmolality and plasma vasopressin in human subjects, *Am. J. Physiol.* **238:**E313–E317.

22. Weitzman, R. E., Fisher, D. A., DiStefano, J. H., III, and Bennett, C. M., 1977, Episodic secretion of arginine vasopressin, *Am. J. Physiol.* **233:**E32–E36.

23. Robertson, G. L., Athar, S., and Shelton, R. L., 1977, Osmotic control of vasopressin function, in: *Disturbances in Body Fluid Osmolality* (T. E. Andreoli, J. J. Grantham, and F. C. Rector, Jr., eds.), pp. 125–148, The American Physiological Society, Bethesda.

24. Baylis, P. H., and Robertson, G. L., 1980, Plasma vasopressin response to hypertonic saline infusion to assess posterior pituitary function, *J. R. Soc. Med.* **73:**255–260.

25. Brimble, M. J., and Dyball, R. E. J., 1977, Characterization of the responses of oxytocin- and vasopressin-secreting neurones in the supraoptic nucleus to osmotic stimulation, *J. Physiol. (London)* **271:**253–271.

26. Zerbe, R., Vinicor, F., and Robertson, G. L., 1978, Vasopressin (VP) secretion in man is stimulated by urea and suppressed by glucose, *Clin. Res.* **26:**315A.

27. McKinley, M. J., Denton, D. A., and Weisinger, R. S., 1978, Sensors for antidiuresis and thirst—Osmoreceptors or CSF sodium detectors?, *Brain Res.* **141:**89–103.

28. Thrasher, T. N., Brown, C. J., Keil, L. C., and Ramsay, D. J., 1980, Thirst and vasopressin release in the dog: An osmoreceptor or sodium receptor mechanism?, *Am. J. Physiol.* **238:**R333–R339.

29. Olsson, K., and Kolmodin, R., 1974, Dependence of basic secretion of antidiuretic hormone on cerebrospinal fluid [Na], *Acta Physiol. Scand.* **91:**286–288.

30. Rundgren, M., Eriksson, S., and Appelgren, B., 1979, Urea-induced inhibition of antidiuretic hormone (ADH) secretion, *Acta Physiol. Scand.* **106:**491–492.

31. Zerbe, R. L., Miller, J. Z., and Robertson, G. L., 1980, Reproducibility and heritability of vasopressin osmoregulation in humans, *Endocrinology* **106**(Suppl.):78, Abstract 13.

32. Helderman, J. H., Vestal, R. E., Rowe, J. W., Tobin, J. D., Andres, R., and Robertson, G. L., 1978, The response of arginine vasopressin to intravenous ethanol and hypertonic saline in man: The impact of aging, *J. Gerontol.* **33:**39–47.

33. Durr, J. A., Stamoutsos, B., and Lindheimer, M. D., 1981, Osmoregulation during pregnancy in the rat: Evidence for resetting of the threshold for vasopressin secretion during gestation, *J. Clin. Invest.* **68:**337–346.

34. Hytten, F. E., 1968, Physiological changes in early pregnancy, *J. Obstet. Gynaecol. Br. Commonw.* **75:**1193–1197.

35. Robertson, E. G., and Cheyne, G. A., 1972, Plasma biochemistry in relation to oedema of pregnancy, *J. Obstet. Gynaecol. Br. Commonw.* **79:**769–776.

36. Davison, J. M., Calloton, M. B., and Lindheimer, M. D., 1980, Alterations in plasma osmolality (P_{osm}) during human pregnancy, *Clin. Res.* **28:**442A.

37. Buggy, J., and Johnson, A. K., 1977, Preoptic–hypothalamic periventricular lesions: Thirst deficits and hypernatremia, *Am. J. Physiol.* **233:** R44–R52.

38. Bealer, S. L., Phillips, M. I., Johnson, A. K., and Schmid, P. G., 1979, Anteroventral third ventricle lesions reduce antidiuretic responses to angiotensin II, *Am. J. Physiol.* **236:**E610–E615.

39. Miller, T. R., Handelman, W. A., Arnold, P. E., McDonald, K. M., Molinoff, P. B., and Schrier, R. W., 1979, Effect of central catecholamine depletion on the osmotic and non-osmotic stimulation of vasopressin (ADH) in the rat, *J. Clin. Invest.* **64:**1599–1607.

40. Hoffman, W. E., Phillips, M. I., and Schmid, P., 1977, The role of catecholamines in central antidiuretic and pressor mechanisms, *Neuropharmacology* **16**:563–569.
41. Sladek, C. D., and Joynt, R. J., 1979, Cholinergic involvement in osmotic control of vasopressin release by the organ-cultured rat hypothalamo-neurohypophyseal system, *Endocrinology* **105**:367–371.
42. Sladek, D. C., and Knigge, K. M., 1977, Cholinergic stimulation of vasopressin release from the rat hypothalamo-neurohypophyseal system in organ culture, *Endocrinology* **101**:411.
43. de Weid, D., and Laszlo, F. A., 1967, Effect of autonomic blocking agents on ADH-release induced by hyperosmoticity, *J. Endocrinol.* **37**:XVI.
44. Bridges, T. E., and Thorn, N. A., 1970, The effect of autonomic blocking agents on vasopressin release *in vivo* induced by osmoreceptor stimulation, *J. Endocrinol.* **48**:263.
45. Milton, A. S.,and Paterson, A. T., 1974, A microinjection study of the control of antidiuretic hormone release by the supraoptic nucleus of the hypothalamus in the rat, *J. Physiol. (London)* **241**:607.
46. Morris, M., McCann, S. M., and Orias, R., 1977, Role of transmitters in mediating hypothalamic control of electrolyte excretion, *Can. J. Physiol. Pharmacol.* **55**:1143.
47. Gann, D. S., Ward, D. G., and Carlson, D. E., 1978, Neural control of ACTH: A homeostatic reflex, *Recent Prog. Horm. Res.* **34**:357–396.
48. Sawchenko, P. E., and Swanson, L. W., 1981, Central noradrenergic pathways for the integration of hypothalamic neuroendocrine and autonomic responses, *Science* **214**:685–687.
49. Thames, M. D., and Schmid, P. G., 1979, Cardiopulmonary receptors with vagal afferents tonically inhibit ADH release in the dog, *Am. J. Physiol.* **237**:H299–H304.
50. Fumoux, F., Czernichow, P., Arnauld, E., Du Pont, J., and Vincent, J. D., 1978, Effect of hypotension induced by sodium nitrocyanoferrate (III) on the release of arginine vasopressin in the unanaesthetized monkey, *J. Endocrinol.* **78**:449–450.
51. Wood, C. E., Shinsako, J., Keil, L. C., Ramsay, D. J., and Dallman, M. F., 1981, Hormonal and hemodynamic responses to 15 ml/kg hemorrhage in conscious dogs: Responses correlate to body temperature, *Proc. Soc. Exp. Biol. Med.* **167**:15–19.
52. Robertson, G. L., and Rowe, J., 1980, The effect of aging on neurohypophyseal function, *Peptides* **1**(Suppl. 1):159–162.
53. Kannan, H., and Yagi, K., 1978, Supraoptic neurosecretory neurons: Evidence for the existence of converging inputs both from carotid baroreceptors and osmoreceptors, *Brain Res.* **145**:385–390.
54. Bark, H., Le Roith, D., Nyska, M., and Glick, S. M., 1980, Elevations in plasma ADH levels during PEEP ventilation in the dog: Mechanisms involved, *Am. J. Physiol.* **239**:E474–E481.
55. Wiggins, R. C., Basar, I., Slater, J. D. H., Forsling, M., and Ramage, C. M., 1977, Vasovagal hypotension and vasopressin release, *Clin. Endocrinol.* **6**:387–393.

56. Kendler, K. S., Weitzman, R. E., and Fisher, D. A., 1978, The effect of pain on plasma arginine vasopressin concentrations in man, *Clin. Endocrinol.* **8**:80–94.

57. Husain, M. K., Manger, W. M., Rock, T. W., Weiss, R. J., and Frantz, A. G., 1979, Vasopressin release due to manual restraint in the rat: Role of body compression and comparison with other stressful stimuli, *Endocrinology* **104**:641–644.

58. Rowe, J. W., Shelton, R. L., Helderman, J. H., Vestal, R. E., and Robertson, G. L., 1979, Influence of the emetic reflex on vasopressin release in man, *Kidney Int.* **16**:729–735.

59. Coutinho, E. M., 1969, Oxytocic and antidiuretic effects of nausea in women, *Am. J. Obstet. Gynecol.* **105**:127–131.

60. Eversmann, T., Guttsmann, M., Uhlich, E., Ulbrecht, G., von Werder, K., and Scriba, P. C., 1978, Increased secretion of growth hormone, prolactin, antidiuretic hormone, and cortisol induced by the stress of motion sickness, *Aviat. Space Environ. Med.* January 1978:53–57.

61. Baylis, P. H., and Heath, D. A., 1977, Plasma-arginine-vasopressin response to insulin-induced hypoglycaemia, Lancet **2**:428–430.

62. Baylis, P. H., Zerbe, R. L., and Robertson, G. L., 1981, Arginine vasopressin response to insulin-induced hypoglycemia in man, *J. Clin. Endocrinol. Metab.* **53**:935–940.

63. Baylis, P. H., and Robertson, G. L., 1980, Rat vasopressin in response to insulin-induced hypoglycemia, *Endocrinology* **107**:1975–1979.

64. Thompson, D. A., Campbell, R. G., Lilavivat, U., Welle, S. L., and Robertson, G. L., 1981, Increased thirst and plasma arginine vasopressin levels during 2-deoxy-D-glucose-induced glucoprivation in humans, *J. Clin. Invest.* **67**:1083–1093.

65. Baylis, P. H., and Robertson, G. L., 1980, Vasopressin response to 2-deoxy-D-glucose in the Rat, *Endocrinology* **107**:1970–1974.

66. Granberg, P.-O., 1962, Effect of acute hypoxia on renal haemodynamics and water diuresis in man, *Scand. J. Clin. Lab. Invest.* **14**(Suppl. 63) :5–62.

67. Forsling, M. L., and Rees, M., 1975, Effects of hypoxia and hypercapnia on plasma vasopressin concentration, *J. Endocrinol.* **67**:62P–63P.

68. Anderson, R. J., Pluss, R. G., Berns, A. S., Jackson, J. I., Arnold, P. E., Schrier, R. W., and McDonald, K. M., 1978, Mechanism of effect of hypoxia on renal water function, *J. Clin. Invest.* **62**:769–777.

69. Baylis, P. H., Stockley, R. A., and Heath, D. A., 1977, Effect of acute hypoxaemia on plasma arginine vasopressin in conscious man, *Clin. Sci. Mol. Med.* **53**:401–404.

70. Claybaugh, J. R., Hansen, J. E., and Wozniak, D. B., 1978, Response of antidiuretic hormone to acute exposure to mild and severe hypoxia in man, *J. Endocrinol.* **77**:157–160.

71. Heyes, M. P., Farber, M. O., Manfredi, F., Robertshaw, D., Weinberger, M., Fineberg, N., and Robertson, G., 1982, Acute effects of hypoxia on renal and endocrine function in normal humans, *Am. J. Physiol.* **243**:R265–R270.

72. de Bodo, R. C., 1944, The antidiuretic action of morphine and its mechanism, *J. Pharmacol. Exp. Ther.* **82**:74–85.

73. Duke, H. N., Pickford, M., and Watt, J. A., 1951, The antidiuretic action of morphine: Its site and mode of action in the hypothalamus of the dog, *Q. J. Exp. Physiol.* **36:**149–158.

74. Giarman, N. J., Mattie, L. R., and Stephenson, W. F., 1953, Studies on the antidiuretic action of morphine, *Science* **117:**225–226.

75. Giarman, N. J., and Condouris, G. A., 1954, The antidiuretic action of morphine and some of its analogues, *Arch. Int. Pharmacodyn.* **97:**28–33.

76. Schnieden, H., and Blackmore, E. K., 1955, The effect of nalorphine on the antidiuretic action of morphine in rats and men, *Br. J. Pharmacol.* **10:**45–50.

77. Inturrisi, C. E., and Fujimoto, J. M., 1968, Studies on the antidiuretic action of morphine in the rat, *Eur. J. Pharmacol.* **2:**301–307.

78. Handley, C. A., and Keller, A. D., 1950, Changes in renal function produced by morphine in normal dogs and dogs with diabetes insipidus, *J. Pharmacol. Exp. Ther.* **99:**33–37.

79. Fujimoto, J. M., 1971, The kidney, in: *Narcotic Drugs: Biochemical Pharmacology* (D. H. Clouet, ed.), pp. 366–393, Plenum Press, New York.

80. Hayward, J. N., 1974, Effects of drugs of abuse on motivated behavior and magnocellular neuroendocrine cells, in: *Narcotics and the Hypothalamus* (E. Zimmermann and R. George. eds.), pp. 83–93, Raven Press, New York.

81. Miller, M., 1975, Inhibition of ADH release in the rat by narcotic antagonists, *Neuroendocrinology* **19:**241–251.

82. Weitzman, R. E., Fisher, D. A., Minick, S., Ling, N., and Guillemin, R., 1977, β-Endorphin stimulates secretion of arginine vasopressin *in vivo*, *Endocrinology* **101:**1643–1646.

83. Bisset, G. W., Chowdrey, H. S., and Feldberg, W., 1978, Release of vasopressin by enkephalin, *Br. J. Pharmacol.* **62:**370–371.

84. Tseng, L.-F., Loh, H. H., and Li, C. H., 1978, $β_h$-Endorphin: Antidiuretic effects in rats. *Int. J. Pept. Protein Res.* **12:**173–176.

85. Catlin, D. H., George, R., and Li, C. H., 1978, β-Endorphin: Pharmacologic and behavioral activity in cats after low intravenous doses, *Life Sci.* **23:**2147–2154.

86. Goldstein, A., 1976, Opioid peptides (endorphines) in pituitary and brain, *Science* **193:**1081–1086.

87. Sar, M., Stumpf, W. E., Miller, R. J., Chang, K.-J., and Cuatrecasas, P., 1978, Immunohistochemical localization of enkephalin in rat brain and spinal cord, *J. Comp. Neurol.* **182:**17–37.

88. Rossier, J., Battenberg, E., Pittman, Q., Bayon, A., Koda, L., Miller, R., Guillemin, R., and Bloom, F., 1979, Hypothalamic enkephalin neurones may regulate the neurohypophysis, *Nature (London)* **277:**653–655.

89. Miller, M., 1980, Role of endogenous opioids in neurohypophysial function of man, *J. Clin. Endocrinol. Metab.* **50:**1016–1020.

90. Kamoi, K., White, K., and Robertson, G. L., 1979, Opiates elevate the osmotic threshold for vasopressin (VP) release in rats, *Clin. Res.* **27:**254A.

91. van Wimersma, Greidanus, T. B., Thody, T. J., Verspaget, H., de Rotte, G. A., Goedemans, H. J. H., Croiset, G., and van Ree, J. M., 1979, Effects of morphine and β-Endorphin on basal and elevated plasma levels of α-MSH and vasopressin, *Life Sci.* **24:**579–586.

92. Lord, J. A. H., Waterfield, A. A., Hughes, J., and Kosterlitz, H. W., 1977, Endogenous opioid peptides: Multiple agonists and receptors, *Nature (London)* **267**:496–499.

93. Chang, K.-J., and Cuatrecasas, P., 1979, Multiple opiate receptors: Enkephalins and morphine bind to receptors of different specificity, *J. Biol. Chem.* **254**:2610–2618.

94. Kosterlitz, H. W., Lord, J. A. H., Paterson, S. J., and Waterfield, A. A., 1980, Effects of changes in the structure of enkephalins and of narcotic analgesic drugs on their interactions with μ- and δ-receptors, *Br. J. Pharmacol.* **68**:333–342.

95. Egan, T. M., and North, R. A., 1981, Both μ and δ opiate receptors exist on the same neuron, *Science* **214**:923–925.

96. Aziz, L. A. Forsling, M. L., and Woolf, C. J., 1980, The action of morphine on vasopressin release in the rat, *J. Physiol. (London)* **300**:24P–25P.

97. Brownell, J., del Pozo, E., and Donatsch, P., 1980, Inhibition of vasopressin secretion by a Met-enkephalin (FK 33-824) in humans, *Acta Endocrinol. (Copenhagen)* **94**:304–308.

98. Grossman, A., Besser, G. M., Milles, J. J., and Baylis, P. H., 1980, Inhibition of vasopressin release in man by an opiate peptide, *Lancet* **2**:1108–1110.

99. Summy-Long, J. Y., Keil, L. C., Deen, K., and Severs, W. B., 1981, Opiate regulation of angiotensin-induced drinking and vasopressin release, *J. Pharmacol. Exp. Ther.* **217**:630–637.

100. Iversen, L. L., Iversen, S. D., and Bloom, F. E., 1980, Opiate receptors influence vasopressin release from nerve terminals in rat neurohypophysis, *Nature (London)* **284**:350–351.

101. Clarke, G., Lincoln, D. W., and Wood, P., 1980, Inhibition of vasopressin neurones by intraventricular morphine, *J. Physiol (London)* **303**:59P:–60P.

102. Knepel, W., Nutto, D., Anhut, H., and Hertting, G., 1980, Naloxone promotes stimulus-evoked vasopressin release in vivo, *Eur. J. Pharmacol.* **65**:449–450.

103. Lightman, S. L., and Forsling, M. L., 1980, Evidence for endogenous opioid control of vasopressin release in man, *J. Clin. Endocrinol. Metab.* **50**:569–571.

104. Oiso, Y., and Robertson, G. L., 1982, Role of endogenous opiates in mediating ethanol-induced suppression of vasopressin, *Proceedings of the 64th meeting of the Endocrine Society* **Abst. 751**:267.

105. Huidobro-Toro, J. P., 1980, Antidiuretic effect of β-endorphin and morphine in Brattleboro rats: Development of tolerance and physical dependence after chronic morphine treatment, *Br. J. Pharmacol.* **71**:51–56.

106. Cadnapaphornchal, P., Boykin, J. L., Berl, T., McDonald, K. M., and Schrier, R. W., 1974, Mechanism of effect of nicotine on renal water excretion, *Am. J. Physiol.* **227**:1216–1220.

107. Bisset, G. W., Feldberg, W., Guertzenstein, P. G., and Silva, M. R. E., Jr., 1975, Vasopressin release by nicotine: The site of action, *Br. J. Pharmacol.* **54**:463–474.

108. Cates, J. E., and Garrold, O., 1951, The effect of nicotine on urinary flow in diabetes insipidus, *Clin. Sci.* **10**:145.

109. Lewis, A. A. G., and Chalmers, T. M., 1951, A nicotine test for the investigation of diabetes insipidus, *Clin. Sci.* **10**:137.

110. Dingman, J. F., Benirschke, K., and Thorn, G. W., 1957, Studies of neurohypophyseal function in man, *Am. J. Med.* **23:**226.

111. Pullen, Q. T., Clappison, B. H., and Johnston, C. I., 1979, Plasma vasopressin and human neurophysin in physiological and pathological states associated with changes in vasopressin secretion, *J. Clin. Endocrinol. Metab.* **49:**580.

112. Robinson, A. G., 1975, Isolation, assay and secretion of individual human neurophysins, *J. Clin. Invest.* **55:**360.

113. Rowe, J. W., Kilgore, A., and Robertson, G. L., 1980, Evidence in man that cigarette smoking induces vasopressin release via an airway-specific mechanism, *J. Clin. Endocrinol. Metab.* **51:**170–172.

114. Pokracki, F. J., Robinson, A. G., and Seif, S. M., 1981, Chlorpropamide effect: Measurement of neurophysin and vasopressin in humans and rats, *Metabolism* **30:**72–78.

115. Stephens, W. P., Coe, J. Y., and Baylis, P. H., 1978, Plasma arginine vasopressin concentrations and antidiuretic action of carbamazepine, *Br. Med. J.* **1:**1445–1447.

116. Thomas, T. H., Ball, S. G., Wales, J. K., and Lee, M. R., 1978, Effect of carbamazepine on plasma and urine arginine-vasopressin, *Clin. Sci. Mol. Med.* **54:**419–424.

117. Meinders, A. F., Cejka, V., and Robertson, G. L., 1974, The antidiuretic action of carbamazepine in man, *Clin. Sci. Mol. Med.* **47:**289–299.

118. Smith, N. J., Espir, M. L. E., and Baylis, P. H., 1977, Raised plasma arginine vasopressin concentration in carbamazepine-induced water intoxication, *Br. Med. J.***1:**804.

119. Miller, P. D., Dubovsky, S. L., McDonald, K. M., Katz, F. H., Robertson, G. L., and Schrier, R. W., 1979, Central, renal and adrenal effects of lithium in man, *Am. J. Med.* **66:**797–803.

120. Padfield, P. L., Park, S. J., Morton, J. J., and Braidwood, A. E., 1977, Plasma levels of antidiuretic hormone in patients receiving prolonged lithium therapy, *Br. J. Psychiatry* **130:**144–147.

121. Humphreys, M. H., Reid, I. A., and Chou, L. Y. N., 1975, Suppression of antidiuretic hormone secretion by clonidine in the anesthetized dog, *Kidney Int.* **7:**405–412.

122. Reid, I. A., Nolan, P. L., Wolf, J. A., AND Keil, L. C. 1979, Suppression of vasopressin secretion by clonidine: Effect of α-adrenoceptor antagonists, *Endocrinology* **104:**1403–1406.

123. Kimura, T., Share, L., Wang, B. C., and Crofton, J. T., 1981, The role of central adrenoreceptors in the control of vasopressin release and blood pressure, *Endocrinology* **108:**1829–1836.

124. Sowers, J. R., Hershman, J. M., Skowsky, W. R., and Carlson, H. E., 1976, Effect of TRH on serum arginine vasopressin in euthyroid and hypothyroid subjects, *Horm. Res.* **7:**232–237.

125. Oliver, C., Eskay, R. I., Ben-Jonathan, N., and Porter, J. C., 1974, Distribution and concentration of TRH in the rat brain, *Endocrinology* **95:**540–546.

126. Jackson, I. M. D., and Reichlin, S., 1974, Thyrotropin-releasing hormone (TRH): Distribution in hypothalamic and extrahypothalamic brain tissues of mammalian and submammalian chordates, *Endocrinology* **95:**854–861.

127. Skowsky, W. R., Swan, L., and Smith, P., 1979, Effects of sex steroid hormones on arginine vasopressin in intact and castrated male and female rats, *Endocrinology* **104:**105–108.

128. Legros, L. L., Govaerts, A., Demoulin, A., and Franchimont, P ., 1973, Interactions entre un Derive Progestalif et l'Ethinyl Oestradiol sur l'Elimination Urinaire de Neurophysine d'Ocytocine et de Vasopressine Immunoreactives et sur le Taux de Neurophysine Serique l et ll chez l'Homme Normal, *C. R. Soc. Biol.* **167:**1668.

129. Ukai, M., Nagase, T., Hirohashi, M., and Yanaihara, N., 1981, Antidiuretic activities of substance P and its analogs, *Experientia* **37:**521–523.

130. Jamison, R. L., and Robertson, C. R., 1979, Recent formulations of the urinary concentrating mechanism: A status report, *Kidney Int.* **16:**537–545.

131. Handler, J. S., and Orloff, J., 1981, Antidiuretic hormone, *Annu. Rev. Physiol.* **43:**611–624.

132. Dousa, T. P., and Valtin, H., 1976, Cellular actions of vasopressin in the mammalian kidney, *Kidney Int.* **10:**46–63.

133. Bia, M. J., DeWitt, S., and Forrest, J. N., Jr., 1979, Dissociation between plasma, urine and renal papillary cyclic AMP content following vasopressin and DDAVP, *Am. J. Physiol.***237:**F218–F225.

134. Bell, N. H., Clark, C. M., Jr., Avery, S., Sinha, T., Trygstad, C. W., and Allen, D. O., 1974, Demonstration of a defect in the formation of adenosine 3', 5'-monophosphate in vasopressin resistant diabetes insipidos, *Pediatr. Res.* **8:**223–230.

135. Beck, T. R., and Dunn, M. J., 1981, The relationship of antidiuretic hormone and renal prostaglandins, *Miner. Electrolyte Metab.* **6:**46–59.

136. Beck, T. R., Hassid, A., and Dunn, M. J., 1980, The effect of arginine vasopressin and its analog on the synthesis of prostaglandin E_2 by rat renal medullary interstitial cells in culture, *J. Pharmacol. Exp. Ther.* **215:**15–19.

137. Dunn, M. J., Kinter, L. B., Reinier, B., III, Shier, D., Greeley, H. P., and Valtin, H., 1980, Interaction of vasopressin and renal prostaglandins in the homozygous diabetes insipidus rat, *Adv. Prostaglandin Thromboxane Res.* **7:**1009–1015.

138. Burch, R. M., Knapp, D. R., and Halushka, P. V., 1979, Vasopressin stimulates thromboxane synthesis in the toad urinary bladder: Effects of imidazole, *J. Pharmacol. Exp. Ther.* **210:**344–348.

139. Carretero, O. A., and Scicli, A. G., 1976, Renal kallikrein: Its localization and possible role in renal function, *Fed. Proc.* **35:**194–198.

140. Levinsky, N. G., 1979, The renal kallikrein–kinin system, *Circ. Res.* **44:**441–451.

141. Scicli, A. G., Gandolfi, R., and Carretero, O. A., 1978, Site of formation of kinins in the dog nephron, *Am. J. Physiol.***234:**F36–F40.

142. Robertson, G. L., and Conder, M. L., 1980, The regulation of urinary kinin excretion, in: *Hormonal Regulation of Sodium Excretion* (B. Lichardus, R. W. Schrier, and J. Ponev, eds.), pp. 239–248, Elsevier/North-Holland, Amsterdam.

143. Carvounis, C. P., Carvounis, G., and Abbett, L. A., 1981, Role of the endogenous kallikrein–kinin system in modulating vasopressin-stimulated

water flow and urea permeability in the toad urinary bladder, *J. Clin. Invest.* **67:**1792–1796.

144. Furtado, M. R. F., 1971, Inhibition of the permeability response to vasopressin and oxytocin in the toad bladder: Effect of bradykinin, kallidin, eleodosin and physalamine, *J. Membr. Biol.* **4:**167–178.

145. Zusman, R. M., and Keiser, H. R., 1977, Prostaglandin biosynthesis by rabbit renomedullary interstitial cells in tissue culture: Stimulation by angiotensin II, bradykinin, and arginine vasopressin, *J. Clin. Invest.* **60:**215–233.

146. Humes, H. D., Simmons, C. F., Jr., and Brenner, B. M., 1980, Effect of verapamil on the hydroosmotic response to antidiuretic hormone in toad urinary bladder, *Am. J. Physiol.* **239:**F250–F257.

147. Levine, S. D., Kachadorian, W. A., Levin, D. N., and Schlondorff, D., 1981, Effects of trifluoperazine on function and structure of toad urinary bladder, *J. Clin. Invest.* **67:**662–672.

148. Beauwens, R., and Rentmeesters, M., 1981, Rose of calmodulin in antidiuretic hormone mediated water transport, *Biochem. Biophys. Res. Commun.* **99:**491–495.

149. Humes, H. D., Simmons, C. F., Jr., and Brenner, B. M., 1980, Interaction between antidiuretic and parathyroid hormones on urine concentration, *Am. J. Physiol.* **239:**F244–F249.

150. Reid, I. A., and Rose, J. C., 1977, An intrarenal effect of somatostatin on water excretion, *Endocrinology* **100:**782–785.

151. Forrest, J. N., Jr., Reichlin, S., and Goodman, D. B. P., 1980, Somatostatin: An endogenous peptide in the toad urinary bladder inhibits vasopressin-stimulated water flow, *Proc. Natl. Acad. Sci. USA* **77:**4984–4987.

152. Sawyer, W. H., Pang, P. K. T., Seto, J., McEnroe, M., Lammek, B., and Manning, M., 1981, Vasopressin analogs that antagonize antidiuretic responses by rats to the antidiuretic hormone, *Science* **212:**49–51.

153. Edwards, B. R., Gellai, M., and Valtin, H., 1980, Concentration of urine in the absence of ADH with minimal or no decrease in GFR, *Am. J. Physiol.* **239:**F84–F91.

154. Rowe, L. W., 1929, Studies on oxytocin and vasopressin: Pressor action, *Endocrinology* **13:**205.

155. Grabiel, A., and Glendy, R. E., 1951, Circulatory effects following the intravenous administration of pitressin in normal persons and in patients with hypertension and agina pectoris, *Am. Heart J.* **21:**481.

156. Wagner, H. N., and Braunwald, E., 1956, The pressor effect of the antidiuretic principle of the posterior pituitary in orthostatic hypotension, *J. Clin. Invest.* **35:**1412.

157. Laycock, J. F., Penn, W., Shirley, D. G., and Walter, S. J., 1979, The role of vasopressin in blood pressure regulation immediately following acute haemorrhage in the rat, *J. Physiol. (London* **296:**267–275.

158. Altura, B. M., 1980, Evidence that endogenous vasopressin plays a protective role in circulatory shock: Role for reticuloendothelial system using Brattleboro rats, *Experientia* **36:**1080–1082.

159. Cowley, A. W., Jr., Switzer, S. J., and Guinn, M. M., 1980, Evidence and quantification of the vasopressin arterial pressure control system in the dog, *Circ. Res.* **46:**58–67.

160. Montani, J.-P., Liard, J.-F., Schoun, J., and Mohring, J., 1980, Hemodynamic effects of exogenous and endogenous vasopressin at low plasma concentrations in conscious dogs, *Circ. Res.* **47**:346–355.
161. Cowley, A. W., Jr., Monos, E.,and Guyton, A.C., 1974, Interaction of vasopressin and the baroreceptor reflex system in the regulation of arterial blood pressure in the dog. *Circ. Res.* **24**:505–514.
162. Malayan, S. A., Ramsay, D. J., Keil, L. C., and Reid, I. A., 1980, Effects of plasma increases in plasma vasopressin concentration on plasma renin activity, blood pressure, heart rate, and plasma corticosteroid concentration in conscious dogs, *Endocrinology* **107**:1899–1904.
163. Mohring, J., Glanzer, K., Maciel, J. A., Jr., Dusing, R., Kramer, H. J., Arbogast, R., and Koch-Weser, J., 1980, Greatly enhanced pressor response to antidiuretic hormone in patients with impaired cardiovascular reflexes due to idiopathic orthostatic hypotension, *J. Cardiovasc. Pharmacol.* **2**: 367–378.
164. Ciriello, J., and Calaresu, F. R., 1980, Role of paraventricular and supraoptic nuclei in central cardiovascular regulation in the cat, *Am. J. Physiol.* **81**:R137–R142.
165. Hems, D. A., Whitton, P. D., and Ma, G. Y., 1975, Metabolic activities of vasopressin, glucagon and adrenalin in the intact rat, *Biochim. Biophys. Acta* **411**:155.
166. Whitton, P. A., Rodriques, L. M., and Hems, D. A., 1978, Stimulation by vasopressin, angiotensin and oxytocin of gluconeogenesis in hepatocyte suspensions, *Biochem. J.* **176**:893–898.
167. Williamson, D. H., Ilic, V., Tordoff, A. F. C., and Ellington, E. V., 1980, Interactions between vasopressin and glucagon on ketogenesis and oleate metabolism in isolated hepatocytes from fed rats, *Biochem. J.* **186**: 621–624.
168. Schapiro, H., and Britt, L. G., 1972, The action of vasopressin on the gastrointestinal tract: A review of the literature, *Am. J. Dig. Dis.* **17**:649–667.
169. Schapiro, H., 1975, Inhibitory action of antidiuretic hormone on canine pancreatic exocrine flow, *Am. J. Dig. Dis.* **20**:853–857.
170. Dornhorst, A., Carlson, D. E., Seif, S. M., Robinson, A. G., Zimmerman, E. A., and Gann, D. S., 1981, Control of adrenocorticotropin and vasopressin by the supraoptic and paraventricular nuclei, *Endocrinology* **108**:1420–1424.
171. Arimura, A., Saito, T., Bowers, C. Y., and Schally, A. V., 1967, Pituitary–adrenal activation in rats with hereditary hypothalamic diabetes insipidus, *Acta Endocrinol. (Copenhagen)* **54**:155–165.
172. McCann, S. M., Antunes-Rodrigues, J., Nallar, R., and Valtin, H., 1966, Pituitary adrenal function in the absence of vasopressin, *Endocrinology* **79**:1058–1064.
173. Karteszi, M., Stark, E., Rappay, G., Laszlo, F. A., and Makara, G. B., 1981, Corticoliberin activity of rat neurohypophysis is distinct from vasopressin, *Am. J. Physiol.* **240**:E689–E693.
174. Buckingham, J. C., and Leach, J. H., 1980, Hypothalamo-pituitary-adrenocortical function in rats with inherited diabetes insipidus, *J. Physiol. (London)* **305**:397–404.
175. Knepel, W., Anhut, H., Nutto, D., and Hertting, G., 1980, Evidence that

vasopressin is involved in the isoprenaline-induced β-endorphin release, *Eur. J. Pharmacol.* **68:**359–363.

176. Raichle, M. E., and Grubb, R. L., Jr., 1978, Regulation of brain water permeability by centrally-released vasopressin, *Brain Res.* **143:**191–194.

177. Barker, J. L., 1977, Physiological roles of peptides in the nervous system, in: *Peptides in Neurobiology* (A. Gainer, ed.), pp. 295–343, Plenum Press, New York.

178. de Wied, D., 1976, Hormonal influences on motivation, learning, and memory processes, *Hosp. Pract.* January 1976:123–131.

179. Walter, R., Hoffman, P. L., Flexner, J. B., and Flexner, L. B., 1975, Neurohypophyseal hormones, analogs, and fragments; Their effect on puromycin-induced amnesia, *Proc. Natl. Acad. Sci. USA* **72:**4180–4184.

180. Gold, P. W., Goodwin, F. K., Ballenger, J. C., Post, R. M., Weingartner, H., and Robertson, G. L., 1981, Central vasopressin function in affective illness, *Int. J. Ment. Health* **9:**91–107.

181. Miller, M., Dalakos, T., Moses, A. M., Fellerman, H., and Streeten, D. H. P., 1970, Recognition of partial defects in antidiuretic hormone secretion, *Ann. Intern. Med.* **73:**721–729.

182. Streeten, D. H. P., Moses, A. M., and Miller, M., 1980, Disorders of neurohypophysis, in: *Harrison's Principles of Internal Medicine* (K. J. Isselbacher, R. D. Adams, E. Braunwald, R. G. Petersdorf, and J. D. Wilson, eds.) 9th ed., pp. 1684–1694, McGraw–Hill, New York.

183. Shimizu, S., and Hoshimo, M., 1978, Application of vasopressin radioimmunoassay to clinical study: Role of vasopressin in hypo- and hypernatremia and some other disorders of water metabolism, *Contrib. Nephrol.* **9:**42–60.

184. Baylis, P. H., Gaskill, M. B., and Robertson, G. L., 1981, Vasopressin secretion in primary polydipsia and cranial diabetes insipidus, *Q. J. Med.* **50:**345–358.

185. Zerbe, R. L., Baylis, P. H., and Robertson, G. L., 1981, Vasopressin function in clinical disorders of water balance, in: *Butterworth's International Medical Review Series, Clinical Endocrinology*, Volume 1 (G. L. Robertson and C. G. Beardwell, eds.), pp. 297–329, Butterworths, London.

186. Zerbe, R. L., and Robertson, G. L., 1981, A comparison of plasma vasopressin measurements with a standard indirect test in the differential diagnosis of polyuria, *N. Engl. J. Med.* **305:**1539–1546.

187. Block, L. H., Locher, R., Tenscheri, W., Siegenthaler, W., Hofmann, T., Mettler, R., and Vetter, W., 1981, ^{125}I-8-Larginine vasopressin binding to human mononuclear phagocytes, *J. Clin. Invest.* **68:**374–381.

188. Laczi, F., Mezel, G., Julesz, J., and Laszlo, F. A., 1980, Effects of vasopressin analogues (DDAVP, DVDAVP) in the form of sublingual tablets in central diabetes insipidus, *Int. J. Clin. Pharmacol. Ther. Toxicol.* **18:**63–68.

189. Zusman, R. W., Keiser, H. R., and Handler, J. S., 1977, Inhibition of vasopressin-stimulated prostaglandin E biosynthesis by chlorpropamide in the toad urinary bladder, *J. Clin. Invest.* **60:**1348–1353.

190. Halter, J. B., Goldberg, A. P., Robertson, G. L., and Porte, D., Jr., 1977, Selective osmoreceptor dysfunction in the syndrome of chronic hypernatremia, *J. Clin. Endocrinol. Metab.* **44:**609–616.

191. Nandi, M., and Harrington, A. R., 1978, Successful treatment of hypernatremic thirst deficiency with chlorpropamide, *Clin. Nephrol.* **10**:90–95.

192. Schaad, U., Vassella, F., Zuppinger, K., and Oetliker, O., 1979, Hypodipsia–hypernatremia syndrome, *Helv. Paediatr. Acta* **34**:63–76.

193. Kimura, T., Matsui, K., Ota, K., and Yoshinaga, K., 1979, Hypothalamic hypernatremia due to volume-dependent ADH release, and its treatment with carbamazepine and clofibrate, *Tohoku J. Exp. Med.* **127**:101–111.

194. Rosansky, S. J., and Nidus, B. D., 1981, Volume receptor control of ADH release in essential hypernatremia, *NY State J. Med.* March 1981:351–356.

195. AvRuskin, T. W., Tang, S. C., and Juan, C., 1981, Essential hypernatremia, antidiuretic hormone and neurophysin secretion: Response to chlorpropamide, *Accta Endocrinol (Copenhagen)* **96**:145–153.

196. Bode, H. H., and Crawford, J. D., 1969, Nephrogenic diabetes insipidus in North America—The Hopewell hypothesis, *N. Engl. J. Med.* **280**:750–754.

197. Robertson, G. L., and Scheidler, J. A., 1981, A newly recognized variant of familial nephrogenic diabetes insipidus distinguished by partial resistance to vasopressin (type II), *Clin. Res.* **29**:555A.

198. Singer, I., and Forrest, J. N., Jr., 1976, Drug-induced states of nephrogenic diabetes insipidus, *Kidney Int.* **10**:82–95.

199. Barbour, G. L., Straub, K. D., O'Neal, B. L., and Leatherman, J. W., 1979, Vasopressin-resistant nephrogenic diabetes insipidus: A result of amphotericin B therapy, *Arch. Intern. Med.* **139**:86–88.

200. Lee, R. V., Jampol, L. M., and Brown, W. V., 1971, Nephrogenic diabetes insipidus and lithium intoxication—Complications of lithium carbonate therapy, *N. Engl. J. Med.* **284**:94–94, 1971.

201. Forrest, J. N., Jr., Cohen, A. D., Torretti, J., Himmelhoch, J. M., and Epstein, F. H., 1974, On the mechanism of lithium-induced diabetes insipidus in man and the rat, *J. Clin. Invest.* **53**:1115–1122.

202. Dousa, T. P., and Barnes, L. D., 1978, Lithium-induced diuretic effect of antidiuretic hormone in rats, *Am. J. Physiol.* **231**:1754–1759.

203. Christensen, S., 1980, DDAVP (1-desamino-8-D-arginine-vasopressin) treatment of lithium-induced polyuria in the rat, *Scand. J. Clin. Lab. Invest.* **40**:151–157.

204. Hestbech, J., Hansen, H. E., Amdisen, A., and Olsen, S., 1977, Chronic renal lesions following long-term treatment with lithium, *Kidney Int.* **12**:205–213.

205. Feibusch, J., Barbosa-Saldivar, J. L., Bernstein, R. S., and Robertson, G. L., 1980, Tumor-associated nephrogenic diabetes insipidus, *Ann. Intern. Med.* **92**:797–798.

206. Cooke, C. R., Turin, M. D., and Walker, W. G., 1979, The syndrome of inappropriate antidiuretic hormone secretion (SIADH): Pathophysiologic mechanisms in solute and volume regulation, *Medicine (Baltimore)* **58**: 240–251.

207. Zerbe, R., Stropes, L., and Robertson, G. L., 1980, Vasopressin function in the syndrome of inappropriate antidiuresis, *Annu. Rev. Med.* **31**:315–327.

208. Fyhrquist, F., Holmberg, G., Perheentupa, J., and Wallenius, M., 1977, Inappropriate secretion of antidiuretic hormone, hypertension, and hypoplastic corpus callosum, *J. Clin. Endocrinol. Metab.* **45**:691–694.

209. Burgar, P. J., Norenberg, N. D., and Yarnell, P. R., 1977, Hyponatremia and central pontine myelinoysis, *Neurology* **27**:223–228.

210. Whitaker, M. D., McArthur, R. G., Corenblum, B., Davidman, M., and Haslam, R. H., 1979, Idiopathic, sustained, inappropriate secretion of ADH with associated hypertension and thirst, *Am. J. Med.* **67**:511–515.

211. Baylis, P. H., and Robertson, G. L., 1979, Absent baroregulation of vasopressin (VP) with hypertension and inappropriate antidiuresis (SIADH), *Clin. Res.* **27**:447A.

212. Robertson, G. L., 1978, Cancer and inappropriate antidiuresis, in: *Biological Markers of Neoplasia: Basic and Applied Aspects* (R. W. Rudden, ed.) pp. 277–293, Elsevier North-Holland, Amsterdam.

213. Perks, W. H., Crow, J. C., and Green, M., 1978, Mesothelioma associated with the syndrome of inappropriate secretion of antidiuretic hormone, *Am. Rev. Respir. Dis.* **117**:780–791.

214. Robertson, G. L., 1980, Psychogenic polydipsia and inappropriate antidiuresis, *Arch. Intern. Med.* **140**:1574–1575.

215. Raskind, M. A., Orenstein, H., and Christopher, T. G., 1975, Acute psychosis, increased water ingestion and inappropriate antidiuretic hormone secretion, *Am. J. Psychiatry* **132**:907–910.

216. Rose, C. J., and Perez-Cruet, J., 1979, Incidence and morbidity of self-induced water intoxication in state mental hospital patients, *Am. J. Psychiatry* **136**:221–222.

217. Rosenbaum, J. F., Rothman, J. S., and Murray, G. B., 1979, Psychosis and water intoxication, *J. Clin. Psychiatry* **40**:287–291.

218. Jose, C. J., and Evenson, R. C., 1980, Antecedents of self-induced water intoxication, *J. Nerv. Ment. Dis.* **168**:498–500.

219. Smith, W. O., and Clark, M. J., 1980, Self-induced water intoxication in schizophrenic patients, *Am. J. Psychiatry* **137**:1055–1060.

220. Hariprasad, M. K., Eisinger, R. P., Nadler, I. M., Padmanabhan, C. S., and Nidus, B. D., 1980, Hyponatremia in psychogenic polydipsia, *Arch. Intern. Med.* **140**:1639–1642.

221. Rendell, M., McGrane, D., and Cuesta, M., 1978, Fatal compulsive water drinking, *J. Am. Med. Assoc.* **240**:2557–2559.

222. Skowsky, W. R., and Kikuchi, T. A., 1978, The role of vasopressin in the impaired water excretion of myxedema, *Am. J. Med.* **64**:613–621.

223. Waters, A. K., 1978, Increased vasopressin excretion in patients with hypothyroidism, *Acta Endocrinol (Copenhagen)* **88**:285–290.

224. Macaron, C., and Famuyiwa, O., 1978, Hyponatremia of hypothyroidism: Appropriate suppression of antidiuretic hormone levels, *Arch. Intern. Med.* **138**:820–822.

225. Robertson, G. L., 1979, The physiopathology of ADH secretion, in: *Clinical Neuroendocrinology: A Pathophysiological Approach* (G. Tolis, J. B. Martin, F. Naftolin, eds.) pp. 247–260, Raven Press, New York.

226. Bode, U., Seif, S. M., and Levine, A. S., 1980, Studies on the antidiuretic effect of cyclophosphamide: Vasopressin release and sodium excretion, *Med. Pediatr. Oncol.* **8**:295–303.

227. Zusman, R. M., Vinci, J. M., Bowden, R. E., Horwitz, D., and Keiser, H.

R., 1979, Effect of indomethacin and adrenocorticotrophic hormone on renal function in man: An experimental model of inappropriate antidiuresis, *Kidney Int.* **15:**62–70.

228. Nelson, P. B., Seif, S. M., Mardon, J. C., and Robinson, A. G., 1981, Hyponatremia in intracranial disease: Perhaps not the syndrome of inappropriate secretion of antidiuretic hormone (SIADH) *J. Neurosurg.* **55:938–941.**

229. Kleeman, C. R., Maxwell, M. H., and Rockney, R. E., 1958, Mechanisms of impaired water excretion in adrenal and pituitary insufficiency. I. The role of altered glomerular filtration rate and solute excretion, *J. Clin. Invest.* **37:**1799–1808.

230. Green, H. H., Harrington, A. R., and Valtin, H., 1970, On the role of antidiuretic hormone in the inhibition of acute water diuresis in adrenal insufficiency and the effects of gluco- and mineralocorticoids in reversing the inhibition, *J. Clin. Invest.* **49:**1724–1736.

231. Kleeman, C. R., Czaczkes, J. W., and Cutler, R., 1964, Mechanisms of impaired water excretion in adrenal and pituitary insufficiency. IV. Antidiuretic hormone in primary and secondary adrenal insufficiency, *J. Clin. Invest.* **43:**1641–1648.

232. Gill, J. R., Gann, D. S., and Bartter, F. C., 1962, Restoration of water diuresis in Addisonian patients by expansion of the volume of extracellular fluid, *J. Clin. Invest.* **41:**1078–1085.

233. Ackerman, G. L., and Miller, C. L., 1970, Role of hypovolemia in the impaired water diuresis of adrenal insufficiency, *J. Clin. Endocrinol. Metab.* **30:**252–258.

234. Ufferman, R. C., and Schrier, R. W., 1972, Importance of sodium intake and mineralocorticoid hormone in the impaired water excretion in adrenal insufficiency, *J. Clin. Invest.* **51:**1639–1646.

235. Boykin, J., DeTorrente, A., Erickson, A., Robertson, G., and Schrier, R. W., 1978, Role of plasma vasopressin in impaired water excretion of glucocorticoid deficiency, *J. Clin. Invest.* **62:**738–744.

236. Seif, S. M., Robinson, A. G., Zimmerman, E. A., and Wilkins, J., 1978, Plasma neurophysin and vasopressin in the rat: Response to adrenalectomy and steroid replacement, *Endocrinology* **103:**1009–1015.

237. Boykin, J., DeTorrente, A., Robertson, G. L., Erickson, A., and Schrier, R. W., 1979, Persistent plasma vasopressin levels in the hypoosmolar state associated with mineralocorticoid deficiency, *Miner. Electrolyte Metab.* **2:**310–315.

238. Mandell, I. N., DeFronzo, R. A., Robertson, G. L., and Forrest, J. N., Jr., 1980, Role of plasma arginine vasopressin in the impaired water diuresis of isolated glucocorticoid deficiency in the rat, *Kidney Int.* **17:**186–195.

239. Linas, S. L., Berl, T., Robertson, G. L., Aisenbray, G. A., Schrier, R. W., and Anderson, R. J., 1980, Role of vasopressin in the impaired water excretion of glucocorticoid deficiency, *Kidney Int.* **18:**58–67.

240. Robertson, G. L., Aycinena, P. A., and Zerbe, R. L., 1982, Neurogenic disorders of osmoregulation, *Am. J. Med.* **72:**339–353.

241. Bell, N. H., Schedl, H. P., and Bartter, F. C., 1964, An explanation for

abnormal water retention and hypoosmolality in congestive heart failure, *Am. J. Med.* **36**:351–360.

242. Better, O. S., Aisenbrey, G. A., Berl, T., Anderson, R. J., Handelman, W. A., Linas, S. L., Guggenheim, S. J., and Schrier, R. W., 1980, Role of antidiuretic hormone in impaired urinary dilution associated with chronic bile-duct ligation, *Clin. Sci.* **58**:493–500.

243. Linas, S. L. Anderson, R. J., Guggenheim, S. J., Robertson, G. L., and Berl, T., 1981, Role of vasopressin in impaired water excretion in conscious rats with experimental cirrhosis, *Kidney Int.* **20**:173–180.

244. Szatalowicz, V. L., Arnold, P. E., Chaimovitz, C., Bichet, D., Berl, T., and Schrier, R. W., 1981, Radioimmunoassay of plasma arginine vasopressin in hyponatremic patients with congestive heart vailure, *N. Engl. J. Med.* **305**:263–266.

245. Zerbe, R. L., Vinicor, F., and Robertson, G. L., 1979, Plasma vasopressin in uncontrolled diabetes mellitus, *Diabetes* **28**:503–508.

246. Walsh, C. H., Baylis, P. H., and Malins, J. M., 1979, Plasma arginine vasopressin in diabetic ketoacidosis, *Diabetologia* **16**:93–96.

247. Zerbe, R. L., Vinicor, F., and Robertson, G. L., 1978, Demonstration of intact osmotic regulation of vasopressin (VP) in juvenile onset diabetics (JOD), *Endocrinology* **102**:(Suppl.):225.

248. Zerbre, R. L., Robertson, G., Vinicor, F., and Henry, D., 1979, Orthostatic stimulation of vasopressin (VP) is exaggerated in juvenile onset diabetics (JOD), *J. Am. Diabetes Assoc.* **28**:349.

249. Van Houten, M., Posner, B. I., Kopriwa, B. M., and Brawer, J. R., 1979, Insulin-binding sites in the rat brain: In vivo localization to the circumventricular organs by quantitative radioautography, *Endocrinology* **105**:666–673.

250. Möhring, J., Petri, M., Möhring, B., and Haack, D., 1976, Is vasopressin involved in the pathogenesis of malignant desoxycorticosterone hypertension in rats? *Lancet* **1**:170–172.

251. Möhring, J., Möhring, B., Petri, M., and Haack, D., 1977, Vasopressor role of ADH in the pathogenesis of malignant DOC hypertension, *Am. J. Physiol.* **232**:F260–F269.

252. Möhring, J., Kintz, J., and Schoun, J., 1978, Role of vasopressin in blood pressure control of spontaneously hypertensive rats, *Clin. Sci. Mol. Med.* **55**:247s–250s.

253. Möhring, J., Möhring, B., Petri, M., and Haack, D., 1978, Plasma vasopressin concentrations and effects of vasopressin antiserum on blood pressure in rats with malignant two-kidney Goldblatt hypertension, *Circ. Res.* **42**:17–22.

254. Möhring, J., Kintz, J., and Schoun, J., 1979, Studies on the role of vasopressin in blood pressure control of spontaneously hypertensive rats with established hypertension (SHR, stroke-prone-strain), *J. Cardiovasc. Pharmacol.* **1**:593–608.

255. Crofton, J. T., Share, L., Shade, R. E., Allen, C., and Tarnowski, D., 1978, Vasopressin in the rat with spontaneous hypertension, *Am. J. Physiol.* **235**:H361–H366.

256. Pullan, P.T., Johnston, C. I., Anderson, W. P., and Korner, P. I., 1980, Plasma vasopressin in blood pressure homeostasis and in experimental renal hypertension, *Am. J. Physiol.* **239**:H81–H87.

257. Manning, M., Lowbridge, J., Stier, C. T., Jr., Haldar, J., and Sawyer, W. H., 1977, [1-deaminopenicillamine, 4-valine]-8-p-arginine-vasopressin, a highly potent inhibitor of the vasopressor response to arginine vasopressin, *J. Med. Chem.* **20**:1228–1230.

258. Rabito, S. F., Carretero, O. A., and Scicli, A. G., 1981, Evidence against a role of vasopressin in the maintenance of high blood pressure in mineralocorticoid and renovascular hypertension, *Hypertension* **3**:34–38.

259. Padfield, P. L., Brown, J. J., Lever, A. F., and Morton, J. J., 1976, Changes of vasopressin in hypertension: Cause or effect? *Lancet* **1**:1255–1257.

260. Shimamoto, D., Ando, T., Nakahashi, Y., Nakao, T., Tanaka, S., Sakuma, M., and Miyahara, M., 1979, Plasma and urinary ADH levels in patients with essential hypertension, *Jpn. Circ. J.* **43**:43–47.

261. Ganguly, A., Robertson, G. L., and Weinberger, M. H., 1979, Is osmoregulation of vasopressin affected by hypertension? *Clin. Res.* **27**:626A.

262. Ganguly, A., and Robertson, G. L., 1980, Elevated threshold for vasopressin release in primary aldosteronism, *Clin. Res.* **28**:330A.

Index